PHOTODYNAMIC THERAPY OF OCULAR DISEASES

PHOTODYNAMIC THERAPY OF OCULAR DISEASES

Editors

EVANGELOS S. GRAGOUDAS, M.D.

Acting Chairman and Professor
Department of Ophthalmology
Harvard Medical School
Director, Retina Service
Massachusetts Eye & Ear Infirmary
Boston, Massachusetts

JOAN W. MILLER, M.D.

Professor
Department of Ophthalmology
Harvard Medical School
Massachusetts Eye & Ear Infirmary
Boston, Massachusetts

LEONIDAS ZOGRAFOS, M.D.

Professor
Department of Ophthalmology
University Eye Clinic
Chairman
Department of Ophthalmology
Jules Gonin Eye Hospital
Lausanne, Switzerland

LIPPINCOTT WILLIAMS & WILKINS
A **Wolters Kluwer** Company
Philadelphia • Baltimore • New York • London
Buenos Aires • Hong Kong • Sydney • Tokyo

Acquisitions Editor: Jonathan Pine
Developmental Editor: Alyson Forbes
Production Editor: Danielle Power
Manufacturing Manager: Colin Warnock
Cover Designer: Karen Quigley
Compositor: Lippincott Williams & Wilkins Desktop Division
Printer: Walsworth

530 Walnut Street
Philadelphia, PA 19106 USA
LWW.com

Printed in the USA

Library of Congress Cataloging-in-Publication Data

Photodynamic therapy of ocular diseases / [edited by] Evangelos S. Gradoudas, Joan W. Miller, Leonidas Zografos.
p. ; cm.
Includes bibliographical references and index.
ISBN 0-7817-3446-0
1. Eye–Diseases–Photochemotherapy. I. Gragoudas, Evangelos S. II. Miller, Joan W. (Joan Whitten) III. Zografos, Leonidas.
[DNLM: 1. Eye Diseases–therapy. 2. Photochemotherapy–methods. WW 166 P575 2002]
RE992.P5P467 2002
617.7′0631–dc21

2003047482

Care has been taken to confirm the accuracy of the information presented and to describe generally accepted practices. However, the authors, editors, and publisher are not responsible for errors or omissions or for any consequences from application of the information in this book and make no warranty, expressed or implied, with respect to the currency, completeness, or accuracy of the contents of the publication. Application of this information in a particular situation remains the professional responsibility of the practitioner.

The authors, editors, and publisher have exerted every effort to ensure that drug selection and dosage set forth in this text are in accordance with current recommendations and practice at the time of publication. However, in view of ongoing research, changes in government regulations, and the constant flow of information relating to drug therapy and drug reactions, the reader is urged to check the package insert for each drug for any change in indications and dosage and for added warnings and precautions. This is particularly important when the recommended agent is a new or infrequently employed drug.

Some drugs and medical devices presented in this publication have Food and Drug Administration (FDA) clearance for limited use in restricted research settings. It is the responsibility of the health care provider to ascertain the FDA status of each drug or device planned for use in their clinical practice.

10 9 8 7 6 5 4 3 2 1

To Robert Haimovici, M.D., for his scholarly contributions to the field.

CONTENTS

CONTRIBUTING AUTHORS

J. Daniel Arbour, M.D., F.R.C.S.C. Associate Professor, Department of Ophthalmology, University of Montreal; and Vitreo-Retinal Surgeon, Department of Ophthalmology, Notre-Dame Hospital, Montreal, Quebec, Canada

Jennifer Joan Arnold, M.B.B.S. (Hons) F.R.A.N.Z.C.O. Marsden Eye Specialists, Parramatta, Australia

J.P. Ballini Swiss Federal Institute of Technology, Lausanne, Switzerland

Mark S. Blumenkranz, M.D. Professor and Chairman, Department of Ophthalmology, Stanford University School of Medicine, Stanford, California

Antonio P. Ciardella, M.D. Vitreoretina Fellow, Department of Ophthalmology, Manhattan Eye, Ear & Throat Hospital, New York, New York

René-Pierre Copt, M.D. Jules Gonin Eye Hospital, Lausanne, Switzerland

Gabriel Coscas, M.D. Clinique Ophtalmologique, Universitaire de Creteil, Creteil, France

Danny Gauthier, M.D., F.R.C.S.C. Assistant Professor, Department of Ophthalmology, University of Montreal; and Department of Ophthalmology, CHUM, Notre-Dame Hospital, Montreal, Quebec, Canada

Mauro Goldbaum, M.D. Residency Program Coordinator, Department of Ophthalmology, Instituto Suel Abujamra; and Attending Ophthalmologist, Department of Ophthalmology, Hospital Geral de Itap. da Serra, São Paulo, Brazil

Evangelos S. Gragoudas, M.D. Acting Chairman and Professor, Department of Ophthalmology, Harvard Medical School; Director, Retina Service, Massachusetts Eye & Ear Infirmary, Boston, Massachusetts

Kenneth B. Graham, M.D. Assistant Professor, Department of Ophthalmology, Albert Einstein College of Medicine, Bronx, New York; and Active Staff, Department of Ophthalmology, North Shore–Long Island Jewish Health System, Manhasset, New York

Robert Haimovici, M.D. (*deceased*) Assistant Professor, Department of Ophthalmology, Boston University School of Medicine, Boston, Massachusetts

Deeba Husain, M.D. Retina Fellow, Retina Service, Massachusetts Eye & Ear Infirmary, Harvard Medical School, Boston, Massachusetts

Rosa Y. Kim, M.D. Vitreoretinal Consultants, The Methodist Hospital, Houston, Texas

Sean S. Koh, M.D. Vitreoretinal Fellow, Massachusetts Eye & Ear Infirmary, Department of Ophthalmology, Harvard Medical School, Boston, Massachusetts

Michal Kramer, M.D. Instructor, Sackler School of Medicine, Tel-Aviv University; and Faculty, Department of Ophthalmology, Rabin Medical Center, Petah-Tikva, Israel

Eric Logean Engineer, Laboratory of Optics and Biophysics, Institute of Research in Ophthalmology, Sion, Switzerland

Mary E. Malmberg, R.N., C.R.N.A. PDT Clinic Director, Associated Retinal Consultants, P.C., Royal Oak, Michigan

Joan W. Miller, M.D. Professor, Department of Ophthalmology, Massachusetts Eye & Ear Infirmary, Harvard Medical School, Boston, Massachusetts

Jordi M. Monés, M.D. Associate Professor, Cátedra Institut de Microcirurgia Ocular, Universitat Autònoma de Barcelona; and Vitreoretinal Consultant, Macula Unit, Institut de Microcirurgia Ocular de Barcelona, I.M.O., Barcelona, Spain

Darius M. Moshfeghi, M.D. Assistant Professor, Vitreoretinal Surgery and Ophthalmic Oncology, Stanford University Hospital and Clinics, Stanford, California

Akira Obana, M.D., Ph.D. Associate Professor, Department of Ophthalmology and Visual Sciences, Osaka City University Graduate School of Medicine, Osaka City, Osaka, Japan

Gholam A. Peyman, M.D. Professor, Department of Ophthalmology, Tulane University Health Sciences Center; and Co-Director, Vitreoretinal Service, Department of Ophthalmology, Tulane Hospital and Clinics, New Orleans, Louisiana

Constantin J. Pournaras, M.D. "Chargé de Cours" and Senior Consultant, Department of Ophthalmology, University Hospital of Geneva, Geneva, Switzerland

Martin H. Reinke, M.D. Vitreoretinal Service, Key-Whitman Eye Center, Dallas, Texas

Reem Z. Renno, M.D. Department of Ophthalmology, University of California–Los Angeles; and Jules Stein Eye Institute, Los Angeles, California

Charles E. Riva, D.Sc. Professor, Laboratory of Optics and Biophysics, Institute of Research in Ophthalmology, Sion, Switzerland

Philip J. Rosenfeld, M.D., Ph.D. Associate Professor, Department of Ophthalmology, Bascom Palmer Eye Institute, University of Miami School of Medicine; and Associate Professor, Department of Ophthalmology, Anne Bates Leach Eye Hospital, Miami, Florida

Jason S. Slakter, M.D. Clinical Professor, Department of Ophthalmology, New York University School of Medicine; and Surgeon Director, Department of Ophthalmology, Manhattan Eye, Ear & Throat Hospital, New York, New York

Wendy J. Snyder, Ph.D. Senior Manager, Department of Ophthalmology, Miravant Medical Technologies, Santa Barbara, California

Gisèle Soubrane, M.D., Ph.D. Professor, Department of Ophthalmology, Eye University Clinic, Centre Hospitalier Internacommunal, Creteil, France

Yoshiko Terada, M.D., Ph.D. Research Fellow, Angiogenesis Laboratory/Retina Service, Massachusetts Eye & Ear Infirmary, Boston, Massachusetts; and Department of Ophthalmology, Okayama University Graduate School of Medicine and Dentistry, Okayama, Japan

Edgar Lee Thomas, M.D. Co-Director, Clinical Research, Retina-Vitreous Associates, Beverly Hills, California

Hubert Erik van den Bergh, Ph.D. Professor, Institute of Environmental Science and Technology, Swiss Federal Institute of Technology, Lausanne, Switzerland

George A. Williams, M.D. Clinical Professor, Department of Biomedical Sciences, Eye Research Institute, Oakland University, Rochester, Michigan; and Chairmain, Department of Ophthalmology, William Beaumont Hospital, Royal Oak, Michigan

Kathryn Woodburn, Ph.D.

Lawrence A. Yannuzzi, M.D. Professor of Clinical Ophthalmology, Columbia University Medical School; and Manhattan Eye, Ear & Throat Hospital, New York, New York

Shin Yoneya, M.D., Ph.D. Professor and Chairman, Department of Ophthalmology, Saitama Medical School, Moroyama, Iruma, Saitama, Japan

Lucy H. Y. Young, M.D., Ph.D. Associate Professor, Department of Ophthalmology, Harvard Medical School; and Department of Ophthalmology, Massachusetts Eye & Ear Infirmary, Boston, Massachusetts

Leonidas Zografos, M.D. Professor, Department of Ophthalmology, University Eye Clinic; and Chairman, Department of Ophthalmology, Jules Gonin Eye Hospital, Lausanne, Switzerland

PREFACE

The treatment of neovascular age-related macular degeneration (AMD), with its known devastating effect on central vision in the senior citizen population of developed countries, remains one of the most frustrating problems for the vitreoretinal specialist. During the last three decades, its diagnosis has become highly accurate and several advances in epidemiology, genetics, and angiogenetics have increased our knowledge in understanding the pathophysiology of this disorder.

Only a few years ago, thermal laser photocoagulation was the only available method of treatment and applicable to only a small number of patients with limited success. Several new treatment strategies have revolutionized the potential successful management of neovascular AMD and hopefully will reduce the visual disability in this group of patients. At the present time, the best available treatment of proven benefit for subfoveal neovascular AMD, which unfortunately occurs in the majority of the affected patients, is photodynamic therapy (PDT). Large-scale multicenter randomized Phase III clinical trials using verteporfin PDT have shown that PDT is effective in reducing visual loss in a large number of patients with subfoveal neovascular AMD. Other major clinical trials in Phase II and Phase III are in progress using different photosensitizers, and new dyes are under investigation in animal models.

The goal of this book is to provide the reader with an overview of the history and principles of PDT, the results of preclinical animal studies of different photosensitizing dyes, and the present state of the art in the clinical use of PDT. It has been our privilege to assemble an excellent group of collaborators who have worked extensively in the field of photodynamic therapy. This is an evolving field in ophthalmology and the editors hope that this book will provide the vitreoretinal specialist with a valuable insight into PDT and assist them in the treatment of their patients.

We would like to thank all the authors for their excellent contributions and for making this effort a pleasure rather than a burden. We owe special thanks to Ms. Delois Patterson and Lippincott Williams & Wilkins for their outstanding work in making suggestions, editing the text, and coordinating the efforts of all the contributors.

Evangelos S. Gragoudas, M.D.
Joan W. Miller, M.D.
Leonidas Zografos, M.D.

PHOTODYNAMIC THERAPY OF OCULAR DISEASES

1

HISTORY OF PHOTODYNAMIC THERAPY FOR OCULAR DISORDERS

JOAN W. MILLER
EVANGELOS S. GRAGOUDAS

Photodynamic therapy (PDT) is not a new technique, but has undergone a recent resurgence with the advent of newer photosensitizing dyes and more rigorous investigations into its application. Using an exogenous photosensitizer to achieve a therapeutic effect was described approximately 1,500 years ago, when Psoralen (obtained from the seed of Psoralia Corifolia in India and the leaves of Amnii Majus in Egypt) was used to treat vitiligo (1). Von Tappeiner and Rabb initiated the use of oxygen-dependent photosensitizer reactions in an example of scientific serendipity (1). A thunderstorm occurred during their experiments study of the toxic properties of acridine on paramecium. Paramecia exposed to acridine and the light from the thunderstorm died, leading the scientists to study the effects of acridine and altered light conditions. They found that light combined with even small concentrations of acridine led to increased toxicity to the paramecia (2). Von Tappeiner and Jodbauer demonstrated the oxygen dependence of this reaction and coined the term photodynamic action (3). Von Tappeiner and Jestoniek developed PDT for skin diseases including psoriasis, lupus, condylomata, and cancer using eosin as a photosensitizer (1). Meyer-Betz in 1913 demonstrated the photosensitizing effects of hematoporphyrin and its derivatives in rat tumors (4).

Modern PDT was initiated with the extraction of hematoporphyrin (HPD) derivative by Lipson and colleagues in 1960 (5). Treatment using light and intravenous hematoporphyrin derivative, termed photoradiation, led to long-term cures in animal tumors (6,7). Over the next 20 years these techniques were used to treat malignancies at various sites, including the bladder, lung, head and neck, brain, uterus, and gastrointestinal tract (8,9). Most reports concluded that superficial and minimally invasive disease responds best to PDT. The treatment of large tumors generally required higher light or photosensitizer doses to produce a complete response and were associated with an increased rate of complications. These earlier studies often lacked standardized inclusion criteria, treatment protocols and end points, definition of response rates and length of follow-up, making interpretation of the results difficult. Improved photosensitizers, advances in photosensitizer delivery and light dosimetry, and the adoption of increasingly rigorous study designs allow better comparisons with more established forms of therapy.

MECHANISM OF ACTION, PHOTOSENSITIZER LOCALIZATION, AND TREATMENT PARAMETERS

These topics are reviewed here, but are covered in greater detail in Chapters 2, 3, and 11. Photodynamic therapy requires the administration of a photosensitizing dye, usually intravenously, which localizes to the target tissue. Light irradiation of this tissue at an absorption maximum of the dye, elevates the photosensitizer from its electronic ground state to a higher level (excited) triplet state. The excited photosensitizer quickly returns to the ground state, and, in the process, transfers energy to other molecules. When this energy is transferred to molecular oxygen, in the type II mechanism, singlet oxygen is formed, which then reacts with proteins, nucleic acids, and lipid membranes (10). When the excited photosensitizer transfers energy to other compounds, in the type I mechanism, superoxide, hydroxyl, and other free radicals may be formed (11). These highly reactive molecules cause cellular injury resulting in apoptosis and/or necrosis. Tumor cells may be damaged directly but endothelial cells lining blood vessels also may be damaged, leading to thrombosis. Photodynamic tissue effects are not dependent on increasing the temperature of the target tissues and thus differ from conventional thermal photocoagulation or dye-enhanced thermal photocoagulation.

The factors governing the effectiveness of a given photosensitizer are multiple, and depend in part on its photophysical and physicochemical properties. The absorption spectrum of the photosensitizer dictates the wavelengths of the radiation that may be suitable for PDT. Generally, the wavelength(s) selected coincides with an absorption maximum of the photosensitizer. The absorption spectrum of several photosensitizers that have been used in ophthalmology are superimposed in Figures 11.1 and 11.2. The effective penetration depth of the PDT treatment is dependent on the wavelength of the light and the optical properties of the tissue. Typically, the effective penetration depth is 2 to 3 mm at 630 nm, and increases to 5 to 6 mm at longer wavelengths (700 to 800 nm) (12). These values can be altered by changing the biological and physical characteristics of the photosensitizer. In general, photosensitizers absorbing at longer wavelengths, with higher molar absorption at these wavelengths, are more efficient photodynamic agents (13).

Other important aspects of a particular photosensitizer include the metabolism, pH, and route of administration of the photosensitizer. For most ophthalmic applications, photosensitizers are administered intravenously, either as an intravenous infusion or more rapidly as an intravenous bolus injection. A key consideration in PDT, is the ability of the photosensitizer to localize preferentially in target tissues, which leads to damage of the target tissue, and minimizes collateral damage to surrounding tissues (14). Strategies that have been used to deliver photosensitizers include liposomes, emulsions, precomplexing with lipoproteins, and binding of photosensitizers to targeting antibodies or peptides (15–20).

The subcellular target also may vary among photosensitizers (19). Some photosensitizers cause damage primarily to the plasma membrane and mitochondria, and others cause nuclear or lysosomal damage. Subcellular localization affects the pathway of cellular injury, with mitochondrial localization leading to apoptosis rather than necrosis, whereas localization to plasma membranes or lysosomes more typically leads to necrosis (21). Despite evidence for direct damage to tumor cells under some circumstances, most data suggest that occlusion of tumor vasculature is an important mechanism leading to tumor cell death. Photodynamic therapy–induced damage to endothelial cells results in platelet adhesion and degranulation, leading to stasis and aggregation of blood cells and vascular occlusion. After PDT, there is release of eicosanoids, including thromboxane and histamine, as well as tumor necrosis factor (TNF-α), which may contribute to vascular occlusion (22).

Many light sources can be used for PDT, including broadband light from incandescent or arc lamps, or monochromatic light from tunable argon-pumped dye lasers or diode lasers. Broad light bands may enhance the photodynamic effect if they excite secondary absorption peaks of the photosensitizer. Slit-lamp delivery of laser light allows for spatial confinement and is particularly suited to intraocular applications (23–25). The laser treatment parameters for PDT are important for its selectivity, and include the fluence or J/cm^2, and the irradiance (or fluence rate) in mW/cm^2, which determines the length of time of the treatment at a particular fluence. Although PDT typically has been performed with low irradiances in the range of 150 to 200 mW/cm^2, work in our laboratory demonstrated the utility and safety of higher irradiances (26). Ocular applications using 600 mW/cm^2 have been adopted in preclinical and clinical studies using a variety of photosensitizers (27–29). The timing of irradiation for PDT, or the time after photosensitizer injection that the light is applied, is also critical for the selectivity of treatment. Although photosensitizer fluorescence has been investigated by a number of approaches, ophthalmology is ideally suited for demonstrating photosensitizer spatial and temporal localization by fluorescent angiography. Using standard digital fundus cameras and imaging systems, with filters modified to optimize photosensitizer absorption and fluorescence, one can obtain serial fundus images following intravenous administration of the photosensitizer (30–33). These images can be analyzed using image software, to compare fluorescence in tissues of interest [retinal vessels, choroidal neovascularization (CNV), and normal choroid] over time. One can determine whether a photosensitizer localizes to CNV at a time when it is no longer in retinal vessels, whether it leaks out of CNV into the subretinal space, and one can predict the time window for irradiation during PDT. These approaches are described in more detail in Chapters 11, 21, and 22.

PHOTOSENSITIZERS IN OPHTHALMOLOGY

Several major classes of photosensitizers have been used in vitro and in vivo in animal models for investigations of photodynamic therapy (Table 1.1). The properties and ocular localization of the photosensitizers are discussed in more

TABLE 1.1. THERAPEUTIC PHOTOSENSITIZERS USED FOR THE TREATMENT OF OCULAR NEOVASCULARIZATION

Xanthene derivatives
Rose Bengal
Tetrapyrrole derivatives
Hematoporphyrin derivative
Photofrin (porfimer sodium/dihematoporphyrin ether)
Benzoporphyrin derivative (verteporfin)
Tin etiopurpurin
Lutetium texaphyrin
ATXS10(Na)
Chlorins and bacteriochlorins
Chlorin e6
Bacteriochlorin a
Phthalocyanines
Chloroaluminum sulfonated phthalocyanine
Zinc phthalocyanine

detail in Chapters 2 and 11 and in the chapters describing experimental and clinical studies. To date (3), photosensitizers have been tested in clinical trials in ophthalmology; verteporfin or benzoporphyrin derivative, Purlytin or tin ethyl etiopurpurin, and Lu-Tex or lutetium texaphyrin.

Porphyrin derivatives such as HPD derivative and porfimer sodium (Photofrin) are the most widely studied photodynamic agents. Hematoporphyrin is a complex mixture of porphyrins that is synthesized from hematoporphyrin (34). Photodynamic therapy with HPD is performed with 630-nm wavelength light to increase tissue penetration and decrease absorption by other tissue chromophores. Drawbacks of this agent are its small absorption peak at these longer wavelengths and the prolonged skin photosensitivity lasting 1 month or more after therapy. Porfimer sodium is a partially purified component of HPD that is more potent and produces less skin toxicity than does HPD (35). Porfimer sodium has been approved for human use for certain cancers in a variety of countries.

The chlorins, bacteriochlorins, and benzoporphyrin derivatives are newer porphyrin derivatives with favorable properties that recently have been used for PDT. Chlorin derivatives such as monoaspartyl chlorin e6 or NPe6 are effective photosensitizers in animal tumor models (28,36). Bacteriochlorin a is a chlorin derivative that has an absorption maximum at 760 nm and a higher molar absorption coefficient compared with HPD (37). Verteporfin (or BPD) is another modified porphyrin that has an absorption maximum of about 690 nm and is phototoxic *in vivo.* Verteporfin is rapidly inactivated or cleared from the body with no significant phototoxicity after 24 hours (38). It has been used to treat experimental ocular neovascularization and tumors, and currently is the only photosensitizer approved for use in ophthalmology (39). Purlytin or tin-etiopurpurin (SnET2), which absorbs at 664 nm, has been used to treat experimental CNV, and was investigated in clinical trials for neovascular age-related macular degeneration (AMD) (40). ATX S10Na is a water-soluble porphyrin compound that has a half-life in plasma of approximately 30 minutes and has been studied in experimental CNV (41).

Phthalocyanines are another class of photosensitizers with a strong absorption band at 675 nm (42,43). Central metals such as zinc and aluminum are incorporated into their structure to increase the triplet state and singlet oxygen yields. Their solubility and cellular localization is at least partially determined by the number and charge of their side chains. The phthalocyanines are cleared more rapidly and produce substantially less skin toxicity than HPD, porfimer sodium, or dihematoporphyrin ether (DHE) (43). Phthalocyanines have been investigated in experimental models of ocular neovascularization and ocular tumors, but their safety for use in humans has not yet been determined (44–46).

Texaphyrins are pure, synthetic water-soluble macrocycles that are formulated with central metallic ions. Lutetium texaphyrin contains lutetium, absorbing at 732 nm, and is stable, pure, water-soluble, and shows rapid skin clearance and no skin photosensitization (47). Its efficacy has been demonstrated in the treatment of experimental tumors and atheromatous plaque, and it has been studied in Phase I trials of patients with metastatic cancer (48,49). In addition, Lu-Tex PDT was investigated in experimental CNV and clinical trials (50,51). Xanthene derivatives also have photosensitizing properties (52,53). Rose Bengal is a halogenated fluorescein derivative with increased singlet oxygen yields and photosensitizing ability that has been used to produce photochemically mediated vascular damage of ocular vessels (54–56).

EXPERIMENTAL AND CLINICAL USE

Ocular Tumors

Iris and Ciliary Body Melanoma

Clinical Studies

There have been several case reports describing PDT for the treatment of human iris and ciliary body melanoma. As early as 1984, Tse and coworkers (57) treated two ciliary body melanomas and one iris melanoma with HPD and transcorneal red light (xenon arc lamp or argon pumped dye laser at 630 nm), with low irradiances (18 to 200 mW/cm^2) and high fluences (1,400 J/cm^2 and 2,566 J/cm^2). There was incomplete necrosis of both tumors as shown by histopathologic examination, but the tumor treated with the higher fluence showed an increased depth of necrosis. The iris melanoma received 1,080 J/cm^2 and showed a complete clinical response. Sery and coworkers (58) treated a patient with diffuse multinodular iris melanoma with HPD given at 2.5 mg/kg and 632-nm red light from an argon-pumped dye laser delivered by a fiberoptic probe and found no response. A combined photodynamic and photothermal approach for the treatment of iris melanoma has also been reported with variable results (35,59).

Some complications were noted with PDT of human iris and ciliary body melanomas, including iris neovascularization and neovascular glaucoma, but these also can occur with other treatment modalities (57,60). Severe uveitis is associated with high fluences and photosensitizer doses and may be the result of sudden and extensive necrosis of neoplastic tissues (35,46). This complication might be minimized by the treatment of large tumors in multiple sessions.

These early pilot human studies were inconclusive regarding the efficacy of PDT and indicated the need for an improved understanding of light dosimetry and other factors limiting photodynamic injury. Accordingly, investigators pursued PDT research using experimental models. The simplest tumor model is the Greene hamster melanoma model, in which Greene hamster melanoma cells are grown in culture and injected into the anterior chamber of rabbits (61–65). Tumor nodules rapidly proliferate, filling the anterior chamber, and, if untreated, eventually lead to ocular perforation. The photosensitizer is injected intravenously and the anterior segment tumors are treated with laser light using an optical fiber, or with the slit-lamp.

Studies using the Greene hamster model and HPD or DHE typically showed no discernible change in the tumor or surface hemorrhages and vascular occlusion. Anterior chamber inflammation was noted and fluorescein angiography (FA) demonstrated occlusion of the tumor vessels (63). Histopathologic examination has shown only partial tumor necrosis, similar to results reported in patients (65). Complete necrosis has been reported in small tumors of up to 4 mm in height with HPD, 2.5 mg/kg, and a fluence of 102 J/cm^2 or greater (irradiance: 71 mW/cm^2) (62,64). When using this model, high doses of HPD (7.5 to 10 mg/kg) or energy levels of more than 180 J/cm^2 caused unacceptable ocular toxicity, including corneal and conjunctival edema, and intraocular hemorrhage and inflammation (62). Histopathologic study of eyes after experimental anterior chamber melanoma with HPD phototherapy suggests that occlusion of tumor vessels is the predominant mechanism responsible for tumor necrosis, although direct PDT effects on tumors have also been reported (66).

This anterior chamber model has been used to study the feasibility of PDT with newer-generation photosensitizers such as chloroaluminum sulfonated phthalocyanine (CASPc) or benzoporphyrin derivative monoacid (BPD-MA) (46,67). Panagopoulos and coworkers performed PDT 24 hours after the intravenous administration of CASPc, 5 mg/kg, using 675-nm red light at nonthermal power densities (63 to 216 mW/cm^2). Tumors treated with light or dye alone showed continued growth. Four eyes treated with 3 to 10 J/cm^2 (10 to 48 mW/cm^2) after intravenous CASPc administration, experienced tumor regrowth after initial growth arrest. Eyes that received 20 J/cm^2 or greater had permanent growth arrest, which was confirmed histopathologically. Those that received the highest light doses (57 to 60 J/cm^2) or very high doses of CASPc (16 to 30 mg/kg) showed permanent growth arrest but developed corneal edema, hyphema, and severe anterior segment inflammation.

Others used the same model to perform PDT using BPD-MA precomplexed with low-density lipoprotein (67). After irradiation with 692 nm of red light using energies of 100 J/cm^2 (150 mW/cm^2), necrosis of anterior chamber tumors was seen histopathologically. Photodynamic therapy using newer photosensitizers such as CASPc and BPD appears to be effective in the treatment of Greene hamster melanoma tumors, but it is recognized that this model has limitations. Physical damage to adjacent structures such as the cornea and lens, which has been observed with this model, may be related in part to the abnormal location of these tumors as well as to the effects of PDT. Tumor cells that are not visible at the time of PDT remain untreated and continue to grow and preclude long-term follow-up of affected eyes. The Greene hamster models, which also have been criticized as a melanoma model because of their lack of pigmentation, may make these tumors more susceptible to PDT-mediated injury. Newer models with pigmented melanoma cells may address this criticism.

Choroidal Melanoma

Clinical Studies

The treatment of choroidal melanoma with PDT in patients has been described in a few reports. Tse and coworkers (57) treated three patients with choroidal melanoma using HPD, 3 to 5 mg/kg, and transcorneal red light delivered via a xenon arc lamp or an argon pumped dye laser (630 nm). Two patients treated with 64 or 850 J/cm^2 showed no histologic evidence of tumor necrosis. A third patient received a higher fluence (2,160 J/cm^2) and showed limited tumor necrosis to a depth of 2 to 3 mm. Between 1982 and 1985, Bruce (68,69) treated 24 patients with choroidal melanoma using HPD, 2.5 mg/kg, followed 72 hours later by transcorneal and transscleral exposure to 630 nm red light (200 to 6,800 J/cm^2) from an argon pumped dye laser. Skin photosensitivity, chemosis, iritis, and vision loss occurred in all 24 patients. Subsequent improvement in vision occurred in patients with tumors greater than 4 mm from the macula. Exudative retinal detachment, vitreitis, and choroidal detachment were less common complications. Although patients with small- and medium-sized tumors responded best, no definitive statement was made regarding the numbers of patients cured (69).

Murphree and coworkers (70) treated seven patients with choroidal melanoma using HPD, 2.5 mg/kg, and transcorneal and transscleral red light, and reported only one complete response in a patient with an amelanotic melanoma who was treated twice. More recently, Favilla and coworkers (71) treated 19 patients with choroidal melanoma using HPD, 5 to 7.5 mg/kg, and transpupillary laser light of 620 to 630 nm. Three patients also received transscleral application. All tumors were less than 10 mm in height and all but one were less than 7 mm in height. Complete response was recorded in six patients who had light or moderately pigmented tumors. No regression was seen in eight patients, five of whom had darkly pigmented tumors.

In general, these clinical studies indicate that small melanomas or those that are nonpigmented or lightly pigmented may respond favorably to PDT, whereas large melanomas are not responsive. Increased light absorption by chromophores such as melanin or hemoglobin may contribute to the incomplete eradication of large tumors (58). Other possible factors include the choice of photosensitizer, low or inhomogeneous oxygen concentrations within the tumor, or inadequate distribution or quenching of the photosensitizer. The results of these studies indicate that PDT for choroidal melanoma has not yet proved to be as effective as existing methods of treatment, such as charged-particle and plaque radiotherapy (72).

Experimental Studies

Several investigators have treated experimental choroidal melanoma with newer-generation photosensitizers. These studies are described in more detail in Chapter 13 (73–77). In these experiments, tumor cells such as the Greene hamster melanoma are injected into the suprachoroidal space and growth is monitored by indirect ophthalmoscopy, fundus photography, and, in some cases, echography, and color Doppler imaging (75). Tumors then are treated with laser light delivered via the slit-lamp. Schmidt-Erfurth and coworkers (73) treated experimental subchoroidal Greene hamster melanoma with BPD-MA, 2 mg/kg, precomplexed with lipoprotein and 692 nm red light. Complete necrosis of tumors was confirmed by histopathologic examination after treatment with 100 J/cm^2. Complications included transient vitreitis and a self-limited exudative retinal detachment in 50% of treated eyes, which largely resolved within 48 hours.

In order to study the efficacy of PDT for pigmented tumors, Hu and coworkers (78) established a pigmented choroidal melanoma model in the rabbit. Tumor-bearing rabbits were injected with CASPc, 5 mg/kg, and 24 hours later tumors were irradiated with 675 nm of red light from an argon pumped dye laser. Complete tumor arrest was accomplished with light doses of 35 to 60 J/cm^2 (74). Photodynamic therapy using BPD also was effective in treating experimental pigmented choroidal melanoma (77). In 18 rabbit eyes treated with PDT using BPD, regression was seen in all tumors treated with 60 J/cm^2. Histologic examination showed acute vascular damage through the full thickness of the tumor (up to 4.6 mm) (79). These experimental studies suggest that PDT with newer photosensitizing agents and modified treatment strategies holds promise for the treatment of human choroidal melanoma.

Retinoblastoma

Clinical Studies

A few investigators have treated patients with retinoblastoma using PDT. Murphree and coworkers (70) treated six patients with recurrent retinoblastoma with HPD and subthermal threshold 630 nm red light. Despite initial response, there was recurrence of tumor growth in all six patients. Ohnishi and coworkers (80) performed PDT using HPD, 2.5 and 5 mg/kg, and argon laser (488 to 514.5 nm) in five children with retinoblastoma, four of whom had received previous ionizing radiation treatment. In the case treated primarily with PDT using HPD, 5 mg/kg (300 mW/cm^2, 270 J/cm^2), angionecrosis, thrombus formation, and tumor cell death were seen to a depth of about 6 mm. Complications in the five patients included choroidal hemorrhage and tractional retinal detachment. Using a similar approach, Murphree (81) successfully treated two patients with recurrent retinoblastoma using HPD followed by continuous-wave argon green laser photocoagulation. Although PDT of retinoblastoma may prove clinically effective, it is probably not a reasonable consideration in eyes with vitreous seeding where the absence of tumor vasculature hinders photosensitizer uptake (82).

Experimental Studies

Photodynamic therapy has been tested in animal models of retinoblastoma, with successful tumor necrosis, but high photosensitizer doses may be associated with complications such as retinal edema, detachment, and choroidal hemorrhage (82–85). Pending further reports, the treatment of human retinoblastoma with PDT remains investigational.

OCULAR NEOVASCULARIZATION

The rationale for using PDT to occlude pathologic neovascularization arose from observations first recognized in treating tumors. Porphyrin photosensitizing dyes preferentially localize to neovascular tissue in tumors, and tumor damage from PDT occurs secondary to vascular occlusion. The mechanism of vascular thrombosis in the eye is similar to that previously described for ocular tumors and its rate also is directly related to light intensity, photosensitizer doses, and oxygen concentration (54–56). The potential for PDT to produce selective closure of ocular neovascularization with decreased collateral damage to other structures has been investigated in several experimental studies, and subsequently in clinical trials in macular degeneration.

Corneal Neovascularization

Experimental corneal neovascularization (induced by intrastromal injection of interleukin-2) was treated with PDT using intravenous DHE and irradiation 72 hours later with 514 nm light (86). Significant reduction in corneal neovascularization was observed but complicated by blepharitis, and iris injury. Pallikaris and colleagues (87,88) treated experimental corneal neovascularization induced by intrastromal silk sutures in rabbit eyes using phthalocyanine and 675 nm light (87). Neovascular vessels were thrombosed histologically in the first few days after PDT, although some larger vessels appeared patent by postoperative day 20. Some thrombosis of normal iris vessels was noted, although the iris appeared to have recovered by 1 month following PDT. Additional studies demonstrated that closure of corneal neovascularization was more effective with increasing phthalocyanine dose and irradiation early after drug administration (88). Using topically administered ATX-S10 (Na), Gohto and colleagues successfully treated experimental corneal neovascularization when light was applied with 20 minutes of drug administration (89). They have also shown effective closure with intravenous photosensitizer administration (90). Schmidt-Erfurth and colleagues used verteporfin PDT to occlude experimental corneal neovascularization, although they found better results with irradiation was performed 60 to 90 minutes after drug administration. (91). Clinical PDT of corneal neovascularization has not been reported.

Iris Neovascularization

Photodynamic therapy has been used successfully to treat experimental iris neovascularization. Experimental iris neovascularization may be produced in primates by photothermal or thermal occlusion of major retinal veins leading to retinal schemia and VEGF production (92,93). Using this model, Packer and coworkers treated iris neovascularization with PDT using HPD, 3 mg/kg, and 675 nm red light (200 mW/cm^2, 540 J/cm^2) (94). Twenty-four hours after PDT there was marked reduction in fluorescein staining as seen by iris angiography, but also a substantial inflammatory anterior chamber reaction. Iris neovascularization later recurred in one eye, which was then retreated. Using a similar model, Miller and coworkers treated experimental iris neovascularization with intravenous CASPc, 0.5 to 1.0 mg/kg, and 675 nm red laser light (200 mW, 34 to 102 J/cm^2) and found thrombotic occlusion of iris neovascularization as early as 1 hour after treatment (45). Leaky iris vessels reappeared by day 7 in one treated eye, without evidence for recanalization of PDT-treated vessels. Minimal anterior chamber reaction and a transient rise in intraocular pressure occurred after treatment. Experimental iris neovascularization also has been successfully treated with PDT using verteporfin and 689 nm light (95). The treatment of clinical iris neovascularization with PDT may have a role as adjunctive therapy in combination with standard retinal ablation. A recent report described preliminary data in a pilot clinical trial of verteporfin PDT of iris neovascularization in patients. Iris neovascularization was successfully occluded using PDT without injury to normal iris vessels or other normal tissue (96).

Choroidal Neovascularization

Photodynamic therapy has been shown to be a relatively selective therapy for CNV, depending on the photosensitizer characteristics, drug dose, light dose, and timing of light application. Preliminary studies examined closure of normal choroidal vessels, including work by Nanda and colleagues that used PDT with Rose Bengal to occlude the medullary ray and choroidal vessels in the rabbit (54). They used 10 mg/kg of Rose Bengal, with irradiation 1 to 2 minutes after Rose Bengal injection using a 300 W xenon-arc lamp with filters to provide light at 550 + 10 nm, using 30 J or 1,695 J/cm^2 and 125 mW/cm^2 (at the cornea).

In 1987, Thomas and Langhofer investigated PDT of experimental CNV using dihematoporphyrin ether (DHE) (97). They used 8 mg/kg of DHE, with irradiation 12 hours after DHE injection, using a single 200-μm burn of 514-nm argon green light of 100 mW for 0.1 seconds. They demonstrated occlusion of CNV, but their laser parameters are consistent with thermal laser photocoagulation (318 W/cm^2), rather than PDT. Ben and Hevda Miller used Rose Bengal to occlude experimental CNV in the monkey (23). They used 40 mg/kg of Rose Bengal, and irradiated the retina with slit-lamp illumination using filters to provide light at wavelengths between 510 and 750 nm, with irradiance of 12.7 mW/cm^2 and fluence of 1.5 to 7.6 J/cm^2. They demonstrated occlusion of CNV with sparing of retinal vessels if irradiation was applied between 40 and 70 minutes after Rose Bengal injection. Kliman and colleagues treated experimental CNV in the monkey with PDT using CASPc. They achieved closure of CNV using 0.5 mg/kg of CASPc with an irradiation of 675 nm light 5 to 30 minutes after CASPc injection, at 283 mW/cm^2 and 34 J/cm^2. Although they did not specifically address the selectivity of their effect, they did note retinal hemorrhages after treatment, suggesting some nonselective effects on retinal vessels (44).

All of these investigators, and others, postulated the use of PDT in AMD. With the exception of Ben and Hevda Miller, the investigators did not study the selectivity of the PDT effects on the surrounding retinal tissue, especially retinal vessels. Without evidence of selectivity, PDT of CNV would not offer any clinical advantage over thermal laser photocoagulation. These studies also were limited by the characteristics of the available dyes. The first-generation photosensitizers had clinical limitations. Hematoporphyrin derivative is an impure compound, leading to some variability in treatment effect. It causes prolonged cutaneous photosensitivity as well as having poor absorption in the longer wavelengths (which provide better tissue penetration). CASPc also is an impure compound, and along with Rose Bengal has potential systemic toxicity. Miller and colleagues demonstrated relatively selective occlusion of experimental CNV using verteporfin PDT, studies that led to clinical trials and subsequent adoption of verteporfin PDT into clinical practice. These experimental and clinical studies are discussed in Chapter 5 and Section III. Photodynamic therapy of experimental CNV also has been shown to be efficacious using lutetium texaphyrin (Chapter 8), ATX-S10(Na) (Chapter 6), and Purlytin (Chapter 7). Both Purlytin and lutetium texaphyrin were studied subsequently in clinical trials (Chapters 19 and 20).

RECENT ADVANCES IN OPHTHALMIC PHOTODYNAMIC THERAPY

Early studies of PDT in ophthalmology were limited in part by the available photosensitizers. Advances in ophthalmic

PDT could be made with the development of photosensitizers with better attributes, including more rapid clearance. Several photosensitizers have been studied more thoroughly for ophthalmic application; they include verteporfin, Purlytin, and Lu-Tex, with studies in PDT in experimental models as well as clinical trials for PDT of CNV. Verteporfin PDT was approved by health authorities in the United States and abroad for clinical use in 2000, and remains the only photosensitizer approved for clinical use in ophthalmology to date. Currently, it is approved for treating CNV secondary to AMD and other disorders. There have been published reports of verteporfin PDT being used with some success to treat choroidal hemangiomas, retinal angiomas, and central serous choroidopathy. Additional applications include neovascular glaucoma, proliferative retinopathy, and other tumors, including choroidal melanoma and retinoblastoma. We are in the early stages of a new era in ophthalmic PDT. Additional work needs to be carried out to improve our understanding of cellular mechanisms and improve our results in clinical treatment.

REFERENCES

1. Spikes J. Historical review. Photodynamic action: from paramecium to photochemotherapy. *Photochem Photobiol* 1997;65S: 142S–147S.
2. Rabb C. Uber die Wirkung Fluroeszierenden Stoffe auf Infusoria. *Z Biol* 1900;39:524–526.
3. von Tappeiner H, Jensionek A. Therapeutische Versuche mit fluorescierenden Stoffen. *Munch Med Wochenschr* 1903;47: 2042–2044.
4. Meyer-Betz F. Untersuchengen uber die biologische (photodynamische) Wirkung des Hamatopophyrins und anderer Derivative des Blut-und Gallenfarbstoffs. *Dtsch Arch Klin Med* 1913; 112:476–503.
5. Lipson R, Blades E. The photodynamic properties of a particular hematoporphyrin derivative. *Arch Dermatol* 1960;82:508–516.
6. Diamond I, McDonagh A, Wilson C, et al. Photodynamic therapy of malignant tumors. *Lancet* 1972;2:1175–1177.
7. Dougherty T, Grindley G, Fiel R, et al. Photoradiation therapy II: cure of animal tumors with hematoporphyrin derivative and light. *J Natl Cancer Inst* 1975;55:115–121.
8. Dougherty T, Lawrence G, Kaufman J, et al. Photoradiation in the treatment of recurrent breast carcinoma. *J Natl Cancer Inst* 1979;62:231–237.
9. Dougherty T. Photosensitization of malignant tumors. *Semin Surg Oncol* 1986;2:24–37.
10. Weishaupt K, Gomer C, Dougherty T. Identification of singlet oxygen as the cytotoxic agent in photo-inactivation of murine tumor. *Cancer Res* 1976;36:2326–2329.
11. Buettner G, Oberly L. The apparent production of superoxide and hydroxyl radicals by hematoporphyrin and light as seen by spin-trapping. *Fed Biol Sci Letts* 1980;121:161–164.
12. Svaasand L, Ellingson R. Optical properties of human brain. *Photochem Photobiol* 1983;38:283–289.
13. Hasan T, Parish J. Photodynamic therapy of cancer. In: Holland JEA, ed. *Cancer medicine*, vol 1, 4th ed. Baltimore: Williams & Wilkins, 1997:739–751.
14. Figge F, Weiland G, Manganiello L, et al. Cancer detection and therapy. Affinity of neplastic, embryonic and traumatized tissues for porphyrins and metalloporphyrins. *J Proc Soc Exp Biol Med* 1948;68:640–641.
15. Jori G, Tomio L, Reddi E, et al. Preferential delivery of liposome-incorporated porphryin to neoplastic cells in tumour-bearing rats. *Br J Cancer* 1983;48:307–309.
16. Allison BA, Waterfield E, Richter AM, et al. The effects of plasma lipoproteins on in vitro tumor cell killing and in vivo tumor photosensitization with benzoporphyrin derivative. *Photochem Photobiol* 1991;54:709–715.
17. Jori G. Low density lipoprotein-liposome delivery system for tumor photosensitizers in vivo. In: Henderson B, Dougherty T, eds. *Photodynamic therapy: basic principles and clinical applications.* New York: Marcel Dekker, 1992:173–186.
18. Kessel D. Porphyrin-lipoprotein association as a factor in porphyrin localization. *Cancer Letts* 1986;33:183–188.
19. Jiang F, Allison B, Liu D, Levy J. Enhanced photodynamic killing of target cells by either monoclonal antibody or low density lipoprotein mediated delivery systems. *J Controlled Rel* 1992; 19:41–58.
20. Renno RZ, Miller JW. Photosensitizer delivery for photodynamic therapy of choroidal neovascularization. *Adv Drug Deliv Rev* 2001;52:63–78.
21. Kessel D, Luo Y. Mitochondrial photodamage and PDT-induced apoptosis. *J Photochem Photobiol B Biol* 1998;42:89–95.
22. Fingar V. Vascular effect of photodynamic therapy. *J Clin Laser Med Surg* 1996;14:323–328.
23. Miller H, Miller B. Photodynamic therapy of subretinal neovascularization in the monkey eye. *Arch Ophthalmol* 1993;111: 855–860.
24. Miller JW, Walsh AW, Kramer M, et al. Photodynamic therapy of experimental choroidal neovascularization using lipoprotein-delivered benzoporphyrin. *Arch Ophthalmol* 1995;113:810–818.
25. Kramer M, Miller J, Michaud N, et al. Liposomal BPD verteporfin photodynamic therapy: selective treatment of choroidal neovascularization in monkeys. *Ophthalmology* 1996;103: 427–438.
26. Moulton RS, Walsh AW, Miller JW, et al. Response of retinal and choroidal vessels to photodynamic therapy using benzoporphyrin derivative monoacid. *Invest Ophthal Vis Sci* 1993;34:1169.
27. Husain D, Miller J, Michaud N, et al. Intravenous infusion using liposomal benzoporphyrin derivative verteporfin for photodynamic therapy of experimental choroidal neovascularization. *Arch Ophthalmol* 1996;114:978–985.
28. Mori K, Ohta M, Katagiri T. Photodynamic therapy (PDT) with a combination of a new photosensitizer: NPe6 and a diode laser emitting at 664 nm. *Invest Ophthal Vis Sci* 1996;37:S3177.
29. Miller J, Schmidt-Erfurth U, Sickenberg M, et al. Photodynamic therapy with verteporfin for choroidal neovascularization caused by age related macular degeneration. Results of a single treatment in a Phase 1 and 2 study. *Arch Ophthalmol* 1999;117: 1161–1173.
30. Arbour J, Connolly E, Palmer J, et al. Digital angiography of CNV in the monkey using benzoporphyrin, phthalocyanine, and rose bengal. *Invest Ophthal Vis Sci* 1998;39:S590.
31. Graham K, Arbour J, Connolly E, et al. Digital angiography using lutetium texaphyrin in a monkey model of choroidal neovascularization. *Invest Ophthal Vis Sci* (ARVO Abstract) 1999; 40:S402.
32. Kramer M, Kenney A, Delori F, et al. Imaging of experimental choroidal neovascularization (CNV) using liposomal benzoporphyrin derivative monoacid (BPD-MA) angiography. *Invest Ophthal Vis Sci* 1995;36:S236.
33. Blumenkranz M, Woodburn K, Verdooner S. Lutex texaphyrin angiography: a new method for the evaluation and treatment of retinal and choroidal vascular disorders. *Invest Ophthal Vis Sci* 1998;39:S468.

34. Bonnet R, Ridge R, Scourides P, et al. On the nature of hematoporphyrin derivative. *J Chem Soc Perkins Trans* 1981;1:3135–3140.
35. Davidorf J, Davidorf F. Treatment of iris melanoma with photodynamic therapy. *Ophthal Surg* 1992;23:522–527.
36. Nelson J, Roberts W, Berns MW. In vivo studies on the utilization of mono-l-aspartyl chlorin (NPe6) for photodynamic therapy. *Cancer Res* 1987;47:4681–4685.
37. Schuitmaker J, van Best J, van Delft J, et al. Bacteriochlorin a, a new photosensitizer in photodynamic therapy. *Invest Ophthal Vis Sci* 1990;31:1444–1450.
38. Richter AM, Waterfield E, Jain AK, et al. Photosensitising potency of structural analogues of benzoporhyrin derviative (BPD) in a mouse tumour model. *Br J Cancer* 1991;63:87–93.
39. Treatment of Age-related Macular Degeneration with Photodynamic Therapy (TAP) Study Group. Photodynamic therapy of subfoveal choroidal neovascularization in age-related macular degeneration with verteporfin. Two-year vision results of two randomized clinical trials. *Arch Ophthalmol* 2001;119:198–207.
40. Baumal C, Puliafito C, Pieroth L, et al. Photodynamic therapy (PDT) of experimental choroidal neovascularization with tin ethyl etiopurpurin. *Invest Ophthal Vis Sci* 1996;37:S122.
41. Obana A, Gohto Y, Miki T, et al. Photodynamic therapy of choroidal vessels using a newly developed chlorin derivative (ATX-S10). *Invest Ophthal Vis Sci* 1996;37:S549.
42. Kreimer-Birnbaum M. Modified porphyrins, chlorins, phthalocyanines, and purpurins: second-generation photosensitizers for photodynamic therapy. *Semin Hematol* 1989;26:157–173.
43. Morgan A, Skalkos D. Second generation sensitizers: where are we and where should we be going? *Proc SPIE* 1990;6:87–106.
44. Kliman G, Puliafito C, Stern D, et al. Phthalocyanine photodynamic therapy: new strategy for closure of choroidal neovascularization. *Lasers Surg Med* 1994;15:2–10.
45. Miller JW, Stinson WG, Gregory WA, et al. Phthalocyanine photodynamic therapy of experimental iris neovascularization. *Ophthalmology* 1991;98:1711–1719.
46. Panagopoulos JA, Svitra PP, Puliafito CA, et al. Photodynamic therapy for experimental intraocular melanoma using chloraluminum sulfonated phthalocyanine. *Arch Ophthalmol* 1989;107:886–890.
47. Young S, Woodburn K, Wright M, et al. Lutetium texaphyrin (PCI-0123): a near-infrared, water-soluble photosensitizer. *Photochem Photobiol* 1996;63:892–897.
48. Woodburn K, Fan Q, Kessel D, et al. Phototherapy of cancer and atheromatous plaque with texaphyrins. *J Clin Laser Med Surg* 1996;14:343–348.
49. Woodburn K, Fan Q, Miles D, et al. Localization and efficacy analysis of the phototherapeutic lutetium texaphyrin (PCI-0123) in the murine EMT6 sarcoma model. *Photochem Photobiol* 1997;65:410–415.
50. Arbour J, Graham K, Carson D, et al. Photodynamic therapy of experimental choroidal neovascularization in a monkey model using intravenous infusion of lutetium texaphyrin. *Invest Ophthalmol Vis Sci* (ARVO Abstract) 1999;40:S401.
51. Blumenkranz MS, Woodburn KW, Qing F, et al. Lutetium texaphyrin (Lutex): a potential new agent for ocular fundus angiography and photodynamic therapy. *Am J Ophthalmol Mar* 2000;129:353–362.
52. Yoshikawa K, Kurata H, Iwahara S, et al. Photodynamic action of fluorescein dyes in DNA-damage and in vitro inactivation of transforming DNA in bacteria. *Mutat Res* 1978;56:359–362.
53. Gandin E, Lion Y, Van De Vorst A, et al. Quantum yield of singlet oxygen production by xanthene derivatives. *Photochem Photobiol* 1983;37:271–278.
54. Nanda S, Hatchell D, Tiedeman J, et al. A new method of vascular occlusion. *Arch Ophthalmol* 1987;105:1121–1124.
55. Wilson C, Hatchell D. Photodynamic retinal vascular thrombosis. *Invest Ophthal Vis Sci* 1991;32:2357–2365.
56. Royster A, Nanda S, Hatchell D, et al. Photochemical initiation of thrombosis. *Arch Ophthalmol* 1988;106:1608–1614.
57. Tse D, Dutton J, Weingeist T, et al. Hematoporphyrin photoradiation therapy for intraocular and orbital malignant melanoma. *Arch Ophthalmol* 1984;102:833–838.
58. Sery T, Shields J, Augsburger J, et al. Photodynamic therapy of human ocular cancer. *Ophthal Surg* 1987;18:413–418.
59. Chambers R, Arnson D, Davidorf F, et al. Treatment of iris melanoma with dihematoporphyrin ether and an ophthalmic laser delivery system. *Contemp Ophthal For* 1986;4:70–84.
60. Lewis R, Tse D, Phelphs C, et al. Neovascular glaucoma after photoradiation therapy for uveal melanoma. *Arch Ophthalmol* 1984;102:839–842.
61. Gomer CJ, Jester JV, Razum NJ, et al. Photodynamic therapy of intraocular tumors: examination of hematoporphyrin derivative distribution and long-term damage in rabbit ocular tissue. *Cancer Res* 1985;45:3718–3725.
62. Sery T, Dougherty T. Photoradiation of rabbit ocular malignant melanoma sensitized with hematoporphyrin derivative. *Curr Eye Res* 1984;3:519–528.
63. Franken K, van Delft J, Dubelman T, et al. Hematoporphyrin derivative photoradiation treatment of experimental malignant melanoma in the anterior chamber of the rabbit. *Curr Eye Res* 1985;4:641–654.
64. Gomer C, Murphree A, Doiron D, et al. *Preclinical evaluation of ocular photoradiation therapy.* Paper presented at: Proceedings of the international symposium on porphyrins in tumor phototherapy, New York, 1984.
65. Liu H, Chuo N. Hematoporphyrin phototherapy for experimental intraocular malignant melanoma. *Arch Ophthalmol* 1983;101:901–903.
66. Franken N, Vrensen G, van Delft J, et al. Early morphological changes induced by photodynamic therapy in amelanotic Greene melanoma implanted in the anterior eye chamber of rabbits. *Laser Surg Med* 1988;3:27–34.
67. Schmidt-Erfurth U, Flotte T, Gragoudas ES, et al. Benzoporphyrin-lipoprotein-mediated photodestruction of intraocular tumors. *Exp Eye Res* 1996;62:1–10.
68. Bruce RJ. Evaluation of hematoporphyrin photoradiation therapy to treat choroidal melanoma. *Lasers Surg Med* 1984;4:59–64.
69. Bruce RJ. Photoradiation therapy for choroidal malignant melanoma. In: McCaughan JJ, ed. *A clinical manual: photodynamic therapy of malignancies.* Austin: RG Landes, 1993.
70. Murphree A, Cote M, Gomer C. The evolution of photodynamic therapy techniques in the treatment of intraocular tumors. *Photochem Photobiol* 1987;46:919–923.
71. Favilla I, Barry W, Gosbell A, et al. Phototherapy of posterior uveal melanomas. *Br J Ophthalmol* 1991;75:718–721.
72. Lingua R, Parel J. Photodynamic therapy for ocular tumors. *J Photochem Photobiol B Biol* 1991:119–122.
73. Schmidt-Erfurth U, Bauman W, Gragoudas E, et al. Photodynamic therapy of experimental choroidal melanoma using lipoprotein-delivered benzoporphyrin. *Ophthalmology* 1994;101:89–99.
74. Gonzalez V, Hu L, Theodossiadis P, et al. Photodynamic therapy of pigmented choroidal melanomas. *Invest Ophthal Vis Sci* 1995;36:871–878.
75. Phillips A, Browne B, Allan D. Haematoporphyrin photosensitisation treatment of experimental choroidal melanoma. *Eye* 1987;1:680–685.
76. Ozler S, Nelson S, Liggett P, et al. Photodynamic therapy of experimental subchoroidal melanoma using chloraluminum sulfonated phthalocyanine. *Arch Ophthalmol* 1992;110:555–561.
77. Young L, Howard M, Hu L, et al. Photodynamic therapy of pig-

mented choroidal melanomas using a liposomal preparation of benzoporphyrin derivative. *Arch Ophthalmol* 1996;114:186–192.
78. Hu L, Huh K, Gragoudas E, et al. Establishment of pigmented choroidal melanomas in a rabbit model. *Retina* 1994;14: 264–269.
79. Kim R, Hu L, Foster S, et al. Photodynamic therapy of pigmented choroidal melanomas of greater than 3 mm thickness. *Ophthalmology* 1996;103:2029–2036.
80. Ohnishi Y, Yamana Y, Minei M. Photoradiation therapy using argon laser and a hematoporphyrin derivative for retinoblastoma: a preliminary report. *Jpn J Ophthalmol* 1986;30:409–419.
81. Murphree A. Retinoblastoma. In: Ryan S, Ogden T, eds. *Retina,* vol 1. St Louis: CV Mosby, 1989:544.
82. White L, Gomer C, Doiron D, et al. Ineffective photodynamic therapy (PDT) in a poorly vascularized xenograft model. *Br J Cancer* 1988;57:455–458.
83. Winther J. Porphyrin photodynamic therapy in an experimental retinoblastoma model. *Ophthal Paedatr Gen* 1987;8:49–52.
84. Winther J, Ehlers N. Histopathological changes in an intraocular-like tumour following photodynamic therapy. *Acta Ophthalmol* 1988;66:69–78.
85. Winther J, Overgaard J. Photodynamic therapy of experimental intraocular retinoblastomas: dose-response relationships to light energy and photofrin II. *Acta Ophthalmol* 1989;67:44–50.
86. Epstein R, Hendricks R, Harris D. Photodynamic therapy of corneal neovascularization. *Cornea* 1991;10:424–432.
87. Pallikaris I, Miltiades M, Iliaki O, et al. Effectiveness of corneal neovascularization photothrombosis using phthalocyanine and a diode laser (675 nm). *Lasers Surg Med* 1993;13:197–203.
88. Tsilimbaris M, Pallikaris I, Naoumidi I, et al. Phthalocyanine mediated photodynamic thrombosis of experimental corneal neovascularization: effect of phthalocyanine dose and irradiation onset time on vascular occlusion rate. *Lasers Surg Med* 1994;15:19–31.
89. Gohto Y, Obana A, Kanai M, et al. Photodynamic therapy for corneal neovascularization using topically administered ATX-S10 (Na). *Ophthal Surg Lasers* 2000;31:55–60.
90. Gohto Y, Obana A, Kanai M, et al. Treatment parameters for selective occlusion of experimental corneal neovascularization by photodynamic therapy using a water soluble photosensitizer, ATX-S10 (Na). *Exp Eye Res* 2001;72:13–22.
91. Schmidt-Erfurth U, Hasan T, Schomacker K, et al. In vivo uptake of liposomal benzoporphyrin derivative and photothrombosis in experimental corneal neovascularization. *Lasers Surg Med* 1995;17:178–188.
92. Virdi PS, Hayreh SS. Ocular neovascularization with retinal vascular occlusion. I. Association with experimental retinal vein occlusion. *Arch Ophthalmol* 1982;100:331–341.
93. Miller JW, Adamis AP, Shima D, et al. Vascular endothelial growth factor/vascular permeability factor is temporally and spatially correlated with ocular angiogenesis in a primate model. *Am J Pathol* 1994;145:574–584.
94. Packer AJ, Tse DT, Gu X-Q, et al. Hematoporphyrin photoradiation therapy for iris neovascularization. A preliminary report. *Arch Ophthalmol* 1984;102:1193–1197.
95. Husain D, Miller J, Kenney A, et al. Photodynamic therapy and digital angiography of experimental iris neovascularization using liposomal benzoporphyrin derivative. *Ophthalmology* 1997;104: 1242–1250.
96. Muller V, Ruokonen P, Schellenbeck M, et al. Treatment of rubeosis iridis with photodynamic therapy with verteporfin: a new therapeutic and prophylactic option for patients with the risk of neovascular glaucoma? *Ophthal Res* 2003;35:60–64.
97. Thomas EL, Langhofer M. Closure of experimental subretinal neovascular vessels with dihematoporphyrin either augmented argon green laser photocoagulation. *Photochem Photobiol* 1987; 46:881–886.

2

PRINCIPLES OF PHOTODYNAMIC THERAPY

HUBERT ERIK VAN DEN BERGH
J.P. BALLINI

Photodynamic therapy (PDT) is a medical technology that has been developed mainly to treat cancer (1,2). It consists of the systemic or topical application of a substance (a dye or dye precursor) that localizes more or less selectively in a tumor at concentrations at which this substance is not toxic. Light is then applied at a light dose, which by itself is not harmful to the tissue, and which is absorbed by the dye. This light absorption leads to energized dye molecules, which then initiate a cascade of chemical reactions that can finally lead to tissue destruction, that is, to phototoxicity. In this chapter we outline some of the fundamentals of this process, together with several of the molecules being used. We also describe some of the drug delivery strategies, and discuss PDT as applied clinically to treat choroidal neovascularization (CNV) associated with age-related macular degeneration (AMD).

THE MOLECULES: FIRST- AND SECOND-GENERATION PHOTOSENSITIZERS

The types of dye molecules being used in PDT, also called photosensitizers (PS), are often porphyrins. These were among the first PS studied, and are often derived from blood products or related compounds. Figure 2.1 shows the five-member ring known as pyrrole. Four pyrrole molecules linked together by methine bridges give the tetrapyrrole structure, which is basically the unsubstituted porphyrin macrocycle.

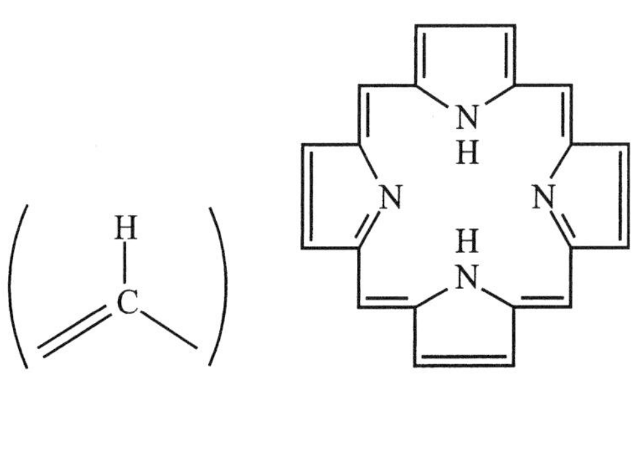

This structure for the porphyrin family of molecules was first proposed as long ago as 1912. Many porphyrins are purple. They are key molecules in nature, playing roles as diverse as:

1. *Oxygen transport* in blood (heme is an iron porphyrin).
2. *Oxygen storage* in muscle tissue (myoglobin).
3. Functioning as redox enzymes in metabolic processes. For instance, the central iron atom in the porphyrin of cytochrome C cycles between Fe^{2+} and Fe^{3+} while performing the electron transfer reaction in *cell respiration.*
4. *Photosynthesis,* which is controlled by chlorophyll, a reduced magnesium porphyrin.

The biosynthesis of heme in mammalian tissue takes place in eight enzyme-catalyzed steps, which are shown in Figure 2.2. Part of these reactions take place in the mitochondria and part in the aqueous phase of the cytoplasm (i.e., the cytosol). The first step is the condensation of succinyl coenzyme A with glycine to form 5-aminolevulinic acid (ALA), which is catalyzed by the enzyme ALA-synthase (Fig. 2.3A). The second step is the condensation of two molecules of ALA catalyzed by ALA dehydrase to give the pyrrole called porphobilinogen (PBG) (Fig. 2.3B). The next step is the condensation of four PBG molecules to uroporphyrinogen III (a reduced porphyrin), also called uro'gen III, in two steps requiring two enzymes: PBG deaminase and uro'gen III cosynthetase (Fig. 2.3C). Next, the acetic acid side chains are decarboxylated by uro'gen III decarboxylase to methyl groups. After this, two of the propionic acid side chains are decarboxylated to vinyl groups, resulting in proto'gen IX, which is oxidized to protoporphyrin IX by proto'gen oxidase (Fig. 2.3D). Finally, Fe^{2+} is inserted into the center of the macrocycle by an enzyme called ferrochelatase.

The spontaneous association of these porphyrin macrocycles to proteins is mostly via noncovalent binding (e.g., hemoglobin, myoglobin, cytochrome P-450, catalase). However, this step also can be catalyzed in such a way as to form a covalently bound heme, as is the case for cytochrome C. It is interesting to note that uro'gen III synthesis, via

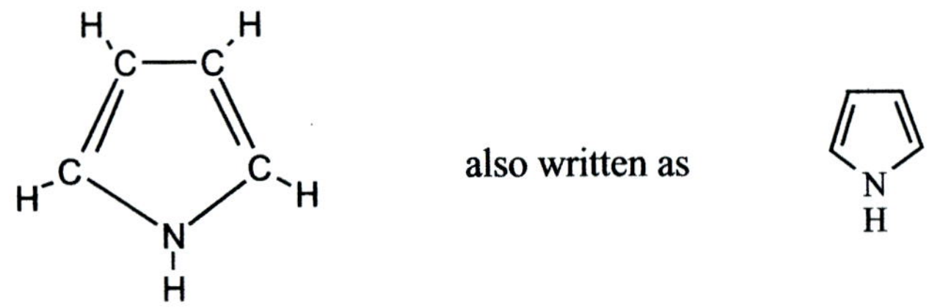

FIGURE 2.1. The five-member heterocycle called pyrrole.

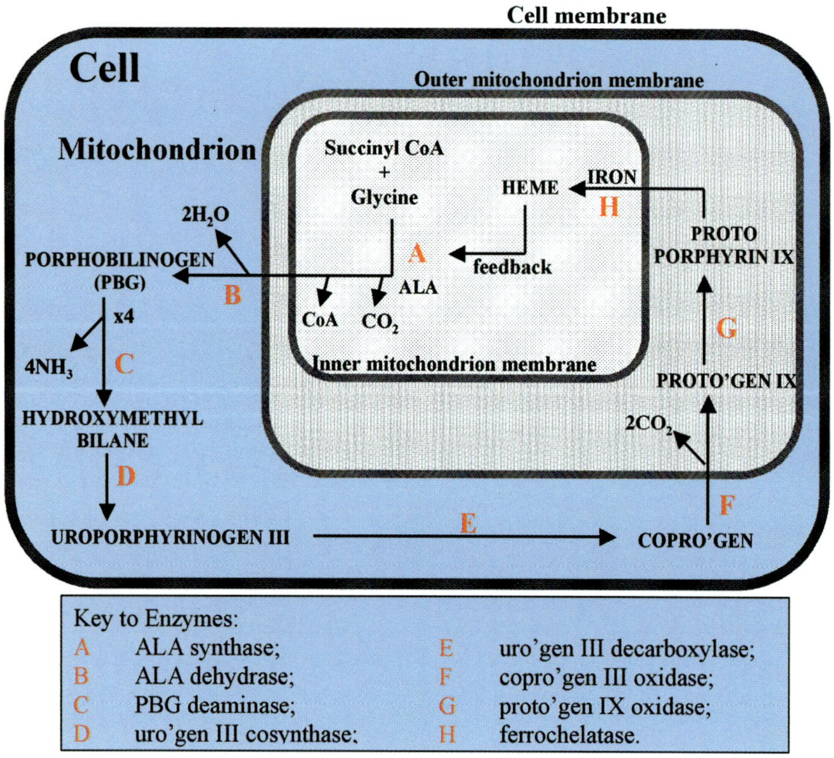

FIGURE 2.2. A schematic overview of the heme biosynthesis in mammalian tissue, together with a list of the enzymes that catalyze this pathway, and the cellular locations where each synthetic step takes place. Steps **A** and **H** occur within the mitochondrion, steps **B** through **F** take place in the cytosol, and step **G** takes place in the space between the inner and outer mitochondrial membranes. Note that the mitochondrion is not drawn to scale.

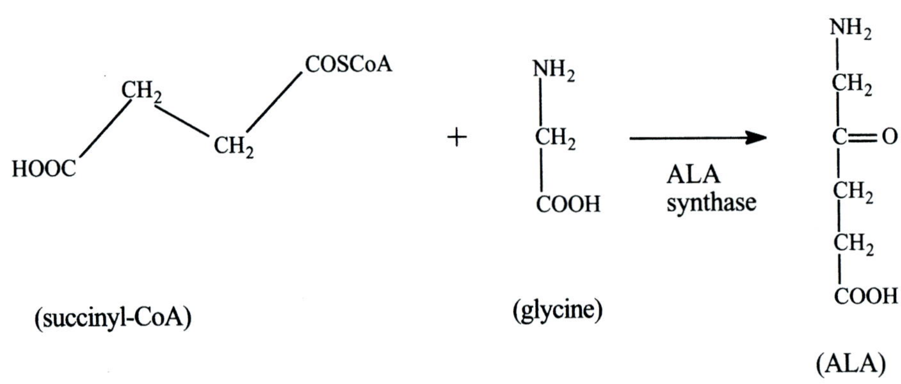

A

FIGURE 2.3. **A:** The formation of 5-aminolevulinic acid.

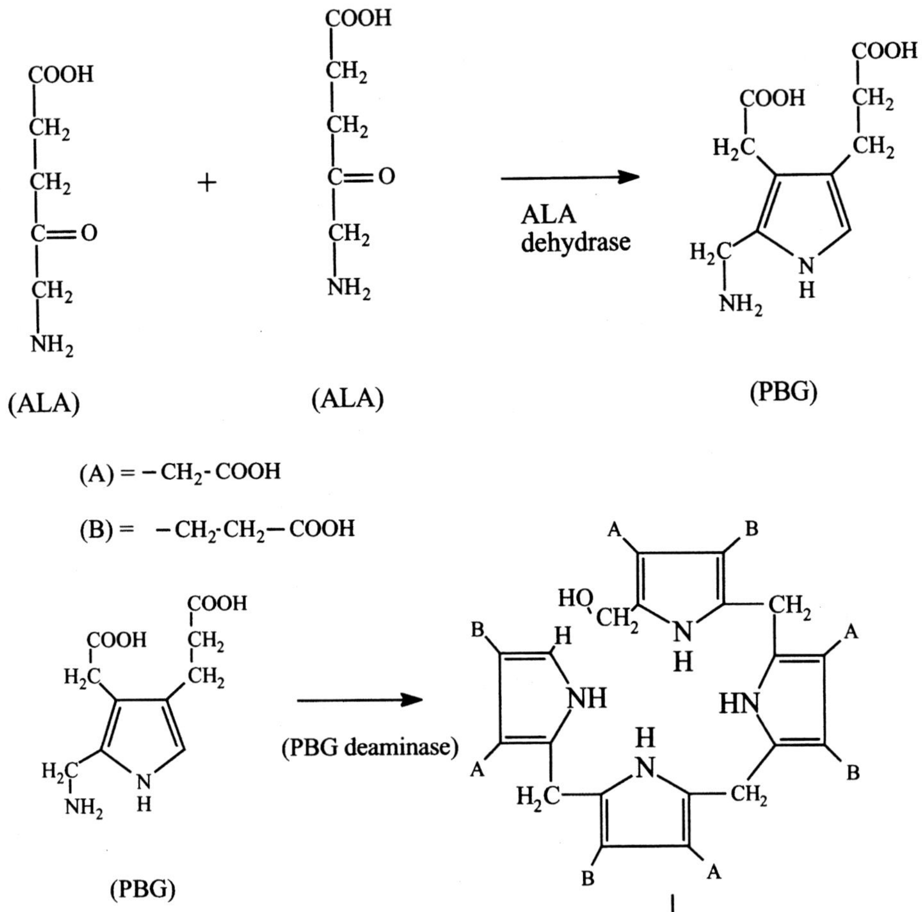

B

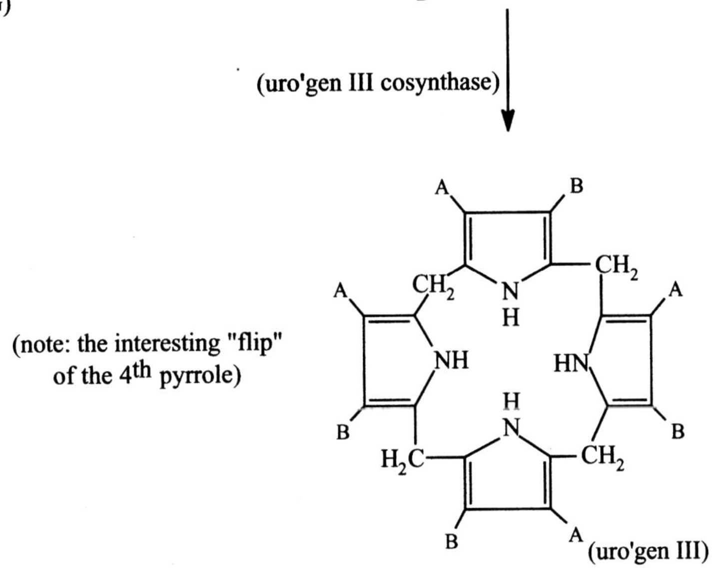

C

FIGURE 2.3. ***(continued)*** **B:** The formation of porphobilinogen. **C:** The two-step condensation to a macrocycle where A = –CH_2-COOH and B = –CH_2-CH_2-COOH.

(continued on next page)

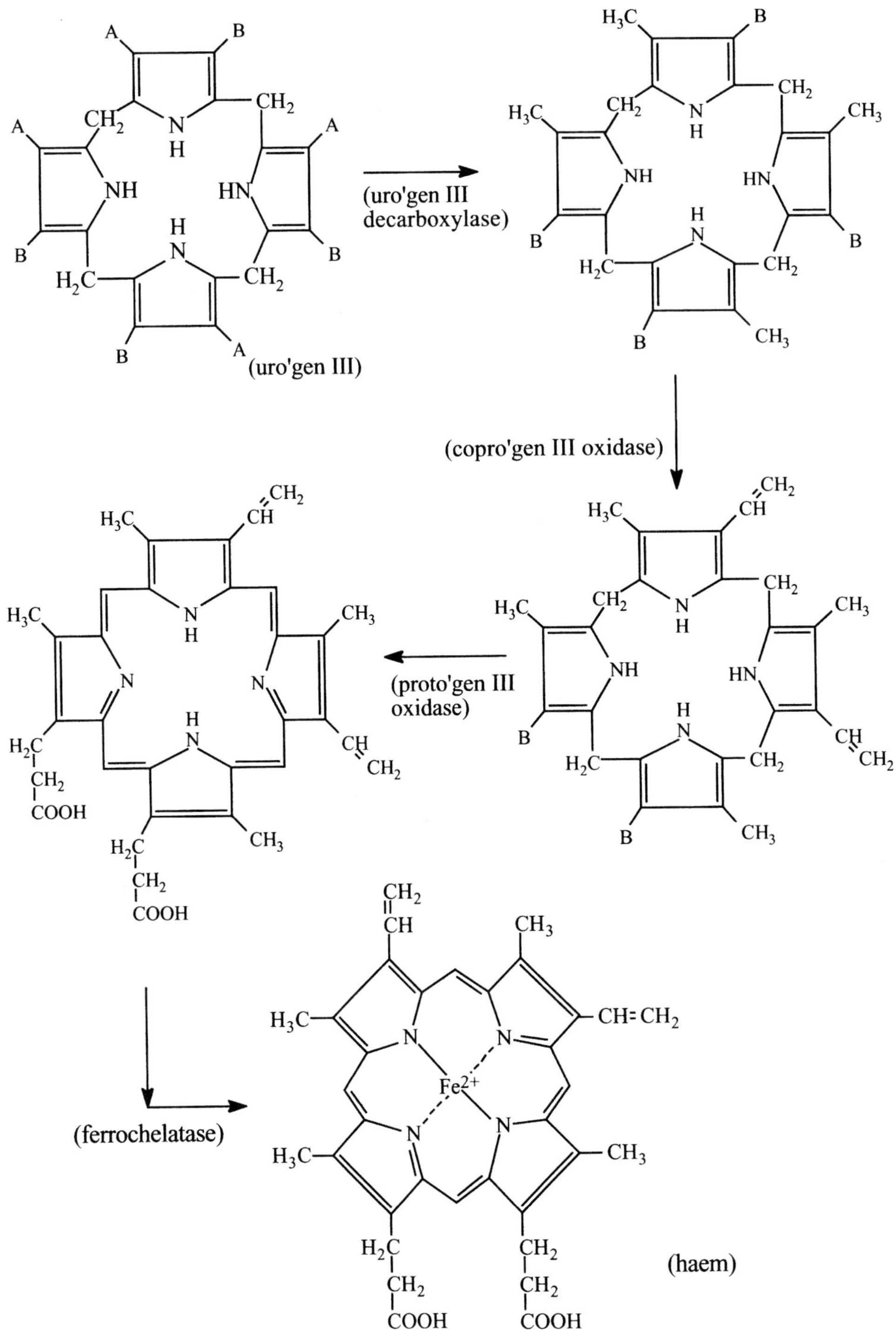

D

FIGURE 2.3. *(continued)* D: Trimming the side chains by decarboxylation, as well as creating the methine bridges and thus the full ring aromaticity.

Mg^{2+} insertion, also can lead to chlorophyll formation. Furthermore, uro'gen III is an intermediate in the production of vitamin B_{12}.

In order to obtain porphyrin-based photosensitizers, one can either follow the complex route of complete chemical synthesis or start with animal blood and derive the desired chemical from a purified blood component. For example, after some purification blood can be added to hot CH_3COOH in the presence of NaCl. This leads to hematoporphyrin IX synthesis (Fig. 2.4).

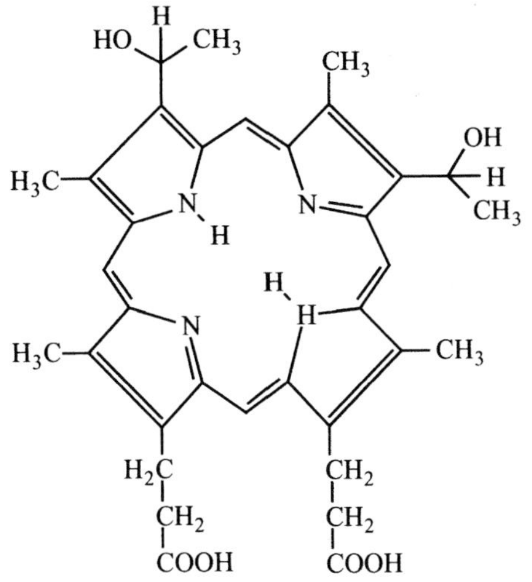

FIGURE 2.4. Hematoporphyrin.

Because hematoporphyrin did not localize optimally in tumors, in the last four decades PDT often was done with the photosensitizer hematoporphyrin derivative (Hpd) (3–12). This was obtained by treatment of hematoporphyrin with acetic and sulfuric acid. The mixture was dissolved in alkali in order to make it injectable. This yields a complex mixture of monomeric, dimeric, and oligomeric porphyrins connected among others by ether and ester linkages. The tumor localizing fraction was thought to consist mainly of oligomeric material, which was later purified and commercialized under the name Photofrin (QLT Inc., Vancouver, BC, Canada). The complex and not particularly well-defined mixture Photofrin was effective in clinical PDT (13–15). It was the first Food and Drug Administration (FDA)–approved PDT drug for a number of clinical applications, among which are certain types of lung cancer, esophageal cancer, and head and neck cancer. However, it demonstrated rather long and variable skin photosensitization as well as somewhat limited effectiveness in treating thick lesions because of its modest absorption at 635 nm. Most treatments were at 48 hours after intravenous (iv) injection. Hence, new photosensitizers were developed, which often were single substances or well-defined simple mixtures with stronger optical absorption in the far red or near infrared spectra for better tissue penetration. High quantum yields of long-lived triplet states were sought, in order to produce high yields of the phototoxic singlet oxygen intermediate. The absence of dark toxicity, a high selectivity of the PS for the tumor relative to the surrounding (underlying) tissue, and a short body half-life were some of the other properties desired in this second-generation of PS. Photosensitizers that fluoresced reasonably well are easier to localize in tissue or cell culture. This simplifies pharmacokinetics (16–18) and makes possible the fluorescence microscopy necessary for detailed localization (19,20). The search for improved selectivity and more specific tissue localization often was approached by changing the molecules' hydrolipoamphiphilicity as well as their charge and other chemical properties. Thus, one finds a number of different substances in the second generation of PS, such as chlorin, bacteriochlorin, phthalocyanine, naphthalocyanine, pheophorbide, purpurin, benzoporphyrin, texaphyrin, phenothiazine compounds, cyanine, acridine, rhodamine, etc., often with different chemical groups on the periphery of the macrocycle to make them more hydrophilic and/or lipophilic. Some of these substances actually made it into clinical trials. They are listed in Figure 2.5 together with some of their properties.

It should be noted that the spectra are difficult to compare directly because they are reported in various solvents. The values of ε reported on the vertical axis are the molar extinction coefficients (21–30). Thus, when looking at the molecules in Figure 2.5, one observes a number of attempts of structure–activity optimization, which we discuss briefly. In Figure 2.5A, a chlorin (mono-L-aspartyl chlorin e6, or NPe6) is shown with an absorption maximum at 654 nm and a fairly large extinction coefficient near 40,000 $l\ mol^{-1}\ cm^{-1}$. The four -COOH groups make it water soluble. Interestingly, as all four COOH groups are on one side of the molecule, it thus has both a hydrophilic and hydrophobic side, which may help passive transport across cell membranes. This substance shows good tumor uptake and rather rapid body clearance (31,32). Hypericin shown in Figure 2.5B is a naturally occurring extended quinone obtained from a plant called St. John's Wort. At its absorption maximum near 590 nm it has an extinction coefficient of about 42,000 $l\ mol^{-1}\ cm^{-1}$. It is not very soluble in water, where it probably aggregates at higher concentrations. Hypericin has been used with some success for the photodetection of early cancer of the urinary bladder (33,34).

Protoporphyrin IX (PPIX) (24,35–37), shown in Figure 2.5C, generally is not directly applied as a sensitizer itself. It is applied in the form of aminolevulinic acid (ALA or an ALA-ester), which is converted to PPIX by the natural heme biosynthesis shown in Figure 2.3 A through D. As can be deduced from Figure 2.2, the addition of systemic or topical 5-ALA to mammalian tissue can lead to the temporary short-circuiting of the slow negative feedback control of heme on the 5-ALA synthase catalyzed step. This results in accumulation of PPIX for a period of several hours because of the rather slow Ferrochelatase-induced insertion of Fe^{2+} in the PPIX macrocycle. This insertion of Fe^{2+} tends to both decrease PPIX fluorescence and decrease PPIX photodynamic activity. Two other interesting features seem to play a role in this process of temporary ALA-induced enhancement of PPIX. First, PBG deaminase activity is enhanced and ferrochelatase activity is decreased in some cancers. Both of these phenomena lead to increased PPIX in tumors for a few hours after 5-ALA application, and hence to the possibility of tumor-selective PDT, and also the effective fluorescence detection of small superficial cancers. It

A) mono-L-aspartyl chlorin e6 (Npe6)

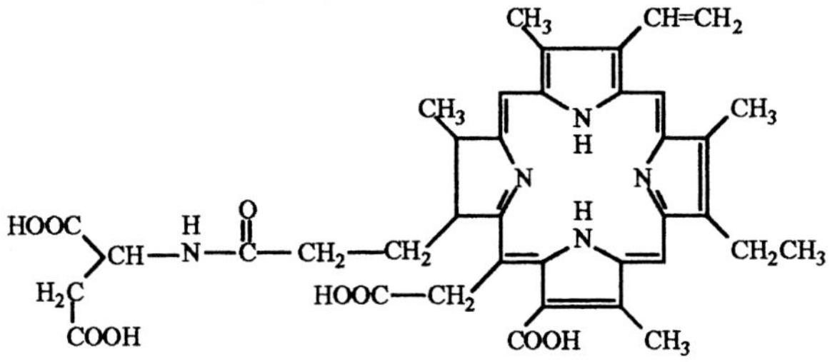

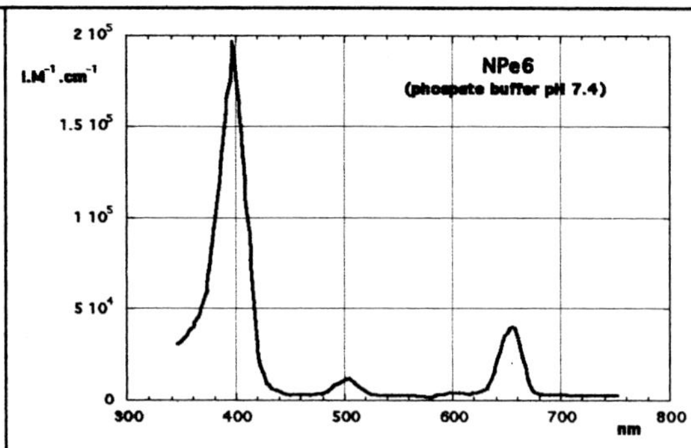

ε(654 nm) = 40000 l mole^{-1}cm^{-1}.
Water soluble amphiphilic compound

B) Hypericin

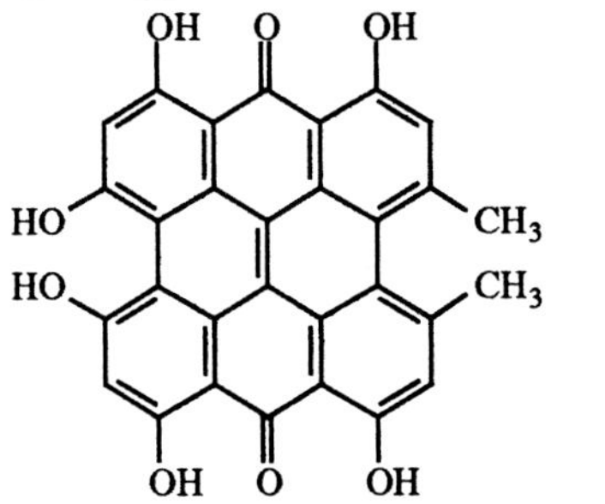

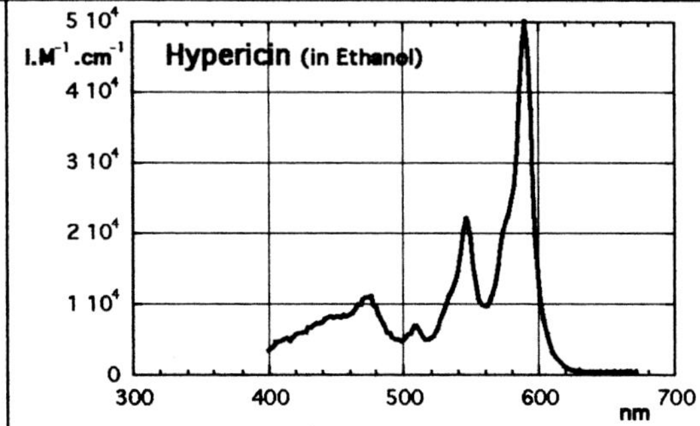

ε(588 nm) = 50000 l mole^{-1}cm^{-1}.
Natural compound, hydrophobic.

C) Protoporphyrin IX

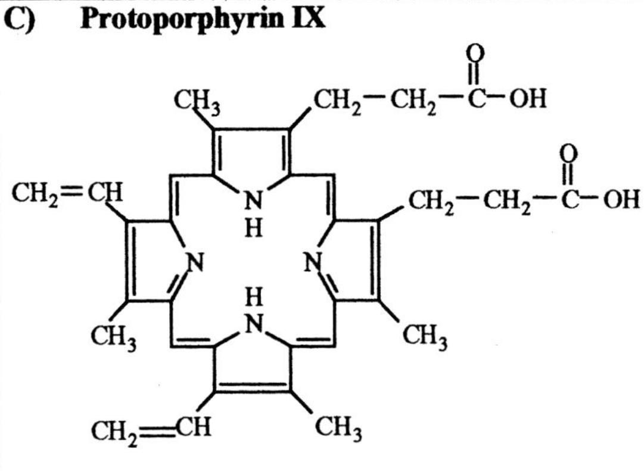

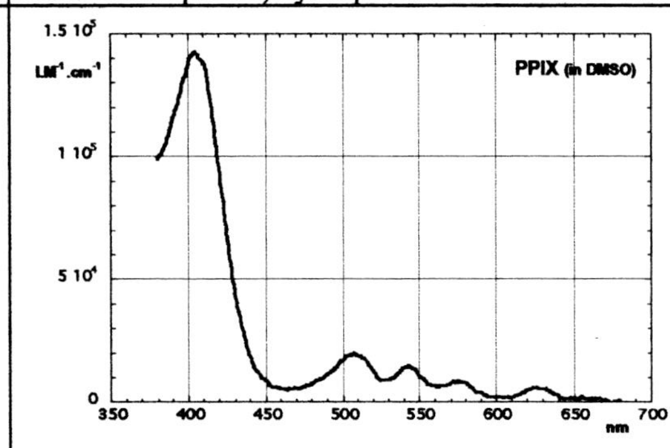

ε(630 nm) = 4600 l mole^{-1}cm^{-1}. ε_{max} is at 407 nm.
Lipophilic compound.
Applied as ALA or ALA ester.

D) Verteporfin (BPD-MA)

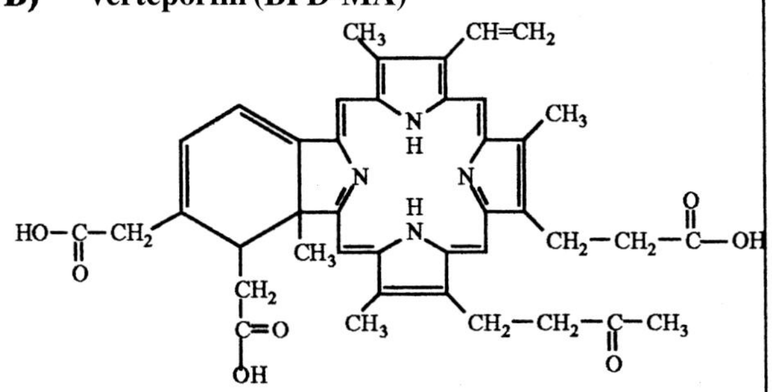

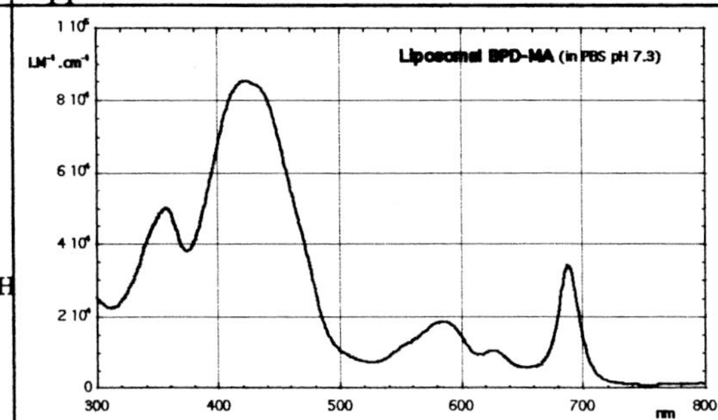

ε(687 nm) = 34000 l mole^{-1}cm^{-1}.
Hydrophobic compound injected in liposomes.

FIGURE 2.5. A–G: Structures and some properties of seven clinically tested second-generation photosensitizers for photodynamic therapy.

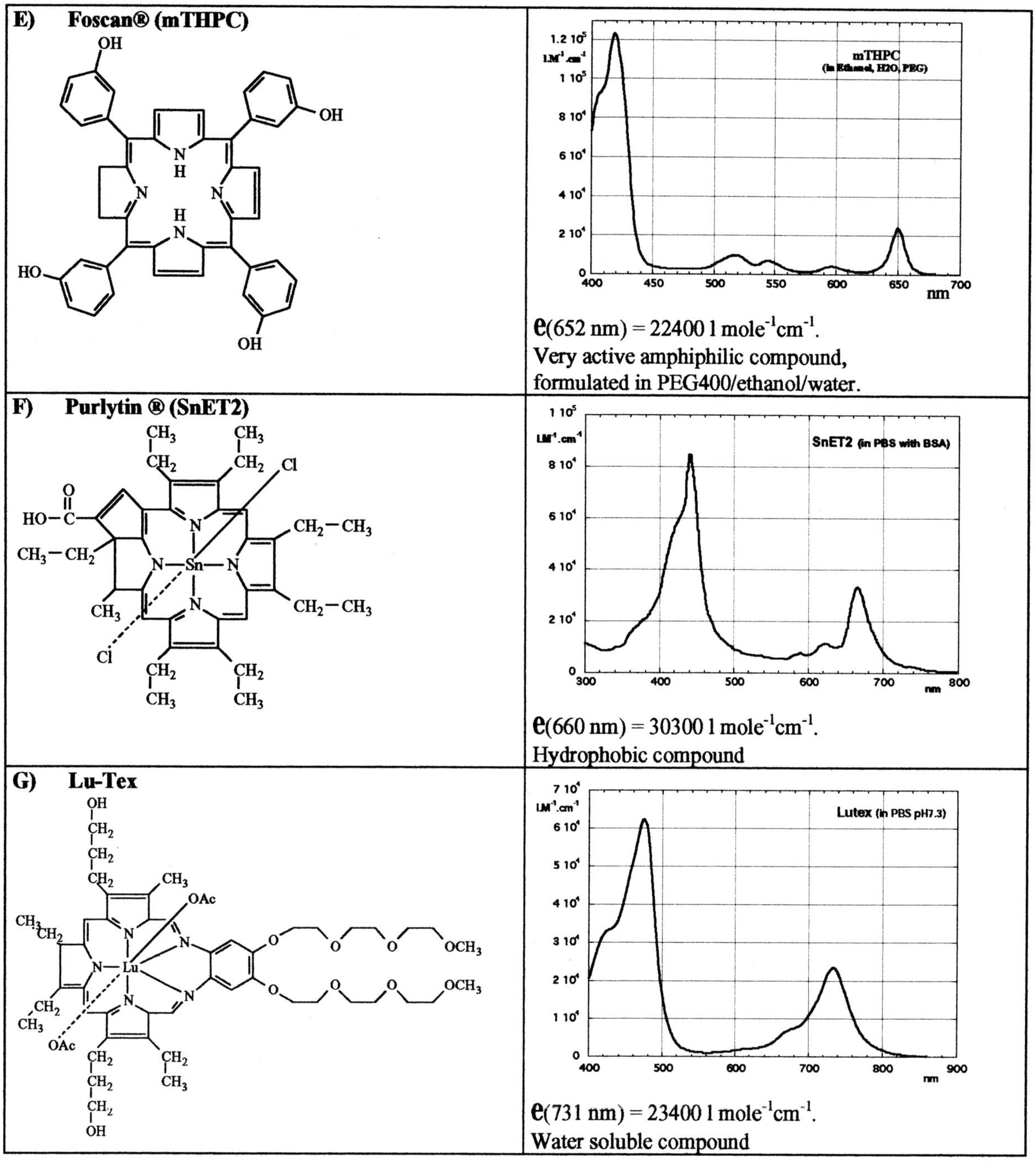

FIGURE 2.5. ***(continued)***

also has been mentioned as an additional reason for enhanced PPIX in tumors that 5-ALA applied to the skin penetrates into malignant superficial lesions more efficiently than through the normal skin stratum corneum. The detection of small early-stage cancers is now in phase III trials for bladder cancer with ALA-hexyl ester (Hexvix, PhotoCure, Oslo, Norway), an ALA precursor (27,38). An example of the early detection of "invisible" superficial cancers is shown in Figure 2.6. Here ALA-hexyl ester 8 mM was applied for 4 hours topically in the bladder prior to fluorescence photodetection. The neoplasms, which are invisible under white light cystoscopy become clearly visible under PPIX fluorescence detection. ALA-induced PDT is approved by the US FDA for the treatment of actinic keratosis, and also is being used as well as the ALA methyl ester precursor (Metvix, PhotoCure, Oslo, Norway) to treat superficial basal cell carcinomas. The optimum therapeutic ratio is reached within 1 to 4 hours after ALA or ALA-ester

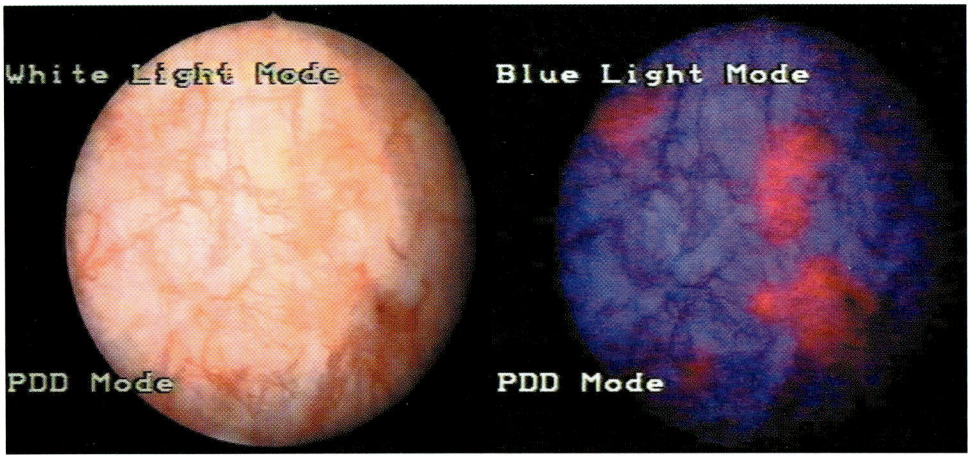

FIGURE 2.6. Bladder carcinoma *in situ* (CIS) photodetection with topical ALA hexyl ester 8 mM application for 4 hours prior to fluorescence photodetection. The CIS, which is invisible under white light cystoscopy, becomes clearly visible under PPIX fluorescence detection ("blue light mode").

administration. The rapid PPIX clearance (<24 hours) that follows helps to decrease skin photosensitivity. PPIX photobleaches quite rapidly; however, the exact influence this has on PDT remains to be established.

Verteporfin or benzoporphyrin derivative monoacid ring A (BPD-MA) (Fig. 2.5D) is a hydrophobic benzochlorin type compound that has to be injected in liposome-like particles. Its main absorption in the red is near 690 nm with ε max (690) of about 34,000 l $mole^{-1}$ cm^{-1}. Rapid body clearance is a main advantage of this mixture, which also is synthesized from blood-derived hematoporphyrin. It is an effective photosensitizer that does not covalently bind to lipoproteins, as do almost all PS, but that associates with them shortly after iv injection. The majority of BPD-MA associates with high-density lipoproteins (HDL), but a large extent associates with low-density lipoproteins (LDL). It has been shown in some animal models that this binding to LDL may lead to enhanced uptake in lesions (39), presumably because of the higher activity of LDL receptors. This substance is now being used in more than 50 countries to treat CNV associated with AMD. Other applications of BPD-MA such as immunomodulation for the treatment of rheumatoid arthritis are under study. Foscan, or meta-tetra hydroxyphenyl chlorin (mTHPC) (shown in Fig. 2.5E), is a chlorin with its red absorption maximum at 652 nm with ε (652) at about 22,400 l $mole^{-1}$ cm^{-1}. It should be noted that the absorption data listed in Figure 2.5 depend to some extent on the surroundings; that is, on the solvent and/or presence of proteins. It is interesting to compare ε (max) in the red of the second-generation compounds of Figure 2.5—which range from 22,400 l $mole^{-1}$ cm^{-1} for FOSCAN to over 40,000 l $mole^{-1}$ cm^{-1} for hypericin and NPe6—with Photofrin—which has ε (630) of about 1,200 l $mole^{-1}$ cm^{-1}. Meta-tetra hydroxyphenyl chlorin has an extremely high photodynamic efficacy. The reason for this is not completely understood, but it has been suggested that it results from its localization near a specific ultrasensitive target in the tissue. Meta-tetra hydroxyphenyl chlorin is delivered in a polyethylene glycol (PEG)–ethanol–water solvent or in propylene glycol–ethanol. More recently, mTHPC has been covalently linked to PEG. Further reduction of such chlorins leads to bacteriochlorins. This process produces a strongly red-shifted optical absorption near 730 to 740 nm, where deep tissue penetration of light is even more enhanced.

Figure 2.5G shows an example of a Lutetium Texaphyrin (Lu-Tex). These compounds have an expanded coordination for the central metal species of five nitrogen atoms. Such molecules have the advantage of being able to include metal ions with a larger ionic radius in the macrocycle. With Lutetium III and two acetate axial ligands, two ethyl groups, two *n*-propanol groups, and two short water-soluble PEG chains, this yields a fairly water-soluble molecule that absorbs at 732 nm with ε max (732 nm) at 42,000 l $mole^{-1}$ cm^{-1}. This substance is being tested among others for prevention of restenosis after balloon angioplasty and the photodynamic removal of atherosclerotic plaque.

Some photosensitizers have a diamagnetic metal atom incorporated in the macrocycle. These metal atoms can be used in macrocycles, resulting in long triplet state lifetimes as in the case of Zn or Al, or to attach axial ligands that help to avoid clustering of the PS. The close contact of stacked PS molecules leads to predominant internal conversion of the clustered macrocycles (see the following). However, inserting paramagnetic metals in the macrocycle leads to shorter lifetimes of the triplet state (e.g., in the case of Cu, Co, or Fe), which then strongly reduces phototoxicity.

Some tentative general conclusions that may be drawn on structure–activity relationships of second-generation compounds follow.

1. For the hydrophilic (i.e., water-soluble) sensitizers, a significant net cationic charge on the PS causes it to localize predominantly in the mitochondria. The charge-to-mass ratio also may play a role in the localization. Photodynamic therapy has a tendency to lead to apoptosis in this case, under not too extreme experimental conditions, as has been shown in cell culture experiments (40–43).
2. The hydrophilic sensitizers with a significant net anionic charge on the PS tend to localize in the lysosomes. The charge-to-mass ratio and the number of negative charges are thought to play a role here. In this case PDT often results in necrosis in cell culture tests, under given experimental conditions.
3. The hydrophobic sensitizers have a tendency to aggregate. This can be avoided by dilution or by using bulky axial ligands, which have been specifically selected for targeting neoplastic tissue in some cases (44), as was the case when two cholesterol moieties were ligated to Ge IV phthalocyanine.
4. Considering all the second-generation compounds tested, the amphiphilic sensitizer mTHPC (45–47) (meta-tetrahydroxyphenylchlorin) was the most active on a "per activated molecule" basis. It has been proposed that this may be related to a particularly optimal microscopic localization of this sensitizer.

A major point to be made after looking at the results obtained with these second-generation photosensitizers is that a systematic comparison between the pharmacokinetics and pharmacodynamics of the individual hydrophobic and amphiphilic sensitizers is rendered particularly difficult by the use of different delivery vehicles, which tend to significantly influence the outcome of these tests. Furthermore, different animal models are used, which also makes comparison of the different PS difficult. Thus, the scientists of the PDT world should adopt common screening protocols for the testing of sensitizers. Such common screening protocols already have been adopted in other fields of oncology.

SENSITIZER SELECTIVITY

There are different approaches for finding more selective agents for PDT. Before entering into details of the specific molecular conjugates that can be designed for this purpose and the targets that might be selected, it is useful to briefly repeat some of the arguments that have been given in the literature for the "tumor selectivity" of PDT with photosensitizers such as HpD, Photofrin, and second-generation compounds such as those listed in Figure 2.5. Different notions are encompassed by the word selectivity as used in PDT and elsewhere in medicine. For the sake of simplicity, we define a selective PS in the case of cancer PDT to mean a molecule with which one can destroy a neoplasm while not significantly damaging the surrounding normal tissues. The arguments that have been used to explain this PDT selectivity imply that to a large extent it results from PS localizing preferentially in the tumor. The latter may be divided somewhat arbitrarily into selective uptake and selective retention/removal in the neoplastic tissue; for instance, see the following.

Selective Uptake

1. Leaky tumor neovessels permit sensitizers, bound largely to blood proteins in certain cases, to pass through the tumor microvessel fenestration (48).
2. In order for rapidly proliferating tissue to take up more cholesterol for lipid synthesis, there is a greater activity of LDL receptors in tumors. Thus, lipophilic PS molecules associated to LDL may be taken up selectively by rapidly proliferating tissue (49–52).

Selective Retention

1. Korbelik and coworkers (53,54) have pointed out that tumor-associated macrophages accumulate PS by phagocytosis of aggregated lipophilic PS. Hamblin and associates have argued along similar lines, implicating the enhanced phagocytosis of lipoproteins with strongly altered characteristics owing to the uptake of numerous PS molecules (55) per lipoprotein molecule.
2. It has been widely argued that some of the normally negatively charged porphyrins have no net charge, and thus become less water soluble in advanced tumors, in which in principle the pH can be significantly lowered. Thus, they are less likely to escape from the neoplastic tissue.
3. Finally, removal of PS (which, with the exception of PPIX, are not natural compounds) from tissue normally takes place by lymphatic drainage, among other mechanisms. The latter can be impaired in a neoplasm, thus inducing enhanced retention in these abnormal tissues (56).

Clearly, other reasons for selective PDT of neoplasms cannot be neglected. For instance, tumors may just be more sensitive to PDT than the surrounding normal tissue. However, it is not our purpose to enter into such detail here.

Unfortunately, in practice, one must conclude that for the case of second-generation PS in early-stage superficial cancers of the hollow organs (i.e., a case proven to be particularly favorable to clinical PDT) (47), the preceding arguments do not lead to selective PDT. Effectively, in most cases encountered in clinical PDT of carcinoma *in situ* or microinvasive carcinomas (e.g., in the lungs and the esophagus), one has found that the PS concentration selectivity, most often measured between neoplastic and normal mucosa, is nearly nonexistent.

In the hollow organs, the selectivity between the destruction of the mucosa that contains the neoplasm on the one hand, and that of the underlying muscle tissue on the other hand, often are key clinical parameters. For example, Foscan (Scotia Pharmaceuticals, Stirling, Scotland) (mTHPC) is significantly taken up by smooth muscle and not by striated muscle. This fact significantly influences PDT in different parts of the esophagus, which is surrounded by either the one or the other type of muscle. Thus, in this case, the risk of fistulae may well depend critically on what type of muscle tissue lies *below* the mucosa being treated by PDT. In practice, for early-stage cancers of the hollow organs, the selectivity of PDT in destroying neoplastic mucosa while conserving surrounding normal mucosa is often simply determined by the limits of the light application.

There are cases in which second-generation sensitizers apparently show good selectivity in a clinical context. One example of this is the "fluorescence intensity selectivity" of mTHPC (Foscan) observed in advanced squamous cell cancers of the buccal cavity (57) as compared to the surrounding "normal" mucosa. Another example concerns the selectivity in the fluorescence intensity of ALA-induced PPIX between carcinoma *in situ* in the bladder and surrounding normal bladder urothelium (26). In both examples, the apparent selectivity has been observed to be better than 10:1. Still, many groups were not satisfied with the therapeutic selectivities attained in PDT with the second-generation PS, and thus started searching for improved approaches to PS targeting. Different approaches were tried in PDT of cancer, including the following.

1. Premixing PS with LDL in order to target tissue with increased LDL receptor activity (49–52)
2. Packaging the PS in liposomes, which transfer the PS to LDL on breaking up (49–52)
3. Conjugating PS with water-soluble polymers in order to decrease liver uptake rates and increase serum half-life. In some cases this appeared to lead to an increased concentration of PS in neoplastic tissue, as was shown for a number of such polymers. For example, one may mention the covalent linkage of mTHPC to polyethylene glycol (58).
4. Conjugating PS with monoclonal antibodies, antibody fragments, small peptides, or oligonucleotides (59–65). The antibodies are targeted to antigens selectively expressed by certain tumors, such as the case of dye-labeled Mab35, which was targeted to carcinoembryonic antigen (CEA) in colon tumors (66–68). Another promising target is thought to be the neovasculature, which for instance expresses selectively $\alpha V\beta 3$ integrins that recognize the Arg-Gly-Asp (RGD) sequence, known to be present in the extracellular matrix components fibronectin, vitronectin, collagen, fibrinogen, and von Willebrand factor (69). One such an approach has been followed by Neri and coworkers who developed an antibody fragment for fibronectin, chemically coupled to a PS, which selectively localizes to newly formed blood vessels, to be used in PDT treatment of neovascularization of the eye (70).

PHOTOSENSITIZER DELIVERY TECHNIQUES

In photodynamic therapy, one of the problems that is often underestimated is how to find a good pharmaceutical formulation for the sensitizer. The formulation should depend on at least three factors.

1. The molecular properties of the PS (Is it hydrophilic or hydrophobic?)
2. The mode of application (Is it applied topically or injected systemically?)
3. What and where is the target (a brain tumor, skin tumor, neovascularization, or another site in the body)?

When the PS is water soluble, it may be formulated in phosphate buffered saline (PBS). Various strategies can be tried for hydrophobic PS, among which are oil-based emulsions, liposomes, inclusion complexes, organic solvents; and serum lipoproteins, among which are LDLs, polymeric nanoparticles, hydrophilic polymer–PS conjugates, monoclonal antibodies (Mab) or antibody fragments, and peptides.

We discuss both active targeting vehicles (e.g., Mab, LDL) and passive targeting vehicles (e.g., oil dispersions, liposomes) in the following.

Organic Solvents

The iv injection of mTHPC (Foscan) is an example in which the four hydroxy groups on the PS are not sufficient to make this chlorin hydrophilic enough to be easily dissolved in PBS. Thus, it has to be dissolved in H_2O, polyethylene glycol 400, and ethanol (5:3:2 vol) or in propylene glycol and ethanol (6:4 vol/vol). Also, BPD-MA has been injected in dimethyl sulfoxide (DMSO), in a mouse tumor model in order to compare the biodistribution and clearance properties of liposomal benzoporphyrin derivative (BPD) to aqueously formulated material (71).

Liposomes

Delivery may be by the use of liposomes for even more lipophilic PS. In a first approximation a detergent-like molecule can be used at a high enough concentration (critical micelle concentration, CMC) to enable transport of the lipophilic PS in the center of a micelle-like structure. The amphiphilic molecules that form a micelle have a structure, where P is a cationic, anionic, or neutral polar end, and A is an apolar tail.

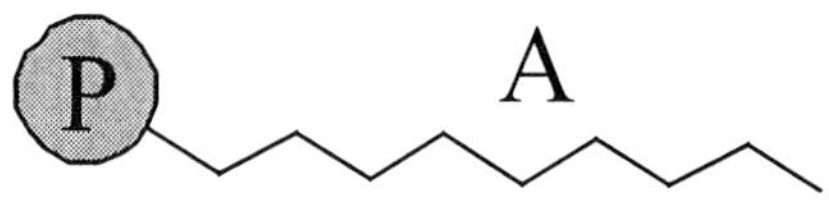

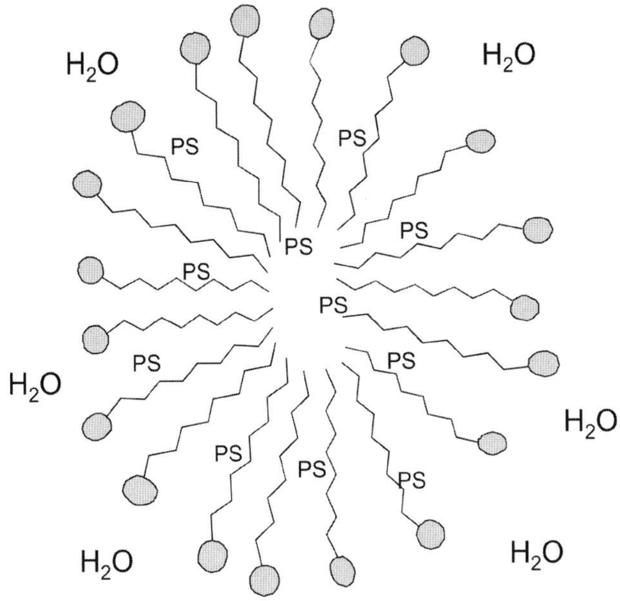

FIGURE 2.7. A schematic picture of a micelle with lipophilic photosensitizer molecules.

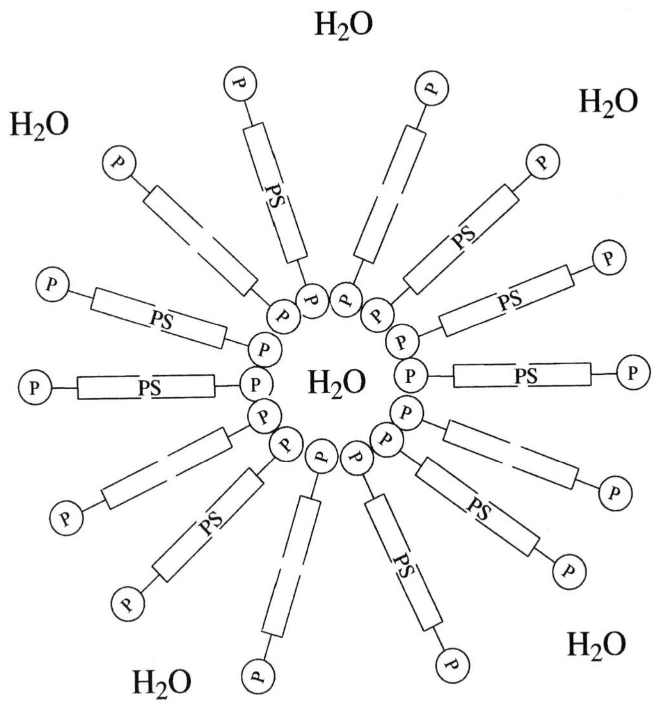

FIGURE 2.9. A liposome schematically.

Thus, a micelle with incorporated PS looks schematically as is shown in Figure 2.7.

Such micelle particles can be quite small, well below 1 μm in diameter. Liposomes themselves are slightly more complicated vehicles in which the application of ultrasound to a solution of phospholipids with two lipophilic hydrocarbon chains such as dipalmitoylphosphatidylcholine (DPPC) (Fig. 2.8) or palmitoyloleylphosphatidylcholine (POPC) leads to the formation of a more or less spherical bilayered structure.

Vesicles made from DPCC, POPC, or other molecules lead to liposomes such as shown in Figure 2.9, with different transition temperatures between the solid or gel-like phase and the liquid phase. Several groups have tested this liposomal delivery (71–73). This also is the way in which BPD-MA (verteporfin) is formulated for delivery in patients with choroidal neovascularization associated with AMD (74). The way in which the lipophilic drugs are stored in a liposome (monomeric or multimeric form) and the permeability of the vesicle (which can depend on added cholesterol) are not easy to control. Nevertheless, some excellent results in PDT have been obtained in this way, even in the clinical context, and there is some interesting speculation on the mechanism of the transfer of the PS from liposomal surroundings to LDL (44).

Oil-Based Emulsions

Oil-based emulsions have been used extensively in PDT as delivery vehicles for hydrophobic photosensitizers. One particularly well-known example of this is Cremophor-EL. (There are many types of Cremophores, with widely varying physicochemical properties.) Cremophor-EL (BASF Aktiengesellschaft, Ludwigschafen, Germany) can be made from ricinoleic acid (Fig. 2.10) and oxirane.

It is not a pure compound. One of the main differences between detergents such as Cremophor, Triton X100, and

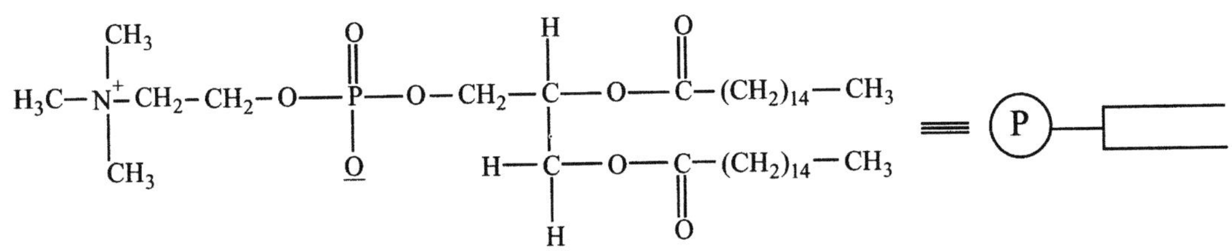

FIGURE 2.8. DPCC shown on the left as a chemical formula and a symbolic representation on the right, and as well as in Figure 2.9, where a liposome made up of DPPC molecules is shown schematically.

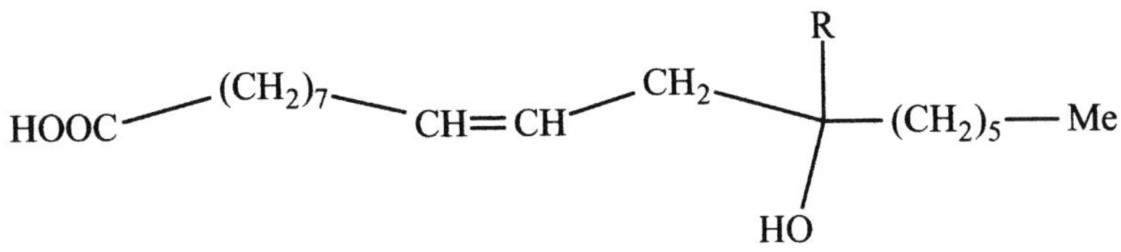

FIGURE 2.10. Ricinoleic acid is not a pure compound and serves as a base for Cremophor-EL.

Tween 80 (polyethylene sorbitan monoleate) (Sigma-Aldrich), on the one hand, and molecules such as DPPC and POPC on the other hand, is that the former are neutral and the latter are charged. The presence or absence of charge may have a significant influence on properties such as membrane crossing. Many PS such as Tin Ethyl Etiopurpurin ($SnET_2$) and the Palladium bacteriochlorophyll derivative TOOKAD ($C_{35}H_{36}N_4O_6Pd$) (Steba Biotech, Toussus-Le-Noble, France) have been formulated with Cremophor for preclinical testing (28,75–78). The pharmacology and toxicology of Cremophor has been studied in some detail (79) and susceptibility to such compounds at the concentrations used is suspected in some cases.

Biodegradable Polymeric Nanospheres

Initial results of delivering lipophilic PS with biodegradable microparticles and nanoparticles have been encouraging (80–82). Polymeric materials used include poly(ethylbutylcyanoacrylate) polyisohexylcyanoacrylate, or poly(D,L-lactic acid) (83–85). In some cases nanospheres were found to be responsible for improved uptake in tumor cells, and influenced the localization of the PS in tissue as well. One of the main advantages of this type of delivery vehicle is the high PS loading that can be achieved. Another advantage is that the nanoparticles (or nanocapsules) can be taken up by phagocytosis, thus delivering the lipophilic PS inside the cell, whereas a lipophilic PS could well get stuck in the cell's plasma membrane by other delivery pathways.

Attaching Photosensitizers Covalently to Polymers

Lipophilic PS have been covalently coupled to hydrophilic polymers such as PEG (58), charged or neutral poly-L-lysin (86) and polyvinyl-alcohol (87). Pegylation often lengthens the time that the photosensitizers remain in circulation and decreased uptake in the liver. In some cases (58) it also leads to higher uptake of PS in neoplastic tissue *in vivo*. It appears that the enveloping action of the long hydrophilic polymer chain around a hydrophobic PS influences the biodistribution of the PS favorably in general.

Inclusion Complexes

Inclusion complexes also have been used for transporting hydrophobic PS. These consist of small cyclic sugar (β-glucose) oligomers of six to eight sugar units, also called cyclodextrins. The ring of sugar molecules has a structure in which the inside is hydrophobic (the lipophilic PS can be located, or partially located here), and the outside of the cyclodextrin is hydrophilic. Thus, the complex between the lipophilic PS and the cyclodextrin can be fairly stable even in an aqueous medium.

Active Delivery with Monoclonal Antibodies, Antibody Fragments, Lipoproteins, or Peptides

To attain simultaneously both the role of lipophilic PS transport *and* improved specific targeting, PS conjugates are created with monoclonal antibodies, antibody fragments, certain lipoproteins, and small peptides (88). This implies that there exists a higher expression of certain receptors, antigens, oncoproteins, or integrins at the site of a lesion (89). The higher specificity of this type of PS delivery should not only lead to more effective therapy with fewer side effects but also to smaller injected PS doses.

The approach of using Mab-dye conjugates was pioneered by Mew and coworkers (90), who attached hematoporphyrin molecules (randomly) to Mabs. In the first clinical application of these studies, Folli and associates (66) actually tested chimerized antibody–dye complexes in a small number of patients. In that case, the Mab-35 was targeted against CEA in colon cancers, and was found *in vivo* to target in general with good but highly variable efficacy. Tissue concentrations of up to 0.06% of the injected dose were found per gram of tumor, and about 10 times less for normal mucosa.

In these and other studies it became clear that more than one PS molecule could be attached to a single Mab. The ratio was about 10 dye molecules per Mab (66). At higher ratios the PS molecules may lose some of their efficacy by interacting with one another. Furthermore, the surface of the antibody may be sufficiently modified to alter its properties, or else dye molecules may start to interfere directly with the active site of the Mab by blocking the Mab–antigen chemical interaction sterically (91). Some of these problems can be avoided by using more sophisticated ways of attaching dye molecules to the Mab (92). Other approaches include attaching multiple Mabs to the surface of particles containing PS, as was the case with targeted liposomes (93), and antibody fragments also can be used.

It is possible or even likely that antigen profiles change between patients as well as within tumor staging, thus leading to a large variability in uptake and selectivity. Finally, great care must be taken to avoid activating the human immune system against Mabs of murine origin (66).

In the PDT literature, quite some attention has been focused on lipoprotein-mediated delivery, and in particular transport of PS by LDL (94). Cancers can be targeted in principle by PS–LDL complexes because like most rapidly proliferating tissue, increased synthesis of biological membranes requires additional LDL, part of which may be taken up by enhanced receptor activity (39,95–97). This is an attractive approach, as the hydrophobic PS can be incorporated in significant quantity in the lipid core of the LDL molecule, without causing major changes in either the recognition of LDL by its receptors or LDL circulation lifetime in the plasma.

It also has been stated in the PDT of CNV associated with AMD that the choroidal neovasculature involved has higher LDL receptor activity. Thus, in the case of BPD-MA, the PS is delivered somewhat selectively to the CNV, a significant fraction of which attaches to LDL. This was shown for BPD-MA first dissolved in DMSO, then complexed with human LDL prior to injection, in a rabbit model (39), where the normal choriocapillary layer in the eye was better targeted, and in laser-induced experimental choroidal neovascularization in the eyes of cynomolgus monkeys (98). Some caution is required at this point. First, not all animals have similar distributions of blood proteins as humans, so that pharmacokinetic data taken with low LDL expression (e.g., in mice), may not directly extrapolate to the clinical context. Furthermore, in bolus-like injections, the original distribution of hydrophobic PS over the different blood proteins may be determined by the kinetics (overload) rather than the thermodynamics (equilibrium), so that a gradual redistribution of the PS may take place with time.

Finally, it should be mentioned that PS has been attached to small oligonuleotides (99), in order to induce a sequence-specific DNA cleavage, and that indocyanine green (ICG) has been attached to peptides (59) in a rat tumor model for a tumor-targeting image. Presumably, the field of PDT will see a lot more of this selective active targeting in the near future, targeting neovasculature via the integrin receptor $\alpha V\beta 3$.

THE PHOTOPHYSICS AND PHOTOCHEMISTRY OF PHOTOSENSITIZATION IN PHOTODYNAMIC THERAPY

In photosensitization reactions the first step is the absorption of light by the PS. Thus, after the energy of the photon is taken up by the PS, a series of physical energy redistribution processes takes place within the PS. This is followed by a chain of chemical and biochemical reactions, which finally may lead to the destruction of tissue.

Photophysics: Photon Absorption Plus Energy Redistribution

The early processes of photon energy absorption by a PS molecule, and the internal energy redistribution in the PS, are shown schematically in a so-called Jablonski diagram (Fig. 2.11). This is an energy level diagram representing the internal energy levels in a PS. The diagram shows that the energy of a molecule is quantized; that is, it can only have certain discrete values. These values are different from molecule to molecule (each molecule has an individual mass). A molecule's energy comes in four types of energy quanta.

1. *Electronic energy.* The electronic energy quanta are generally the biggest energy quanta. Electronic energy is related to how the electrons are arranged in space around the nuclei of the molecule. Thus, the interaction of a PS with an ultraviolet or visible photon, in which the photon is absorbed by the PS, leads to a much more energetic PS.
2. *Vibrational energy.* These are medium-size energy quanta. This type of energy has to do with the atoms of a PS moving periodically relative to one another. Typically when one heats a molecule, it vibrates more. If one heats it enough, it vibrate so much that the atoms fly apart and the molecule decomposes.
3. *Rotational energy.* These are small quanta. This type of energy has to do with the molecule rotating in space. Heating a molecule makes it rotate faster.
4. *Translational energy.* These quanta are very small indeed. When one heats a molecule, it moves faster in space from one point to another.

In order to understand the Jablonski diagram in detail one must realize that the electrons around the atoms of the PS molecule are said to be constrained to certain regions of space called orbitals. There are at most two electrons in each orbital. These electrons have a property called spin. Each electron can have two orientations of spin (up and down). Most orbitals contain electrons with paired spins; that is, with one spin pointing up and one pointing down. If this is the case for all orbitals, we say the molecule is in a singlet state, indicated by ($\uparrow\downarrow$). If the two electrons are pointing in the same direction in one of the orbitals, we call this a triplet state, indicated by ($\uparrow\uparrow$). A PS molecule has multiple singlet and triplet states generally, each of which has its particular electronic energy. The lowest (ground) electronic state is usually a singlet state, which is called S_0.

When a photon is absorbed, energy is added to the PS and it goes from S_0 to S_1, S_2, or another singlet state depending on the photon energy. A blue photon (i.e., a relatively energetic photon) may cause an $S_0 \rightarrow S_2$ transition,

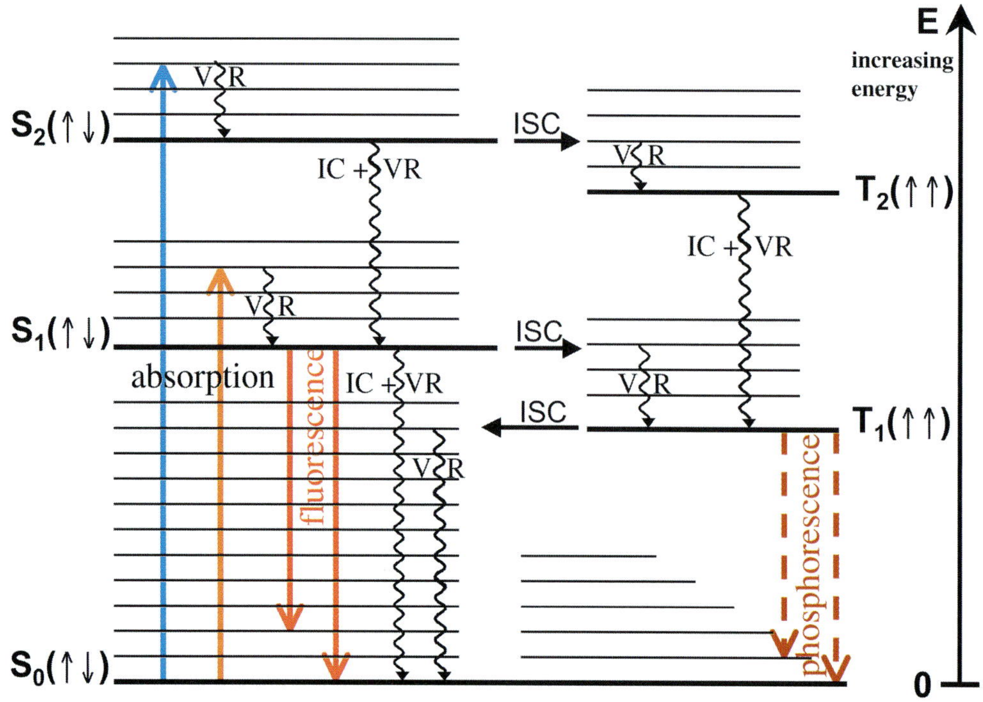

FIGURE 2.11. The Jablonski diagram. The thick horizontal lines indicate electronic energy levels. S_0, S_1, and S_2 are singlet electronic energy levels of the PS; T_1 and T_2 are triplet electronic energy levels. The thin horizontal lines represent the vibrational energy levels associated with each electronic state. (Rotations are not shown for the sake of clarity.) The blue arrow represents light absorption of a blue (i.e., energetic) photon. The red upward pointing arrow represents red (less energetic) light absorption. The red (down pointing) arrows represent fluorescence (i.e., loss of energy) at two different wavelengths. The horizontal arrows labeled ISC (intersystem crossing) represent radiation-less processes in which the PS goes from a singlet to triplet electronic state or vice versa. This process is generally fast relative to vibrational energy loss by energy exchange with the surrounding molecules. The latter, indicated by VR (vibrational relaxation) are also radiation-less processes and indicate energy loss by the PS in the form of heat to the surroundings. The arrows labeled with IC (internal conversion) represent a change in an electronic state (between two singlet or two triplet states), which is generally followed by vibrational relaxation. Thus, the overall IC process is conversion of electronic energy into vibrational energy. This is followed by vibrational relaxation of the PS molecule and the corresponding heating of the environment. Finally, the dashed red vertical arrows represent a low probability energy loss process of the PS by emitting phosphorescent photons in the infrared. This is accompanied by a change from the T_1 electronic state to the S_0 ground state. (From: van den Bergh H. Photodynamic therapy of age related macular degeneration: history and principles. *Semin Ophthalmol* 2002;16:181–200, with permission).

whereas absorption of a red photon (i.e., a less energetic photon) may only be able to induce $S_0 \rightarrow S_1$. Photon-induced (radiative) changes accompanied by a flip of spin, that is $S_0 \rightarrow T_2$, or $T_1 \rightarrow S_2$ are "forbidden," which means these are processes that have an extremely low probability of occurring.

We now describe a typical sequence of some of the processes indicated in the Jablonski diagram. Light absorption by a PS is instantaneous essentially. Often it implies changing from the ground electronic state (S_0) (e.g., the lowest energy arrangement possible for the electrons around the PS molecule) to an electronically excited state (e.g., S_1). This S_1 state has another distribution of the electron cloud around the nuclei of the PS, which corresponds to more energy of the PS molecule in this case. The absorption spectrum corresponding to this process is broad and looks continuous, as can be seen for instance in most of the examples given in Figure 2.5. This is because the photon can induce a transition to different vibrational and rotational energy levels in S_1, and the latter are closely spaced in such a large molecule. Furthermore, there are many different vibrational energy spacings (modes) in a large molecule such as a PS. All this adds up to the fact that the optical absorption appears to be a continuum. Please note that the energy levels corresponding to only one of the vibrational modes are indicated in the Jablonski diagram. We have drawn the case of absorption to S_1 in Figure 2.11 (the red arrow pointing upward) in such a way that the PS in the S_1 state contains some vibrational excess energy on top of its electronic excitation energy. For the sake of simplicity we have not drawn the rotational energy levels in Figure 2.11, nor do we discuss rotational energy here. The PS molecule excited with the red photon now undergoes a number of processes on different time scales. In general, vibrational relaxation (VR) (represented by the black wiggled arrow) takes place very rapidly, that is, on the order of 10^{-12} seconds. This implies that the PS immediately loses some vibrational energy, which it gives off as heat when colliding with the surrounding molecules. The molecule in the vibrational ground state of the S_1 electronically excited state can then undergo one of three processes.

First, it can emit a photon (red arrow pointing downward); this is called fluorescence. This generally takes place on a time scale of the order of $10^{-8} - 10^{-9}$ seconds. This is quasicontinuous broadband emission. Because one considers a large number of molecules, the photon emission results in the formation of different vibrational levels of the electronic ground state (depending on properties called Franck-Condon factors). The length of the arrow representing the fluorescence photon is shorter than the absorbed photon; that is, represents a smaller energy change in the molecule. This difference in wavelength is called a Stokes shift. Thus, PS fluorescence in biological surroundings is always shifted to the red (less energy) from the absorption wavelength.

The second possibility for the photosensitizer molecule in the ground vibrational state of the S_1 state is to follow a pathway in which it converts to a so-called triplet state (T_1) by a process called intersystem crossing (ISC). How probable each of the three pathways is depends on the PS, and it can be influenced by chemically modifying the PS, for instance by adding a central metal atom of a particular kind to a porphyrin, or by substituting heavy atoms such as iodine for the peripheral hydrogen. ISC is a radiation-less process—no photon is absorbed or emitted—and it is indicated by the horizontal black arrow. This ISC implies a change (flip) in the electron spin. Intersystem crossing from S_1 to the lowest triplet state (T_1) results in a T_1 state with excess vibrational energy. This is because the change between electronic states generally is fast compared with vibrational relaxation. This behavior follows a rule known as the Franck-Condon principle. Simplified it means in this case that the light electrons can move around faster than the heavier nuclei. Because T_1 lies lower in energy than S_1, the energy difference must show up as T_1 vibrational energy following the rapid change in electronic states. The T_1 triplet state then proceeds to lose this excess of vibrational energy in collisions with surrounding molecules. This is again a radiation-less process and is shown by a wiggled black arrow. As mentioned, in most cases T_1 can now not just give off a photon and return to the S_0 ground state. This is a so-called "spin-forbidden" radiative process, as it involves a spin flip. Such forbidden radiative processes have a very small probability; thus, this process (emitting a photon to go from $T_1 \rightarrow S_0$), which is called phosphorescence, is very slow, and hence does not occur significantly in most PS. Thus, the T_1 state hangs around for a while and is called metastable.

The third possible pathway for the S_1 state is to undergo internal conversion (IC) to the S_0 ground electronic state. This means that all the electronic excess energy of S_1 is converted in a fast process to vibrational excess energy of the ground state molecule. This vibrational energy in S_0 is then rapidly degraded, in collisions, thus heating the surrounding molecules. To summarize, starting from vibrationally relaxed S_1, the sum of the probabilities of fluorescence, IC, and ISC is unity. Either one or the other of these three processes must happen. The relative probability of fluorescence, IC, and ISC occurring in each PS is different. Thus, molecules such as fluorescein (FA) or ICG are chosen in ophthalmology for their high probability of fluorescence, which is useful in angiography. On the contrary, photosensitizers used in PDT are chosen so that they have a significant ISC probability and hence a high triplet yield. If the T_1 triplet state does not phosphoresce now, and it does not significantly undergo ISC back to S_0, then we have what is called a long-lived (metastable) triplet state. This state (owing to its long lifetime) can induce the chemical reactions described in the following, because it "hangs around" long enough to react or collides with molecular oxygen. The long-lived triplet state T_1 is an important intermediate in photodynamic therapy. Finally, the Jablonski diagram of Figure 2.11 contains higher lying (i.e., more energetic) singlet and triplet states. This means that there are even more electronic states or spatial arrangements of the electron cloud of the sensitizer. For example, if a porphyrin sensitizer absorbs in the blue (i.e., a more energetic photon than in the red), this may give rise to an S_2 singlet state rather than S_1, as shown by the upward pointing long blue arrow in Figure 2.11. Following rapid vibrational relaxation, this S_2 state may then undergo IC to give vibrationally excited S_1, which then relaxes to the lowest S_1 vibrational level. This is followed by one of exactly the same three processes described in the preceding for S_1 (fluorescence, ISC, or IC). The difference, in the case of the porphyrins, is that at the blue wavelengths the absorption coefficient (near 400 nm this is the so-called Soret band), is much larger than in the red (near 630 nm). Thus, using blue photons will in principle cause more PDT, because the probability of absorption of these photons is larger, and finally leads to more of the reactive metastable triplet states. However, because of light absorption (e.g., by blood and light scattering), the penetration of blue light into most tissues is less deep than for red light, so that only superficial cancers can be treated. The absorption coefficient ε of the PS controls the probability of absorption of a photon of a given wavelength by a sample containing a concentration c of the PS. It is defined by the Beer-Lambert equation as $^{10}\log(I_0/I)=\varepsilon.c.l.$ where I_0 = the light intensity at a given wavelength incident on a sample; I = the transmitted light intensity; c = the concentration of the absorbing species (mole/cm^3); l = the thickness of the sample traversed by the light (in cm); ε = the decadic molar absorption or extinction coefficient (cm^3/mole.cm). Strictly speaking, this equation holds for samples that do not have significant losses owing to light scattering.

The Jablonski diagram of Figure 2.11 describes the energy flow in the PS subsequent to photon absorption. Whereas the fluorescence is important for photodetection of cancers or angiography in the eye, the production of long-lived metastable triplet states T_1 is essential for PDT. Not all triplet states of PS are effective in PDT. Another essential requirement is that the triplet state of the PS has enough energy (relative to S_0) to be able to excite ground state di-oxygen ($O_2{}^3\Sigma$) to its lowest electronically excited state ($O_2{}^1\Delta$). Note: The symbols $^3\Sigma$ and $^1\Delta$ refer to a triplet and a singlet state with different geometries of distribution of the electron clouds around the nuclear frame, respectively. Σ and Δ in molecules correspond to s and d orbitals in atoms, where s represents a spherically symmetric distribution.

Photodetection with Fluorescent Photosynthesizers

The fluorescent properties of most of the first- and second-generation PS used in PDT can be used to both localize and dose these sensitizers *in vivo.* This can help to carry out pharmacokinetics (PK) in a clinical context (57), as well as look at the microscopic localization of the PS in cell cultures or tissue biopsies using fluorescence microscopy (19). This domain has recently been reviewed by Wagnières and associates (101). The only remarks made here concerning the fluorescent properties of PS pertain to their use in the PDT of CNV in AMD. Clearly, both in preclinical and clinical tests it is helpful for PK studies and PS dosing to have a compound that fluoresces. The relative concentration of the PS in the various compartments in the eye can be measured semi-quantitatively as a function of time (102). Such measurements may be helpful in finding the optimal treatment time, although the fluorescence in tissue is never quite quantitative, nor may enough be known about the detailed PS localization from the PS angiography to deduce much about real PDT efficacy. A question often asked is: Is imaging of PS using flash cameras really safe? i.e. not causing any significant PDT effect. For BPD-MA, the therapeutic light dose is 50 J/cm^2, and within one flash from a retinal camera through a specific excitation filter for BPD fluorescence imaging, the amount of light is $\approx$50 mJ/flash on the whole retina (about 2 cm^2 for 50° illumination), this gives $\approx$0.5 J/cm^2 for the recording of 20 images, 1% of the therapeutic light dose: This is the sub-threshold of any therapeutic effect.

Useful information also is obtained from fluorescence on leakage out of CNV, and inter-patient variability in PK. Finally, in fluorescence angiography with fluorescein and/or ICG part of the neovasculature ("occult" CNV) may not be easy to see because it lies below the strongly visible light-absorbing retinal pigment epithelium in the case of fluorescein. In the case of ICG, which is excited and emits in the near infrared, the large choroidal vessels below the CNV fluoresce so strongly that they blot out the weak fluorescence from the small neovessels at short times after injection. Thus, because the often weak and poorly demarcated "occult" CNV is hard to spot precisely at times, it may be interesting to have a second- or third-generation PS that strongly fluoresces, that can be excited at wavelengths both in the visible and near infrared range (in order to distinguish between more superficial CNV—above the RPE—and deeper lying CNV—below the RPE), and that localizes predominantly in neovasculature. Because the latter property may not be obvious in second-generation compounds, coupling of a highly fluorescent molecule to a molecule that selectively targets neovasculature may be a solution for the next generation of these compounds. It should be noted here that "occult" CNV by definition does not only refer to CNV below the RPE, but also may result from reduced leakage in "less aggressive" neovasculature.

Primary Photochemical Processes

As mentioned, photosensitizing reactions most often start with the production of a metastable triplet state (T_1) of the PS, following light absorption and intersystem crossing. The triplet state of a photosensitizer also may be written as ^{3}PS, instead of T_1. ^{3}PS is used in the following discussion on photochemistry. Ideally, in PDT the photosensitizer "catalyzes" the destruction of a biological substrate; that is, the PS is not destroyed itself in the photochemical process, and the S_0 state is regenerated in the sensitizing process. This is done by the energy transfer between ^{3}PS and $^3O_2$, which completes the recycling of the PS to the S_0 state while creating reactive oxygen molecules in the $^1\Delta$ state. We see in the following that this may not always be the case, and that some fraction of the sensitizer may be consumed by a phenomenon called photobleaching. Finally, it should be noted that tissue oxygen is consumed in most cases of PDT, and the availability of oxygen depends on the rate of PDT and may even become rate limiting.

We now discuss the steps in the initial photochemistry of the sensitizing process. There are essentially two mechanisms of photosensitization: Types I and II.

Type I Processes

As mentioned, for the sake of simplicity in the following discussion T_1 is replaced by ^{3}PS, and S_0 is replaced by PS. ^{3}PS is formed from PS as shown in the Jablonski diagram following photon absorption and ISC. ^{3}PS then undergoes either electron transfer reactions (see reactions 1 and 2) with a substrate molecule (M) or hydrogen atom transfer (reactions 3 and 4). Thus, because electron transfer may cause either oxidation (loss of an electron) or reduction (the substrate M transfers an electron to the sensitizer), we have

$$^3PS + M \rightarrow PS^{\cdot -} + M^{\cdot +} \quad [1]$$

$$^3PS + M \rightarrow PS^{\cdot +} + M^{\cdot -} \quad [2]$$

The dots indicate that the species are radicals; that is, they have an odd total number of electrons, the −/+ signs indicate net charge. The fact that a molecular species has an uneven number of electrons (i.e., it is a radical) does not necessarily imply that it has an electrical net charge.

Likewise, the transfer of hydrogen atoms can occur

$$^3PS\text{-}H + M \rightarrow PS^{\cdot} + MH^{\cdot} \quad [3]$$

In reaction [3], ^{3}PS-H just is another way of writing ^{3}PS. The −H symbolizes just that one of the many hydrogen atoms in ^{3}PS, which is going to be abstracted in the H atom transfer reaction.

$$^3PS + M\text{-}H \rightarrow PS\text{-}H^{\cdot} + M^{\cdot} \quad [4]$$

In reaction [4], M-H is identical to M. The triplet state photosensitizer (^{3}PS) abstracts one of the many hydrogen atoms of the molecule M, to become $^{\cdot}$PS-H, whereas the radical $M^{\cdot}$ is actually the original substrate molecule M minus one of its hydrogen atoms, and PS-H$^{\cdot}$ is PS with a hydrogen atom added to it.

Radical species, which have one unpaired electron, are generally more reactive than molecules, which have an even number of electrons.

If molecular oxygen is available in the tissue, reactions [3] and [4] are followed by a rapid addition reaction that takes place between the radical species and molecular O_2, thus forming peroxyl radicals:

$$PS^{\cdot} + O_2 \rightarrow PS - O_2^{\cdot} \quad [5]$$

and

$$M^{\cdot} + O_2 \rightarrow M - O_2^{\cdot} \quad [6]$$

where the peroxyl radicals can then start a chain of reactions, which in the case of reaction [6] can continue like

$$M - O_2^{\cdot} + M - H \rightarrow M^{\cdot} + M - O_2 - H \quad [7]$$

A well-known laboratory example of the hydrogen transfer reaction shown in the preceding is the photolysis of benzophenone in the presence of an alcohol. This is shown in detail in Appendix 1.

The radical anions formed in reactions [1,2] can react further to form another not very reactive intermediate the superoxide radical anion ($O_2^{\cdot -}$) by

$$PS^{\cdot -} + O_2 \rightarrow PS + O_2^{\cdot -} \quad [8]$$

$$M^{\cdot -} + O_2 \rightarrow M + O_2^{\cdot -} \quad [9]$$

$O_2^{\cdot -}$ can then induce a number of reactions such as

$$O_2^{\cdot -} + H^+ \leftrightarrow HO_2^{\cdot} \quad [10]$$

at high radical concentrations, these radicals can combine by $^{\cdot}HO_2 + {}^{\cdot}HO_2 \rightarrow H_2O_2 + O_2$. H_2O_2 is toxic and is destroyed by catalase or other enzymes. Another pathway that leads to H_2O_2 is

$$HO_2^{\cdot} + O_2^{\cdot -} + H^+ \rightarrow H_2O_2 + O_2 \quad [11]$$

H_2O_2 catalyzed by iron in a so-called Fenton reaction can give rise to the extremely reactive $OH^{\cdot}$ radical

$$H_2O_2 + F_e^{2+} \rightarrow OH^{\cdot} + OH^- + F_e^{3+} \quad [12]$$

$OH^{\cdot}$ radicals can then abstract hydrogen or add to double bonds. In the absence of sufficient oxygen, the termination reactions such as [13,14] dominate.

$$PS^{\cdot -} + M^{\cdot +} \rightarrow PS - M \quad [13]$$

$$M^{\cdot} + M^{\cdot} \rightarrow M - M \quad [14]$$

To summarize the type I processes: O_2 does not take part in the first step, which consists of electron or hydrogen atom transfer. However, if enough O_2 exists, its presence can lead to reactive oxygen containing species such as hydrogen peroxide (H_2O_2), and the hydroxyl radical ($OH^{\cdot}$). These reactive intermediates can then react with a multitude of biomolecules, possibly leading to apoptosis and/or necrosis of the tissue. If PS is destroyed or chemically modified in reactions such as those shown in equations 1 through 14, this is called photobleaching; and the optical absorption or fluorescence specific to the presence of PS disappears. If there is not enough molecular oxygen in the tissue, some of the reactive oxygen-containing intermediates are not generated. This may limit the overall efficacy of the photosensitizing process.

Type II Processes

Type II processes require oxygen in the first step, which start (as the type I processes) from the metastable triplet state of the photosensitizer ^{3}PS:

$$^3PS + O_2\,(^3\Sigma) \rightarrow PS + O_2\,(^1\Delta) \text{ or } (^1\Sigma) \quad [15]$$

Here the $^3\Sigma$, $^1\Delta$ and $^1\Sigma$ are symbols that indicate the triplet ground states of O_2 and the first and second excited singlet states, respectively. Oxygen is exceptional in nature, having a triplet ground state. Most molecules have a singlet ground state. If the triplet metastable state of the photosensitizer (because of its relatively long lifetime) is present long enough, then molecular oxygen in the tissue (which is diffusing around) collides with it. If the energy of the triplet state (relative to the ground singlet state of PS) is near to or above the excitation energy of one of the two lowest excited oxygen singlet states, collisional energy transfer can take place, leading to the formation of O_2 ($^1\Delta$); that is, excited molecular oxygen. It is thought that in some cases, O_2 ($^1\Sigma$), a higher lying singlet state may be populated first, but this rapidly converts internally to the $^1\Delta$ state. Reaction (15) is generally fast. Reaction (15) represents a so-called triplet–triplet annihilation, which results in energy transfer to yield singlet oxygen ($^1O_2$). In terms of simplified molecular orbitals, it may be depicted as an *electron exchange* mechanism, as shown in the following (103):

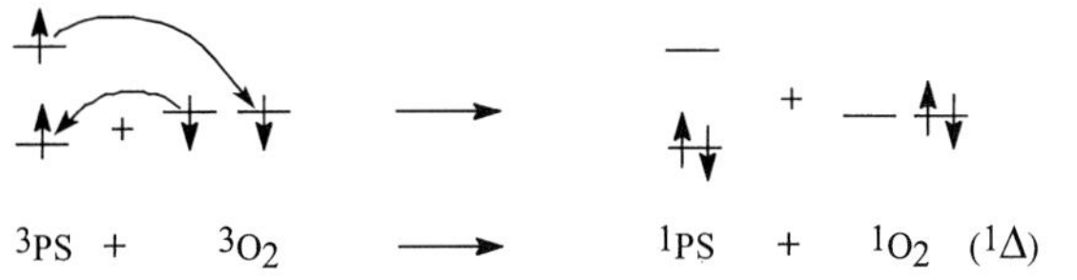

[16]

Other mechanisms for creating $^1O_2$ from ^3PS include *electron transfer*:

$$^3PS + {^3O_2} \rightarrow PS^{\dot{+}} + O_2^{\dot{-}} \rightarrow PS + {^1O_2} \quad [17]$$

and diradical formation:

$$^3PS + {^3O_2} \rightarrow P\dot{S}-O-O^{\cdot} \rightarrow PS + {^1O_2} \quad [18]$$

It should be noted that in the process of creating singlet oxygen by collisional electronic energy transfer from ^3PS, as shown in equation [15], we regenerate singlet ground state PS (i.e., S_0), which can absorb light again. Thus, a single PS molecule can go through such a cycle many times: Each time, after absorbing a photon and undergoing ISC to ^3PS, it converts one unreactive O_2 ($^3\Sigma$) to a much more reactive $O_2(^1\Delta)$. The latter is metastable also. (It can slowly emit an infrared photon or undergo ISC.) However, because of its high reactivity it does not diffuse very far before reacting, probably on the order of a few tens of nanometers in biological surroundings (104). Typical reactions of $O_2(^1\Delta)$ are shown in reaction [19a] with an unsaturated lipid, and in [19b] in a ring opening reaction.

It should be carefully noted that the short diffusion distance of $O_2(^1\Delta)$ prior to reaction implies that PDT damage is located nearly exactly at the position of the dye molecules themselves. Oxygen is consumed and the PS is regenerated in processes [15] and [19a,b]. A situation may also exist in this type of photochemistry in which the production of singlet oxygen is limited by the diffusion of oxygen molecules to the region where the PS is localized. This implies that for a given concentration of PS it may not be effective to keep increasing the photon flux to the tissue, because the tissue destruction rate will not increase further; that is, O_2 diffusion becomes the rate-limiting step. Finally, it should be realized that $O_2(^1\Delta)$ occasionally reacts with the PS itself, thus changing its optical properties. This is a photobleaching event. The presence of reactive intermediates generated by type I and/or II mechanism can be invoked by direct measurement of infrared radiation for the case of $O_2(^1\Delta)$ (although this is very difficult *in vivo*), or by electron spin resonance for a paramagnetic species (105) such as $OH^{\cdot}$, and/or by adding reactive chemical traps such as furfuryl alcohol for $O_2(^1\Delta)$.

The relative importance of type I versus type II mechanisms is hard to determine in complex biological systems. However, if oxygen is depleted faster than it can diffuse to the region of PDT (e.g., because of high concentrations of PS and high light fluence rates), then the lack of oxygen may cause the type I mechanism to become predominant at some point. Another way to try to estimate the relative contribution of type II chemistry is to add singlet oxygen quenchers such as 1,4-diazabicyclo [2,2,2] octane (DABCO), β-carotene, or sodium azide (105), and observe the change in PDT efficacy. One can also substitute heavy water (D_2O) for normal water in the sample, because in D_2O the $O_2(^1\Delta)$ lives longer and thus is more reactive. Similarly, quenchers also exist for the type I intermediates (catalase for H_2O_2, mannitol for $OH^{\cdot}$, and superoxide dismutase for $O_2^{\cdot -}$). It should be noted that most of these methods are not completely free of interference between species because of lack of complete chemical selectivity.

Several authors affirm that most of the evidence appears to point to a predominant type II mechanism under many of the conditions encountered in preclinical and clinical PDT (106).

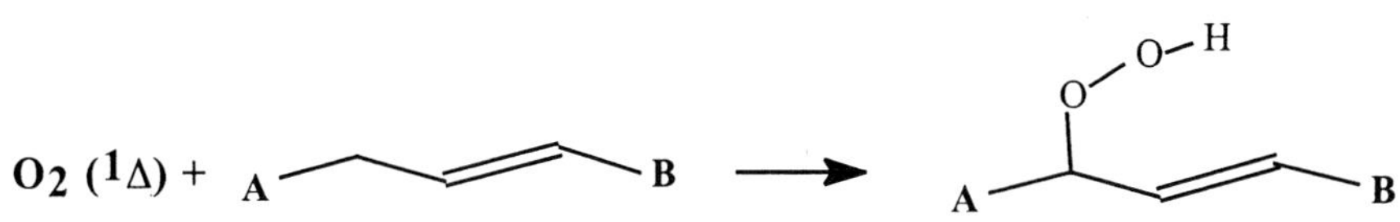

[19a]

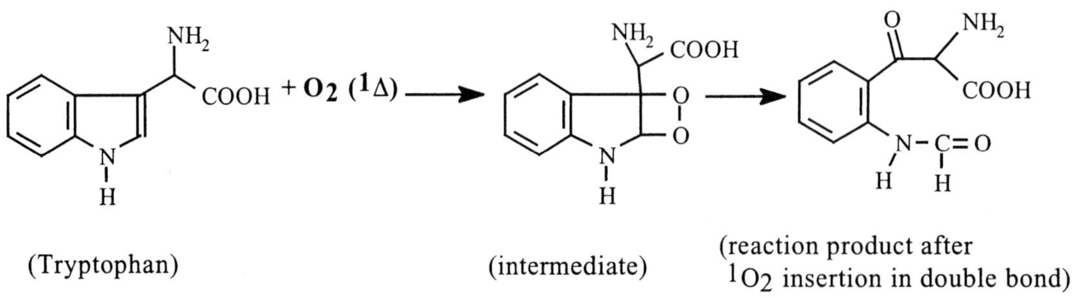

[19b]

PHOTODYNAMIC THERAPY–INDUCED BIOMOLECULAR PATHWAY CHANGES

One current focal point in PDT is the understanding of how photooxidative stress induced by various photosensitizers in different tissue locations, and at different conditions, induces biomolecular cascades that lead to given physiological responses such as necrosis and/or apoptosis. A more complete understanding of these PDT-induced pathway changes should lead to a more quantitative control of the therapy. Jori and Spikes (107) have reviewed the photobiochemistry of porphyrins. They discussed the primary reactions in the photooxidation of lipids, steroids, purines, pyrimidines, nucleic acids, proteins, and amino acids, among the possible biological targets.

When these and other biomolecules in cells are exposed to the oxidative stress associated with PDT, pathways are changed that regulate gene expression, cell cycle, and cell death. For instance, PDT-induced cell death, via apoptosis and/or necrosis, is thought to be influenced by the localization of the sensitizer as well as the PDT conditions such as the time delay between drug and light application, light intensity and dose, drug dose, and so on (42,108,109).

It is difficult to prove in clinical PDT today if tissue destruction is caused mainly by necrotic or apoptotic factors. Here, we take a short look at apoptosis as an example of a PDT-induced cascade. Apoptosis is an ordered process, which takes place in normal tissue where cells need to be replaced, or when cells are exposed to an external stress such as PDT, and are damaged beyond the possibility of repair. The cells then induce their own destruction. This apoptosis requires a multitude of active cellular processes, with the complete uptake of the cell by macrophages or neighboring cells as the final outcome. Whereas tissue necrosis is known to provoke inflammatory responses, removal of apoptotic cells by macrophages is considered to be physiologically inert. Thus, no debris is left in apoptosis, as is the case in the less controlled process of necrosis. Apoptotic cells shrink and are rapidly "eaten" by neighboring cells, thus limiting the leakage of intracellular components to the surroundings, and hence reducing the probability of undesired tissue inflammation, which is caused by necrotic cells that swell and burst, spilling their content over neighboring cells. Because apoptosis is often induced at less severe PDT conditions than necrosis, it may be a preferred pathway in the treatment of some types of disease. Consequently, studying how to optimize apoptosis induced by PDT is highly desirable. The main hydrolytic protein degrading reactions induced in apoptosis are catalyzed by a group of enzymes called caspases. These caspases are produced in the form of proenzymes that are activated either by apoptosis-related proteins or through cleavage by other caspases. All caspases have the amino acid cysteine in their active catalytic site and cleave the target protein at given aspartic acids; hence, the name caspase. Thus, each caspase consists of an inactive precursor called a procaspase, which is often itself activated by cleavage at an aspartic acid site by another caspase. Consequently, a significant part of apoptosis is a cascade of caspases. Activation of a caspase is by cleavage at two aspartic acid sites. The so-called prodomain is discarded, leaving two large and two small subunits as the activated enzyme. Apoptosis can be induced by several parallel pathways, which are not completely independent; that is, they can interfere with one another. These pathways are dependent on the sites where the PDT-induced photooxidation takes place, that is, on photosensitizer localization. As mentioned, the localization of lipophilic PS or hydrophilic cationic PS in the mitochondria, followed by light application under the right conditions for PDT, can lead to the release of cytochrome C (41,110–115), which may be related to the loss in mitochondrial membrane potential and/or the opening of the permeability transition pore complex (PTPC). This in way can affect respiration (110,111, 113–115), and the formation in the cytosol of the apoptosome complex by binding of cytochrome C to the apoptosis activating factor-1 (APAF-1), which induces the release of caspase 9. The latter then activates caspase 3 (116,117). Apoptosis also may be induced via a group of receptors called "death receptors," which are found at the cell surface, among which are those of the well-known tumor necrosis factor (TNF) family. The caspases are activated by an oligomerization process at these sites. Parallel to the mentioned caspase 3 activation, PDT-induced damage at other cell locations (e.g., the TNF death receptor at the cell membrane) can lead to the activation of procaspase 8 (i.e., release of caspase 8), which in turn also leads to active caspase 3. The biomolecular components of these different pathways may interact with one another (110, 111,113–115), thus complicating the picture. Activated caspase 8 also cleaves Bid (a protein of the Bcl-2 family) (108,109), which yields the proapoptic protein fragment called tBid. tBid in turn interacts with the mitochondria increasing cytochrome C release.

Caspase 3 (118) then initiates the cleavage and activation of several other caspases, among them caspase 6, which cleaves to nuclear lamina. The latter are cytoskeletal proteins that form the nuclear structure; thus, this process leads to breakdown of the cell nucleus. Caspases 3 and 7 cleave PARP (Poly [ADP-ribose] polymerase), a DNA repair protein, as well as ICAD/DFF45, an inhibitor of CAD caspase-activated DNase.

Alternatively, PDT damage can be located in the lysosomes for some photosensitizers (119), which results in the release of proteins cleaving cathepsins. This is complicated in that it can cause both the Bid → tBid cleavage, thus increasing apoptosis; and caspase 3 cleave, thus inhibiting apoptosis.

Finally, PDT with certain sensitizers can cause damage to the endoplasmic reticulum that induces release of Ca^{2+}, which in turn regulates the mitochondrial membrane permeabilization and hence apoptosis. Some PDT-induced biomolecular pathways may promote or inhibit apoptosis depending on the amount of damage done to: (a) the cell membrane; (b) the mitochondrion; (c) lysosomes; and (d) the endoplasmic reticulum. Because many proteins of the Bcl-2 group have a hydrophobic tail, they can bind to the mitochondria as shown. Consequently, in the end it may be the ratio of *apoptosis suppressors* such as Bcl-2 and Bcl-x to *apoptosis promoters* such as Bax that determine a cell's sensitivity to apoptosis. Finally, the caspase cascade causes the relocation of the negatively charged phospholipid phosphatidylserine from the inner surface of the cell membrane to the outer surface. This identifies the cell to neighboring cells and macrophages as one that is to be digested.

The situation of proapoptotic and antiapoptotic reactions induced by PDT is summarized in a simplified way in Figure 2.12. The balance among all these reactions finally leads to cell survival or cell death. Also shown in Figure 2.12 are several other proapoptotic and antiapoptotic members of the Bcl-2 family of proteins, among which Bcl-2 and Bcl-xL downregulate apoptosis, whereas Bax is proapoptotic.

Several groups are studying the details of how the caspase cleavage products lead to cell shrinking, membrane blebbing, DNA fragmentation (and repair), and finally apoptosis, the ultimate goal being to find a quantitative relation between PDT conditions and the optimal mechanism of inducing cell death.

In a novel approach along these lines several research groups (118) have focused on sublethal PDT experiments, which may be advantageous for studying the PDT-induced biomolecular cascades in many cases. Examples of this are growth arrest (e.g., interruption of the cell cycle) (120) and the induction of cytokines (e.g., molecules of the interleukin family), which may be useful when using PDT to induce immune modulation.

In conclusion, by studying sublethal PDT, it is possible to extract important information on the modulation of pathways that interfere with gene expression, cell cycle, and cell death. The outcome of PDT, either in terms of survival

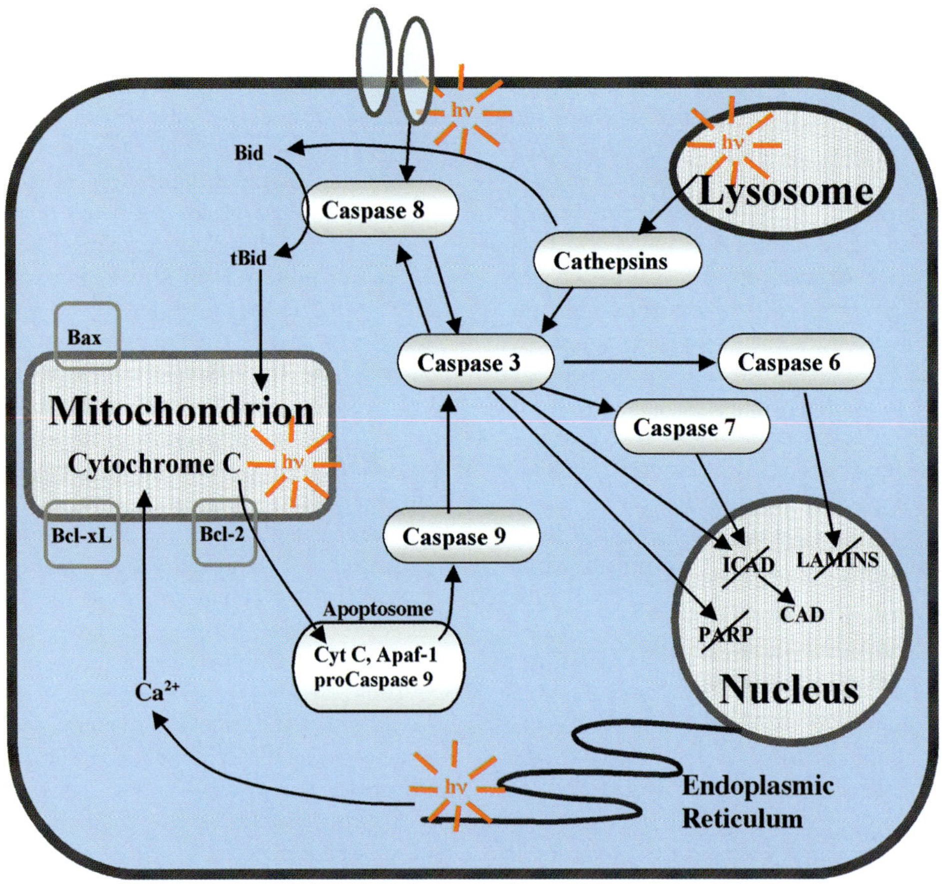

FIGURE 2.12. A schematic summary of part of the biomolecular cascade induced by photodynamic therapy at different sites, which may lead to apoptosis. (From: Oleinick NL, et al. The role of apoptosis in response to photodynamic therapy: what, where, why, and how. *Photochem Photobiol Sci* 2002;1:1–21, with permission.)

or death by apoptosis and/or necrosis, is the result of an extremely complicated series of parallel and sequential events, with pathways that can cross and interfere with one another. It is hoped that the improved understanding of the details of these processes may help to optimize PDT in areas that range from the total destruction of a cancer by necrosis/apoptosis to "softer" processes like the modulation of the immune system. It should be noted that most of the investigations on the biomolecular cascades involved in apoptosis were done on cancer cell lines. The extrapolation of this information to vascular therapy (mostly involving endothelial cells, which is of particular interest here) (121) has to be further investigated.

VASCULAR EFFECTS OF PHOTODYNAMIC THERAPY

This chapter is of direct interest to the application of PDT in the treatment of CNV in AMD and other diseases involving neovasculature. The subject has been reviewed by Henderson (122) and more recently by Fingar (123,124). The vascular effect induced by photodynamic therapy was found quite early on in solid tumors. Vascular damage and blood flow stasis have become well-established phenomena in the PDT of cancer with many different PS. The vascular PDT effects are probably initiated to a large extent by damage to the endothelial cells, involving some of the usual PDT cellular targets (e.g., the plasma membrane, lysosomes, or mitochondria) depending on the photosensitizer and applied conditions. Most PDT sensitizers show vascular damage during or after light exposure of the tissue containing the photosensitizer, in particular if high enough serum levels of the PS are attained. Some PS show a delayed vascular PDT effect. In solid tumors, PDT disruption of the blood flow can be synergistic to the direct cell-kill mechanism, by causing a lack of oxygen and nutrients, as well as the build-up of cellular refuse (125,126). Hausmann (127) was probably the first to report on the vascular effect in PDT. This was followed by observations by Levy (128) in 1929, Castellani and associates (129), and later McGovern (130). More recently, Bicher and colleagues (131) measured oxygen decrease after PDT, suggesting vascular damage, and Selman and coworkers reported on the measurement of blood flow changes induced by PDT by observing the movement of microspheres (70,132,133). They also recorded morphologic changes in microvessels (134). After that, Star and coworkers (135) reported on an elegant experiment in a transparent chamber animal model where they could directly observe tumor growth, and then the PDT-induced morphologic changes in the vasculature. Another attractive experimental approach to measurements of PDT-induced vascular changes was taken by Reed and coworkers (136), who observed blood flow by laser Doppler velocimetry, a technique that has also been applied to measure PDT effects on choroidal blood flow in the eye (137–139). Finally, Henderson and coworkers (125,140) demonstrated the importance of the "strangulation effect" of PDT-induced blood stasis by an *in vivo-ex vivo* cell transplantation technique. Here PDT was done on animal tumors followed by transplantation after different time intervals, and vitality assay of the transplanted cells *in vitro*. The longer the cells were left in place in the animal model after PDT, the less survival was observed. This result was interpreted as mainly resulting from PDT-induced vascular effects causing anoxia and deprivation of nutrients.

Let us now consider second-generation photosensitizers as they are currently being used to treat CNV associated with AMD in the clinic and in clinical tests. The scenario is iv injection of the PS followed within 1 hour (sometimes minutes) by light application. Most PDT experiences in animal models where vascular effects were studied point to the preferred use of amphiphilic and lipophilic PS when there was a short time delay between drug injection and light application. Studies with hydrophilic PS were done by B and H Miller with Rose Bengal on laser-induced choroidal CNV on cynomolgus monkeys (141), and by JW Miller on laser-induced iris CNV on monkeys with phthalocyanine (142). At present there are some unconfirmed reports that hydrophilic PS also could be effective in closing neovessels a short time after injection. This finding would be interesting if confirmed, because packaging in liposomes (which is used in the case of some of the more lipophilic drugs) could be avoided. In these preclinical data, there was generally a reasonable correlation between the PS level in the plasma and the PDT-induced vascular effect (125,143); that is, the higher the plasma level, the more effective the PDT-induced stasis. This may be related to the relatively rapid uptake of this type of PS in endothelial cells. It is more difficult to discern the mechanism in the case of PDT of CNV used in the eye with hydrophilic sensitizers. It may be that in some such cases, the slower uptake by—and removal from—endothelial cells implies that the plasma level of PS may have reduced significantly beyond its maximum concentration at the longer time delays when light is applied. To explain the increase in PDT-induced stasis of blood flow at these longer time delays, one must speculate that it takes so long for the optimal targets in the endothelial cells to be reached by the PS. It also may be noted that migration of PS to the subendothelial capillary wall (where the connective tissue is known to bind porphyrins and thus may be a good PDT target), may be slower in the case of hydrophilic sensitizers.

Taking into account the little hard evidence that exists, it currently appears that the primary target of vascular PDT is the endothelium (144–146). Photodynamic therapy damage to endothelial cells can result in the release of von Willebrand factor (147) and other blood clotting agents. Thromboxane and prostacyclin also can be released (144,145). Damaged endothelium results in calcium level modulation as well, which in turn can modulate the smooth muscle cell calcium balance, with vessel contraction as a possible consequence (147). Photodynamic therapy causes changes in the cytoskeleton in addition. This has been investigated in some detail (148–152). Perturbation of the cytoskeleton can lead to alteration of cell shape. Both endothelial cell rounding (122–124) and contraction have been observed, as was the case in PDT-induced apoptosis. The change in shape of endothelial cells leads to the interruption of the tight junctions between the endothelial cells and a decrease in interendothelial cell communication, and causes exposure of the subendothelial basement membrane proteins, as shown in Figure 2.13.

The released clotting factors such as thromboxane activate circulating platelets, among others. Some of the circulating platelets may have been damaged themselves directly by PDT (153–155), although this probably does not play a major part in the blood clotting mechanism. The activated platelets now stick to the gaps between the damaged rounded endothelial cells, and further aggregation of platelets takes place at these sites (150,156), thus starting to plug the vessel. Polymorphonuclear leukocytes start to adhere to the damaged vessel wall, and are probably also involved in increasing vascular permeability via their action on endothelial cells. In addition, increased vascular permeability may be expected following the release of histamine, which is a vasodilator. The consequences of this scenario are vascular leakage and edema (157–159). Increased vessel wall permeability is observed in PDT with many different sensitizers (158–161). Another part of the mechanism is associated with the PDT-induced damage to membrane lipids. This can cause the release of arachidonic acid, which can react with cyclooxygenase in a cascade of processes, thus inducing the release of prostaglandin endoperoxides and, in the end, producing the vasoconstrictor thromboxane, which acts on the surrounding smooth muscle cells. Consequently, the PDT-induced modulation of compounds, among which those described in the preceding (eicosanoids, cytokines, clotting factors, histamine, etc.) causes an increase of aggregating and vasodilating compounds, thus destroying the normally existing balance between dilating and constricting agents and aggregating and disaggregating compounds among others. The results of this are twofold: (a) a temporary increase in vessel permeability and leakage; followed by (b) vessel constriction and blood clotting with the consequent blood flow stasis. Smaller vessels can be closed by PDT more easily than larger vessels. This also is evident in the human choroid. Thus, in PDT of CNV in the human eye it is fortunate

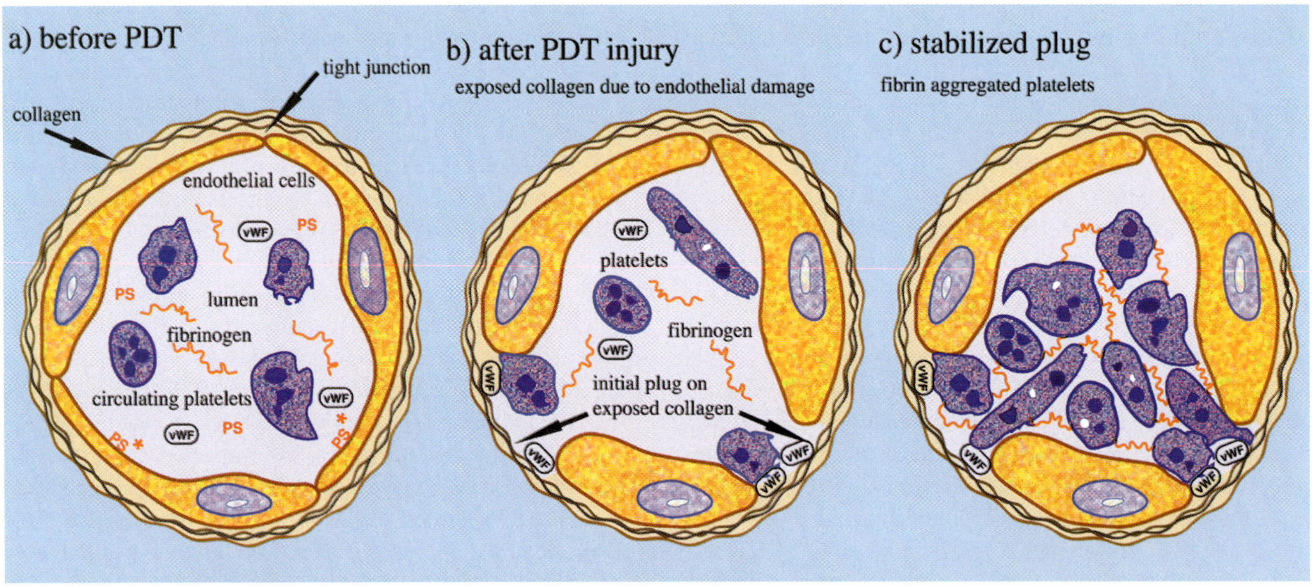

FIGURE 2.13. A simplified sequence describing PDT damage response to the endothelium. **A:** The blood vessel wall prior to PDT. Endothelial cells lining the vessel wall are flat and linked by tight junctions. **B:** Photodynamic therapy-induced oxidative stress to the endothelium causes changes in the cytoskeleton and rounding and retraction of endothelial cells, thus exposing parts of the subendothelial connective tissue. von Willebrand and other clotting factors are released at the exposed site, which leads to platelet activation. **C:** The activated platelets release eicosanoids, causing platelet aggregation at the damaged surface as well as arteriole constriction. Polymorphonuclear leukocytes also stick to the damaged surface and activate platelets, and induce vascular leakage.

that apparently only part of the choriocapillaries are occluded by PDT and not also the larger choroidal vessels at the applied conditions.

This behavior, as well as many other aspects observed in clinical PDT, is quite well reproduced in the CAM model. Generally, the larger the PDT "dose" (161) (in terms of "light dose" and "drug dose"), the larger the diameter of the vessels that can be occluded. The larger diameter vessels in which stasis is observed have a tendency to open up again, so that blood flow can be reestablished. A final aspect that may play a role in the PDT of blood vessels is that the increased pressure in the perivascular region caused by PDT-induced leakage may also help to induce vasoconstriction.

For the work concerning closure of choroidal vessels in the monkey, the authors refer the reader to Chapter 5.

The following summarizes the preceding discussion in the form of a simplified mechanism for blood flow stasis induced by PDT.

1. The injected photosensitizer arrives at the endothelial cells in which it is partially internalized.
2. Light application causes oxygen radical mediated damage to the endothelial cell.
3. Cytoskeletal changes and endothelial cell rounding are observed, which cause widening of junctions between endothelial cells. This leads to exposure of the vascular basement membrane, and/or the perivasculature.
4. Platelets are activated and start to aggregate at the damaged sites. This and other PDT-induced damage causes the release of eicosanoids that induce: (a) increased vascular permeability and leakage; and (b) clotting (thromboxane).
5. In a parallel process, polymorphonuclear leukocytes start to adhere to the PDT-damaged surface, also helping platelet activation and inducing vascular permeability.

SCREENING FOR VASCULAR EFFECTS OF PHOTODYNAMIC THERAPY WITH THE CHORIOALLANTOIC MEMBRANE MODEL

Screening drugs for a particular application remains one of the toughest problems in medicine. The multiple procedures and models used to screen PDT compounds for their tumor eradicating efficiency probably can not be used optimally as screening techniques for PDT of CNV-associated with AMD. Hence, we developed a model that is thought to be better adapted for early screening of photosensitizers for this application. With this model, we have evaluated a number of photosensitizers as possible candidates for the

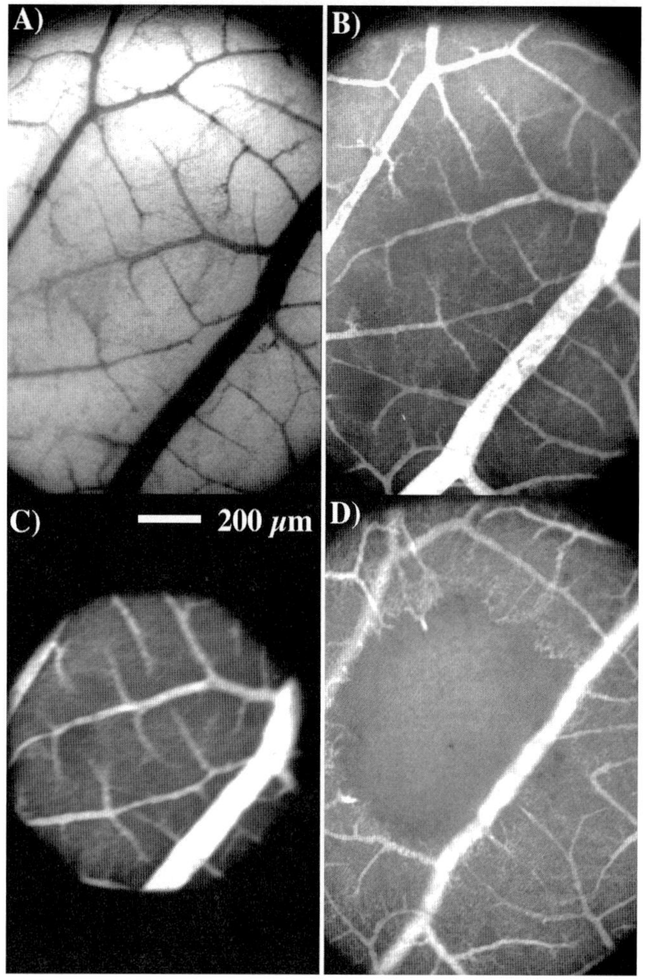

FIGURE 2.14. PDT on chorioallantoic membrane (CAM) blood vessels using intravenously injected benzoporphyrin derivative monoacid ring A (BPD-MA) (4 μg/embryo). **A:** Autofluorescence image (λex = 390–440 nm; λem : 540–580 nm). Note the strong absorption of blood at the excitation wavelength. **B:** Benzoporphyrin derivative fluorescence angiography fluorescence angiography (BPD-FA) prior to PDT, that is, before irradiation (λex = 390–440 nm; λem : > 610 nm, exposure time 1 s), 45 seconds after the injection of 0.3 mg/kg (embryo) BPD-MA in liposomes. **C:** Benzoporphyrin derivative monoacid ring A fluorescence angiography (λex = 390–440 nm; λem : > 610 nm, exposure time 1 s) during therapy. Diameter of the irradiation area: 1.4 mm; therapeutic irradiation conditions: 25 J/cm^2. The irradiation was started 60 seconds after BPD-MA infusion of 0.3 mg/kg (embryo) BPD-MA in liposomes. **D:** Fluorescence angiography of the CAM using iv injection of Rhodamine 101 (R101-FA) (λex = 390–440 nm; λem : > 610 nm, exposure time 1 s) 24 hours after PDT. One can see that smaller blood vessel become occluded because of BPD-MA–mediated PDT, whereas the bigger diameter blood vessels remain perfused, or have undergone reperfusion. The dark spot shows important similarities with the 1 week post-PDT early fluorescein angiography.

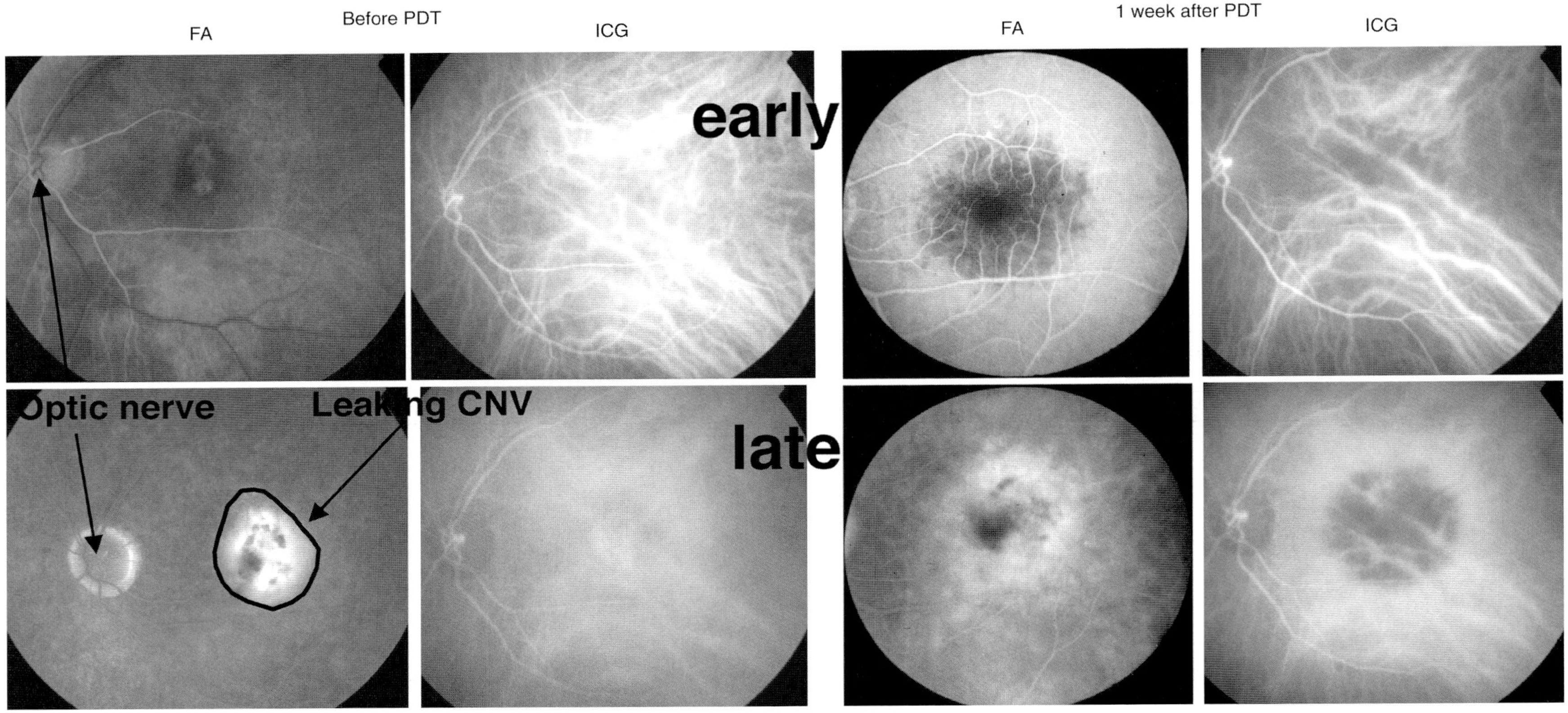

FIGURE 2.15. The early phase (1 min after iv) and late phase (5 min after iv) of fluorescein and indocyanine green angiograms obtained in clinical tests before and 1 week after photodynamic therapy with benzoporphyrin derivative monoacid ring A in liposomes. Figure 2.15 shows early and late FA and ICG angiograms of the retina of a patient before PDT with predominantly "classic" CNV, as demonstrated by the strong well-demarcated hyperfluorescent region near the center of the macula. Figure 2.15 also shows the same eye *1 week after PDT* with 12 mg/m^2 of BPD-MA in liposomes and 50 J/cm^2 of light at 689 nm given at 600 mW/cm^2 about 15 minutes after the start of the slow iv injection (162). The early-phase FA and late-phase ICG angiograms 1 week after PDT show the dark hypofluorescent spot, indicating that both the CNV and choriocapillaries remain closed on this time scale. The dark spot also helps to demonstrate that the retinal capillaries near the macula are still patent. The lack of oxygen, and possibly also the inflammation caused by the PDT response, may cause a reopening of some of the occluded blood vessels and/or possible regrowth of new leaky vessels on a shortened time scale. This probably implies that the next retreatment will have to take place soon. The closure of the normal choriocapillaries invoked from the absence of FA leakage has been confirmed by indocyanine green angiography at near infrared wavelengths where blood absorption is strongly reduced.

next generation in the photodynamic treatment of CNV in AMD. The model was developed in the chick CAM (160,161). Extrapolations of observations in the CAM model on vascular leakage, closure of blood vessels, and pharmacokinetics are now facilitated by having closely compared several compounds in the CAM and the clinical context.

We have obtained extensive clinical experience with the PDT of CNV in AMD by participating in the design and the execution of phase I, II, and III trials with BPD-MA (74,162–164) and the phase I and II trials with Lutetium Texaphyrin (165). The BPD-MA phase I and II trials were carried out at first in three clinical centers, among them Lausanne, Switzerland. The Lutetium Texaphyrin phase I and II trials (the first 70 patients) were carried out exclusively in Lausanne. This clinical experience is completed with FA and ICG tests on these patients, some of which were part of an attempt to render fluorescence assays in the eye fundus more quantitative (102). Hence, we have access to data obtained with two quite different compounds that can be compared between the human eye and the CAM model for PDT-induced closure of CNV, and four compounds that have been tested for leakage kinetics and general pharmacokinetics. An example of such a comparison is shown in Figures 2.14 and 2.15, which demonstrate the similarities in the observations between the CAM model and the clinical context. Clearly, further testing is required of the compounds that appear promising in the CAM model, and assays of Ryan's cynomolgus monkey model (166–168) probably will be the final step in such a preclinical development.

HOW SELECTIVE IS PHOTODYNAMIC THERAPY OF CHOROIDAL NEOVASCULARIZATION IN PRACTICE?

The vascular effects discovered in the PDT of solid tumors described earlier in the chapter led a number of groups to consider PDT of other diseases involving neovasculature. Among these were the treatment of rheumatoid arthritis (169–172) of choroidal neovessels in AMD. The latter has been discussed in several articles (173,174), and its development as well as the preclinical experiments are reviewed by J Miller and others elsewhere in this volume. We limit ourselves here to a few remarks considering the "selectivity" of PDT in this application in the retina. By selectivity we mean that blood flow stasis is induced in the leaky choroidal neovessels by PDT, while trying to avoid closure of the retinal capillaries and choriocapillaries, as well as avoiding damage to the retinal pigmented epithelium, the photoreceptors, and other parts of the neural retina. The choriocapillaries provide for a significant fraction of the oxygen, nutrients, and transport of fluids in the normal retina. The fenestrated choriocapillaries are the major blood supply to be found at a short distance from the photoreceptors in the region of the fovea. Other differences between retinal and choroidal capillaries include the fact that retinal capillaries are part of the central artery system and have a relatively high internal pressure and flow rate. Furthermore, the blood retinal barrier is considered to be part of the blood–brain barrier (175). Also, oxygen regulation is quite different in the retinal capillaries compared to the choroidal capillaries. The latter might be used to change the selectivity and efficacy of the PDT treatment when using carbogen gas (5% carbon dioxide and 95% oxygen) inhalation. Finally, the structure and morphology of the tortuous choroidal neovessels may be significantly different from one patient to another and thus could show different resistance to PDT and different selectivity for the photosensitizer. For example, the "aggressive classic" CNV is thought to be quite different in morphology, structure, and receptor activity from the "less aggressive" occult CNV.

We have observed a certain degree of selectivity in the PDT-induced blood flow stasis in the clinical treatment of CNV in AMD with BPD-MA in liposomes and light at 689 nm applied about 5 minutes after completion of iv injection. A typical example can be found in Figure 2.15, which shows early phase (1 min after iv) and late phase (5 min after iv) of FA and ICG angiograms, for a patient before and 1 week after PDT. The leakage shown in late FA before PDT by the strong well-demarcated hyperfluorescence in the center of FA angiograms indicates a case of mostly "classic" CNV. The dark round spot in early FA shown 1 week after PDT, which corresponds closely to the area of the retina exposed to 689 nm light, indicates strongly reduced fluorescein fluorescence from both the classic CNV (the leakage of which is no longer visible at all) and the normal choriocapillaries, as can be seen in this "early" fluorescein angiogram. It should be noted that the "background" diffuse fluorescence of fluorescein, shown outside of the dark hypofluorescent central area, is mostly owing to normal leakage from the fenestrated choriocapillaries. Thus, PDT has apparently caused blood flow stasis in the leaking neovessels—which is desirable—as well as some degree of stasis in the normal choriocapillaries—which is undesirable, because it reduces oxygen and nutrient supply to all of the PDT-treated regions and possibly increases PDT-induced inflammation. Furthermore, the way the treatment is carried out at present, that is, exposure of a circular area with fairly wide treatment margins, implies that this region of choriocapillary closure is much bigger than the region of neovasculature.

In Figure 2.15, one further observes a large amount of ICG fluorescence from the larger choroidal vessels at "early" times after injection (prior to PDT). This strong fluorescence essentially blots out the weaker fluorescence that may be present from the choriocapillaries that are situated above the larger choroidal vessels. The "late" ICG angiogram taken before PDT shows some ICG leakage in the macular region. Indocyanine green, which is mostly attached to serum albumin, leaks more slowly than fluorescein. The "late-stage" fluorescein angiogram taken 1 week after PDT shows some degree of leakage reappearing, indicating that some of the choriocapillaries may be leaking again in the area of PDT, or that some small degree of neovascularization is already forming. Because the CNV have apparently not opened up to the same degree as before, some apparent selectivity appears to be established in the treatment. The fact that the choriocapillaries have been closed to some extent during PDT may be seen 1 week after PDT, where the "late-stage" ICG angiograms show a circular area of hypofluorescence that corresponds to the irradiated choriocapillaries that are still closed.

One may conclude that the selectivity of the PDT of CNV with BPD-MA in liposomes is not complete at the applied conditions, because the normal choriocapillaries are not sufficiently spared. However, the observed selectivity in closure of small choroidal vessels (neovessels and capillaries), as compared to the apparent total absence of blood flow stasis in the retinal capillaries, appears to be essentially perfect at these conditions. This is most fortunate, because closure of the retinal capillaries that lie just outside the macular region has been shown to lead to immediate and significant loss of visual acuity (163). Thus, in PDT of CNV associated with AMD, three types of selectivity are needed in CNV closure, sparing: (a) retinal capillaries; (b) normal choroidal capillaries; and (3) the RPE and other close lying parts of the neural retina. Closing the retinal capillaries close to the macula implies loss of eyesight; and closing the choriocapillaries implies depriving the fovea with its associated area of retinal pigment epithelium, photoreceptors, and neural retina of oxygen, fluids, and nutrients.

Figure 2.16 schematically shows what is meant by this selective closure of CNV. Briefly, one wants to close the neovessels without significant occlusion of either the choriocapillaries or the retinal capillaries and no significant damage to RPE, photoreceptors, nerve layers, or Bruch's membrane. Part of this desired selectivity is not currently completely attained. As the photoreceptor outer segments (OS) undergo some oxidative damage under light exposure, up to 10% of the OS must be replaced per day, and these fragments must be degraded by the RPE cells. The RPE also has other important functions. For instance, it controls the concentration of the retinal molecules that are responsible for light absorption in the photoreceptors. It controls the ionic composition around the photoreceptors as well (176), and filters the fluids being transported between photoreceptors and choroidal blood supply. Because each RPE cell serves about 50 photoreceptors in this capacity it must phagocytose the equivalent of several outer segments per day. It is the build-up of debris in the RPE cells and the underlying Bruch's membrane (BM) caused by the failing of this digestive process that is thought to be part of the etiology of the age-related degenerative process in the macula.

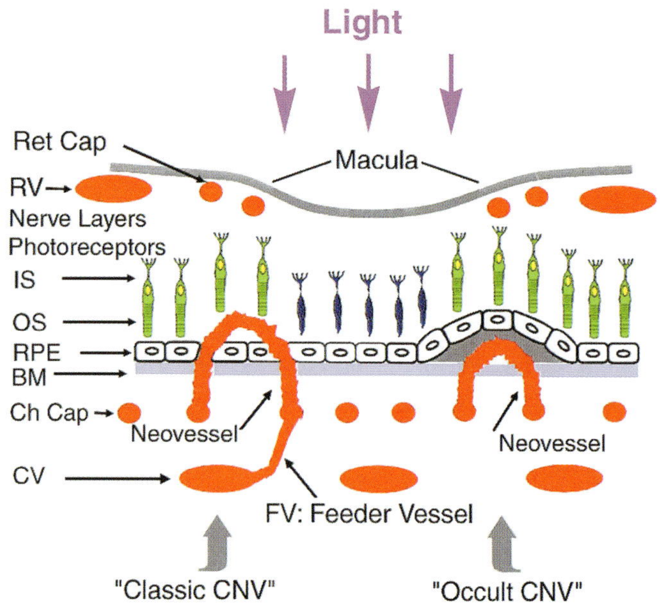

FIGURE 2.16. A simplified schematic diagram of the central part of the retina. In the middle of the macula one finds the fovea (not indicated), which is the zone responsible for the high visual acuity of the human eye. The retinal pigment epithelium and Bruch's membrane form a barrier between the neural retina and the choroidal blood supply. The photoreceptors consist of rods, and in the center of macula mainly cones—the outer and inner segments of which are indicated. The horizontal, bipolar, amacrine, and ganglion cells in the nerve layers that "preprocess" the vision signals coming from the photoreceptor inner segments are not shown in detail. The vision signals then are transferred via axons and the optic nerve to the brain. Light comes in from the top side of the drawing downward and the vision signals in the neural retina move up in the opposite direction, prior to following the axons near the surface of the retina to the optic nerve. One needs to focus on the three types of small capillaries: (a) The retinal capillaries (ret cap), which are fed by the larger retinal vessels, and which in turn are part of the retinal blood barrier. These can be seen clearly in Figure 2.15, early fluorescein 1 week after photodynamic therapy. (b) The fenestrated choriocapillaries (ch cap), which normally provide most of the oxygen, nutrients, and liquid exchange with the neural retina. (c) The very leaky choroidal neovessels, which grow out of the choriocapillaries and are fed by feeder vessels from the larger choroidal vessels. (From: van den Bergh H, et al. PDT of choroidal neovascularisation associated with age-related macular degeneration. *Photodynam News* 2001;4:4–8, with permission.)

The amount of leakage of the PS from the neovessels as well as the choriocapillaries should be carefully studied in order to avoid PDT damage to all the important and sensitive elements of the retina lying close to the leaky CNV. Photosensitizer leakage should be quite low prior to and during light application. Most second-generation PS used in clinical studies up to now at short times after injection are bound to blood proteins to a large extent. These PS–protein complexes apparently are large enough to significantly reduce the PS leakage, even from the neovessels, on the time scale of interest (<30 minutes). Extremely water-soluble dyes may leak out of the CNV on a much shorter time scale and hence may not be desirable compounds in PDT of CNV. All the preceding leads to the fact that an improved photodynamic treatment of CNV in AMD should target the neovasculature as selectively as possible. Hence, receptor-mediated delivery of PS conjugates may well be an excellent solution, either using antibody fragments that tag onto molecules such as fibronectin, which in turn selectively target the αVβ3 integrins, which are thought to be found at high concentrations in the neovasculature. Another solution is to attach dyes to small peptides such as "RGD" to directly target integrins such as αVβ3 or αVβ5 in the CNV (59–65). It should be noted that one can not completely rule out that a small amount of leakage of PS, followed by rapid and more-or-less selective phagocytosis by the RPE prior to PDT, may result in selective PDT damage and oxidative stress to the RPE cells. It is not yet clear at this point in time if such damage will be detrimental to short- and long-term visual acuity and contrast.

CONCLUSIONS

We have reviewed some of the relevant photophysics and photochemistry underlying PDT of AMD in view of understanding the basic processes as well as some of the biomolecular cascades induced by photooxidative stress. The relationship among structure, activity, and selectivity of some of the second-generation photosensitizers is mentioned, and a sequence of PDT-induced processes leading to blood flow stasis in small vessels is outlined. The chapter concludes with a proposed screening model used in the search of new sensitizers (which involves CAM), and a discussion of the present partial lack in selectivity of PDT in the closure of CNV. Some suggestions are included on how to make PDT treatment even more successful.

APPENDIX 1

An example of H-transfer in the photolysis of benzophenone in the presence of an alcohol:

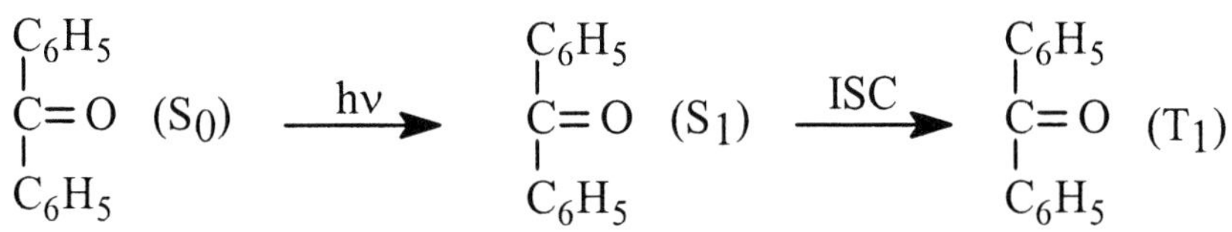

(photophysics)

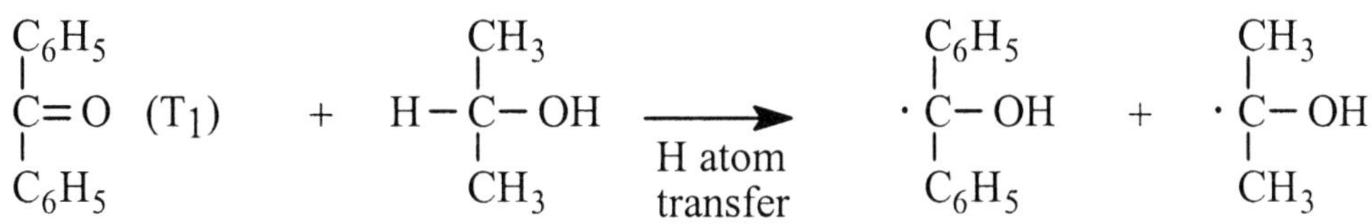

(radical initiation)

This can be followed by radical reactions such as:

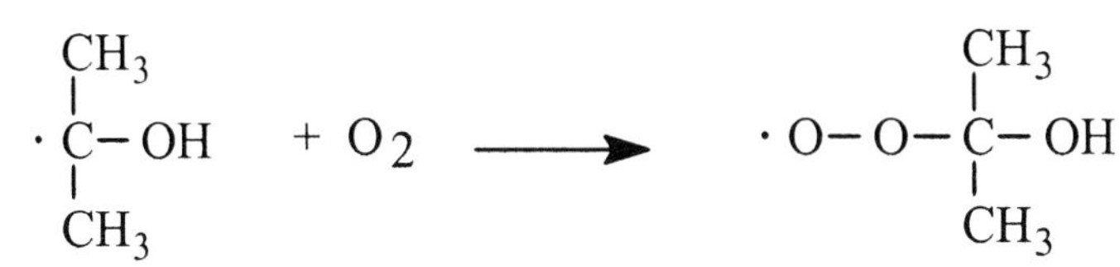

(propagation of the radical reaction chain)

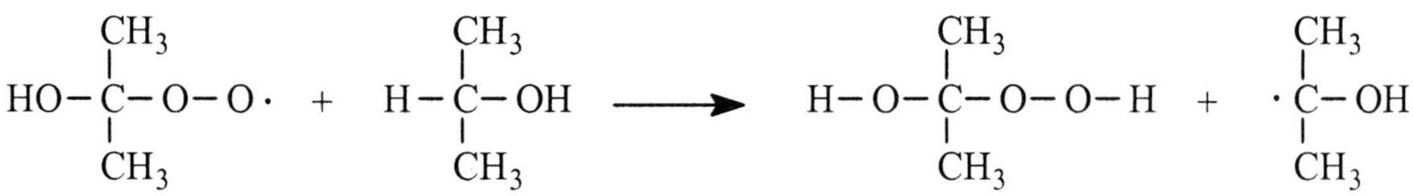

The hydroxy hydroperoxide is unstable and decomposes to hydrogen peroxide and acetone by:

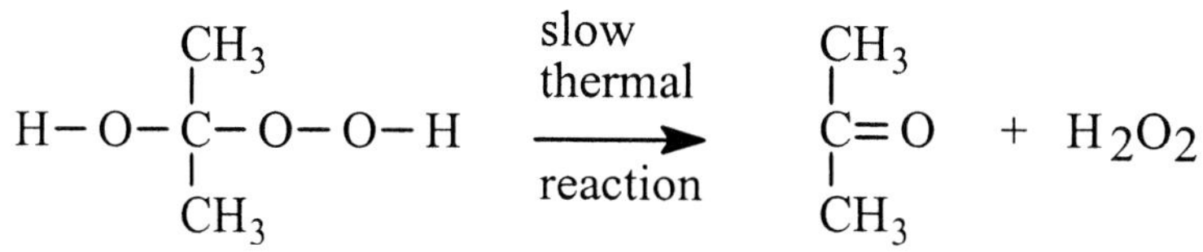

The remaining radicals will combine at some point, thus ending the radical chain reactions:

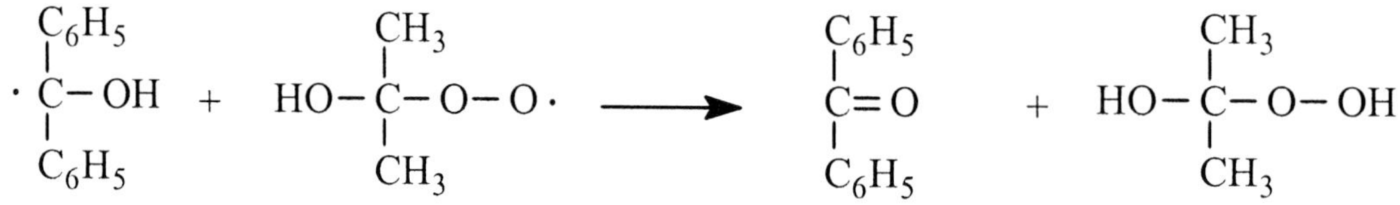

The overall reaction is:

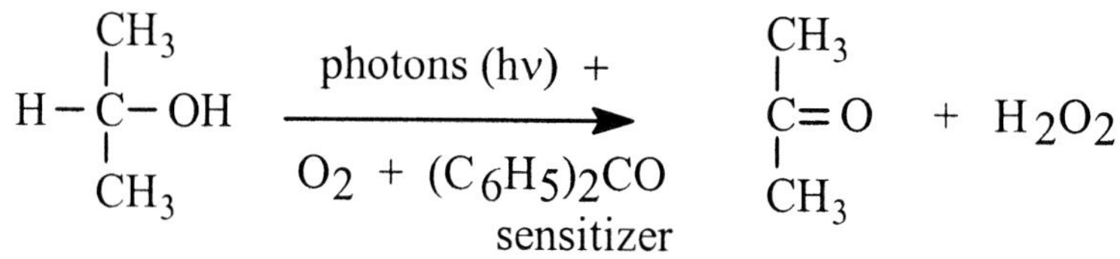

It should be noted that the sensitizer benzophenone acts here as a catalyst (i.e., it is not consumed).

ACKNOWLEDGMENTS

The authors are grateful to N. Oleinick, J. Miller, M. Sickenberg, R. Gurny and coworkers, and R. Bonnett for helpful and stimulating discussions.

Many sources were consulted in writing this chapter; however, the authors are particularly indebted to Yvette Konan (83) and Nancy L. Oleinick (118), and to R. Bonnett (177) and Lionel R. Milgrom (178).

REFERENCES

1. Fuchs R. Hippokrates Sämtliche Werke. In: Fuchs R, ed. *Hippokrates Sämtliche Werke.* Munich: 1895–1900:354–355.
2. Regan JD, Parrish JA. *The science of photomedicine.* New York: Plenum, 1982.
3. Diamond I, Granelli SG, McDonagh AF, et al. Photodynamic therapy of malignant tumours. *Lancet* 1972;2:1175–1177.
4. Dougherty TJ. Activated dyes as antitumor agents. *J Natl Cancer Inst* 1974;52:1333–1336.
5. Dougherty TJ, Grindey GB, Fiel R, et al. Photoradiation therapy. II. Cure of animal tumors with hematoporphyrin and light. *J Natl Cancer Inst* 1975;55:115–121.
6. Dougherty TJ, Kaufman JE, Goldfarb A, et al. Photoradiation therapy for the treatment of malignant tumors. *Cancer Res* 1978;38:2628–2635.
7. Dougherty TJ, Gomer CJ, Henderson BW, et al. Photodynamic therapy. *J Natl Cancer Inst* 1998;90:889–905.
8. Kelly JF, Snell ME, Berenbaum MC, et al. Photodynamic destruction of human bladder carcinoma. *Br J Cancer* 1975;31: 237–244.
9. Kelly JF, Snell ME. Hematoporphyrin derivative: a possible aid in the diagnosis and therapy of carcinoma of the bladder. *J Urol* 1976;115:150–151.
10. Lipson RL, et al. Hematoporphyrin derivative: a new aid for endoscopic detection of malignant disease. *J Thorac Cardiovasc Surg* 1961;42:623–629.
11. Lipson RL, et al. Further evaluation of the use of hematoporphyrin derivative as a new aid for the endoscopic detection of malignant disease. *Dis Chest Field* 1964;46:676–679.
12. Schwartz SK, et al. Some relationships of porphyrins, x-rays and tumours. *Univ Minn Med Bull* 1955;27:7–13.
13. Monnier P, et al. Photodetection and photodynamic therapy of "early" squamous cell carcinomas of the pharynx, oesophagus and tracheo-bronchial tree. *Lasers Med Sci* 1990;5:149–169.
14. Monnier P, et al. Further appraisal of PDI and PDT of early squamous cell carcinomas of the pharynx, oesophagus and bronchi. In: Spinelli P, et al, eds. *Photodynamic therapy and biomedical lasers.* Amsterdam: Elsevier, 1992:7–14.
15. Savary JF, Grosjean P, Monnier P, et al. Photodynamic therapy of early squamous-cell carcinomas of the esophagus: a review of 31 cases. *Endoscopy* 1998;30:258–265.
16. Braichotte D, et al. Clinical pharmacokinetic studies of Photofrin II by fluorescence spectroscopy. In: Spinelli P, et al, eds. *Photodynamic therapy and biomedical lasers.* Amsterdam: Elsevier, 1992:883–887.

17. Braichotte D, et al. Clinical pharmacokinetic studies of photofrin by fluorescence spectroscopy in the oral cavity, the esophagus, and the bronchi. *Cancer* 1995;75:2768–2778.
18. Braichotte D, Savary JF, Glanzmann T, et al. Clinical pharmacokinetic studies of tetra(meta-hydroxyphenyl)chlorin in squamous-cell carcinoma by fluorescence spectroscopy at 2 wavelengths. *Int J Cancer* 1995;63:198–204.
19. Andrejevic S, Savary JF, Monnier P, et al. Measurements by fluorescence microscopy of the time-dependent distribution of meso-tetra-hydroxyphenyl chlorin in healthy tissues and chemically induced "early" squamous cell carcinoma of the Syrian hamster cheek pouch. *J Photochem Photobiol B* 1996;36: 143–151.
20. Andrejevic-Blant S, Hadjur C, Ballini JP, et al. Photodynamic therapy of early squamous cell carcinoma with tetra(m-hydroxyphenyl)chlorin: optimal drug-light interval. *Br J Cancer* 1997; 76:1021–1028.
21. Aveline BM, Hasan T, Redmond RW, et al. The effects of aggregation, protein binding and cellular incorporation on the photophysical properties of benzoporphyrin derivative monoacid ring A (BPD-MA). *J Photochem Photobiol B* 1995;30:161–169.
22. Bilgin MD, al Akhras MA, Khalili M, et al. Photosensitization of red blood cell hemolysis by lutetium texaphyrin. *Photochem Photobiol* 2000;72:121–127.
23. Bonnett R, White RD, Winfield UJ, et al. Hydroporphyrins of the meso-tetra(hydroxyphenyl)porphyrin series as tumour photosensitizers. *Biochem J* 1989;261:277–280.
24. Kennedy JC, Pottier RH. Endogenous protoporphyrin IX, a clinically useful photosensitizer for photodynamic therapy. *J Photochem Photobiol B* 1992;14:275–292.
25. Kloek J, Beijersbergen van H. Prodrugs of 5-aminolevulinic acid for photodynamic therapy. *Photochem Photobiol* 1996;64: 994–1000.
26. Lange N. personal communication.
27. Lange N, Jichlinski P, Zellweger M, et al. Photodetection of early human bladder cancer based on the fluorescence of 5-aminolevulinic acid hexyl ester-induced protoporphyrin IX: a pilot study. *Br J Cancer* 1999;80:185–193.
28. Morgan AR, Garbo GM, Keck RW, et al. New photosensitizers for photodynamic therapy: combined effect of metallopurpurin derivatives and light on transplantable bladder tumors. *Cancer Res* 1988;48:194–198.
29. Roslaniec M, Weitman H, Freeman D, et al. Liposome binding constants and singlet oxygen quantum yields of hypericin, tetra hydroxy helianthrone and their derivatives: studies in organic solutions and in liposomes. *J Photochem Photobiol B* 2000;57: 149–158.
30. Spikes JD, Bommer JC. Photosensitizing properties of mono-L-aspartyl chlorin e6 (NPe6): a candidate sensitizer for the photodynamic therapy of tumors. *J Photochem Photobiol B* 1993;17: 135–143.
31. McMahon KS, Wieman TJ, Moore PH, et al. Effects of photodynamic therapy using mono-L-aspartyl chlorin e6 on vessel constriction, vessel leakage, and tumor response. *Cancer Res* 1994;54:5374–5379.
32. Taber SW, Fingar VH, Coots CT, et al. Photodynamic therapy using mono-L-aspartyl chlorin E(6) (Npe6) for the treatment of cutaneous disease: a phase-I clinical study. *Clin Cancer Res* 1998;4:2741–2746.
33. D'Hallewin MA, De Witte PA, Waelkens E, et al. Fluorescence detection of flat bladder carcinoma *in situ* after intravesical instillation of hypericin. *J Urol* 2000;164:349–351.
34. Zupko I, Kamuhabwa AR, D'Hallewin MA, et al. In vivo photodynamic activity of hypericin in transitional cell carcinoma bladder tumors. *Int J Oncol* 2001;18:1099–1105.
35. Malik Z, et al. Topical application of 5-aminolevulinic acid, DMSO and EDTA: protoporphyrin IX accumulation in skin and tumours of mice. *J Photochem Photobiol B* 1995;28:213–218.
36. Schoenfeld N, et al. Protoporphyrin biosynthesis in melanoma B16 cells stimulated by 5-aminolevulinic acid and chemical inducers: characterization of photodynamic inactivation. *Int J Cancer* 1994;56:106–112.
37. Kennedy JC, et al. Photodynamic therapy with endogenous protoporphyrin IX: basic principles and present clinical experience. *J Photochem Photobiol B Biol* 1990;6:143–148.
38. Marti A, et al. Optimisation of the formation and distribution of protoporphyrin IX in the urothelium: an in vitro approach. *J Urol* 1999;162:546–552.
39. Schmidt-Erfurth U, et al. Vascular targeting in photodynamic occlusion of subretinal vessels. *Ophthalmology* 1994;101: 1953–1961.
40. Kessel D, Luo Y. Mitochondrial photodamage and Pdt-induced apoptosis. *J Photochem Photobiol B Biol* 1998;42:89–95.
41. Kessel D, Luo Y. Photodynamic therapy: a mitochondrial inducer of apoptosis. *Cell Death Diff* 1999;6:28–35.
42. Oleinick NL, Evans HH. The photobiology of photodynamic therapy: cellular targets and mechanisms. *Radiat Res* 1998; 150:S146–156.
43. Oleinick NL. Apoptosis in response to photodynamic therapy. *Photodynam News* 1998;1:6–9.
44. Segalla A, et al. CGP 55398, a liposomal Ge(IV) phthalocyanine bearing two axially ligated cholesterol moieties: a new potential agent for photodynamic therapy of tumours. *Br J Cancer* 1994;69:817–825.
45. Braichotte D, et al. Preliminary clinical results on a second generation photosensitizer: mTHPC. In: Spinelli P, et al, eds. *Photodynamic therapy and biomedical lasers.* New York: Elsevier Science, 1992:461–465.
46. Braichotte D, et al. A clinical comparison of the pharmacokinetics of m-THPC and photofrin II as observed by light induced fluorescence. *Proc SPIE* 1994;2081:62–73.
47. Radu A, et al. Photodynamic therapy for 101 early cancers of the upper aerodigestive tract, the esophagus, and the bronchi: a single-institution experience. *Diagn Ther Endoscop* 1999; 5:145–154.
48. Yuan F, et al. Microvascular permeability of albumin, vascular surface area, and vascular volume measured in human adenocarcinoma LS174T using dorsal chamber in SCID mice. *Microvasc Res* 1993;45:269–289.
49. Allison BA, et al. Evidence for low-density lipoprotein receptor-mediated uptake of benzoporphyrin derivative. *Br J Cancer* 1994;69:833–839.
50. Hamblin MR, Newman EL. Photosensitizer targeting in photodynamic therapy. II. Conjugates of haematoporphyrin with serum lipoproteins. *J Photochem Photobiol B* 1994;26:147–157.
51. Jori G, Reddi E. The role of lipoproteins in the delivery of tumour-targeting photosensitizers. *Int J Biochem* 1993;25: 1369–1375.
52. Schmidt-Erfurth U, et al. Photodynamic targeting of human retinoblastoma cells using covalent low-density lipoprotein conjugates. *Br J Cancer* 1997;75:54–61.
53. Korbelik M, et al. Photofrin uptake by murine macrophages. *Cancer Res* 1991;51:2251–2255.
54. Korbelik M, Krosl G. Photofrin accumulation in malignant and host cell populations of a murine fibrosarcoma. *Photochem Photobiol* 1995;62:162–168.
55. Hamblin MR, Newman EL. On the mechanism of the tumour-localising effect in photodynamic therapy. *J Photochem Photobiol B* 1994;23:3–8.
56. Roberts WG, Hasan T. Role of neovasculature and vascular permeability on the tumor retention of photodynamic agents. *Cancer Res* 1992;52:924–930.

57. Braichotte D, et al. Clinical pharmacokinetic studies of tetra(meta-hydroxyphenyl)chlorin in squamous cell carcinoma by fluorescence spectroscopy at 2 wavelengths. *Int J Cancer* 1995;63:198–204.
58. Westerman P, et al. Long circulating half-life and high tumor selectivity of the photosensitizer meta-tetrahydroxyphenylchlorin conjugated to polyethylene glycol in nude mice grafted with a human colon carcinoma. *Int J Cancer* 1998;76:842–850.
59. Achilefu S, et al. Novel receptor-targeted fluorescent contrast agents for in vivo tumor imaging. *Invest Radiol* 2000;35:479–485.
60. Duska LR, et al. Biodistribution of charged F(ab')2 photoimmunoconjugates in a xenograft model of ovarian cancer. *Br J Cancer* 1997;75:837–844.
61. Friedlander M, et al. Involvement of integrins alpha v beta 3 and alpha v beta 5 in ocular neovascular diseases. *Proc Natl Acad Sci USA* 1996;93:9764–9769.
62. Gijsens A, De Witte P. Photocytotoxic action of EGF-PVA-Sn(IV)chlorin e6 and EGF-dextran-Sn(IV)chlorin e6 internalizable conjugates on A431 cells. *Int J Oncol* 1998;13: 1171–1177.
63. Hamblin MR, et al. Effect of charge on the interaction of site-specific photoimmunoconjugates with human ovarian cancer cells. *Cancer Res* 1996;56:5205–5210.
64. Tsuchida T, et al. Correlation between site II-specific human serum albumin (HSA) binding affinity and murine in vivo photosensitizing efficacy of some Photofrin components. *Photochem Photobiol* 1997;66:224–228.
65. Vrouenraets MB, et al. Development of meta-tetrahydroxyphenylchlorin-monoclonal antibody conjugates for photoimmunotherapy. *Cancer Res* 1999;59:1505–1513.
66. Folli S, et al. Immunophotodiagnosis of colon carcinomas in patients injected with fluoresceinated chimeric antibodies against carcinoembryonic antigen. *Proc Natl Acad Sci USA* 1992;89:7973–7977.
67. Folli S, et al. Antibody-indocyanine conjugates for immunophotodetection of human squamous cell carcinoma in nude mice. *Cancer Res* 1994;54:2643–2649.
68. Pèlegrin A, et al. Antibody-fluorescein conjugates for photoimmunodiagnosis of human colon carcinoma in nude mice. *Cancer* 1991;67:2529–2537.
69. Ruoslahti E, Pierschbacher MD. New perspectives in cell adhesion: RGD and integrins. *Science* 1987;238:491–497.
70. Birchler M, et al. Selective targeting and photocoagulation of ocular angiogenesis mediated by a phage-derived human antibody fragment. *Nat Biotechnol* 1999;17:984–988.
71. Richter AM, et al. Liposomal delivery of a photosensitizer, benzoporphyrin derivative monoacid ring A (BPD), to tumor tissue in a mouse tumor model. *Photochem Photobiol* 1993;57: 1000–1006.
72. Isele U, et al. Large-scale production of liposomes containing monomeric zinc phthalocyanine by controlled dilution of organic solvents. *J Pharm Sci* 1994;83:1608–1616.
73. Jori G, et al. Controlled targeting of different subcellular sites by porphyrins in tumour-bearing mice. *Br J Cancer* 1986;53: 615–621.
74. Miller JW, et al. Photodynamic therapy with verteporfin for choroidal neovascularization caused by age-related macular degeneration: results of a single treatment in a phase 1 and 2 study. *Arch Ophthalmol* 1999;117:1161–1173.
75. Garbo GM. The use of liposomes, emulsions or inclusion complexes may potentiate in vivo effects of SnET2. *SPIE Photodyn Ther* 1990;1203:118–125.
76. Kessel D, et al. Sites and efficacy of photodamage by tin etiopurpurin in vitro using different delivery systems. *Photochem Photobiol* 1991;54:193–196.
77. Kongshaug M, et al. Binding of drugs to human plasma proteins, exemplified by Sn(IV)-etiopurpurin dichloride delivered in Cremophor and DMSO. *Int J Biochem* 1993;25: 739–760.
78. Woodburn K, Kessel D. The alteration of plasma lipoproteins by Cremophor EL. *J Photochem Photobiol B* 1994;22:197–201.
79. Dorr RT. Pharmacology and toxicology of Cremophor EL diluent. *Ann Pharmacother* 1994;28:S11–14.
80. Bachor R, et al. Photosensitized destruction of human bladder carcinoma cells treated with chlorin e6-conjugated microspheres. *Proc Natl Acad Sci USA* 1991;88:1580–1584.
81. Bourdon O, et al. A comparative study of the cellular uptake, localization and phototoxicity of meta-tetra(hydroxyphenyl) chlorin encapsulated in surface-modified submicronic oil/water carriers in HT29 tumor cells. *J Photochem Photobiol B* 2000;55: 164–171.
82. Couvreur P. Polyalkylcyanoacrylates as colloidal drug carriers. *Crit Rev Ther Drug Carrier Syst* 1988;5:1–20.
83. Konan YN, et al. State of the art in the delivery of photosensitizers for photodynamic therapy. *J Photochem Photobiol B* 2002; 66:89–106.
84. Konan YN, et al. Preparation and characterization of sterile and freeze-dried sub-200 nm nanoparticles. *Int J Pharmacol* 2002; 233:239–252.
85. Konan YN, et al. Preparation and characterisation of strerile sab-200 nm meso-tetra(4-hydroxyphenyl) porphyrine-loaded nanoparticles for potential use in photodynamic therapy. *Eur J Pharmacol Biopharmacol* 2003;55:115–124.
86. Hamblin MR, et al. In vivo fluorescence imaging of the transport of charged chlorin e6 conjugates in a rat orthotopic prostate tumour. *Br J Cancer* 1999;81:261–268.
87. Brasseur N, et al. Water-soluble aluminium phthalocyanine-polymer conjugates for PDT: photodynamic activities and pharmacokinetics in tumour-bearing mice. *Br J Cancer* 1999; 80:1533–1541.
88. Hasan T. Photosensitizer delivery mediated by macromolecular delivery systems. In: Henderson BW, Dougherty TJ, eds. *Photodynamic therapy: basic principles and clinical applications.* New York: Marcel Dekker, 1992:187–200.
89. Pietersz GA, Krauer K. Antibody-targeted drugs for the therapy of cancer. *J Drug Target* 1994;2:183–215.
90. Mew D, et al. Photoimmunotherapy: treatment of animal tumors with tumor-specific monoclonal antibody-hematoporphyrin conjugates. *J Immunol* 1983;130:1473–1477.
91. Klyashchitsky BA, et al. Approaches to targeted photodynamic tumor therapy. *J Control Rel* 1994;29:1–16.
92. Del Governatore M, et al. Targeted photodestruction of human colon cancer cells using charged 17.1A chlorin e6 immunoconjugates. *Br J Cancer* 2000;82:56–64.
93. Liu D, Huang L. Immunoloposome targeting to pulmonary endothelium. In: Gregoriadis G, et al, eds. *Liposomes in drug delivery.* Newark, NJ: Harwood Academic, 1993:111–121.
94. Jori G. Low-density lipoproteins-liposome delivery systems for tumor photosensitizers in vivo. In: Henderson BW, Dougherty TJ, eds. *Photodynamic therapy: basic principles and clinical applications.* New York: Marcel Dekker, 1992:173–186.
95. Duncan R. Drug targeting: where are we now and where are we going? *J Drug Target* 1997;5:1–4.
96. Reddi E, et al. Liposome- or LDL-administered Zn (II)-phthalocyanine as a photodynamic agent for tumours. I. Pharmacokinetic properties and phototherapeutic efficiency. *Br J Cancer* 1990;61:407–411.
97. Shaw JM, et al. Delivery of lipophilic drugs using lipoproteins. *Ann NY Acad Sci* 1987;507:252–271.
98. Miller JW, et al. Photodynamic therapy of experimental cho-

roidal neovascularization using lipoprotein-delivered benzoporphyrin. *Arch Ophthalmol* 1995;113:810–818.
99. Boutorine AS, et al. Chlorin-oligonucleotide conjugates: synthesis, properties, and red light-induced photochemical sequence-specific DNA cleavage in duplexes and triplexes. *J Am Chem Soc* 1996;118:9469–9476.
100. van den Bergh H. Photodynamic therapy of age related macular degeneration: history and principles. *Semin Ophthalmol* 2002;16:181–200.
101. Wagnieres GA, Wilson BC, Star WM. In vivo fluorescence spectroscopy and imaging for oncological applications. *Photochem Photobiol* 1998;68:603–632.
102. Sickenberg M, et al. A computer-based method to quantify the classic pattern of choroidal neovascularization in order to monitor photodynamic therapy. *Graefes Arch Clin Exp Ophthalmol* 1999;237:353–360.
103. Turro NJ. *Modern molecular photochemistry.* Sausalito, CA: California University Science Books, 1991.
104. Peng Q, et al. Correlation of subcellular and intratumoral photosensitizer localization with ultrastructural features after photodynamic therapy. *Ultrastruct Pathol* 1996;20:109–129.
105. Hadjur C, et al. EPR and spectrophotometric studies of free radicals (O-2 center dot(–), center dot OH, BPD-MA center dot(–)) and singlet oxygen (O-1(2)) generated by irradiation of benzoporphyrin derivative monoacid ring A. *Photochem Photobiol* 1997;65:818–827.
106. Bonnett R. The overall mechanistic picture. In: Bonnett R, ed. *Chemical aspects of photodynamic therapy.* New York: Gordon and Breach, 2000:83–87.
107. Jori G, Spikes D. Topics in photomedicine. In: Smith-Kendric C, ed. Topics in photomedicine. New York: Plenum Press, 1984:183–318.
108. Moor AC. Signaling pathways in cell death and survival after photodynamic therapy. *J Photochem Photobiol B* 2000;57:1–13.
109. Moor AC, Ortel B. Photodynamic therapy and fluorescence diagnosis in dermatology. In Calzavara-Pinton P, et al, eds. *Photodynamic therapy and fluorescence diagnosis in dermatology.* New York: Elsevier Science, 2001:39–54.
110. Carthy CM, et al. Early release of mitochondrial cytochrome c and expression of mitochondrial epitope 7A6 with a porphyrin-derived photosensitizer: Bcl-2 and Bcl-xL overexpression do not prevent early mitochondrial events but still depress caspase activity. *Lab Invest* 1999;79:953–965.
111. He J, et al. The induction of partial resistance to photodynamic therapy by the protooncogene BCL-2. *Photochem Photobiol* 1996;64:845–852.
112. Luo Y, Kessel D. Initiation of apoptosis versus necrosis by photodynamic therapy with chloroaluminum phthalocyanine. *Photochem Photobiol* 1997;66:479–483.
113. Oleinick NL. *9th ESP meeting.* Lillehammer, Norway: 2001.
114. Varnes ME, et al. Photodynamic therapy-induced apoptosis in lymphoma cells: translocation of cytochrome c causes inhibition of respiration as well as caspase activation. *Biochem Biophys Res Commun* 1999;255:673–679.
115. Zhang WG, et al. Antisense bcl-2 retrovirus vector increases the sensitivity of a human gastric adenocarcinoma cell line to photodynamic therapy. *Photochem Photobiol* 1999;69:582–586.
116. Nunez G, et al. Caspases: the proteases of the apoptotic pathway. *Oncogene* 1998;17:3237–3245.
117. Thornberry NA, Lazebnik Y. Caspases: enemies within. *Science* 1998;281:1312–1316.
118. Oleinick NL, et al. The role of apoptosis in response to photodynamic therapy: what, where, why, and how. *Photochem Photobiol Sci* 2002;1:1–21.
119. Stoka V, et al. Lysosomal protease pathways to apoptosis. Cleavage of bid, not pro-caspases, is the most likely route. *J Biol Chem* 2001;276:3149–3157.
120. Ahmad N, et al. Photodynamic therapy results in induction of WAF1/CIP1/P21 leading to cell cycle arrest and apoptosis. *Proc Natl Acad Sci USA* 1998;95:6977–6982.
121. Renno RZ, et al. Photodynamic therapy using Lutex induces apoptosis in vitro, and its effect is potentiated by angiostatin in retinal capillary endothelial cells. *Invest Ophthalmol Vis Sci* 2000;41:3963–3971.
122. Henderson BW, Owczarczak B, Sweeney J, et al. Effects of photodynamic treatment of platelets or endothelial cells in vitro on platelet agregation. *Photochem Photobiol* 1992;56:513–521.
123. Fingar VH. Vascular effects of photodynamic therapy. *J Clin Laser Med Surg* 1996;14:323–328.
124. Fingar VH, et al. Vascular damage after photodynamic therapy of solid tumors: a view and comparison of effect in pre-clinical and clinical models at the University of Louisville. *In Vivo* 2000; 14:93–100.
125. Henderson BW, Dougherty TJ. How does photodynamic therapy work? *Photochem Photobiol* 1992;55:145–157.
126. Moan J, Berg K. Photochemotherapy of cancer: experimental research. *Photochem Photobiol* 1992;55:931–948.
127. Hausmann W. Die sensibilisierende Wirkung des Hämatoporphyrins. *Biochem Z* 1911;30:276–316.
128. Levy AG. *J Pathol Bacteriol* 1926;32:387–399.
129. Castellani A, et al. Photodynamic effect of hematoporphyrin on blood microcirculation. *J Pathol Bacteriol* 1963;86:99–102.
130. McGovern VJ. The mechanism of photosensitivity. An experimental study. *AMA Arch Dermatol* 1961;83:40–51.
131. Bicher HI, Bruley DF. Changes in tissue oxygenation and acidity induced by localized microwave hyperthermia and hematoporphyrin phototherapy, an update. *Adv Exp Med Biol* 1983; 159:623–630.
132. Selman SH, et al. Acute blood-flow changes in transplantable fanft-induced urothelial tumors treated with hematoporphyrin derivative and light. *Surg Forum* 1983;34:676–678.
133. Selman SH, et al. Blood flow in transplantable bladder tumors treated with hematoporphyrin derivative and light. *Cancer Res* 1984;44:1924–1927.
134. Chaudhuri K, et al. Morphological changes of tumor microvasculature following hematoporphyrin derivative sensitized photodynamic therapy. *Photochem Photobiol* 1987;46:823–827.
135. Star WM, et al. Destruction of rat mammary tumor and normal tissue microcirculation by hematoporphyrin derivative photoradiation observed in vivo in sandwich observation chambers. *Cancer Res* 1986;46:2532–2540.
136. Reed MW, et al. A comparison of the effects of photodynamic therapy on normal and tumor blood vessels in the rat microcirculation. *Radiat Res* 1989;119:542 552.
137. de Gottrau P, et al. Regulation of subfoveolar choroidal blood flow in age-related macular degeneration. *Invest Ophthalmol Vis Sci* 2000;41:S159.
138. Petrig BL, et al. Subfoveal blood flow in choroidal neovascularization compared to normal fovea as measured by Tops-based laser Doppler flowmeter. *Invest Ophthalmol Vis Sci* 1999;40: 29–62.
139. Petrig BL, et al. Subfoveal blood flow in choroidal neovascularization before and after photodynamic therapy as measured by Tops-based confocal laser Doppler flowmeter. *Retina* in press.
140. Henderson BW, et al. Tumor destruction and kinetics of tumor cell death in two experimental mouse tumors following photodynamic therapy. *Cancer Res* 1985;45:572–576.
141. Miller H, Miller B. Photodynamic therapy of subretinal neovascularization in the monkey eye. *Arch Ophthalmol* 1993;111: 855–860.

142. Miller JW, et al. Phthalocyanine photodynamic therapy of experimental iris neovascularization. *Ophthalmology* 1991;98: 1711–1719.
143. Bellnier DA, Dougherty TJ. The time course of cutaneous porphyrin photosensitization in the murine ear. *Photochem Photobiol* 1989;49:369–372.
144. Ben-Hur E, et al. Release of clotting factors from photosensitized endothelial cells: a possible trigger for blood vessel occlusion by photodynamic therapy. *FEBS Lett* 1988;236:105–108.
145. Schuster A, et al. Simultaneous arterial calcium dynamics and diameter measurements: application to myoendothelial communication. *Am J Physiol Heart Circ Physiol* 2001;280: H1088–1096.
146. West CM, et al. A comparison of the sensitivity to photodynamic treatment of endothelial and tumour cells in different proliferative states. *Int J Radiat Biol* 1990;58:145–156.
147. Foster TH, et al. Photosensitized release of von Willebrand factor from cultured human endothelial cells. *Cancer Res* 1991;51: 3261–3266.
148. Boekelheide K, et al. Microtubule assembly inhibition by porphyrins and related compounds. *Photochem Photobiol* 1987;46: 657–661.
149. Dadosh N, Shaklai N. Impaired of red cell membrane cytoskeleton by protoporphyrin-IX: light and dark effects. *Photochem Photobiol* 1988;47:689–697.
150. Nelson JS, et al. Tumor destruction in photodynamic therapy. *Photochem Photobiol* 1987;46:829–835.
151. Sporn LA, Foster TH. Photofrin and light induces microtubule depolymerization in cultured human endothelial cells. *Cancer Res* 1992;52:3443–3448.
152. Wieman TJ. *Photochem Photobiol* 1991;53S:965–975.
153. Henderson B. Effects of photodynamic treatment of platelets or endothelial cells in vitro on platelet aggregation. *Photochem Photobiol* 1992;56:513–521.
154. Zhou CN. Mechanisms of tumor necrosis induced by photodynamic therapy. *J Photochem Photobiol B* 1989;3:299–318.
155. Zieve PD, et al. The effect of hematoporphyrin and light on human platelets. I. Morphologic, functional, and biochemical changes. *J Cell Physiol* 1966;67:271–279.
156. Star WM, et al. Destructive effect of photoradiation on the microcirculation of a rat mammary tumor growing in "sandwich" observation chambers. *Prog Clin Biol Res* 1984;170:637–645.
157. Doukas J, et al. Vasoactive amines and eicosanoids interactively regulate both polymorphonuclear leukocyte diapedesis and albumin permeability in vitro. *Microvasc Res* 1989;37:125–137.
158. Fingar VH, et al. The role of microvascular damage in photodynamic therapy: the effect of treatment on vessel constriction, permeability, and leukocyte adhesion. *Cancer Res* 1992;52: 4914–4921.
159. Reed MW, et al. The microvascular effects of photodynamic therapy: evidence for a possible role of cyclooxygenase products. *Photochem Photobiol* 1989;50:419–423.
160. Lange N, Wagnieres G, van den Bergh H. Unpublished results.
161. Lange N, et al. A new drug-screening procedure for photosensitizing agents used in photodynamic therapy for CNV. *Invest Ophthalmol Vis Sci* 2001;42:38–46.
162. Schmidt-Erfurth U, et al. Photodynamic therapy of subfoveal choroidal neovascularization: clinical and angiographic examples. *Graefes Arch Clin Exp Ophthalmol* 1998;236:365–374.
163. Schmidt-Erfurth U, et al. Photodynamic therapy with verteporfin for choroidal neovascularization caused by age-related macular degeneration: results of retreatments in a phase 1 and 2 study. *Arch Ophthalmol* 1999;117:1177–1187.
164. Sickenberg M, et al. A preliminary study of photodynamic therapy using verteporfin for choroidal neovascularization in pathologic myopia, ocular histoplasmosis syndrome, angioid streaks, and idiopathic causes. *Arch Ophthalmol* 2000;118:327–336.
165. Sickenberg M, et al. Preliminary clinical results of Lutex fluorescence pharmacokinetic and photodynamic therapy to treat choroidal neovascularization. *XII Congress European Society of Ophthalmology (SOE)* Stockholm, Sweden: 1999.
166. Kramer M, et al. Liposomal benzoporphyrin derivative verteporfin photodynamic therapy. Selective treatment of choroidal neovascularization in monkeys. *Ophthalmology* 1996;103:427–438.
167. Reinke MH, et al. Verteporfin photodynamic therapy retreatment of normal retina and choroid in the cynomolgus monkey. *Ophthalmology* 1999;106:1915–1923.
168. Husain D, et al. Effects of photodynamic therapy using verteporfin on experimental choroidal neovascularization and normal retina and choroid up to 7 weeks after treatment. *Invest Ophthalmol Vis Sci* 1999;40:2322–2331.
169. Trauner KB, et al. Photodynamic synovectomy using benzoporphyrin derivative in an antigen-induced arthritis model for rheumatoid arthritis. *Photochem Photobiol* 1998;67:133–139.
170. Trauner K, et al. Influence of light delivery on photodynamic synovectomy in an antigen-induced arthritis model for rheumatoid arthritis. *Lasers Surg Med* 1998;22:147–156.
171. Trauner KB, Hasan T. Photodynamic treatment of rheumatoid and inflammatory arthritis. *Photochem Photobiol* 1996;64: 740–750.
172. Kirdaite G, et al. Protoporphyrin IX photodynamic therapy for synovitis. *Arthritis Rheum* 2002;46:1371–1378.
173. Schmidt-Erfurth U, Hasan T. Mechanisms of action of photodynamic therapy with verteporfin for the treatment of age-related macular degeneration. *Surv Ophthalmol* 2000;45:195–214.
174. van den Bergh H, et al. PDT of choroidal neovascularisation associated with age-related macular degeneration. *Photodynam News* 2001;4:4–8.
175. Bernstein MH, Hollenberg MJ. Fine structure of the choriocapillaris and retinal capillaries. *Invest Ophthalmol* 965;4: 1016–1025.
176. Sun H, Nathans J. The challenge of macular degeneration. *Sci Am* 2001;285:69–75.
177. Bonnett R. *Chemical aspects of photodynamic therapy.* New York: Gordon and Breach, 2000.
178. Milgrom LR. *The colors of life: an introduction to the chemistry of porphyrins and related compounds.* New York: Oxford University Press, 1997.

3

IN VITRO ASSESSMENT AND BIOASSAY OF PHOTOSENSITIZERS FOR OCULAR PHOTODYNAMIC THERAPY

REEM Z. RENNO
YOSHIKO TERADA
EVANGELOS S. GRAGOUDAS
JOAN W. MILLER

Photodynamic therapy (PDT) has been established as a relatively selective therapy for choroidal neovascularization (CNV), sparing retinal and large choroidal vessels while incurring minimal changes in the neurosensory retina (1–6). Nevertheless, repeated PDT treatments can be expected to lead to cumulative damage to the retinal pigment epithelial cells (RPE) and choriocapillaris, which may lead to progressive treatment–related vision loss.

Photodynamic therapy involves a multitude of treatment parameters such as photosensitizer dose, timing of irradiation, light dose, mode of delivery (intravenous or local), duration of delivery (bolus versus infusion), and photosensitizer formulation and stabilization (7). All of these parameters were studied with verteporfin PDT for the treatment of CNV in animal models and clinical trials (1–3,5,8,9) prior to receiving approval as a treatment for patients with wet age-related macular degeneration (6, 10,11).

In vitro cell systems have been used extensively and successfully by investigators to test cutaneous and cardiovascular photodynamic applications prior to proceeding with animal and preclinical testing. An *in vitro* system or simple bioassay for PDT of CNV may speed the development of future photosensitizers as well as test other strategies to improve the therapy in general. We have developed a system using cell lines of relevance to CNV, namely, bovine retinal capillary endothelial cells (BRCE) and human RPE cells to study *in vitro* PDT effects. To date we have studied two of the photosensitizers currently in clinical application and/or trial, verteporfin and Motexafin Lutetium (Lu-Tex, Pharmacyclics, Inc., Sunnyvale, CA). Bovine retinal capillary endothelial cells were used as a representative capillary endothelial cell line of the posterior segment because retinal capillary endothelium is much easier to obtain and perpetuate in culture than choriocapillaris; additionally, many of the differences between choriocapillaris and retinal capillary endothelium are lost in culture.

Obana and colleagues used an *in vitro* system to study the photosensitizer ATX-S10(Na) for CNV (12,13). Recently other investigators developed an *in vivo* bioassay for photosensitizer screening using the chick chorioallantoic membrane (CAM), which is helpful in providing preliminary dosimetry for preclinical testing of vascular occlusion (14).

VERTEPORFIN PHOTODYNAMIC THERAPY FOR CHOROIDAL NEOVASCULARIZATION *IN VITRO*

The uptake of verteporfin by BRCE and RPE cells is rapid, peaking at 15 minutes and 30 minutes in BRCE and RPE, respectively (Fig. 3.1A). Verteporfin achieves a lower maximal concentration in RPE as compared to BRCE (Renno et al., unpublished) and clears rapidly from BRCE and RPE with most of the drug (85%) released within 45 minutes (Fig. 3.1A). These findings at the cellular level further confirm the observed *in vivo* advantageous property of verteporfin over the first-generation photosensitizers regarding its rapid clearance.

The selectivity of verteporfin between BRCE and RPE may result from differences in their modes of uptake. Three possible mechanisms of photosensitizer uptake have been postulated: (a) simple diffusion of lipophilic sensitizers; (b) fluid phase endocytosis of water-soluble sensitizers; and (c) receptor-mediated endocytosis of low-density lipoprotein (LDL)–associated dye (15). Verteporfin is a lipophilic dye that may rely for its incorporation (16) partly on LDL receptors and partly on simple diffusion. The difference in the composition of

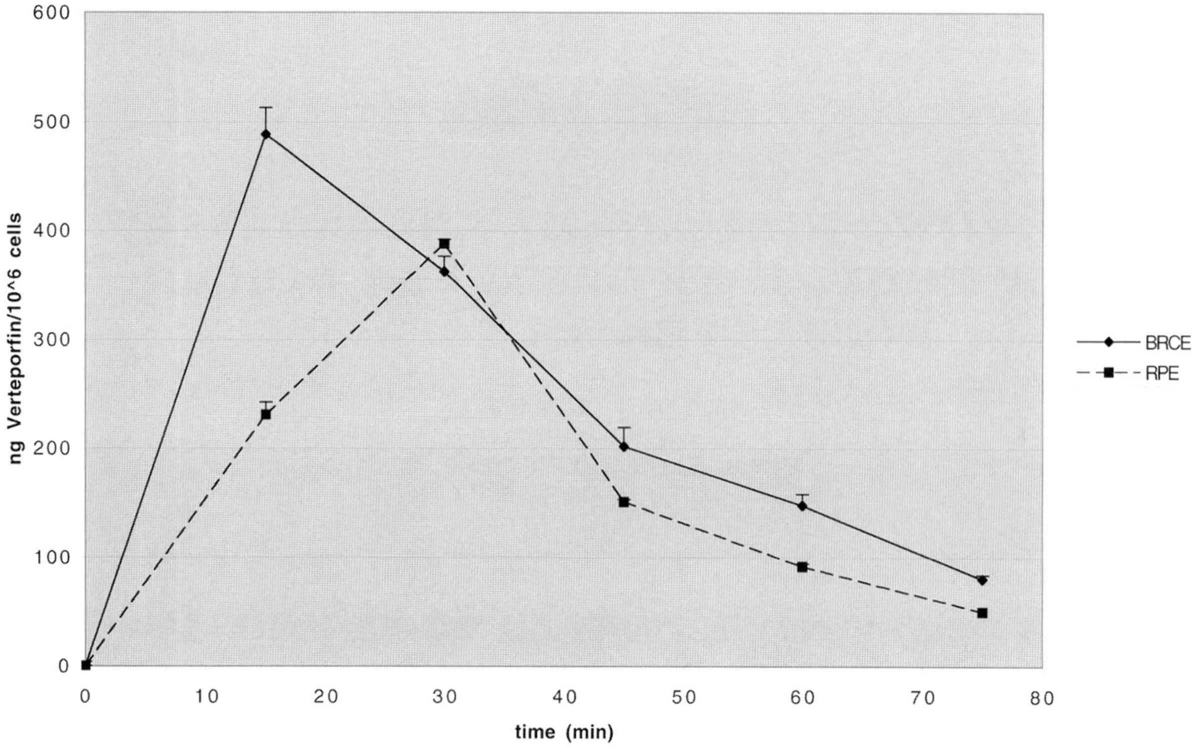

A

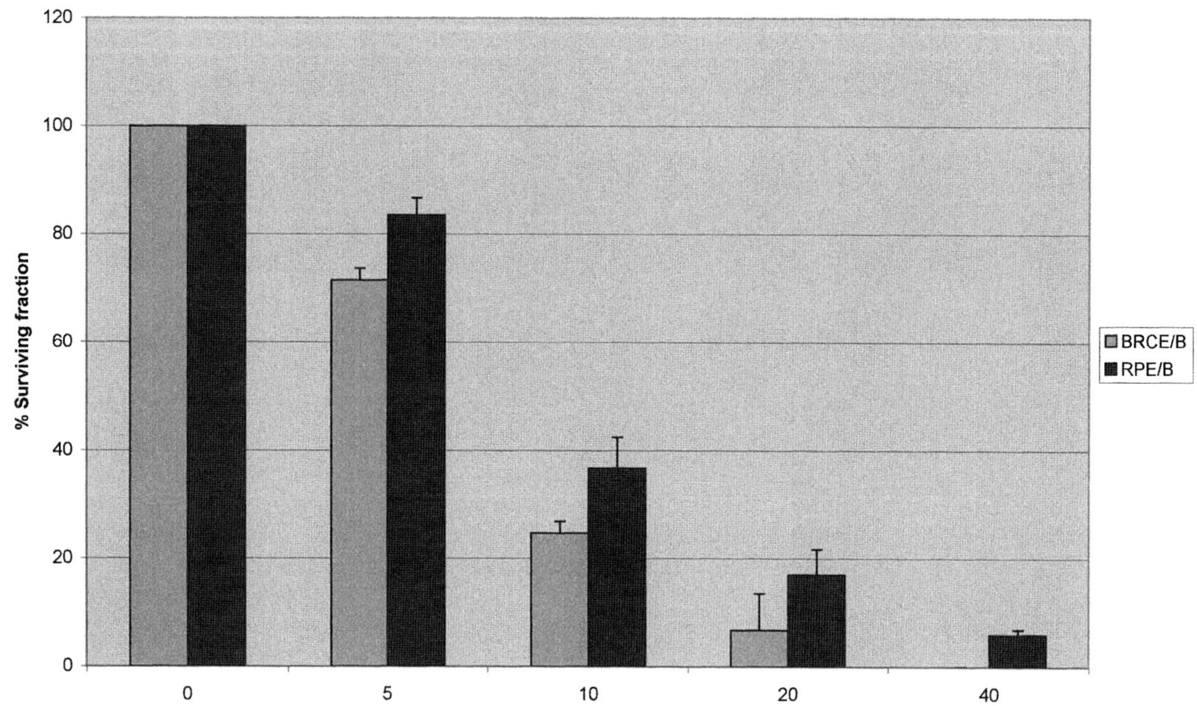

B

FIGURE 3.1. A: Uptake and release of verteporfin by the bovine retinal capillary endothelial cells (BRCE) and retinal pigment epithelial (RPE) cell lines. Cells at 10^7/mL were incubated with verteporfin (3 μg/mL) in Dulbecco's modified eagle medium (DMEM) containing 5% fetal bovine serum (FBS). Cell samples were taken at intervals and tested for verteporfin uptake by fluorescence measurements. Cell samples were removed, washed, and placed in medium devoid of verteporfin after 30 minutes. Cells were assessed for their verteporfin content at various time intervals after this step. Data represent the mean of three separate experiments ±SEM. **B:** Bovine retinal capillary endothelial cells and retinal pigment epithelial cells survival following photodynamic therapy using verteporfin as photosensitizer. Cells were plated and incubated with verteporfin (3 μg/mL) for 15 minutes, after which they were treated with various light doses delivered by a 689-nm light from a coherent ocular photoactivation diode and laser delivery system. Photodamage of the treated samples was assessed by the methylthiazolydiphenyl-tetrazolium bromide (MTT) assay and the surviving fraction was determined. Data represent the mean of three separate experiments ±SEM.

BRCE and RPE cellular membranes might account for the fact that verteporfin achieves a higher intracellular concentration in BRCE as compared to RPE. The potential contribution of LDL receptors in verteporfin cellular uptake could not be assessed in our experiments because fetal calf serum is particularly low in LDL. However, lipophilic dyes (e.g., verteporfin) may concentrate more in CNV than surrounding RPE because CNV is composed of highly proliferating vascular tissue, which may express more LDL receptors than quiescent tissue (17–21).

Verteporfin PDT cytotoxicity in BRCE and RPE exhibits a dose–response curve (Fig. 3.1B) with respect to fluence, which confirms the findings of further investigators in other cell types (22). Photodynamic therapy–induced cytotoxicity in BRCE and RPE using a verteporfin dose of 3 μg/mL was tested by irradiating the cells with various doses of monochromatic red light following incubation with verteporfin and assessing for cell survival using the standard tetrazolium (MTT) assay. The time point chosen for irradiation (30 minutes) corresponded to the time of peak dye concentration in BRCE because those are the target cells for PDT of CNV. The extent of BRCE cytotoxicity induced by verteporfin PDT is significantly more pronounced than that induced in RPE (Renno et al., unpublished).

LU-TEX PHOTODYNAMIC THERAPY FOR CHOROIDAL NEOVASCULARIZATION *IN VITRO*

Rapid saturation of Lu-Tex is achieved in BRCE and RPE cells. Peak Lu-Tex concentration is reached at 30 minutes in both BRCE and RPE (Fig. 3.2A), with a lower maximal concentration in RPE as compared to BRCE (Renno et al., unpublished).

Lu-Tex is water-soluble and depends on the intrinsic property of the lipid bilayer of cells for its uptake. The difference in uptake of Lu-Tex between BRCE and RPE is not surprising because there is a wide variation in the membrane composition of different cell types.

Rapid clearance of Lu-Tex from BRCE and RPE is noted, mirroring the uptake in that most of the drug (85%) is released within 45 minutes (Fig. 3.2A). These findings further confirm the observed *in vivo* advantageous property of Lu-Tex over the first-generation photosensitizers regarding its rapid clearance.

Lu-Tex PDT cytotoxicity in BRCE and RPE exhibits a dose–response curve (Fig. 3.2B) with respect to fluence, confirming the findings of other investigators (22). The extent of BRCE cytotoxicity induced by Lu-Tex PDT is significantly more pronounced than that induced in RPE (Renno et al., unpublished).

ATX-S10(NA) PHOTODYNAMIC THERAPY FOR CHOROIDAL NEOVASCULARIZATION *IN VITRO*

ATX-S10(Na) (13,17-bis (1-carboxy propionyl) carbamoylethyl-8-ethenyl-2-hydroxy-3-hydroxyiminoethylidene-2, 7,12,18-tetramethyl porphyrin sodium) fluorescence in human microvascular endothelial cells is weak up to 15 minutes postincubation with the photosensitizer at concentrations ranging from 0 to 50 μg/mL, and becomes intense at 30 minutes and 1 hour (12). The later time peak of uptake suggests that cellular uptake of ATX-S10(Na) occurs at least partially by endocytosis (23). ATX-S10(Na) uptake by RPE cells occurs more slowly than uptake by endothelial cells. Following laser irradiation with doses of 0 to 100 J/cm^2, cellular viability decreases in a dose-dependent manner with respect to both dye and light dose. Cellular injury is much higher at 30 minutes and 1 hour compared to 5 minutes (see Chapter 6) (12).

CELLULAR PROTECTIVE RESPONSE OF BOVINE RETINAL CAPILLARY ENDOTHELIAL CELLS AND RETINAL PIGMENT EPITHELIAL CELLS AGAINST PHOTODYNAMIC THERAPY

Cell lines of relevance to CNV demonstrate adaptive responses to cellular oxidative stress (Renno et al., unpublished) following PDT *in vitro*. Bovine retinal capillary endothelial and RPE cells normally exhibit a spindle-shaped, spread morphology on tissue culture plates (Fig. 3.3 A and D). Cells round up and lose their contact with each other immediately following PDT at sublethal doses. Swelling and plasma membrane blebbing of damaged cells as well as some densely refractive bodies of dying cells is evident, and the ability to remain attached to the surface also is substantially lost just after treatment (Fig. 3.3 B and E). Although it appears that the majority of the cells have been severely damaged by PDT right after treatment, some cells have disappeared 24 hours later, whereas those that remain regain their spindle shape and ability to attach (Fig. 3.3 C and F).

Comparable findings also were observed in other cell lines using verteporfin/PDT (24). Recovery of cells sustaining injury from PDT is evident from *in vivo* studies and suggested by clinical studies as well (3,6,10,25). Intracellular events associated with photosensitizers and their subsequent activation with light are not fully understood as yet. A thorough understanding of the mechanism(s) of cell death in response to PDT may be valuable in identifying and developing effective and more selective photosensitizers for CNV.

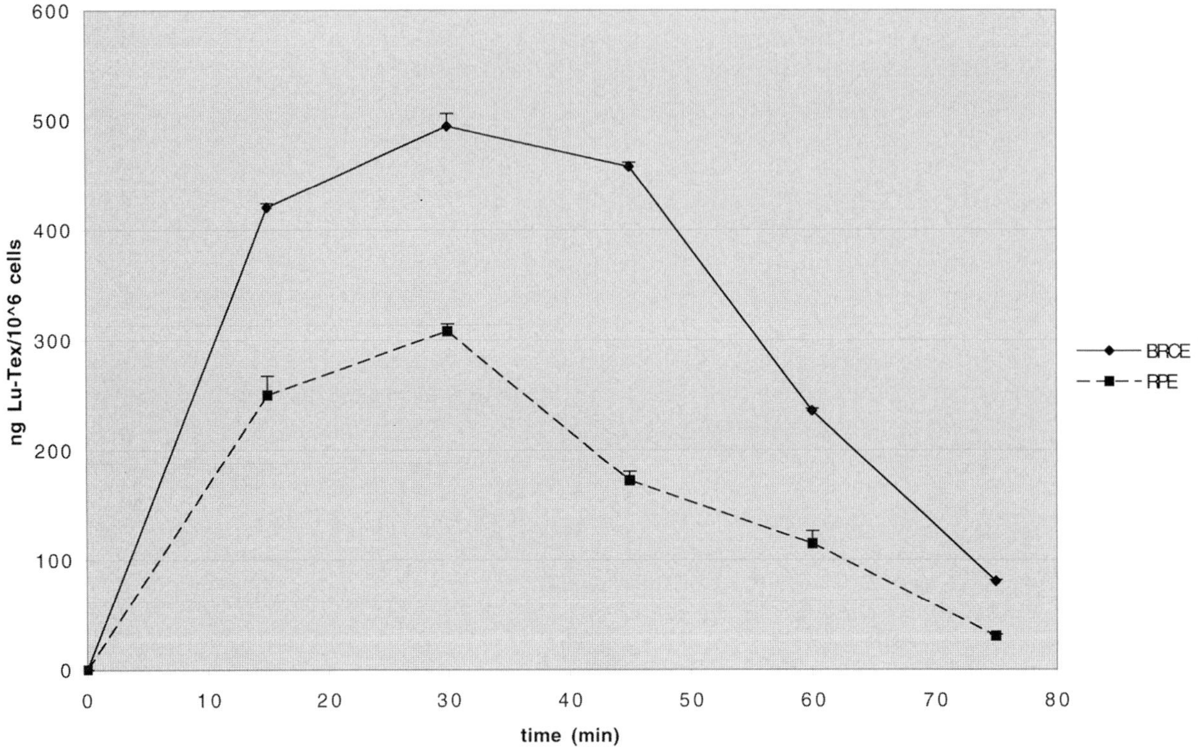
600
500
400
300
200
100
0
ng Lu-Tex/10^6 cells
0
10
20
30
40
50
60
70
80
time (min)
BRCE
RPE

A

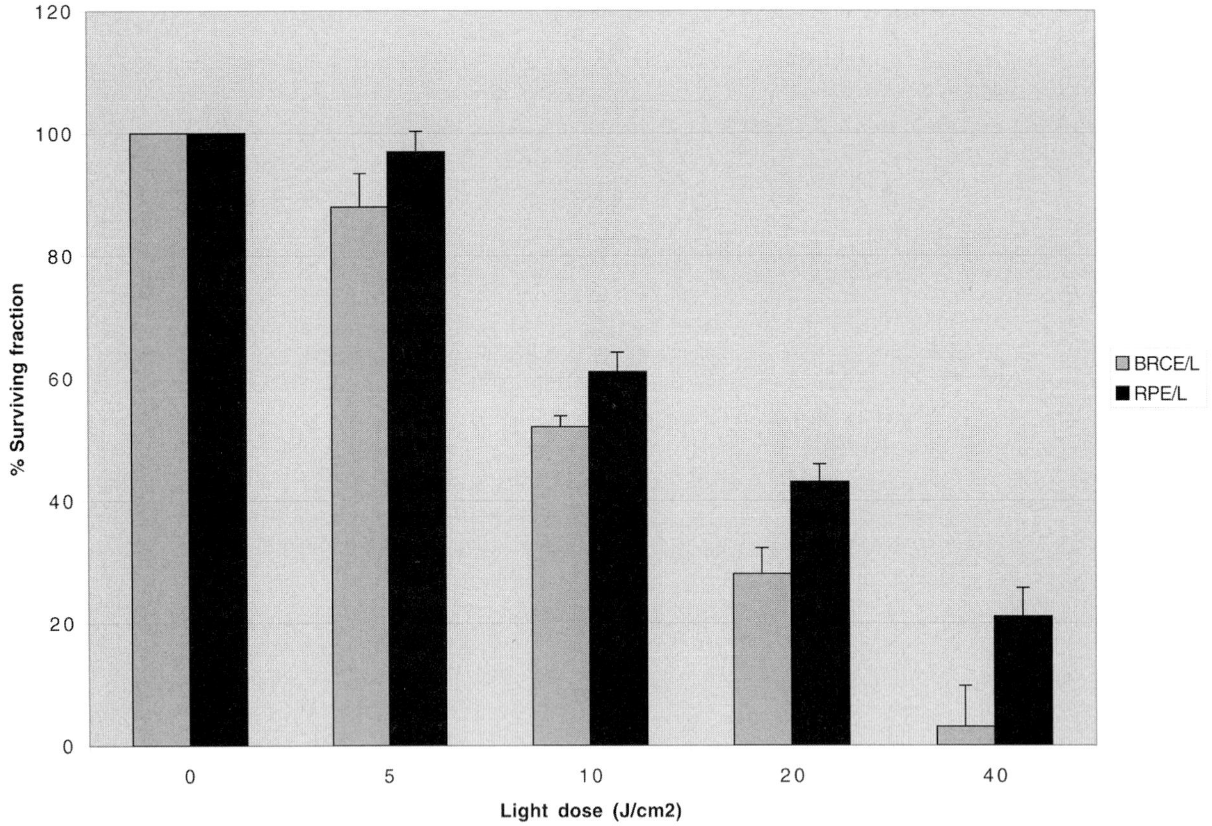
120
100
80
60
40
20
0
% Surviving fraction
0
5
10
20
40
Light dose (J/cm2)
BRCE/L
RPE/L

B

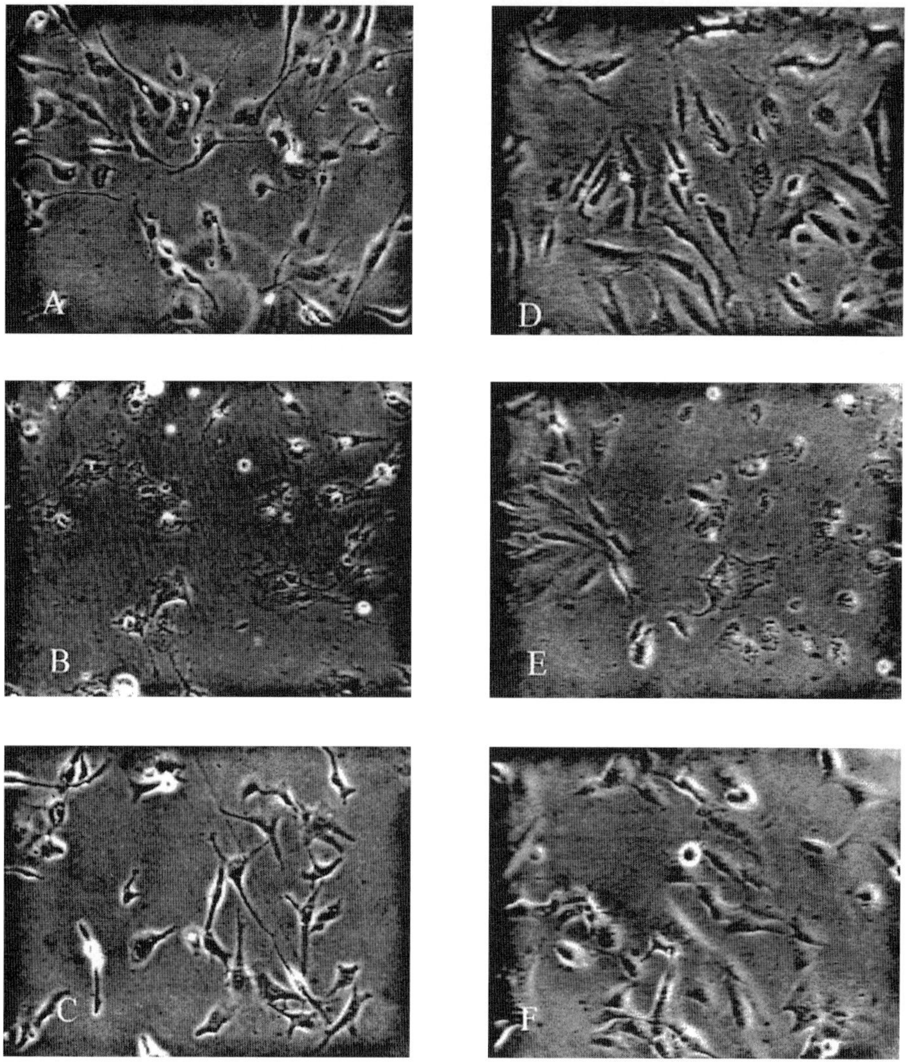

FIGURE 3.3. Bovine retinal capillary endothelial cells (BRCE) and retinal pigment epithelial cell (RPE) morphology following photodynamic therapy (PDT). **A,B,C:** Bovine retinal capillary endothelial cells before, at 0 hour, and 24 hours post–PDT, respectively. **D,E,F:** Retinal pigment epithelial cells before, at 0 hour, and 24 hours post–PDT, respectively.

FIGURE 3.2. A: Uptake and release of Lu-Tex by the bovine retinal capillary endothelial cells (BRCE) and retinal pigment epithelial (RPE) cell lines. Cells at 107/mL were incubated with Lu-Tex (3 μg/mL) in Dulbecco's modified eagle medium (DMEM) containing 5% fetal bovine serum (FBS). Cell samples were taken at intervals and tested for Lu-Tex uptake by fluorescent measurements. Cell samples were removed, washed, and placed in medium devoid of Lu-Tex after 30 minutes. After this step, cells were assessed for their Lu-Tex content at various time intervals. Data represent the mean of three separate experiments ±SEM. **B:** Bovine retinal capillary endothelial cells and retinal pigment epithelial survival following photodynamic therapy using Lu-Tex as a photosensitizer. Cells were plated and incubated with Lu-Tex (3 μg/mL) for 30 minutes, after which they were treated with various light doses delivered by a 732-nm light from a coherent ocular photoactivation diode and laser delivery system. Photodamage of the treated samples was assessed by the MTT assay and the surviving fraction was determined. Data represent the mean of three separate experiments ±SEM.

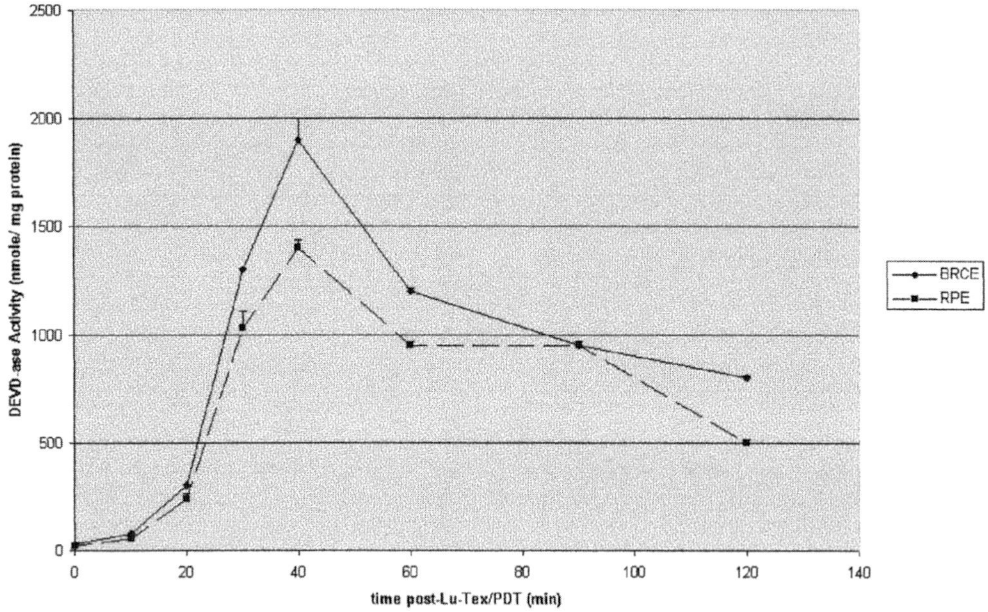

2500
2000
1500
1000
500
0
DEVD-ase Activity (nmole/ mg protein)
0
20
40
60
80
100
120
140
time post-Lu-Tex/PDT (min)
BRCE
RPE

A

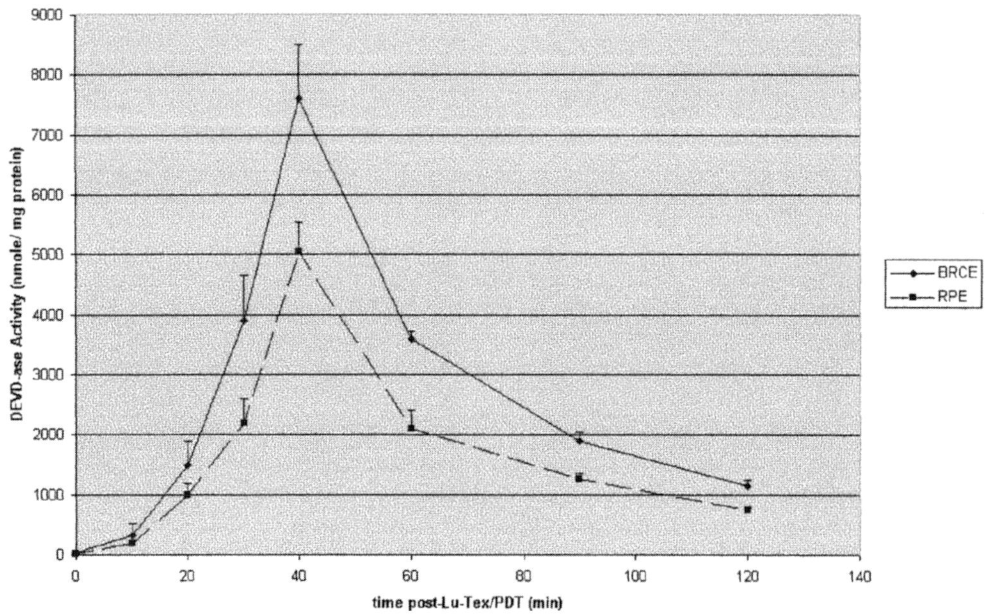

9000
8000
7000
6000
5000
4000
3000
2000
1000
0
DEVD-ase Activity (nmole/ mg protein)
0
20
40
60
80
100
120
140
time post-Lu-Tex/PDT (min)
BRCE
RPE

B

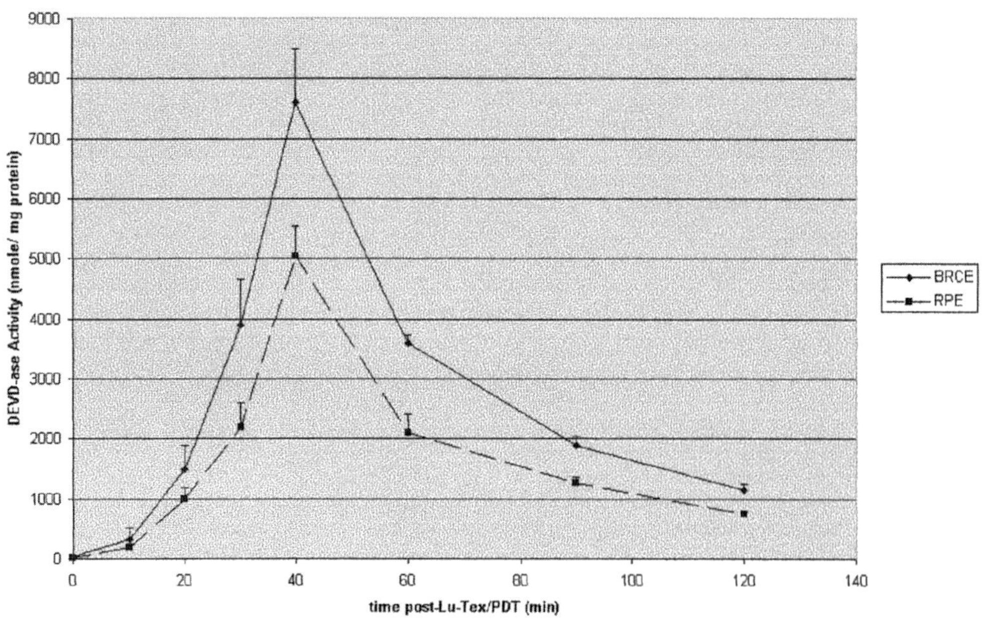

9000
8000
7000
6000
5000
4000
3000
2000
1000
0
DEVD-ase Activity (nmole/ mg protein)
0
20
40
60
80
100
120
140
time post-Lu-Tex/PDT (min)
BRCE
RPE

C

MODE OF CELL DEATH *IN VITRO* BY PHOTODYNAMIC THERAPY

Lu-Tex has been used as a model photosensitizer. PDT using Lu-Tex appears to induce tumor involution in the murine EMT6 sarcoma model by a mixture of apoptosis and necrosis (26). Photophorin/PDT also has been shown to induce apoptosis or necrosis in monkey kidney cell line (CV1), depending on the incubation protocol (13,27). Because PDT-induced apoptosis appears to be a function of the photosensitizer, cell line, and severity of treatment conditions, these findings can not be automatically extended to CNV. Investigators have begun to study these effects in the appropriate systems (24, 27–31).

Apoptosis involves the activation of a genetically determined cell suicide program that results in a morphologically distinct form of cell death characterized by cell shrinkage, nuclear condensation, DNA fragmentation, membrane reorganization, and blebbing (32). It has been suggested that apoptosis is associated with the generation of reactive oxygen species (ROS) and the product of the bcl-2 gene protects against apoptosis by inhibiting the generation or action of ROS (33–36). Bcl-2 belongs to a growing family of apoptosis regulatory gene products, which may be antagonists (bcl-2, bcl-xL, etc.) or death agonists (bax, bak, etc.) (37). Control of cell death appears to be regulated by these interactions and constitutive activities of the various family members (33). It is known that several apoptotic pathways coexist in mammalian cells that are preferentially activated in a stimulus-, stage-, and context-specific and cell-type manner (38). A proper understanding of the specific mechanism(s) involved in Lu-Tex/PDT–induced cytotoxicity in endothelial and RPE cells may permit interventions that enhance the selectivity and effectiveness of this treatment modality for CNV (6,10,25).

Lu-Tex/Photodynamic Therapy Induces Apoptosis in Bovine Retinal Capillary Endothelial Cells and Retinal Pigment Epithelial Cells

Lu-Tex/PDT induces caspase 3–like activation, a hallmark of apoptosis (39), in both BRCE and RPE in a dose- and time-dependent fashion, suggesting that apoptosis is a mediator of Lu-Tex/PDT cytotoxicity in these cell lines. The kinetics of activation were measured spectrofluorometrically by assaying the hydrolysis of a substrate (Ac-DEVD-AFC) that can be cleaved only by the caspase 3–like protease family members (Fig. 3.4). Rapid elevation of caspase 3–like activity is observed as early as 10 minutes post–Lu-Tex/PDT and peaking at 40 minutes in both BRCE and RPE and at all doses used. The rate of entry into apoptosis is time- and dose-dependent in each cell line but the amount of caspase 3–like activation is always significantly higher in BRCE compared to RPE.

Modulation of bcl-2 Family Members in Bovine Retinal Capillary Endothelial Cells and Retinal Pigment Epithelial Cells After Lu-Tex/Photodynamic Therapy

In view of the relationship among bcl-2, PDT, and ROS, investigation of the constitutive expression of antiapoptotic bcl-2 and bcl-xL, and proapoptotic bax and bak; and their modulation post–PDT were carried (39). Differential expression of members of bcl-2 family members in BRCE and RPE is observed: bcl-2 and bax are detected in BRCE, whereas bcl-xL and bak are detected in RPE (Table 3.1). After Lu-Tex/PDT at LD_{50}, downregulation of bcl-2 and upregulation of bax is observed in BRCE, resulting in an increase of the cellular ratio of bax/bcl-2 protein (Fig. 3.5A). In RPE, there is an upregulation of both bcl-xL and bak up to 4 hours post–PDT, following which bcl-xL levels reach a plateau and bak levels start to decline (Fig. 3.5B). The upregulation of bax in BRCE is dose-dependent; however, the upregulation of its proapoptotic counterpart bak in RPE exhibits dose dependence only until 20 J/cm^2; after which it starts to decline (Fig. 3.5C).

Collectively, those results indicate that Lu-Tex/PDT induces apoptosis in BRCE through the modulation of bcl-2 and bax in a dose- and time-dependent fashion; and in RPE through the modulation of bcl-xL and bak. Yet, at all times post–PDT, there is an upregulation of the antiapoptotic bcl-xL levels in RPE; concomitantly, as of 4 hours posttreatment, the levels of the proapoptotic bak start declining following its initial upregulation. Furthermore, following incremental PDT doses, the proapoptotic bak is upregulated in RPE until 20 J/cm^2, following which bak levels start declining despite an increase of PDT dose to 40 J/cm^2. Thus, it is conceivable to think of a protective survival response being mounted in RPE at these lethal doses to counteract the apoptotic trigger. Such a hypothesis is further supported by the histologic evidence of RPE recovery post–PDT *in vivo* (2,3) and by reports from other investigators proving that overexpression of antiapoptotic bcl-2 family members renders cells partially resistant to PDT (40) and inhibits the activation of caspase 3 following

FIGURE 3.4. Kinetics of caspase 3–like activation following Lu-Tex/PDT in bovine retinal capillary endothelial cells (BRCE) and retinal pigment epithelial cells (RPE). BRCE and RPE cells were exposed to Lu-Tex/PDT at fluences of **(A)** 10; **(B)** 20; and **(C)** 40 J/cm^2. At the indicated times thereafter, cells were collected and lysed. Aliquots (50 μg of protein) were incubated with Ac-Asp-Glu-Val-Asp aminofluoro coumarin (DEVD-AFC) at 37°C for 30 minutes. The amount of fluorochrome released was determined by comparison to an AFC standard curve in lysis buffer. Data represent the means from three independent experiments.

TABLE 3.1. SUMMARY OF IMMUNODETECTION OF BCL_2 FAMILY MEMBERS IN BOVINE RETINAL CAPILLARY ENDOTHELIAL CELLS (BRCE) AND RETINAL PIGMENT EPITHELIAL CELLS (RPE)

	Cell Line	
Bcl_2 Family Member	BRCE	RPE
Bcl_2	+	−
Bcl-xL	−	+
Bax	+	−
Bak	−	+

PDT (41); reversibly, antisense bcl-2 retrovirus increases their sensitivity to PDT (42).

MODE OF CELL DEATH FOLLOWING PHOTODYNAMIC THERAPY USING ATX-S10(NA)

Photodynamic therapy performed on cells in medium containing ATX-S10(Na) induces necrosis predominantly, whereas in contrast, PDT performed after longer incubation with ATX-S10(Na) followed by washing resulted in apoptosis. It was concluded that apoptosis is predominantly the mechanism in cells that takes up ATX-S10(Na) into lysosomes, and that necrosis is seen if ATX-S10(Na) is attached to the cell membrane (13).

It has been reported that photosensitizers that localize in mitochondria and lysosomes are likely to induce apoptosis, whereas those that localize to the plasma membrane are likely to cause necrosis (13,43).

THE CHICK CHORIOALLANTOIC MEMBRANE BIOASSAY FOR PHOTOSENSITIZER SCREENING

The chick CAM assay has been used extensively as a simple model for *in vivo* research on angiogenesis research and is used as a simple *in vivo* microvasculature assay for screening of angiogenic factors and inhibitors. The CAM is the major respiratory organ of the chick embryo; its well-vascularized surface is formed by the fusion of the two mesodermal lay-

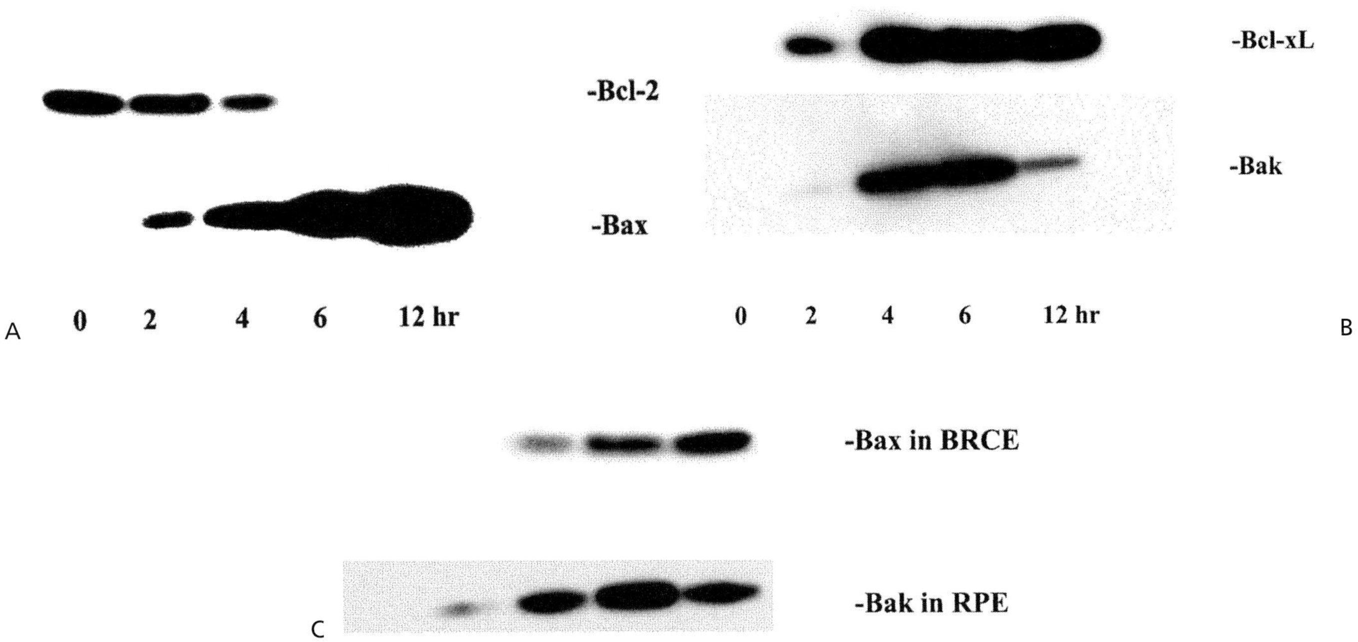

FIGURE 3.5. Expression of bcl-2, bcl-xL, bax, and bak in bovine retinal capillary endothelial cells (BRCE) and retinal pigment epithelial cells (RPE) after Lu-Tex/PDT. **A,B:** BRCE and RPE were treated with Lu-Tex/PDT (LD_{50}). At the indicated time points after photodynamic therapy (PDT), whole cell extracts were obtained and analyzed via sodium dodecyl sulfate (SDS)—page followed by Western blotting using antibodies to bcl-2, bcl-xL, bax, and bak. In BRCE, upregulation of bax and downregulation of bcl-2 are observed over 12 hours. In RPE, upregulation of bcl-xL is observed along with peak upregulation of bak up to 4 hours followed by its progressive decline. **C:** Following incremental doses of PDT, BRCE and RPE cellular lysates were obtained 4 hours after treatment and analyzed via SDS-page followed by Western blotting using antibodies to bax and bak. In BRCE, bax is upregulated in a dose-dependent fashion. In RPE, the level of bak plateaus at 20 J/cm^2.

ers. This extra embryonic membrane is commonly used *in vivo* to study both new vessel formation and its inhibition in response to tissues, cells, or soluble factors (43). The transparency of its superficial layers permits nearly any wavelength in the visible part of the electromagnetic spectrum to be used for fluorescence analysis because it is easily visualized (14).

Three second-generation photosensitizers—5-aminolevulinic acid (ALA), benzoporphyrin derivative monoacid ring A (BPD-MA), and Lu-Tex—have been tested for their ability to produce photodynamic response in the chick CAM when delivered systemically by *intraperitoneal injection*. Exposure of the CAM vasculature to the appropriate laser light results in light–dose-dependent vascular damage with all three compounds (44). The chick CAM model has been used as an *in vivo* assay for BPD-MA following *intravenous injection* of the dye (45–48) and showed strong similarities to results obtained in clinical tests for PDT of CNV. The effect of PDT was assessed by fluorescence angiography 24 hours after PDT. Vascular damage could be induced by varying the PDT parameters. Lipophilic photosensitizers tended to remain confined to the intravascular space, whereas hydrophilic ones extravasated. By variation of PDT parameters, vascular damage could be directed toward closure of vessels with diameters smaller than 10 μm. It is not clear, however, whether the CAM model, unlike cell culture systems, can distinguish between proliferating (e.g., in CNV) and resting (e.g., normal choriocapillaris) blood vessels, nor does it take into account the phenomenon of vascular heterogeneity among different organs (49,50). Additionally, because cellular molecular events following PDT are cell-type specific, the CAM assay can not be used to explore those specific pathways as they relate to CNV—an essential landmark in the endeavor aimed at rationally optimizing PDT. Yet this model, unlike cell culture studies, allows the study of the vasculature photothrombosis phenomenon, which is central to PDT, although other structures of interest (e.g., the RPE and neurosensory retina) are absent in this model. The assay is not expensive when compared to the gold standard of animal testing, requires a certain expertise, and is a useful adjunct to cell cultures for the biochemical screening of photosensitizers.

In summary, we described *in vitro* and *in vivo* systems to study the effect of PDT prior to studies in animal models. These systems might permit a wide range of studies directed toward fully elucidating the mode of PDT–induced death, associated cellular protective mechanisms, and exploration of the potential of combination therapy against CNV.

REFERENCES

1. Miller JW, Walsh AW, Kramer M, et al. Photodynamic therapy of experimental choroidal neovascularization using lipoprotein-delivered benzoporphyrin. *Arch Ophthalmol* 1995;113:810–818.
2. Kramer M, Miller JW, Michaud N, et al. Liposomal benzoporphyrin derivative verteporfin photodynamic therapy: selective treatment of choroidal neovascularization in monkeys. *Ophthalmology* 1996;103(3):427–438.
3. Husain D, Kramer M, Kenny AG, et al. Effects of photodynamic therapy using verteporfin on experimental choroidal neovascularization and normal retina and choroid up to seven weeks after treatment. *Invest Ophthalmol Visl Sci* 1999;40:2322–2331.
4. Husain D, Miller JW. Photodynamic therapy of exudative age-related macular degeneration. *Semin Ophthalmol* 1997;12: 14–25.
5. Husain D, Miller JW, Michaud N, et al. Intravenous infusion of liposomal benzoporphyrin derivative for photodynamic therapy of experimental choroidal neovascularization. *Arch Ophthalmol* 1996;114:978–985.
6. TAP Study Group, Treatment of Age-Related Macular Degeneration with Photodynamic Therapy (TAP) study group. Verteporfin (Visudyne) therapy of subfoveal choroidal neovascularization in age-related macular degeneration. One year results of two randomized clinical trials. *Arch Ophthalmol* 1999;117:1329–1345.
7. Renno RZ, Miller JW. Photosensitizer delivery for photodynamic therapy of choroidal neovascularization. *Adv Drug Deliv Rev* 2001;52:63–78.
8. Miller H, Miller B. Photodynamic therapy of subretinal neovascularization in the monkey eye. *Arch Ophthalmol* 1993;111: 855–860.
9. Kramer M, Kenney AG, DeLori D, et al. Imaging of experimental choroidal neovascularization (CNV) using liposomal benzoporphyrin derivative monoacid (BPD-MA) angiography. *Invest Ophthalmol Vis Sci (Suppl)* 1995;36:S236.
10. Miller JW, Schmidt-Erfurth U, Sickenberg M, et al. Photodynamic therapy for choroidal neovascularization due to age-related macular degeneration with Verteporfin: results of a single treatment in a phase I and II study. *Arch Ophthalmol* 1999;117: 1161–1173.
11. Bressler N, TS Group. Photodynamic therapy of subfoveal choroidal neovascularization in related age macular degeneration with verteporfin: two-year results of randomized clinical trials-tap report 2. *Arch Ophthalmol* 2001;119:198–207.
12. Gohto Y, et al. *Uptake of ATX-S10(Na) by cultured vascular endothelial cells and its photodynamic effect.* Fort Lauderdale, FL: ARVO, 2000.
13. Gohto Y, et al. *In vitro photodynamic effects of ATX-S10(Na) and mode of cell death on vascular endothelial cells.* Fort Lauderdale, FL: ARVO, 2001.
14. Lange N, Ballinni JP, Wagnieres G, et al. A new drug-screening procedure for photosensitizing agents used in photodynamic therapy for CNV. *Invest Ophthalmol Vis Sci* 2001;42:38–46.
15. Berg K, Moan J. Lysosomes and microtubules as targets for photochemotherapy of cancer. *Photochem Photobiol* 1997;65: 403–409.
16. Haimovici R, Kramer M, Miller JW, et al. Localization of lipoprotein-delivered benzoporphyrin derivative in the rabbit eye. *Curr Eye Res* 1997;16:83–90.
17. Gaffney J, West D, Arnold F, et al. Differences in the uptake of modified low density lipoproteins by tissue cultured endothelial cells. *J Cell Sci* 1985;79:317–325.
18. Jori G. Low density lipoprotein-liposome delivery system for tumor photosensitizers in vivo. In: Henderson B, Doughery T, eds. *Photodynamic therapy: basic principles and clinical applications.* New York: Marcel Dekker, 1992:219–268.
19. Kessel D, Woodburn K. Biodistribution of photosensitizing agents. *Int J Biochem* 1993;25:1377–1383.
20. Netland PA, Zetter BR, Via DP, et al. In situ labelling of vascular endothelium fluorescent acetylated low density lipoprotein. *Histochem J* 1985;17:1309–1320.

21. West CM, West DC, Kumar S, et al. A comparison of the sensitivity to photodynamic treatment of endothelial and tumor cells in different proliferative states. *Int J Radiat Biol* 1990;58:145–156.
22. Richter A, et al. Kinetics of cellular uptake and retention of the benzoporphyrin derivative (BPD): relevance to photodynamic therapy. *SPIE* 1994;2325:189–197.
23. Mori M, Kuroda T, Obana A, et al. In vitro plasma protein binding and cellular uptake of ATX-S10(Na), a hydrophilic chlorin photosensitizer. *Jpn J Cancer Res* 2000;91(8):845–852.
24. Curry P, et al. Intracellular events associated with uptake of a monomeric photosensitizer, benzoporphyrin derivative monoacid ring A (BPD) and its subsequent activation with light. *SPIE* 1993; 1881:262–274.
25. Schmidt-Erfurth U, Miller JW, Sickenberg M, et al. Photodynamic therapy with verteporfin for choroidal neovascularization caused by age-related macular degeneration: results of retreatments in a phase I and II study. *Arch Ophthalmol* 1999;117: 1177–1187.
26. Woodburn KW, Fan Q, Miles DR, et al. Localization and efficacy analysis of the phototherapeutic Lutetium Texaphyrin (PCI-0123) in the murine EMT6 sarcoma model. *Photochem Photobiol* 1997;65:410–415.
27. Dellinger M. Apoptosis or necrosis following photofrin photosensitization: influence of the incubation protocol. *Photochem Photobiol* 1996;64:182–187.
28. Separovic D, Mann KJ, Oleinick NL. Association of ceramide accumulation with photodynamic treatment-induced cell death. *Photochem Photobiol* 1998;68:101–109.
29. He XY, Sikes RA, Thomsen S, et al. Photodynamic therapy with photofrin II induces programmed cell death in carcinoma cell lines. *Photochem Photobiol* 1994;59:468–473.
30. Varnes ME, Chiu SM, Xue LY, et al. Photodynamic therapy-induced apoptosis in lymphoma cells: translocation of cytochrome c causes inhibition of respiration as well as caspase activation. *Biochem Biophys Res Commun* 1999;255:673–679.
31. Kessel D, Luo Y. Photodynamic therapy: a mitochondrial inducer of apoptosis. *Cell Death Diff* 1999;6:28–35.
32. Kerr J, Wyllie A, Currie A. Apoptosis: a basic biological phenomenon with wide ranging implications. *Br J Cancer* 1972;26: 239–257.
33. Hockenbery DM, Oltvai ZN, Yin XM, et al. Bcl-2 functions in an antioxidant pathway to prevent apoptosis. *Cell* 1993;75: 241–251.
34. Kane DJ, Sarafian TA, Anton R, et al. Bcl-2 inhibition of neural death: decreased generation of reactive oxygen species. *Science* 1993;262:1274–1277.
35. Veis DJ, Sorenson CM, Shutter JR, et al. Bcl-2-deficient mice demonstrate fulminant lymphoid apoptosis, polycystic kidneys, and hypopigmented hair. *Cell* 1993;75:229–240.
36. Virgili F, Santini MP, Canali R, et al. Bcl-2 overexpression in the HaCaT cell line is associated with a different membrane fatty acid composition and sensitivity to oxidative stress. *Free Rad Biol Med* 1998;24:93–101.
37. Kroemer G. The proto-oncogene Bcl-2 and its role in regulating apoptosis. *Nat Med* 1997;3:614–620.
38. Hakem R, Hakem A, Duncan GS, et al. Differential requirement for caspase 9 in apoptotic pathways in vivo. *Cell* 1998;94:339–352.
39. Renno RZ, Delori FC, Holzer RA, et al. Photodynamic therapy using Lu-Tex induces apoptosis in vitro and shows potentiate action combined with angio statin in retinal capillary endothelial cells. *Invest Ophthalmol Vis Sci* 2000;41:3963–3971.
40. He J, Agarwal ML, Larkin HE, et al. The induction of partial resistance to photodynamic therapy by the protooncogene BCL-2. *Photochem Photobiol* 1996;64:845–852.
41. Granville DJ, Jiang H, An MT, et al. Overexpression of Bcl-Xl prevents caspase-3-mediated activation of DNA fragmentation factor (DFF) produced by treatment with the photochemotherapeutic agent BPD-MA. *FEBS Letts* 1998;422:151–154.
42. Zhang WG, Ma LP, Wang SW, et al. Antisense Bcl-2 retrovirus vector increases the sensitivity of a human gastric carcinoma cell line to photodynamic therapy. *Photochem Photobiol* 1999;69: 582–586.
43. Ribatti D, Vacca A, Roncali L, et al. The chick embryo chorioallantoic membrane as a model for in vivo research on anti-angiogenesis. *Curr Pharmacol Biotechnol* 2000;1:73–82.
44. Hornung R, Hammer-Wilson MJ, Kimel S, et al. Systemic application of photosensitizers in the chick chorioallantoic membrane model: photodynamic response of CAM vessels and 5-aminolevulinic acid uptake kinetics by transplantable tumors. *J Photochem Photobiol* 1999;49:41–49.
45. Gottfried V, Lindebaum E, Kimel S. Vascular damage during PDT monitored in the chick chorioallantoic membrane. *Int J Radiat Biol* 1991;60:349–354.
46. Roberts W, Hasan T. Role of neovasculature and vascular permeability on the tumor retention of photodynamic agents. *Cancer Res* 1992;25:924–930.
47. Strauss WS, Sailer R, Schneckenburger H, et al. Photodynamic efficacy of naturally occurring porphyrins in endothelial cells in vitro and microvasculature in vivo. *J Photochem Photobiol* 1997; 39:176–184.
48. Toledano H, Edrei R, Kimel S. Photodynamic damage by liposome-bound porphycenes: comparison between in vitro and in vivo models. *J Photochem Photobiol* 1998;42:20–27.
49. Pasqualini R, Ruoslahti E. Organ targeting in vivo using phage display peptide libraries. *Nature* 1996;380:364–366.
50. Rajotte D, Arap W, Hagedorn M, et al. Molecular heterogeneity of the vascular endothelium revealed by in vivo phage display. *J Clin Invest* 1998;102:430–437.

4

COMBINATION OF PHOTODYNAMIC THERAPY AND ANTIANGIOGENIC AGENTS

REEM Z. RENNO
YOSHIKO TERADA
EVANGELOS S. GRAGOUDAS
JOAN W. MILLER

Photodynamic therapy (PDT) for choroidal neovascularization (CNV) has demonstrated promising results despite some observed side effects on the retinal pigment epithelial cells (RPE) and the necessity of repeated treatments (1–7). These limitations of PDT prompted our search for different strategies to improve the efficacy and selectivity of PDT for CNV (Fig. 4.1), including combining antiangiogenic therapy with PDT.

Combination therapy has been investigated *in vitro* by our group and others. Our *in vitro* system, which is described elsewhere in this volume, makes use of cell lines of relevance to CNV; namely, bovine retinal capillary endothelial cells (BRCE) and RPE. Combination therapy has been studied by others in experimental tumor models, and we have investigated therapies in models of experimental CNV.

Antiangiogenic agents that have been examined in one or more systems include angiostatin, anti–vascular endothelial growth factor (VEGF) agents, including antibodies and aptamers, inhibitors of tyrosine kinase receptors, and angiostaxic steroids. Another approach to improve selectivity is to combine PDT with agents that modulate apoptosis, because different pathways may be used by different cells involved. Selective agents may be identified to potentiate or inhibit programmed cell death in endothelial and retinal cells. Finally, ionizing radiation in combination with PDT may be an effective permutation.

IN VITRO PHOTODYNAMIC THERAPY POTENTIATION USING ANGIOSTATIN IN PROLIFERATING RETINAL MICROVASCULATURE

Angiostatin is a proteolytic fragment of plasminogen that was first isolated from the serum and urine of tumor-bearing mice, and inhibits angiogenesis (8,9). *In vitro* and *in vivo* studies showed that radiation and angiostatin have combined cytotoxic effects on endothelial cells; and the combination of those two components produced no increased toxicity to normal tissue (10,11). Using an *in vitro* cell culture system described elsewhere in this volume, we noted a synergistic cytotoxic effect of human angiostatin and Lu-Tex PDT on BRCE compared to RPE (12).

Bovine retinal capillary endothelial cells and RPE survival was assessed after pretreating cells for 18 hours with an angiostatin dose of 500 μg/mL followed by Lu-Tex/PDT at various fluences. Cellular survival was measured using a 1-week cellular proliferation assay in order to determine the lasting cytotoxic effect of the combination treatment of angiostatin/PDT rather than the short-term angiostaxic effect of angiostatin on cellular proliferation. We first demonstrated that human angiostatin inhibits BRCE cells but not RPE: When exposed to angiostatin alone, the proliferation assay demonstrated a 12.61% killing of BRCE at the angiostatin dose used. It also was observed that preexposing BRCE to angiostatin did not interfere with the subsequent cellular uptake of Lu-Tex. In combination with angiostatin, Lu-Tex/PDT produced a synergistic cytotoxic effect on BRCE at all fluences used (5, 10, and 20 J/cm^2), consistently exceeding the cytotoxicity resulting from Lu-Tex/PDT alone, angiostatin alone, or the arithmetic sum of their respective toxicities (Figs. 4.2A and 4.3). When combined with angiostatin, Lu-Tex/PDT has an LD_{100} on BRC of 20 J/cm^2, whereas Lu-Tex/PDT alone has an LD_{100} of 40 J/cm^2. Controls consisted of cells exposed to light only because no dark toxicity was observed at the Lu-Tex concentration used. Furthermore, it was observed that angiostatin did not potentiate Lu-Tex/PDT if delivered after

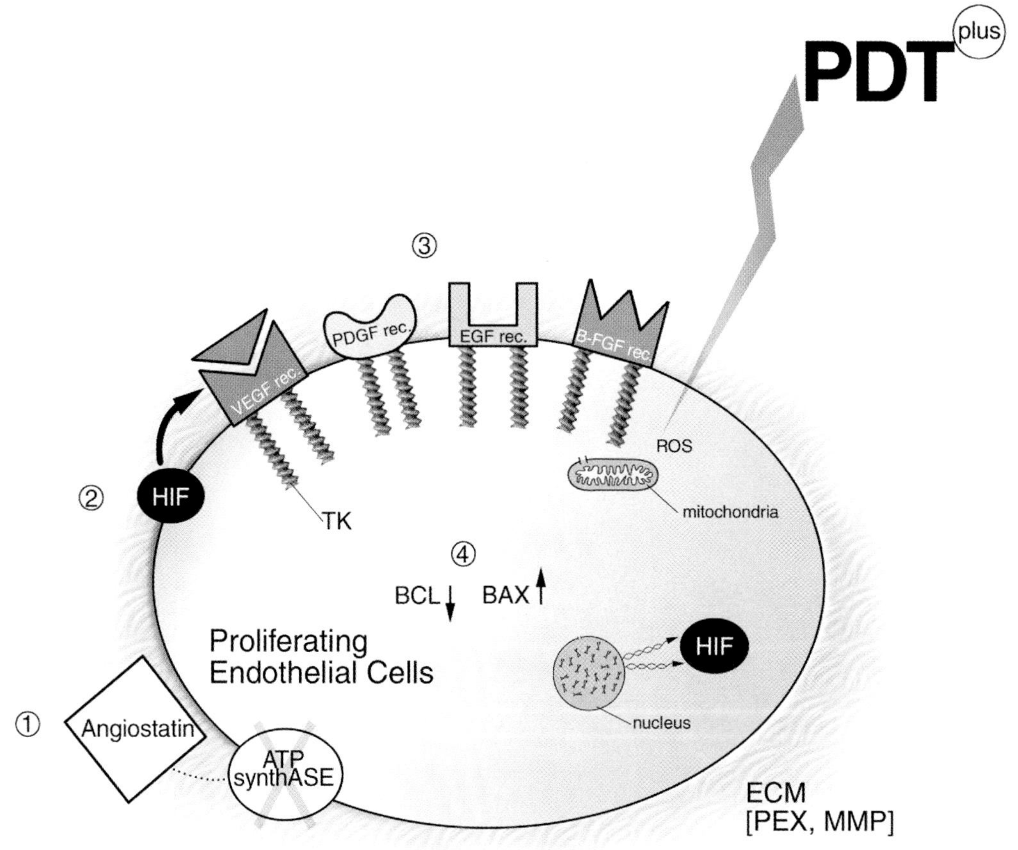

FIGURE 4.1. A schematic representation of the combination of photodynamic therapy and other antiangiogenic drugs.

PDT. In contrast to BRCE, no cytotoxicity was observed when human RPE cells were treated with angiostatin, and no interactive killing was observed following exposure to angiostatin and Lu-Tex/PDT (Figs. 4.2B and 4.3). It appears that a specific antiproliferative effect of angiostatin is exerted on retinal capillary endothelial cells, whereas no effect was observed on RPE.

Angiostatin also was shown to potentiate the effect of verteporfin PDT *in vitro* in retinal microvasculature endothelium while having no effect on the RPE. Verteporfin PDT was performed on cells with or without prior exposure to 100 ng/mL of angiostatin and cellular survival was assessed at 24 hours after PDT. Results showed statistically significant increased cytotoxicity (25% to 50%) to BRCE but not for RPE when angiostatin was combined with verteporfin PDT.

Recently Lai and associates have demonstrated that adeno-associated virus vector expressing angiostatin suppresses CNV in the rat laser-injury model (13). Because angiostatin has a cytostatic rather than cytocidal effect, one might expect it to have a selective effect on proliferating versus resting endothelium. Indeed, using the retinopathy of prematurity model, Drixler and colleagues showed that retinal vessel proliferation secondary to hypoxia is completely inhibited by the systemic administration of angiostatin without affecting normal retinal vascularization (14). Work is currently underway in our laboratory to test the combination of angiostatin and PDT in small animal models of laser-induced CNV.

ANGIOSTATIN AND PHOTODYNAMIC THERAPY: MECHANISM OF SYNERGY

The synergistic effect of angiostatin and PDT on microvascular endothelium was unexpected and we examined the effect of these interventions on cellular apoptosis. We found that the combination of angiostatin and PDT to treat BRCE resulted in a statistically significant increase in caspase 3–like activity (DEVD-ase activity, a hallmark of apoptosis) as compared to the same dose of PDT alone (Fig. 4.4). This suggests that the potentiating effect of angiostatin on PDT of BRCE occurs through apoptosis. The rate of entry into apoptosis by BRCE treated with PDT alone or with the combination of angiostatin/PDT is time-dependent. However, the time course of caspase 3–like activity for angiostatin/PDT differs from that of PDT in that it proceeds faster,

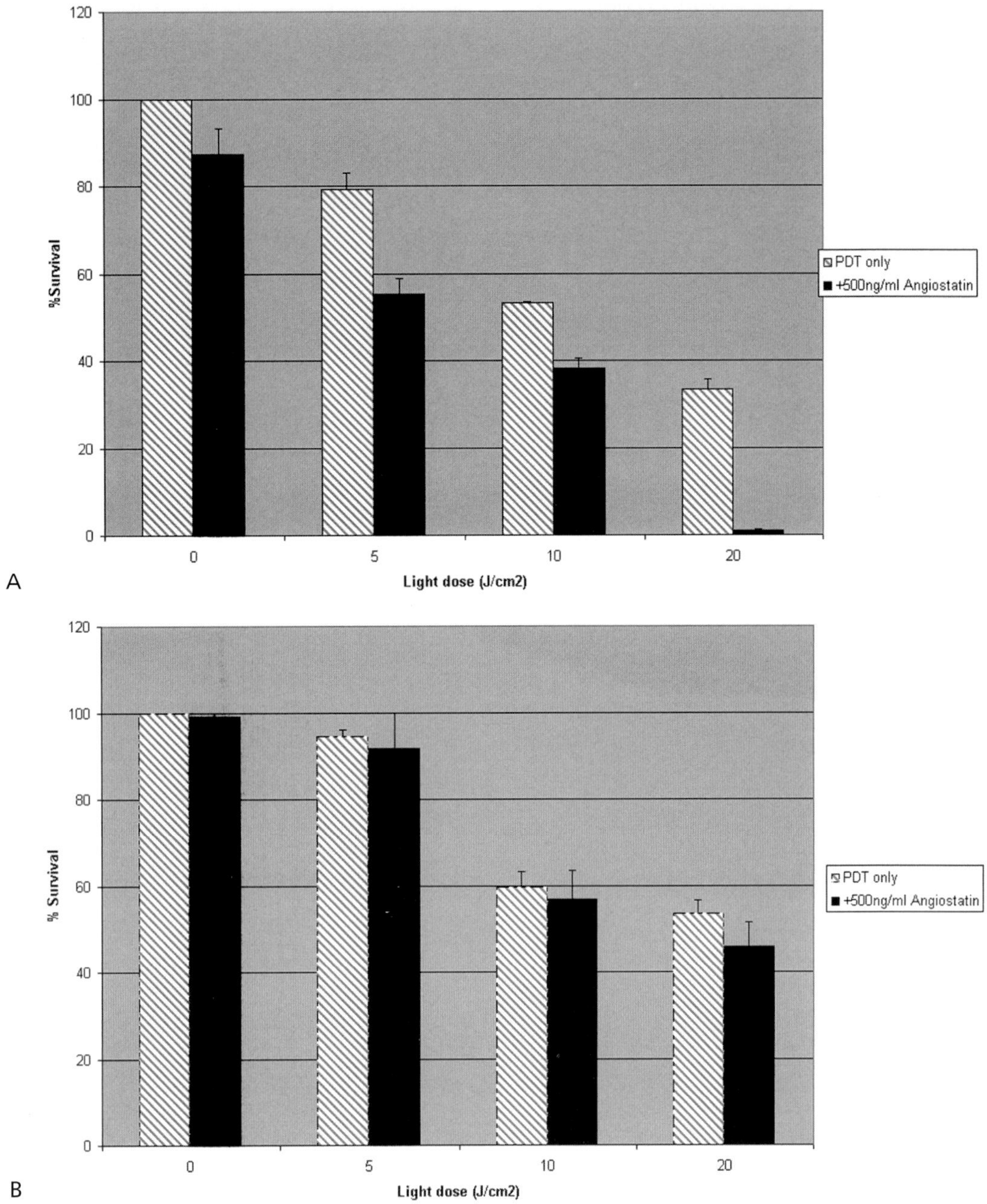

FIGURE 4.2. Bovine retinal capillary endothelial cells (BRCE) and retinal pigment epithelial cells (RPE) survival following Lu-Tex/PDT (photodynamic therapy) ± angiostatin. *In vitro* survival of **(A)** BRCE and **(B)** RPE on exposure to Lu-Tex/PDT in the presence of angiostatin. Cells were plated and exposed to angiostatin 18 hours before Lu-Tex/PDT. A 1-week proliferation assay was used to determine the surviving fraction. Data represent the mean of triplicate experiments ± standard deviation.

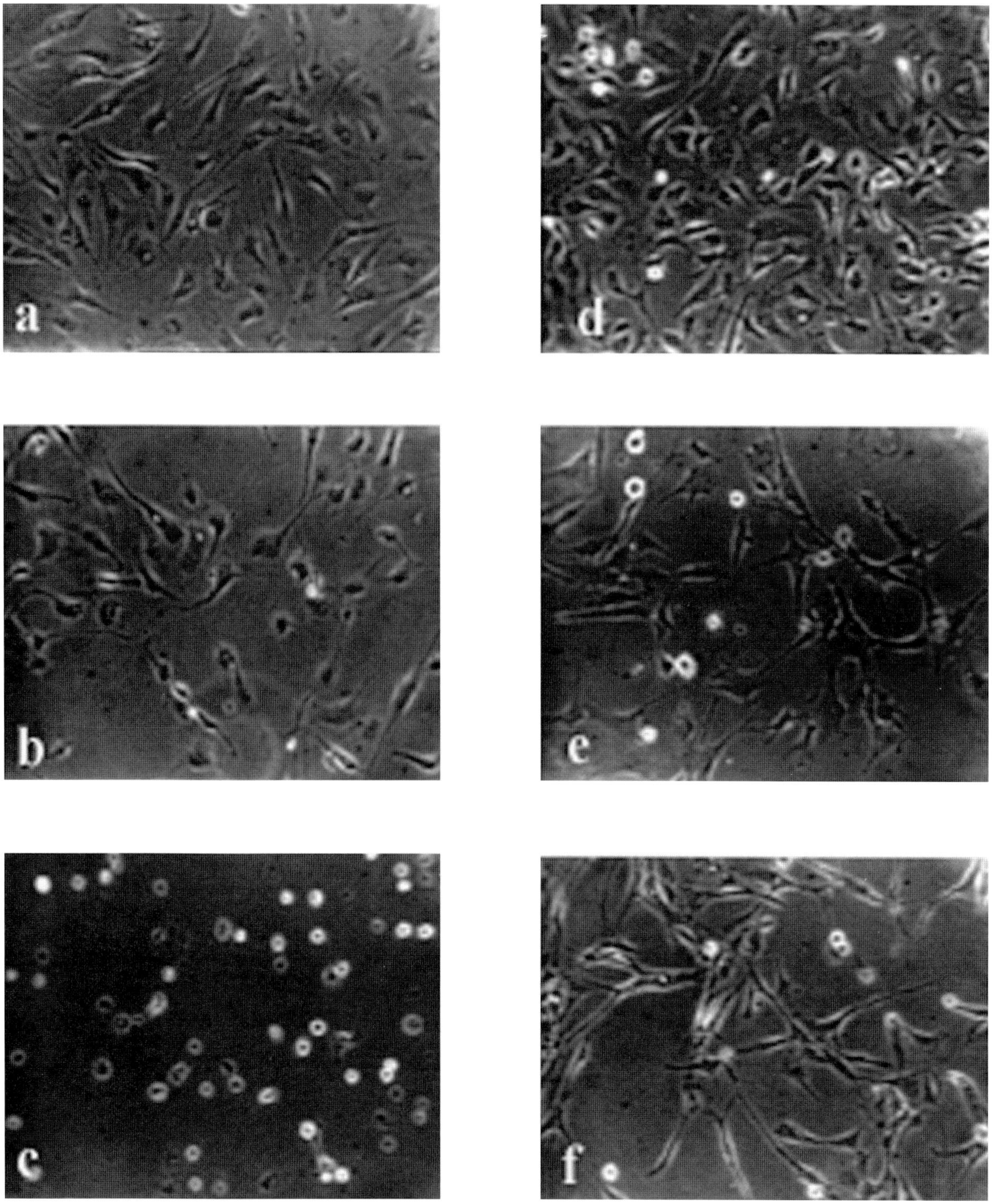

FIGURE 4.3. Bovine retinal capillary endothelial cells (BRCE) and retinal pigment epithelial cells (RPE) morphology following treatment with angiostatin and Lu-Tex/PDT (20 J/cm^2) (original magnification, 16). Micrographs are of representative fields from a 1-week proliferation assay of BRCE and RPE after treatment. **A,B,C:** BRCE treated with angiostatin only, Lu-Tex/PDT only, and (angiostatin + Lu-Tex/PDT), respectively. **D,E,F:** RPE treated with angiostatin only, Lu-Tex/PDT only, and (angiostatin + Lu-Tex/PDT), respectively. One week after PDT, some cells had disappeared, whereas those that remained regained their spindle shape and their ability to attach **(B,E).** However, in BRCE that were first primed with angiostatin followed by PDT, widespread and massive cell death was observed at 1 week. Only remnants of cells and densely refractive bodies of dying ones were seen floating in the medium **(C).** Control BRCE and RPE that were treated with angiostatin alone for 18 hours continued to proliferate and reached confluence **(A,D).** No additive effect of angiostatin to Lu-Tex/PDT was observed in RPE: RPE that were subjected to Lu-Tex/PDT alone or angiostatin and Lu-Tex/PDT appeared unchanged as evidenced by the morphology **(E,F).**

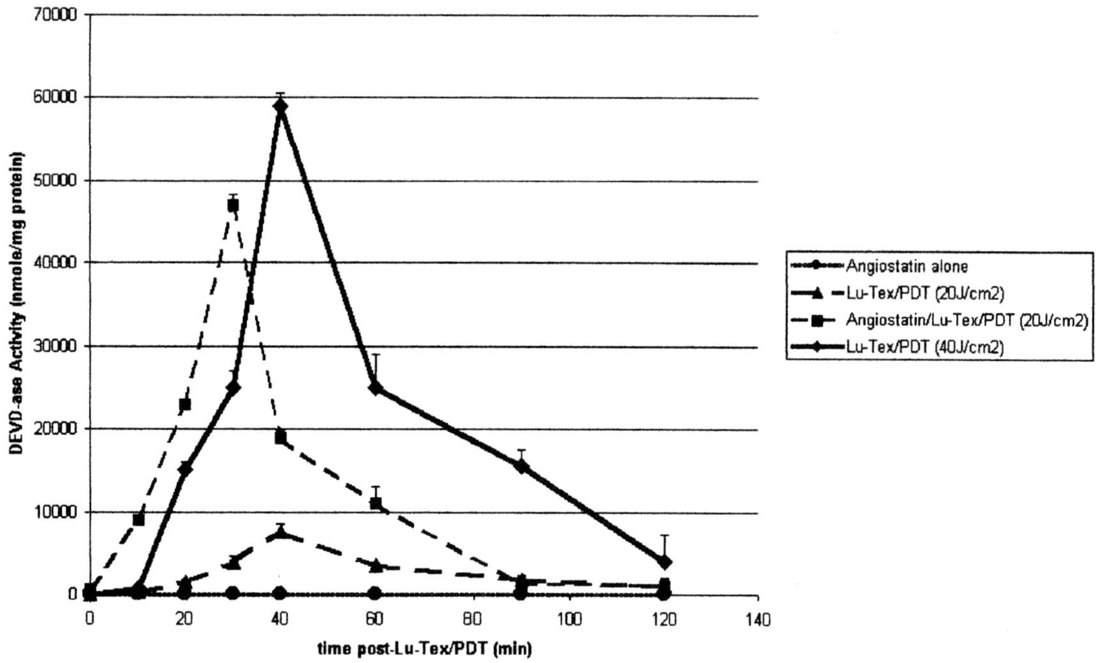

FIGURE 4.4. Caspase 3–like activity in bovine retinal capillary endothelial cells (BRCE) following angiostatin/Lu-Tex/PDT versus Lu-Tex/PDT alone. BRCE were exposed to angiostatin (500 μg/mL) alone, Lu-Tex/PDT (20 J/cm^2, 40 J/cm^2) alone, and combination of angiostatin/Lu-Tex/PDT. At the indicated times thereafter, cells were collected and lysed. Aliquots (50 μg of protein) were incubated with Ac-DEVD-AFC (DEVD-ase substrate) at 37°C for 30 minutes. The amount of fluorochrome released was determined by comparison to an aminofluoro coumarin (AFC) standard curve in lysis buffer. Data represent the means from three independent experiments.

without latency and peaks as soon as 30 minutes following PDT (rather than 40 minutes following PDT alone). One explanation for the latter is that the apoptotic cascade is primed by preincubation with angiostatin, and that the subsequent application of PDT benefited from a lowered threshold of activation to rapidly amplify the apoptotic response. It also is possible that multiple apoptotic pathways are activated by the combination of angiostatin/PDT. Photodynamic therapy is known to initiate cytotoxicity through the generation of reactive oxygen species (ROS) (15), whereas angiostatin was recently shown to act on human endothelial cells by binding to the α-subunit of adenosine triphosphate (ATP) synthase present on the cell surface (16). We also observed that although angiostatin/PDT at 20 J/cm^2 and PDT alone at 40 J/cm^2 results in 100% death of BRCE, the levels of DEVD-ase activation are significantly higher in the combined regimen. This supports the hypothesis that PDT and angiostatin/PDT operate through different apoptotic pathways in BRCE. Finally, because we have previously demonstrated that BRCE and RPE use different apoptotic pathways following PDT, these differences could be exploited to design treatments that selectively augment PDT's effect on BRCE while offering protection to the RPE and other retinal cells.

ANTIANGIOGENIC AGENTS THAT INHIBIT VEGF POTENTIATE PHOTODYNAMIC THERAPY RESPONSIVENESS

VEGF Aptamer as a Candidate Adjuvant to Photodynamic Therapy

VEGF overproduction has been identified as a major factor underlying pathologic angiogenesis *in vivo* in many ocular conditions including neovascular macular degeneration, diabetic retinopathy, retinopathy of prematurity, neovascular glaucoma, and uveitis. Endothelial cell tyrosine kinase receptors, kinase insert domain-containing receptor (KDR) and Flt-1, have been implicated in VEGF responses, including cellular migration, proliferation, and modulation of vascular permeability. Agents have been developed that limit VEGF–cellular interaction to potentially treat these neovascular conditions, particularly agents that block the activity of VEGF165, the VEGF isoforms implicated in pathologic angiogenesis. One agent is a nuclease-resistant, VEGF165-specific aptamer NX1838, EYE 001 (2′-fluoropyrimidine, RNA-based oligonucleotide/40 kDa-polyethylene glycol). Aptamers are synthesized chemically; therefore, they can be readily modified with functional groups that modulate their properties.

Data indicate that EYE 001 inhibits a variety of cellular events associated with VEGF, including dose-dependent binding to KDR and its subsequent phosphorylation and signal transduction, and human umbilical venous endothelial cells (HUVEC) cellular proliferation. Inhibition by EYE 001 was comparable to that observed with anti-VEGF monoclonal antibody, but was ineffective as an inhibitor of VEGF121-induced proliferation. These findings, coupled with nuclease stability of the molecule, suggest that EYE 001 may provide therapeutic utility (17).

The pharmacokinetics and safety of EYE 001 were established following injection into the vitreous humor of rhesus monkeys with no evidence of toxic effects or antibody response (18). Plasma and vitreous humor pharmacokinetics were determined following a single bilateral 0.25, 0.50, 1.0, 1.5, or 2.0 mg/eye and following six biweekly bilateral injections of 0.25 or 0.50 mg per eye, or following biweekly bilateral injections of 0.10 mg/eye followed by two biweekly bilateral injections of 1.0 mg per eye. Plasma and vitreous humor EYE 001 concentrations were linearly related to the dose administered. EYE 001 was cleared intact from the vitreous humor into the plasma with a half-life of approximately 94 hours, which was in agreement with the plasma terminal half-life. The no-observable-effect level was greater than six biweekly bilateral 0.50 mg/eye doses or two biweekly bilateral 1.0 mg/eye doses. These pharmacokinetics and safety data support monthly 1 or 2 mg/eye dose regimens in human clinical trials (18).

Terada and coworkers have shown a significant reduction in CNV leakage in the laser injury CNV mouse model following daily intraperitoneal injections of aptamer (10 to 100 mg aptamer/Kg body weight) initiated at the time of laser induction and continued for 2 weeks of follow-up (unpublished data).

A phase IA safety study of intravitreal EYE 001 was undertaken in 15 patients with neovascular age-related macular degeneration (AMD) and showed no significant safety issues related to the drug. Eighty percent of the patients had stable or improved vision (best corrected visual acuity) 3 months after treatment and 27% of eyes demonstrated a three-line or greater improvement in vision (19).

A phase IB multiple-dose study of intravitreal injection of EYE 001, with or without PDT, was performed on 21 patients with subfoveal CNV secondary to PDT. Results showed no significant safety issues related to the aptamer. Ophthalmic evaluation 3 months after treatment showed that 87.5% of patients who received only the VEGF-aptamer showed stable or improved vision and that 25% demonstrated a three-line or greater improvement in vision on the early treatment diabetic-retinopathy study (ETDRS) chart. A three-line gain at 3 months was observed in 60% of patients who received both the anti-VEGF aptamer and photodynamic therapy (36). Although these results are promising, these early studies were primarily safety studies, with short follow-up and no control groups. A multicenter phase III randomized, controlled clinical trial is in progress to evaluate the vision outcome in neovascular AMD using EYE 001 alone or in combination with PDT.

RhuFab V2, Anti-VEGF Antibody Fragment as a Candidate Adjuvant to Photodynamic Therapy

RhuFab V2 is the Fab portion (the antigen-binding portion) of anti-VEGF monoclonal antibody. It is a recombinant antibody that consists of two parts: a nonbinding human sequence, which makes it less antigenic in primates, and a high-affinity binding epitope derived from the mouse, which serves to bind the antigen. Its molecular weight of 48 kDa makes it a much smaller molecule than the full-length monoclonal antibody with a molecular weight of 148 kDa. Unlike the full length-antibody, rhuFab V2 has been shown to penetrate the internal limiting membrane and access the subretinal space in animal models when injected intravitreously. Therefore, rhuFab V2 potentially offers better retinal and choroidal distribution than its full-length counterpart (20).

Injection of rhuFab V2, a high-affinity recombinant human binding fragment of a monoclonal antibody directed to VEGF, prevented the formation of clinically significant CNV in a monkey model of CNV, and decreased leakage of active CNV. All eyes treated developed acute anterior chamber inflammation within 24 hours that resolved spontaneously (21). RhuFab V2 was evaluated in a clinical trial as a single intravitreal injection in subjects with neovascular AMD and found to be well tolerated (up to 500 μg) with no serious adverse events (22).

Recently we have studied the safety and efficacy of intravitreal injection of rhuFab V2 in combination with verteporfin PDT on experimental CNV in primates. Animals were divided in three groups; at 2 weeks post–laser induction (peak onset of CNV), group I started receiving weekly treatment of PDT alternating with rhuFab V2 injection or vehicle; group II, weekly treatment of rhuFab V2 or vehicle alternating with PDT; group III, bimonthly treatment of both rhuFab V2 or vehicle and PDT for a total of 6 weeks. Eleven of 11 eyes treated with the combination showed no leakage from CNV angiographically up to the 6 weeks of follow up. In those animals treated with placebo injections and PDT only, seven of 11 eyes showed no leakage at 3 weeks; nine of 11 eyes showed no leakage at 6 weeks. The data suggest that intravitreal rhuFab V2 in combination with verteporfin PDT causes greater reduction in angiographic leakage than PDT in experimental CNV (23). Clinical trials testing the long-term efficacy of intravitreal rhuFab with or without PDT are anticipated.

Other Anti-VEGF Agents

Other anti-VEGF agents have been studied in combination with PDT in tumor models. IM862 is a dipeptide of L-glutamyl-L-tryptophan (24), which is shown to inhibit angiogenesis in the chick chorioallantoic membrane bioassay and inhibit VEGF production in cells of monocytic lineage. IM862 inhibits tumor growth in xenograft models but has no direct cytotoxic effect on tumor cells, and probably mediates these effects by inhibiting VEGF production and activating natural killer cells.

Photofrin PDT with and without IM862 was studied in a transplantable BA mouse mammary carcinoma model. Photodynamic therapy treatment parameters produced a moderate cure rate when used alone, and were combined with IM862 administered daily by intraperitoneal injections (25 mg/kg) for 10 days starting 1 hour prior to PDT treatment. The antiangiogenic treatment statistically enhanced the tumoricidal action of PDT as measured by tumor cures. Specifically, Photofrin PDT at 200 J/cm^2 gave a 39% cure rate, whereas Photofrin PDT plus IM862 gave a tumor cure rate of 78%. IM862 used alone did not produce any tumor cures or tumor regression and only slightly modified tumor growth parameters (25).

COMBINING ANTIANGIOGENIC ACTIVITY OF SELECT RECEPTOR TYROSINE KINASE INHIBITORS WITH PHOTODYNAMIC THERAPY FOR TUMOR MODELS

Platelet-derived growth factor (PDGF), basic fibroblast growth factor (bFGF), epidermal growth factor (EGF), and VEGF are all potent, endogenous mitogens of physiologic angiogenesis. All of these factors use receptors that contain a cytoplasmic tyrosine kinase (TK) that initiates signaling pathways affecting endothelial cell proliferation and differentiation (26,27). The roles of these growth factors in coordinating blood vessel development are not clearly understood, but recent reports suggest that these growth factors regulate, although differentially, *de novo* synthesis of blood vessels, vascular remodeling, and angiogenesis (28,29). Another antiangiogenic approach is to target the TK receptors.

PD166285, a broad-spectrum receptor tyrosine kinase (RTK) inhibitor (30,31), and PDI173074, a selective FGFR1 TK inhibitor (32,33), were evaluated for their antiangiogenic activity and antitumor efficacy in combination with Photofrin PDT (32–34). On the day after treatment of murine mammary 16c tumor model with Photofrin-PDT, PD166285 (5 to 10 mg/kg) or PD173074 (30 to 60 mg/kg) were administered orally daily for a period of 28 days. Mice treated with PDT alone showed no significant increase in tumor growth delay when compared with the untreated control group. However, combining PDT and follow-up treatment for 14 days with PD166285 or PD173074 resulted in a dramatic increase in the tumor-free interval. In addition, most animals treated with PDT in combination with PD166285 and PD173074 for 28 days displayed even greater tumor growth delays. In most cases, tumors began to regrow about a week after discontinuing the TK inhibitor whether at 14 or 28 days, confirming the cytostatic nature of those antiangiogenic agents and suggesting the need to employ maintenance-type treatments when utilizing these types of agents (40). To date, the effect of PDT and TK inhibition has not been studied in models of neovascularization.

ANGIOSTATIC STEROIDS IN COMBINATION WITH PHOTODYNAMIC THERAPY

Angiostatic steroids are another class of compounds that have been tested in tumor and neovascularization models. The angiostatic steroid, anecortave acetate (AA), has been shown to inhibit blood vessel growth in multiple preclinical models, including the chick chorioallantoic membrane bioassay, the rabbit corneal pocket, the murine and rat models of oxygen-induced retinopathy (35), and bFGF-induced subretinal neovascularization in the rabbit. Clinical studies using topical administration of anecortave acetate in patients with recurrent pterygium resulted in inhibition of vessel growth. In the subsequent phase III study, 394 patients were treated for more than 1 year, with no clinically significant safety issues. Anecortave acetate has been promised as a treatment for neovascular AMD, and 22 centers are currently evaluating subtenon's retrobulbar anecortave acetate with or without verteporfin/PDT in patients with subfoveal CNV secondary to AMD (36).

PHOTODYNAMIC THERAPY IN COMBINATION WITH IONIZING RADIATION

Ionizing radiation has been proposed as a treatment modality for neovascular AMD. Combined PDT and ionizing radiation has been tested in tumor cell lines. The effect of PDT using aminolevulinic acid (5-ALA), a precursor of the active photosensitizer protoporphyrin IX combined with gamma irradiation, was investigated in several human head and neck tumor cell lines. Results indicate that such a combination has an additive effect (37). We have some limited clinical experience using PDT to treat CNV of patients who were first treated with proton beam radiation (JW Miller, unpublished data), which indicates that such a combination is safe.

SUMMARY

Combination therapy of antiangiogenic agents and PDT may enhance outcomes of therapy for neovascular AMD and other diseases. Work in our laboratory suggests that certain combinations may actually produce a synergistic effect on microvascular endothelium. In addition, antiangiogenic therapy may lead to reduced leakage from CNV and more prolonged closure of CNV. Various candidate agents have been tested *in vitro*, in experimental models, and in clinical studies in some cases. These and additional studies will determine the drugs and methodology of combined therapy to yield the best vision outcomes for patients.

REFERENCES

1. Husain D, Miller JW, Michaud N, et al. Intravenous infusion of liposomal benzoporphyrin derivative for photodynamic therapy of experimental choroidal neovascularization. *Arch Ophtalmol* 1996;114:978–985.
2. Husain D, Miller J. Photodynamic therapy of exudative age-related macular degeneration. *Semin Ophthalmol* 1997;12:14–25.
3. Miller J, Walsh AW, Kramer M, et al. Photodynamic therapy of experimental choroidal neovascularization using lipoprotein-delivered benzoporphyrin. *Arch Ophthalmol* 1995;113: 810–818.
4. Kramer M, Miller JW, Michaud N, et al. Liposomal benzoporphyrin derivative verteporfin photodynamic therapy: selective treatment of choroidal neovascularization in monkeys. *Ophthalmology* 1996;103:427–438.
5. Miller JW, Schmidt-Erfurth U, Sickenberg M, et al. Photodynamic therapy for choroidal neovascularization due to age-related macular degeneration with Verteporfin: results of a single treatment in a phase I and II study. *Arch Ophthalmol* 1999;117:1161–1173.
6. TAP Study Group, Treatment of Age-Related Macular Degeneration with Photodynamic Therapy (TAP) Study Group. Verteporfin (Visudyne) therapy of subfoveal choroidal neovascularization in age-related macular degeneration. One year results of two randomized clinical trials. *Arch Ophthalmol* 1999;117:1329–1345.
7. Bressler N, TS group. Photodynamic therapy of subfoveal choroidal neovascularization in related age macular degeneration with verteporfin: two-year results of randomized clinical trials. *Arch Ophthalmol* 2001;119:198–207.
8. O'Reilly M, Holmgren L, Shing Y, et al. Angiostatin: a novel angiogenesis inhibitor that mediates the suppression of metastases by a Lewis lung carcinoma. *Cell* 1994;79:315–328.
9. O'Reilly M, Holmgren L, Chen C, et al. Angiostatin induces and sustains dormancy of human primary tumors in mice. *Nat Med* 1996;2:689–692.
10. Gorski D, Mauceri HJ, Salloum RM, et al. Potentiation of the antitumor effect of ionizing radiation by brief concomitant exposures to angiostatin. *Cancer Res* 1998;58:5686–5689.
11. Mauceri H, Hanna NN, Beckett MA, et al. Combined effects of angiostatin and ionizing radiation in antitumour therapy. *Nature* 1998;394:287–291.
12. Renno RZ, Delori FC, Holzer RA, et al. Photodynamic therapy using Lu-Tex induces apoptosis in vitro and shows potentiate action combined with angiostatin in retinal capillary endothelial cells. *Invest Ophthalmol Vis Sci* 2000;41:3963–3971.
13. Lai CC, Wu WC, Chen SL, et al. Suppression of choroidal neovascularization by adeno-associated virus vector expressing angiostatin. *Invest Ophthalmol Vis Sci* 2001;42:2401–2407.
14. Drixler T, Rinkes IH, Ritchie ED, et al. Angiostatin inhibits pathological but not physiological retinal angiogenesis. *Invest Ophthalmol Vis Sci* 2001;42:3325–3330.
15. Weishaupt K, Gomer C, Dougherty T. Identification of singlet oxygen as the cytotoxic agent in photoinactivation of a murine tumor. *Cancer Res* 1976;36:2326–2329.
16. Moser TL, Stack MS, Asplin I, et al. Angiostatin binds ATP synthase on the surface of human endothelial cells. *Proc Natl Acad Sci USA* 1999;96:2811–2816.
17. Bell C, Lynam E, Landfair DJ, et al. Oligonucleotide NX1838 inhibits VEGF165-mediated cellular responses in vitro. *In Vitro Cell Dev Biol Anim* 1999;35:533–542.
18. Drolet DW, Nelson J, Tucker CE, et al. Pharmacokinetics and safety of an anti-vascular endothelial growth factor aptamer (NX1838) following injection into the vitreous humor of rhesus monkeys. *Pharmacol Res* 2000;17:1503–1510.
19. The Eyetech Study Group. Preclinical and phase 1A clinical evaluation of an anti-VEGF pegylated aptamer (EYE001) for the treatment of exudative age-related macular degeneration. *Retina* 2002;22:143–152.
20. Mordenti J, Thomsen K, Licko V, et al. Efficacy and concentration-response of murine anti-VEGF monoclonal antibody in tumor-bearing mice and extrapolation to humans. *Toxicol Pathol* 1999;27:14–21.
21. Krzystolik M, Afshari MA, Adamis AP, et al. Prevention of experimental choroidal neovascularization with intravitreal anti-vascular endothelial growth factor antibody fragment. *Arch Ophthalmol* 2002;120:338–346.
22. Schwartz S, Blumenkranz M, Rosenfeld P, et al. Safety of rhuFab V2, an anti-VEGF antibody fragment, as a single intravitreal injection in subjects with neovascular age-related macular degeneration. *ARVO* 2001.
23. Gauthier D, Husain D, Kim I, et al. Safety and efficacy of intravitreal injection of rhuFab VEGF in combination with verteporfin PDT on experimental choroidal neovascularization. *ARVO* 2002.
24. Tulpule A, Scadden DT, Espina BM, et al. Results of a randomized study of IM862 nasal solution in the treatment of AIDS-related Kaposi's sarcoma. *J Cin Oncol* 2000;18:716–723.
25. Ferrario A, von Tiehl KF, Rucker N, et al. Antiangiogenic treatment enhances photodynamic therapy responsiveness in a mouse mammary carcinoma. *Cancer Res* 2000;60:4066–4069.
26. Merenmies J, Parada L, Henkemeyer M. Receptor tyrosine kinase signaling in vascular development. *Cell Growth Diff* 1997;8: 3–10.
27. Tronick S, Aaronson S. Growth factors and signal transduction. In: Mendelsohn J, Howley PM, Israel MA, et al., eds. *The molecular basis of cancer.* Philadelphia: WB Saunders, 1995:114–117.
28. Plate K, Breier G, Weich HA, et al. Vascular endothelial growth factor is a potential tumour angiogenesis factor in human gliomas in vivo. *Nature* 1992;359:843–845.
29. Risau W. Mechanisms of angiogenesis. *Nature* 1997;386:671–674.
30. Connolly C, et al. Discovery and structure-activity studies of a novel series of pyrido(2,3-D)pyrimidine tyrosine kinase inhibitors. *Bioorg Med Chem Letts* 1997;7:2415–2420.
31. Panek RL, Lu GH, Klutchko SR, et al. In vitro pharmacological characterization of PD166285, a new nanomolar potent and broadly active protein kinase inhibitor. *J Pharmacol Exp Ther* 1997;283:1433–1444.
32. Hamby J, Connolly CJ, Schroeder MC, et al. Structure-activity relationships for a novel series of pyrido(2,3-D)pyrimidine tyrosine kinase inhibitors. *J Med Chem* 1997;40:2296–2303.
33. Mohammadi M, Froum S, Hamby JM, et al. Crystal structure of an angiogenesis inhibitor bound to FGF receptor tyrosine kinase domain. *EMBO J* 1998;17:5896–5904.

34. Dimitroff CJ, Klohs W, Sharma A, et al. Antiangiogenic activity of selected receptor tyrosine kinase inhibitors, PD166285 and PD173074: implications for combination treatment with photodynamic therapy. *Invest New Drugs* 1999;17:121–135.
35. Penn JS, Rajaratnam VS, Collier RJ, et al. The effect of an angiostatic steroid on neovascularization in a rat model of retinopathy of prematurity. *Invest Ophthalmol Vis Sci* 2001;42: 283–290.
36. Singerman L, et al. Sub-tenon's retrobulbar anecortave acetate with and without Visudyne photodynamic therapy (PDT) in patients with subfoveal choroidal neovascularization (CNV) in age-related macular degeneration (AMD). *ARVO* 2001.
37. Allman R, Cowburn P, Mason M. Effect of photodynamic therapy in combination with ionizing radiation on human squamous cell carcinoma cell lines of the head and neck. *Br J Cancer* 2000; 83:655–661.

5

VERTEPORFIN PDT FOR EXPERIMENTAL CHOROIDAL NEOVASCULARIZATION

JOAN W. MILLER
EVANGELOS S. GRAGOUDAS

As discussed in Chapter 1, investigations of photodynamic therapy (PDT) of tumors demonstrated that vascular thrombosis played a role in tumor destruction. Studies were undertaken by a number of investigators to test the ability of PDT using various photosensitizers to occlude normal and neovascular vessels, including choroidal neovascularization (CNV) in animal models (1–3). Vascular occlusion was observed using a number of photosensitizers, but the issue of selectivity of CNV occlusion was not addressed. These early studies were limited in part by the characteristics of the available photosensitizers. In the late 1980s, a second-generation porphyrin, benzoporphyrin derivative monoacid (BPD, also known as verteporfin) was developed. Verteporfin is lipophilic, and must be dissolved in an organic solvent such as DMSO or used in a liposomal formulation for intravenous use. It absorbs well at 690 nm and is cleared rapidly from the body. In a series of publications, Allison, Levy, and Richter demonstrated its effectiveness as a photosensitizing agent *in vitro* and *in vivo* (4–9). The first ocular PDT experiments using verteporfin were carried out in a rabbit model of choroidal melanoma by Schmidt, Bauman, and others working under the direction of Dr. Gragoudas (10). Using 2 mg/kg of BPD dissolved in DMSO and complexed to low-density lipoprotein (LDL), they showed effective treatment of tumors with complete necrosis of the tumors, when irradiation was performed 3 hours after BPD injection, using 692 light at 150 mW/cm^2 and 100 J/cm^2. Complications included transient vitreitis and a self-limited exudative retinal detachment in 50% of treated eyes, which largely resolved within 48 hours. Vascular damage was a prominent feature after PDT with verteporfin and a series of experiments were designed to evaluate the effect of PDT on normal choroidal vessels in the rabbit eye (11). Closure of choriocapillaris and some large choroidal vessels was achieved using BPD in DSMO at a dose of 2 mg/kg, with light doses of 10, 50, or 100 J/cm^2 and irradiance of 100 mW/cm^2, and irradiation within 30 minutes or at 3 hours, although choriocapillaris was closed using 10 J/cm^2 and irradiation at 3 hours. Damage throughout the retina was observed in almost all cases. In addition, damage to retinal pigment epithelium (RPE) and photoreceptors was observed in all cases, with the least damage observed with the lowest light dose and irradiation at 3 hours. The experiments were able to demonstrate the ability of PDT with BPD to close choriocapillaris.

Miller and Gragoudas proposed investigating PDT of CNV with verteporfin, in order to test whether PDT using verteporfin could achieve selective occlusion of CNV without damaging retinal vessels, large choroidal vessels, or neurosensory retina. Testing this hypothesis had to be done in a retina with dual circulation, preferably a primate. The well-characterized laser injury model of CNV in the monkey was selected, and collateral damage was assessed by performing PDT in normal eyes.

Studies in CNV were carried out with both BPD dissolved in DMSO and liposomal BPD, also known as verteporfin. The first CNV studies were performed with BPD dissolved in DMSO and mixed with LDL because liposomal BPD or verteporfin was not available for preclinical studies, with only limited quantities being produced for ongoing clinical trials in dermatology. Initial treatment parameters included a drug dose of 1 and 2 mg/kg, fluence of 50, 75, 100, and 150 J/cm^2, and irradiance of 150 mW/cm^2 (Table 5.1) (12). Laser irradiation was performed using a modified argon/dye laser and slit-lamp delivery using a plano contact lens and a spot size of 1250 µm. Irradiation was performed earlier than in the tumor models, because it was hypothesized that this would be more effective in treating neovasculature based on previous work (13). Fluorescein angiography 1 hour after PDT variable of CNV and histology demonstrated fibrin and neutrophils in the vessels of the CNV and choriocapillaris. By 24 hours, angiography demonstrated early hypofluorescence in the area of treatment indicating occlusion of the CNV with late staining beginning at the edge of the treatment spot (Fig. 5.1). In some areas, staining of retinal vessels was observed,

TABLE 5.1. ANGIOGRAPHIC CLOSURE OF CHOROIDAL NEOVASCULARIZATION USING LIPOSOMAL BPD (VERTEPORFIN) AND BPD-LDL IN DMSO

Drug formulation	Intravenous	Dye dose mg/kg	Fluence J/cm²	Irradiance mW/cm²	Number of lesions (CNV)	Time (min) of irradiation after dye injection	Duration of irradiation (min)	CNV closure
BPD-LDL in DMSO	Bolus	2	50	150	2	18 and 38	5.6	2/2
BPD-LDL in DMSO	Bolus	2	75	150	1	81	8.3	1/1
BPD-LDL in DMSO	Bolus	2	100	150	1	22	11.2	1/1
BPD-LDL in DMSO	Bolus	1	50	150	2	5 and 30	5.6	0/2
BPD-LDL in DMSO	Bolus	1	100	150	3	1, 2, and 5	11.2	3/3
BPD-LDL in DMSO	Bolus	1	150	150	4	14, 18, 20, and 43	16.6	3/4
BPD-LDL in DMSO	Bolus	1	150	300	2	5 and 53	8.3	2/2
BPD-LDL in DMSO	Bolus	1	150	600	2	22 and 69	4.2	2/2
Verteporfin (Liposomal BPD)	Bolus	1	150	600	14	5–120	4.2	14/14
Verteporfin	Bolus	0.5	150	600	8	<60	4.2	7/8
Verteporfin	Bolus	0.5	150	600	3	60–80	4.2	0/3
Verteporfin	Bolus	0.375	150	600	20	<50	4.2	17/20
Verteporfin	Bolus	0.375	150	600	11	50–100	4.2	5/11
Verteporfin	Bolus	0.25	150	600	2	<20	4.2	2/2
Verteporfin	Bolus	0.25	150	600	4	Between 20 and 40	4.2	2/4
Verteporfin	Bolus	0.25	150	600	8	≥40	4.2	1/8
Verteporfin	Infusion 32 min	0.375	150	600	8	<50	4.2	8/8
Verteporfin	Infusion 32 min	0.375	150	600	14	Between 50 and 80	4.2	6/14
Verteporfin	Infusion 32 min	0.375	150	600	8	>80	4.2	0/8
Verteporfin	Infusion 10 min	0.375	150	600	1	30	4.2	1/1

From Miller JW, Walsh AW, Kramer M, et al. Photodynamic therapy of experimental choroidal neovascularization using lipoprotein-delivered benzoporphyrin. *Arch Ophthalmol* 1995;113:810–818; Kramer M, Miller JW, Michaud N, et al. Liposomal BPD verteporfin photodynamic therapy: selective treatment of choroidal neovascularization in monkeys. *Ophthalmology* 1996;103:427–438; Husain D, Miller JW, Michaud N, et al. Intravenous infusion using liposomal benzoporphyrin derivative verteporfin for photodynamic therapy of experimental choroidal neovascularization. *Arch Ophthalmol* 1996;114:978–985, with permission.

particularly when irradiation was performed early (within 5 minutes) of BPD injection. Histology at 24 hours after PDT showed necrotic or absent endothelium in the CNV, with fibrin, platelets, neutrophils, and red blood cells (Fig. 5.2). The choriocapillaris was similarly injured, with necrotic or absent endothelium and visible thrombi. The RPE was typically necrotic and some pyknosis of the outer nuclear layer was noted. At the higher drug dose of 2 mg/kg, the larger choroidal vessels showed some loss of endothelium, but this was not seen when a dose of 1 mg/kg was used, except when irradiation was performed in the first 5 minutes after drug administration. Additionally, endothelial cells of the retinal vessels showed vacuolization of the cytoplasm when irradiation was performed within the first 5 minutes. One treated CNV lesion followed for 8 days showed persistent closure of CNV with no vessels noted in the treated CNV but with patent choriocapillaris under the lesion. Because the laser injury model caused significant disruption of retinal architecture, additional studies were performed using the same PDT parameters to treat areas of normal retina/choroid.

The irradiance of 150 mW/cm² was used in the initial studies because PDT had typically been performed at irradiances of less than 200 mW/cm², in order to avoid thermal effect, and in some instances, pain during treatment (14,15). However, it was noted that irradiances at these levels led to treatment times over 10 to 15 minutes, which were judged impractical for ophthalmic clinical practice (12). To test whether higher irradiances led to significant thermal injury, experiments were carried out using BPD in normal primate eyes with irradiances of 150 to 1,800 mW/cm², looking for denaturation of collagen fibrils by electron microscopy (16). These experiments demonstrated no evidence of denaturation even at irradiances as high as 1,800 mW/cm², although some damage to choroidal vessels was noted at 1,200 mW/cm². Photodynamic therapy of CNV using irradiances of 300 and 600 mW/cm², and PDT of normal retina/choroid at 600 mW/cm² was effective and selective (12,17). The mild hyperthermia that may be produced with higher irradiances may act synergistically with PDT to potentiate cell killing (18). Interestingly, investigations of PDT for AMD using other photosensitizers have adopted the higher irradiance of 600 mW/cm² as the standard irradiance parameter (19).

The first experimental work on PDT of CNV using BPD demonstrated effective closure of CNV with several

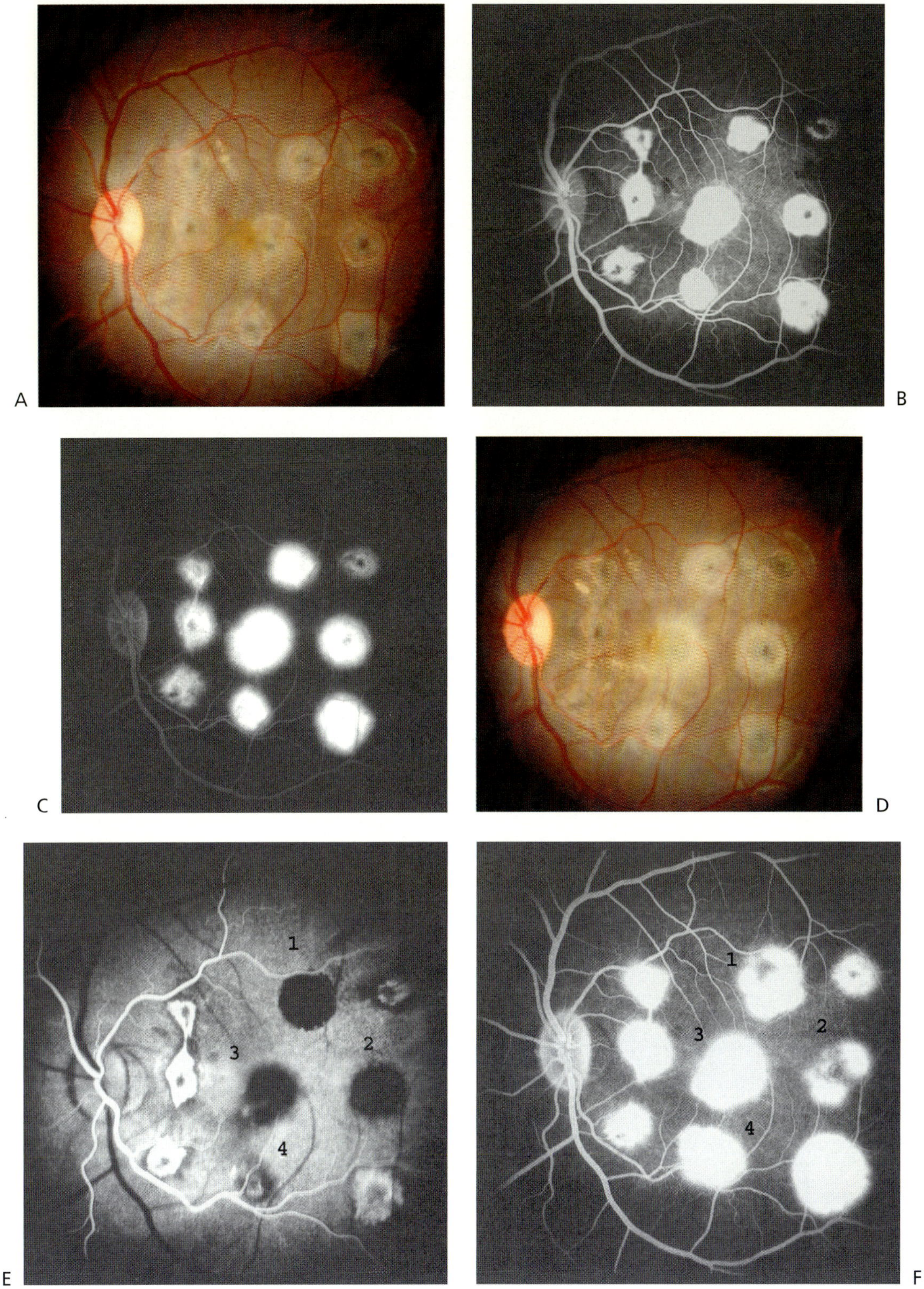

FIGURE 5.1. Photodynamic therapy (PDT) closure of choroidal neovascularization (CNV) using 0.5 mg/kg of liposomal BPD (verteporfin). **A:** Color fundus photograph of CNV before PDT. Argon laser burns were placed 1 month previously. **B and C:** Fluorescein angiogram of CNV before PDT. Areas of CNV show hyperfluorescence in the early frame **(B),** with leakage in the later frame **(C). D:** Color fundus photograph 24 hours after PDT using 0.5 mg/kg verteporfin, 150 J/cm^2 and 600 mW/cm^2. There is mild deep retinal whitening in the treated areas compared with the pre-PDT photograph. **E and F:** Fluorescein angiogram 24 hours after PDT. The time of light application after drug administration was 10 minutes for lesion 1, 20 minutes for lesion 2, 40 minutes for lesion 3, and 50 minutes for lesion 4. Lesion 4 shows some persistent hyperfluorescence in the area corresponding to CNV, whereas lesions 1, 2, and 3 demonstrate hypofluorescence in the early frame of the angiogram and late leakage originating from the rim of the treatment spot. The areas of CNV that were not irradiated appear unchanged with early hyperfluorescence and leakage. (From: Kramer M, Miller JW, Michaud N, et al. Liposomal BPD verteporfin photodynamic therapy: selective treatment of choroidal neovascularization in monkeys. *Ophthalmology* 1996;103:430, with permission.)

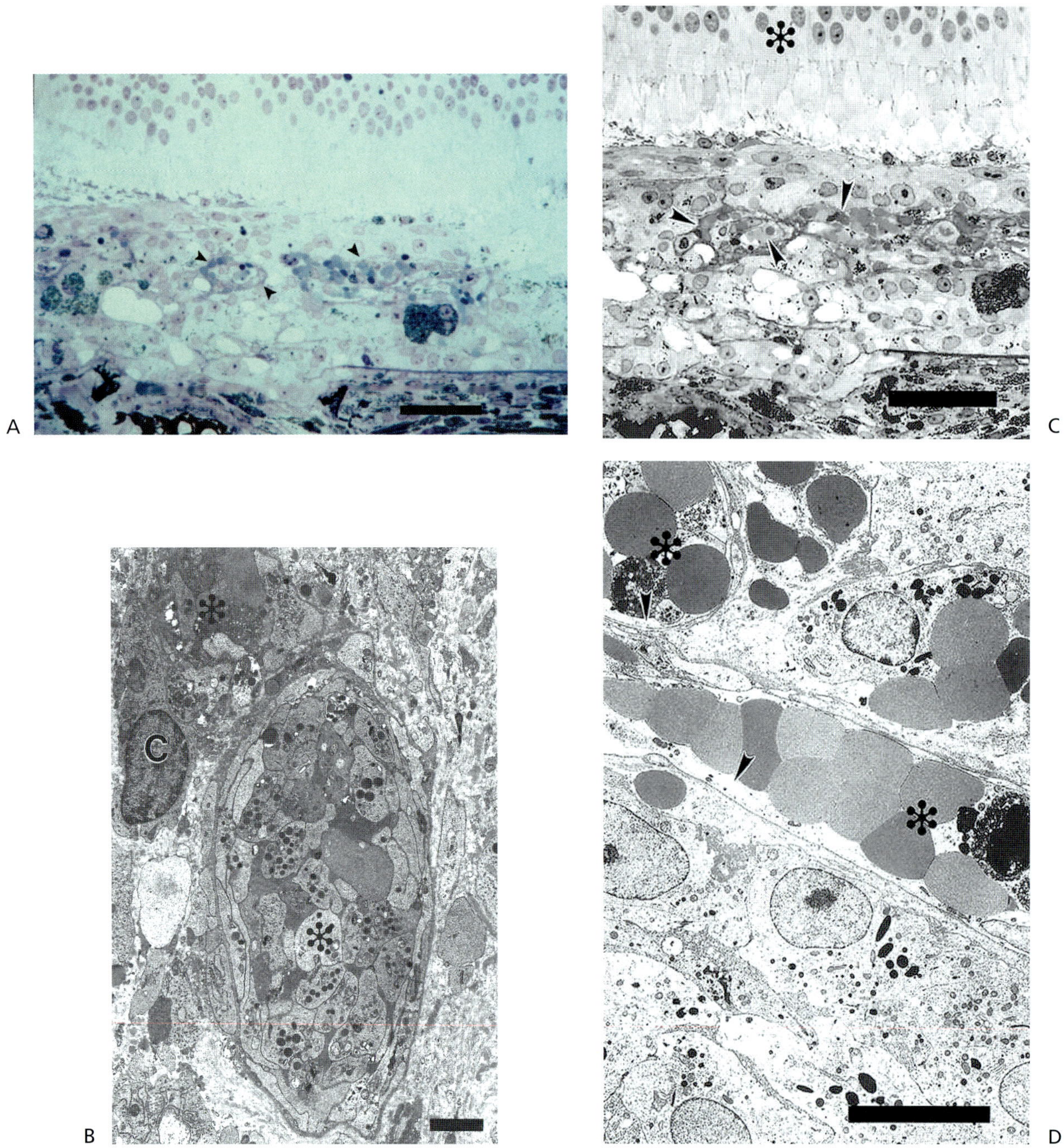

FIGURE 5.2. Photomicrographs of treated choroidal neovascularization (CNV). **A and B:** The CNV was examined 24 hours after photodynamic therapy (PDT) using 0.375 mg/kg verteporfin, irradiated 20 minutes after drug injection, and using 150 J/cm^2 and 600 mW/cm^2. **A:** Light micrograph shows occluded CNV *(arrowheads)* and choriocapillaris; however, the larger choroidal vessels remain patent. Note the lack of damage to other cells and structures (bar = 25 μm). **B:** Electron micrograph of the same occluded CNV shows two vessels *(asterisks)* filled with platelets and erythrocytes. The endothelium has been stripped and there is cellular debris around the vessels as well as a viable cell **(C). C:** Light micrograph of CNV 24 hours after PDT using 0.375 mg/kg verteporfin delivered over 32 minutes with irradiation applied at the end of drug infusion. New vessels in the CNV are closed *(arrowheads)* and there is extravasation of red blood cells. Nonvascular cells are undamaged. Outer nuclear cells also appear undamaged *(asterisk)* (toluidine blue, bar = 50 μm). **D:** Transmission electron micrograph of CNV shown in top panel. Damage to vasculature of CNV is seen as occlusion by red and white blood cells and platelets *(asterisks),* with damage to endothelium *(arrowheads).* Extravasation of red blood cells and survival of metaplastic retinal pigment epithelial cells is seen. (Uranyl acetate, bar = 50 μm) (From: Kramer M, Miller JW, Michaud N, et al. Liposomal BPD verteporfin photodynamic therapy: selective treatment of choroidal neovascularization in monkeys. *Ophthalmology* 1996;103:432; Husain D, Miller JW, Michaud N, et al. Intravenous infusion using liposomal benzoporphyrin derivative verteporfin for photodynamic therapy of experimental choroidal neovascularization. *Arch Ophthalmol* 1996;114:982, with permission.)

treatment regimens. Unlike the findings in tumors, or PDT of experimental CNV with other photosensitizers, no serous retinal detachment, retinal or subretinal hemorrhage, or posttreatment inflammation was noted. The lower drug dose of 1 mg/kg caused less injury to surrounding structures than was noted using 2 mg/kg and irradiation more than 5 minutes after drug injection appeared to avoid damage to retinal vessels. When the drug dose was lowered from 2 to 1 mg/kg, the fluence required to close CNV appeared to increase from 50 to 100 J/cm^2. Higher irradiances of 300 and 600 mW/cm^2 appeared effective and safe and provided a more practical therapy.

Photodynamic therapy using BPD appeared to provide an effective and relatively selective means to treat CNV. Additional studies were undertaken to refine the dosimetry using the liposomal formulation of BPD, or verteporfin that would be used in clinical practice (17). A series of experiments was designed to use verteporfin PDT in experimental CNV and normal eyes, modifying drug dose and timing of irradiation with fluence and irradiance fixed at 150 J/cm^2 and 600 mW/cm^2, respectively. The verteporfin drug doses tested were 0.25, 0.375, 0.5, and 1 mg/kg with irradiation performed between 5 and 120 minutes after drug administration. The spot size used was 1,250 μm, which covered the area of CNV. A total of 69 areas of CNV were treated and effective CNV closure was achieved at all tested drug doses, as determined by angiographic assessment 1 day after PDT. As the drug dose was reduced, the effective time window for irradiation was shortened. For instance, using 1 mg/kg of verteporfin and the light dose specified in the preceding, CNV could be effectively treated with irradiation performed any time between 5 and 120 minutes after drug administration. However, there were some selectivity concerns at this drug dose (see the following). Using 0.5 mg/kg of verteporfin, irradiation had to be performed within 60 minutes to achieve CNV closure, and using 0.375 mg/kg, irradiation had to be performed within 50 minutes. The drug dose of 0.25 mg/kg appeared to be threshold at these light doses, with effective closure occurring only when irradiation was performed within 20 minutes of drug injection. Histologic findings were similar to those described for the BPD in DMSO study.

Because the laser injury model necessarily showed damage to the outer retina secondary to the thermal laser injury, we investigated the selectivity of PDT in normal eyes. We developed a histologic grading scheme based on damage to the outer nuclear layer (ONL), damage to retinal vessels and large choroidal vessels, and neurosensory retina (17) (Table 5.2). We proposed that unacceptable damage was any of the following: pyknosis of the ONL greater than 50%, damage to retinal vessels, or damage to large choroidal vessels. Some damage to RPE was noted even at the lowest treatment doses, and there was associated RPE damage and some disruption of the photoreceptors when closure of choriocapillaris was achieved. A cutoff for acceptable damage was defined and included pyknosis of the ONL of less than 50%, mild disruption of the outer segments, choriocapillaris occlusion, and RPE necrosis. The closure of the choriocapillaris in normal choroid followed a similar pattern as the closure of CNV, in terms of drug and light doses, and timing of irradiation. As with closure of CNV, 0.25 mg/kg seemed to be the threshold dose for closure of choriocapillaris, achieved with almost no effect on the overlying retina. When PDT was performed using drug doses of 0.5, 0.375, and 0.25 mg/kg, the retinal structure was well preserved (Fig. 5.3). In no case was retinal detachment or hemorrhage observed. Reducing the drug dosage resulted in more selective closure of the choriocapillaris with minimal damage to the adjacent tissues. The RPE was typically damaged at all dye doses, and there was mild damage to photoreceptor inner and outer segments at all doses, ranging from minimal swelling to more pronounced vacuolization and disarray. Irradiation within 10 minutes of verteporfin administration at a variety of doses caused damage of retinal vessels, or Grade 5 damage, and was deemed unacceptable. At a verteporfin dose of 0.375 mg/kg, irradiation at 20 minutes or longer after the administration of verteporfin, typically led to closure of choriocapillaris and RPE necrosis, with pyknosis in the ONL of less than 50%, and no damage to retinal or large choroidal vessels, that is, Grade 4 or less. Combining the results of the CNV closure and the effects on normal retina/choroids, optimal treatment parameters appeared to be verteporfin 0.375 mg/kg (approximately 6 mg/m^2), 150 J/cm^2, 600 mW/cm^2, and irradiation between 20 and 50 minutes after administration of verteporfin (Table 5.3).

All of the ocular preclinical work to date had used a bolus intravenous infusion of BPD, either dissolved in DMSO or as the liposomal preparation. However, the clinical trials in dermatology were performed using a 30-minute intravenous infusion, and concerns arose regarding the rapid administration of a liposomal formulation. No systemic effects had been noted in the animals studied to date; nevertheless, studies were undertaken to compare the efficacy of an intravenous infusion (20). An infusion of liposomal verteporfin was administered over 10 minutes (fast infusion) or 32 minutes (slow infusion). The light doses were kept constant at 150 J/cm^2 and 600 mW/cm^2. All CNV were occluded angiographically after PDT when irradiation was performed within 45 minutes of the start of drug infusion, falling off to 50% closure when irradiation was performed between 55 and 75 minutes, after which PDT became ineffective in CNV closure. Only one CNV was treated with the fast infusion and irradiation at 30 minutes after the start of drug infusion with successful occlusion of the CNV. Selectivity was assessed as described. The infusion studies suggested that effective CNV closure could be achieved if irradiation was performed within 55 minutes

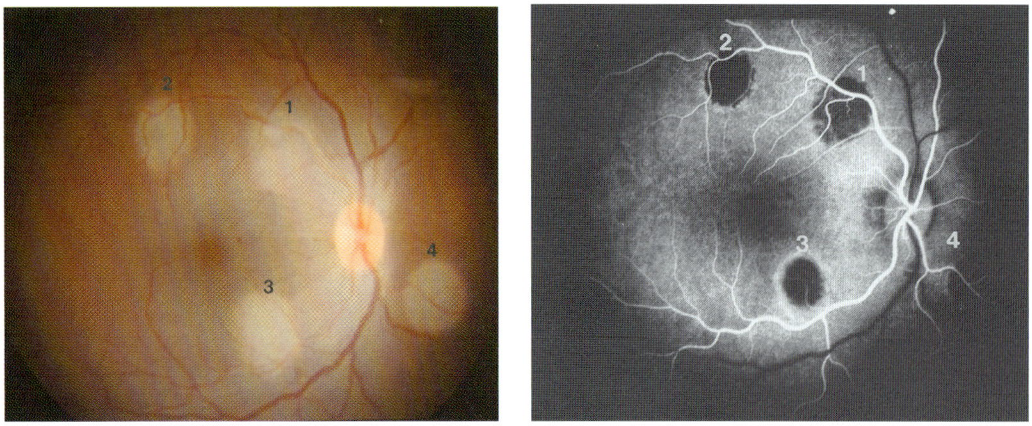

A B

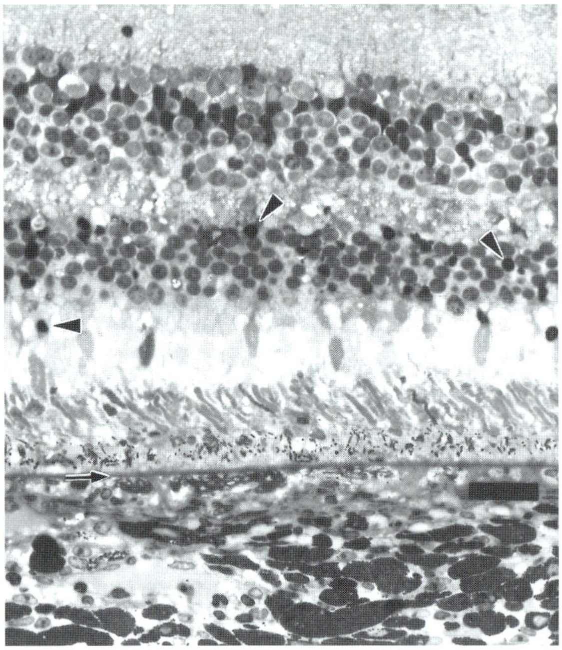

C

FIGURE 5.3. The effect of photodynamic therapy (PDT) on normal retina and choroid. Lesions were irradiated serially after intravenous administration of 0.375 mg/kg verteporfin using 150 J/cm^2 and 600 mW/cm^2. The time of irradiation after drug administration was 10 minutes for lesion 1, 20 minutes for lesion 2, 30 minutes for lesion 3, and 40 minutes for lesion 4. Lesions were processed for histology 24 hours after PDT. **A:** Color fundus photograph 24 hours after PDT of normal retina and choroid. There is mild deep retinal whitening in the irradiated areas. **B:** Early frame fluorescein angiogram 24 hours after PDT, shows hypofluorescence in the treated areas. **C:** Light micrograph of retina and choroid after PDT with the parameters given in the preceding. The lesion shown (grade 2) was irradiated 20 minutes after drug injection. Note the complete closure of the choriocapillaris and the damaged RPE (Bruch's membrane = small arrow). The outer retina shows swelling and some pyknosis of ONL nuclei (arrowheads), and the inner retina shows some swelling and minimal pyknosis. (Bar = 25 μm.) (From: Kramer M, Miller JW, Michaud N, et al. Liposomal BPD verteporfin photodynamic therapy: selective treatment of choroidal neovascularization in monkeys. *Ophthalmology* 1996;103:436, with permission.)

TABLE 5.2. GRADING SCHEME OF PHOTODYNAMIC THERAPY EFFECT ON NORMAL RETINA/CHOROID

Grade	Damaged Retinal/Choroidal Layers
1	RPE only; or RPE + slight photoreceptor changes + occasional pyknosis in the ONL; with or without choriocapillaris closure
2	Choriocapillaris closure + RPE + photoreceptors + 10%–20% pyknosis in the ONL
3	Choriocapillaris closure + RPE + photoreceptors + ONL pyknosis ≤50%
4	Choriocapillaris closure + RPE + photoreceptors + ONL pyknosis >50%
5	Choriocapillaris closure + RPE + photoreceptors + ONL pyknosis >50% or choroidal vessel damage (medium and large), or retinal vessel or inner retinal damage

Unacceptable damage includes damage to retinal vessels, damage to large choroidal vessels, and/or pyknosis of >50% of the ONL. This is a minor modification of the scheme published in Kramer et al., where choroidal vessel damage alone was not sufficient to be considered grade 5. Acceptable damage (grades 1 to 3) could include some distortion of photoreceptor segments and up to 50% pyknosis, with damage to the RPE, choriocapillaris, and medium-sized choroidal vessels feeding the choriocapillaris.
From Kramer M, Miller JW, Michaud N, et al. Liposomal BPD verteporfin photodynamic therapy: selective treatment of choroidal neovascularization in monkeys. *Ophthalmology* 1996;103:427–438, with permission.

TABLE 5.3. HISTOLOGIC GRADING OF PHOTODYNAMIC THERAPY ON NORMAL RETINA/CHOROID

Drug formulation	Intra-venous	Dye dose mg/kg	Fluence J/cm²	Irradiance mW/cm²	Time (min) of irradiation after dye injection	Treated areas no.	No. grade one	No. grade two	No. grade three	No. grade four	No. grade five
Verteporfin	Bolus	1	150	600	<60	6[a]	0	0	0	0	5
Verteporfin	Bolus	1	150	600	60–120	8[a]	0	0	0	6	0
Verteporfin	Bolus	0.5	150	600	<20	1	0	0	0	0	1
Verteporfin	Bolus	0.5	150	600	20–60	3	0	0	0	3	0
Verteporfin	Bolus	0.375	150	600	<20	3	1	1	0	0	1
Verteporfin	Bolus	0.375	150	600	20–50	12[b]	2	3	2	3	0
Verteporfin	Bolus	0.375	150	600	50–100	9	3	2	1	3	0
Verteporfin	Bolus	0.25	150	600	<20	3	1	0	0	0	2
Verteporfin	Bolus	0.25	150	600	20–40	4[c]	3	0	0	0	0
Verteporfin	Bolus	0.25	150	600	>40	2[c]	1	0	0	0	0
Verteporfin	Infusion 32 min	0.375	150	600	32[d]	3	1	0	0	1	1
Verteporfin	Infusion 32 min	0.375	150	600	45–75[d]	12	5	6	0	1	0
Verteporfin	Infusion 32 min	0.375	150	600	85–105[d]	8	4	2	2	0	0
Verteporfin	Infusion 10 min	0.375	150	600	30 and 40[d]	2	0	0	2	0	0

[a]Three lesions irradiated at 40, 100, and 120 minutes were not identified histopathologically; [b]Two lesions at 30 and 40 minutes were not identified histopathologically; [c]Two lesions at 40 and 60 minutes were not identified histopathologically; [d]The time given is the time that light was applied after the start of drug infusion. Some treatments were applied during the period of dextrose infusion, which occurred at 32 to 45 minutes after the start of infusion in the case of slow infusion and at 10 to 11 minutes in the case of the fast infusion.
From Miller JW, et al. *Arch Ophthalmol* 1995;113:810–818; Kramer, et al. *Ophthalmology* 1996;103:427–438; and Husain D, et al. *Arch Ophthalmol* 1996;114:978–985, with permission. See references 12,17, and 20 on p. 71 for complete information.

of the start of drug administration, although the earliest safe time for irradiation was not identified in these studies.

The studies of verteporfin PDT to treat experimental CNV demonstrated the time window for irradiation empirically, by angiographic and histologic outcomes. At the same time angiography using verteporfin and other photosensitizers was being investigated using standard fundus cameras and photosensitizer-specific cameras. This work has led to another methodology for identifying treatment time windows for PDT, by demonstrating the localization of the photosensitizer to the CNV (or lack of it), and the clearance of the photosensitizer from normal retinal and choroidal vessels. This approach is described more fully in Chapters 21 and 22.

Studies also were performed to assess the longer-term effects of PDT using verteporfin on treated CNV as well as normal retina and choroid (21). Persistent closure of CNV (to 4 weeks) was seen in eyes that had been treated with the optimal parameters, and histopathology demonstrated a fibrous scar covered by proliferating RPE, with few open capillaries (Fig. 5.4). In normal eyes treated with PDT, the choriocapillaris was reperfused by 4 weeks, and the RPE appeared to be repopulated with variable pigmentation (Fig. 5.5). Pigmented macrophages were noted overlying the RPE, and there was mild disorganization of the photoreceptor outer segments. It appeared that the damage noted acutely to the RPE and choriocapillaris, recovered by 4 to 7 weeks.

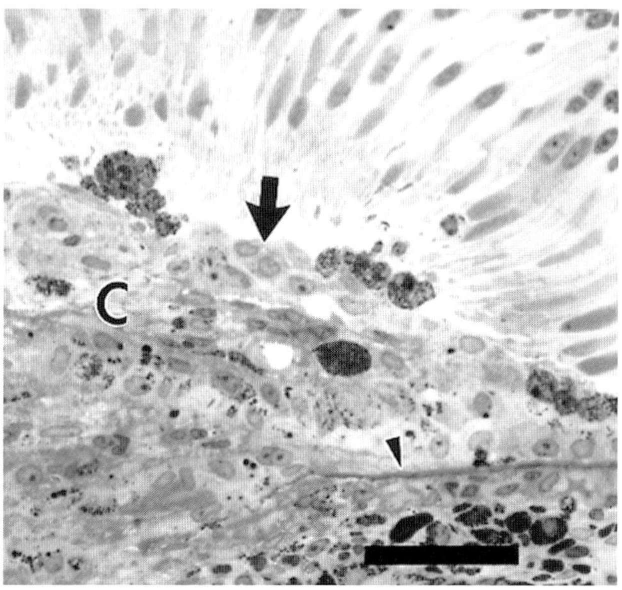

FIGURE 5.4. Light micrograph of choroidal neovascularization (CNV) at 4 weeks after PDT. Choroidal neovascularization is covered by surviving outer nuclear layer, inner segments, and a few rudimentary outer segments. There is a layer of proliferated retinal pigment epithelium (RPE) *(arrow)* enveloping the CNV. Pigment-laden cells are seen overlying the proliferated RPE. The CNV *(C)* extends through Bruch's membrane *(arrowhead)* and has a few capillaries. The spaces seen are acinar structures in RPE cells. (Bar = 50 μm) (From: Husain, et al. *Invest Ophthalmol Vis Sci* 1999;40:2326, with permission. See reference 21 on p. 71.)

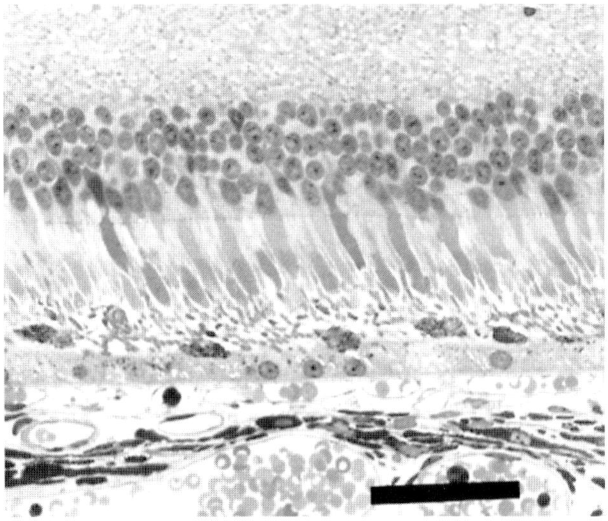
A

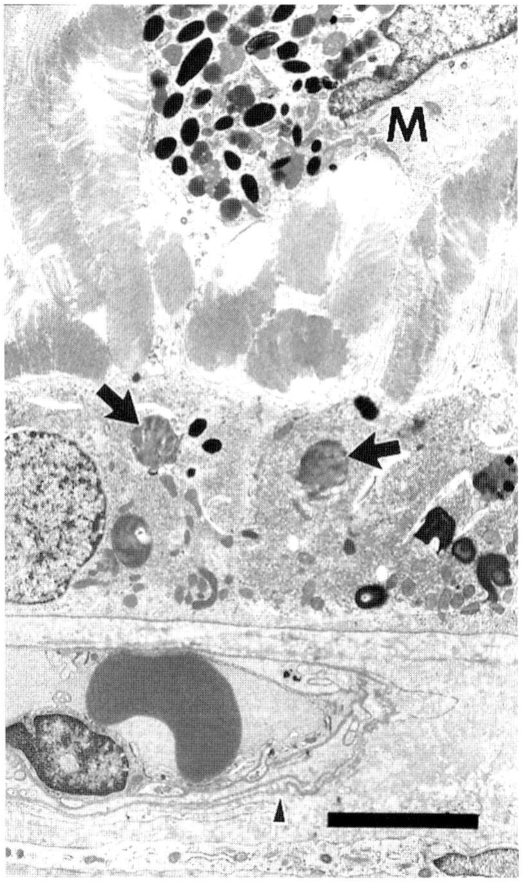

B

FIGURE 5.5. A: Light micrograph of photodynamic therapy (PDT)-treated normal monkey retina and choroid at 6 weeks after treatment. Inner segments appear normal, and outer segments are short and distorted. The retinal pigment epithelium (RPE) is hypopigmented and single layered, with pigment-laden cells overlying the RPE. The choriocapillaris and choroid are patent and appear fully recovered. (Scale bar, 50 μm). **B:** Transmission electron micrograph of normal retina and choroid 4 weeks after PDT. A pigment-laden cell (M) sits between disorganized outer segments on intact RPE. The RPE is lightly pigmented, has rudimentary basal infolding, elongated microvilli, and several lysosomes containing outer segment material *(arrows).* The choriocapillaris is reperfused with reduplication of basement membrane *(arrowhead).* (Scale bar, 5 μm) (From: Husain, et al. Effects of photodynamic therapy using verteporfin on experimental choroidal neovascularization and normal retina and choroid up to seven weeks after treatment. *Invest Ophthalmol Vis Sci* 1999;40:2328, with permission.)

When clinical studies of verteporfin PDT were begun, it became apparent that CNV reperfused and retreatments would be required, and studies were undertaken to assess the recovery following multiple PDT treatments of normal eyes (22). These studies are described more fully in Chapter 10 on repeated PDT treatments by Reinke. Three sequential PDT treatments were performed in the same area of normal retina and choroid. Three doses of liposomal BPD were studied (6, 12, and 18 mg/m^2) with the light doses kept constant (689 nm, 600 mW/cm^2, 100 J/cm^2). Treatments were separated by 2 weeks, and histopathologic examination was performed at 2 and 6 weeks after the third treatment. Minimal damage was seen in the group treated at 6 mg/m^2, with recovery comparable to the single treatment at 0.375 mg/kg (approximately 6 mg/m^2). However, higher dye doses led to significant cumulative damage to the normal retina, choroid and optic nerve, emphasizing that selectivity of PDT with verteporfin is only relative.

In summary, preclinical studies of verteporfin PDT of CNV demonstrated that within certain constraints, the treatment of CNV with PDT was relatively selective, with some damage to choriocapillaris and RPE, but minimal effect on photoreceptors and with preservation of inner retina and retinal and choroidal vessels. Intravenous injection of the verteporfin could be performed rapidly in bolus fashion or in slower infusions with preservation of effect. Higher irradiances were tested and found to be safe and effective, making the treatment more practical. Additionally, it was noted that small changes in drug dose had a more profound effect on CNV and normal structures than changes in light doses, and with decreasing drug doses, the effective time window for light application was shortened. Although a number of treatment parameters could be used, drug and light dose and timing parameters were identified that appeared optimal for subsequent clinical study. Finally, longer-term studies and studies of repeated treatments indicated that the effect on normal structures recovered over time within a range of drug and light doses.

REFERENCES

1. Nanda S, Hatchell D, Tiedeman J, et al. A new method of vascular occlusion. *Arch Ophthalmol* 1987;105:1121-1124.
2. Miller H, Miller B. Photodynamic therapy of subretinal neovascularization in the monkey eye. *Arch Ophthalmol* 1993;111: 855–860.
3. Kliman G, Puliafito C, Stern D, et al. Phthalocyanine photodynamic therapy: new strategy for closure of choroidal neovascularization. *Laser Surg Med* 1994;15:2–10.
4. Allison B, Pritchard P, Richter A, et al. The plasma distribution

of benzoporphyrin derivative and the effects of plasma lipoproteins on its biodistribution. *Photochem Photobiol* 1990;52:501–507.

5. Levy J. Photosensitizers in photodynamic therapy. *Semin Oncol* 1994;21:4–10.
6. Richter AM, Waterfield E, Jain AK, et al. In vitro evaluation of phototoxic properties of four structurally related benzoporphyrin derivatives. *Photochem Photobiol* 1990;52:495–500.
7. Richter AM, Cerruti-Sola S, Sternberg ED, et al. Biodistribution of tritiated benzophorphyrin derivative (3H-BPD-MA), a new potent photosensitizer, in normal and timor-bearing mice. *J Photochem Photobiol B Biol* 1990;5:231–244.
8. Richter AM, Waterfield E, Jain AK, et al. Photosensitising potency of structural analogues of benzoporphyrin derivative (BPD) in a mouse tumour model. *Br J Cancer* 1991;63:87–93.
9. Richter AM, Yip S, Waterfield E, et al. Mouse skin photosensitization with benzoporphyrin derivatives and photofrin: macroscopic and microscopic evaluation. *Photochem Photobiol* 1991;53:281–286.
10. Schmidt-Erfurth U, Bauman W, Gragoudas E, et al. Photodynamic therapy of experimental choroidal melanoma using lipoprotein-delivered benzoporphyrin. *Ophthalmology* 1994;101:89–99.
11. Schmidt-Erfurth U, Hasan T, Gragoudas E, et al. Vascular targeting in photodynamic occlusion of subretinal vessels. *Ophthalmology* 1994;101:1953–1961.
12. Miller JW, Walsh AW, Kramer M, et al. Photodynamic therapy of experimental choroidal neovascularization using lipoprotein-delivered benzoporphyrin. *Arch Ophthalmol* 1995;113:810–818.
13. Miller JW, Stinson WG, Gregory WA, et al. Phthalocyanine photodynamic therapy of experimental Iris Neovascularization. *Ophthalmology* 1991;98:1711–1719.
14. Gomer CJ, Doiron DR, White L, et al. Hematoporphyrin derivative photoradiation induced damage to normal and tumor tissue of the pigmented rabbit eye. *Curr Eye Res* 1984;3:229–237.
15. Gomer CJ, Doiron DR, Jester JV, et al. Hematoporphyrin derivative photoradiation therapy for the treatment of intraocular tumors: examination of acute normal ocular tissue toxicity. *Cancer Res* 1983;43:721–727.
16. Moulton RS, Walsh AW, Miller JW, et al. Response of retinal and choroidal vessels to photodynamic therapy using benzoporphyrin derivative monoacid. *Invest Ophthalmol Vis Sci* 1993;34:1169.
17. Kramer M, Miller JW, Michaud N, et al. Liposomal BPD verteporfin photodynamic therapy: selective treatment of choroidal neovascularization in monkeys. *Ophthalmology* 1996;103:427–438.
18. Waldow S, Dougherty T. Interaction of hyperthermia and photoradiation therapy. *Radiat Res* 1984;97:380–385.
19. Baumal C, Puliafito C, Pieroth L, et al. Phtodynamic therapy (PDT) of experimental choroidal neovascularization with tin ethyl etiopurpurin. *Invest Ophthal Vis Sci* 1996;37:S122.
20. Husain D, Miller JW, Michaud N, et al. Intravenous infusion using liposomal benzoporphyrin derivative verteporfin for photodynamic therapy of experimental choroidal neovascularization. *Arch Ophthalmol* 1996;114:978–985.
21. Husain D, Kramer M, Kenney AG, et al. Effects of photodynamic therapy using verteporfin on experimental choroidal neovascularization and normal retina and choroid up to seven weeks after treatment. *Invest Ophthal Vis Sci* 1999;40:2322–2340.
22. Reinke M, Canakis C, Husain D, et al. Photodynamic therapy (PDT) retreatment of normal retina and choroid in the primate. *Invest Ophthal Vis Sci* 1997;38:S17.

6

PHOTODYNAMIC THERAPY FOR EXPERIMENTAL CHOROIDAL NEOVASCULARIZATION USING ATX-S10(Na)

AKIRA OBANA

ATX-S10(Na): AN AMPHIPHILIC PHOTOSENSITIZER

ATX-S10 was developed by Nakajima and Sakata in 1992 as a new photosensitizer for cancer therapy (1). It was synthesized from protoporphyrin dimethyl ester via photooxidation (2). It became clear that one of the two potent isomers of ATX-S10 exhibited higher affinity and photodynamic effects to tumor cells (3). That isomer was purified and designated ATX-S10(Na) (ATX-S10 · Na(II), Photochemical Co. Okayama, Japan) (Fig. 6.1). ATX-S10(Na) is an iminochlorin aspartic acid derivative and the chemical name is 13,17-bis (1-carboxypropionyl) carbamoylethyl-8-etheny-2-hydroxy-3-hydroxyiminoethylidene-2,7,12,18-tetraethylporphyrin sodium. The molecular weight is 927.79.

This dye has absorption peaks at the wavelength of 401 nm in Soret band and 664 nm in Q band in a water solution. Both absorption peaks shift to the longer wavelengths of 407 and 670 nm in the plasma solution, respectively (Fig. 6.2). The modulus of molar absorption at 670 nm is 16,000, about five times larger than that of photofrin injection (3,000). ATX-S10(Na) in plasma solution emits fluorescence of 680 nm wavelength.

Safety of ATX-S10(Na) is well established in animals. The LD_{50} in rat is more than 1,000 mg/kg. It is rapidly excreted from the body as shown in Figure 6.3 (4). The photosensitivity to the skin is much weaker than photofrin injection and no skin phototoxicity was confirmed at least 1 day after administration in several animal species.

The major difference of ATX-S10(Na) from other sensitizers is its amphiphilicity, which possesses both properties of lipophilicity and hydrophilicity. This unique characteristic possibly induces different biodistribution in the eye and photodynamic effect. Because of its hydrophilic property, a water solution of ATX-S10(Na) can be administered as a bolus intravenous (iv) injection.

PLASMA PROTEIN BINDING OF ATX-S10(Na)

ATX-S10(Na) has high affinity to plasma protein (5). When ATX-S10(Na) was mixed with human plasma at the concentration of 50 μg/mL, which is sufficient for photodynamic therapy (PDT), 97.7 ± 1.6% of ATX-S10(Na) was bound to plasma protein. The binding ratios to several plasma proteins examined by gel filtration chromatography were high-density lipoproteins (HDL) (46%), serum albumin (36%), fibrinogen type I (28%), fibrinogen type III (24%), transferrin (18%), haptoglobin

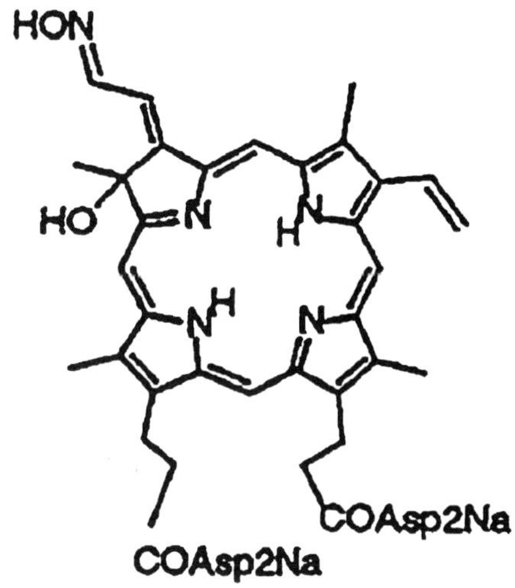

$C_{42}H_{41}N_7Na_4O_{12}$

FIGURE 6.1. The molecular structure of ATX-S10(Na). ($C_{42}H_{41}N_7Na_4O_{12}$).

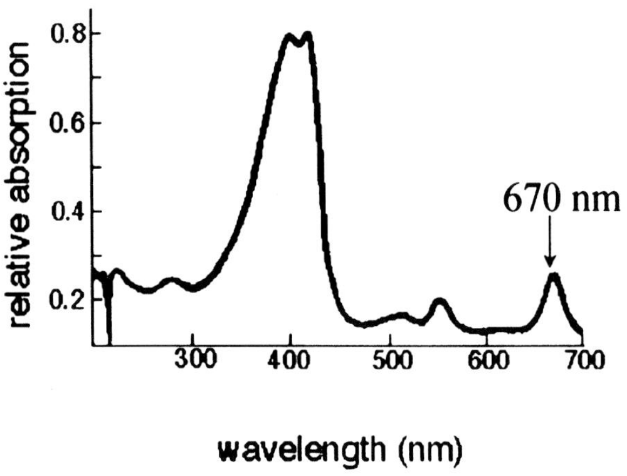

FIGURE 6.2. Absorption spectrum of ATX-S10(Na) in the plasma solution.

(12%), and low-density lipoproteins (10%). Nakajima and colleagues (6) pointed out that water-soluble porphyrin binds to albumin and glycoproteins such as hemopexin. Therefore, a majority of ATX-S10(Na) administrated into the blood is considered to bind to albumin, HDL, and/or other glycoproteins, and transferred to the target tissue.

CELLULAR UPTAKE OF ATX-S10(Na)

It is reported that lipophilic photosensitizers, such as hematoporphyrin derivatives, are taken up into cells by simple diffusion across the plasma membrane and accumulate in membranous organelles such as mitochondria and endoplasmic reticulum. In contrast, hydrophilic photosensitizers are taken up through endocytosis and preferentially accumulate in lysosomes (7). According to the experiments on tumor cells (T.Tn human esophageal cancer) (5), the uptake of ATX-S10(Na) was inhibited by endocytosis inhibitors such as phenylarsine oxide, chloroquine, monensin, and phenylglyoxal, or at the low incubation temperature of 4°C. Therefore, ATX-S10(Na), transferred to the target tissue in a protein-bound form, may be released as the free form in the target tissue and be incorporated into cells by endocytosis. Because small amounts of ATX-S10(Na) are still taken up into cells at 4°C, however, the role of cell-surface proteins, such as transporters, or lipids in the plasma membrane still need to be investigated.

SUBCELLULAR LOCALIZATION OF ATX-S10(Na) IN HUMAN MICROVASCULAR ENDOTHELIAL CELLS AND RETINAL PIGMENT EPITHELIAL CELLS

Because of the limited diffusion distance and short lifetime of singlet oxygen (8), cellular damage in response to PDT largely depends on the intracellular concentration and location of the photosensitizer. We investigated subcellular localization of ATX-S10(Na) in cultured human microvascular endothelial cells and retinal pigment epithelial cells. Both cells were incubated for various times in medium containing ATX-S10(Na) at 2 μg/mL and the fluorescent probe MitoTracker (M-7514, Molecular Probes, Eugene,

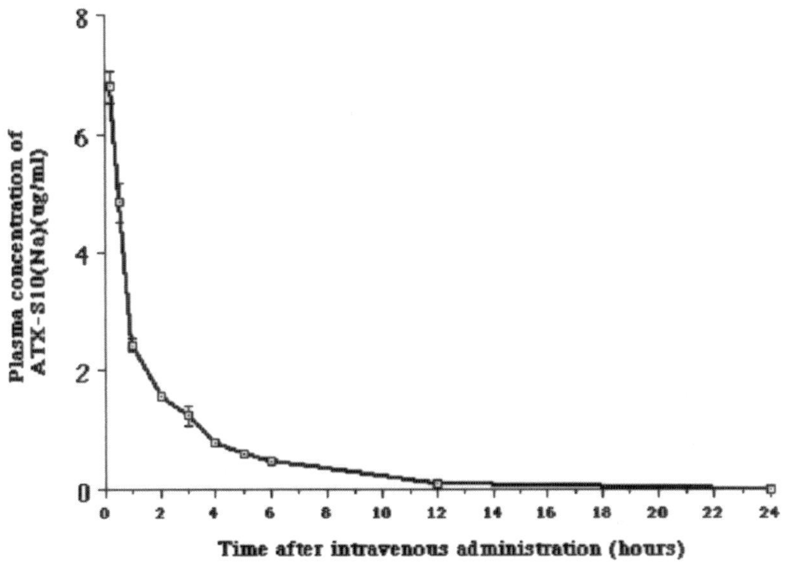

FIGURE 6.3. Time-course of plasma concentration of ATX-S10(Na) in rabbits after injection of 16 mg/kg body weight. Mean ± SEM. (From: Gohto Y, Obana A, Kaneda K, et al. Accumulation of a photosensitizer ATX-S10(Na) to experimental corneal neovascularization. *J Jpn Ophthalmol Soc* 1998;102:724–730, with permission.)

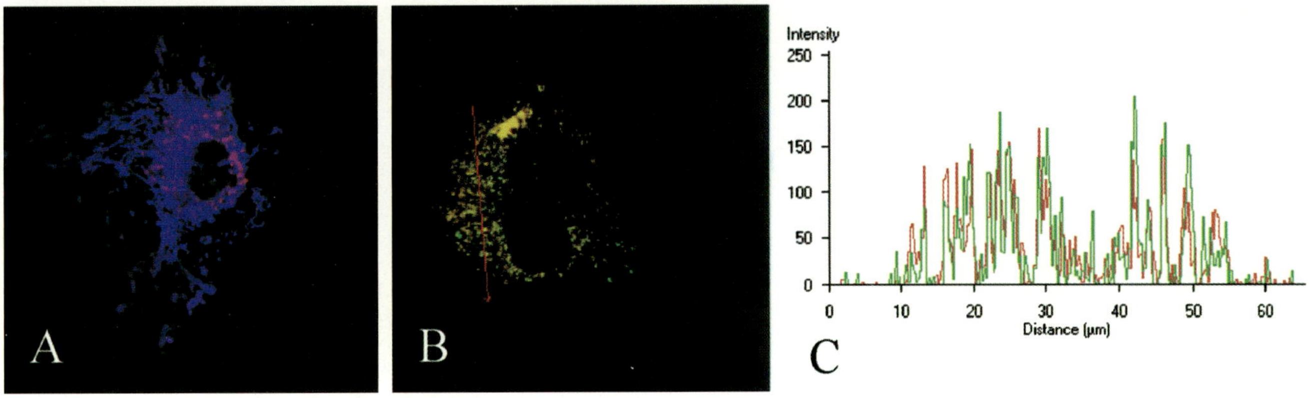

FIGURE 6.4. Confocal image of endothelial cells incubated with ATX-S10(Na) for 2 hours and MitoTracker **(A)** or LysoTracker **(B)**. The red channel represents ATX-S10(Na) fluorescence; the blue channel represents mitochondria, and the green channel represents lysosomes. **C:** The fluorescence profile drawn along the red arrow in **(B)** shows concordance of ATX-S10(Na) and lysosomes.

OR) specific for mitochondria, or LysoTracker (L-7526, Molecular Probes, Eugene, OR) for lysosomes. Intracellular location of fluorescence from the photosensitizer and organelle probes was observed by a confocal laser scanning microscopy.

The results showed that ATX-S10(Na) was taken up by endothelial cells with incubation for 30 minutes or longer, and that most of it was localized in the lysosomes, with a small portion in the mitochondria (Fig. 6.4). This result is consistent with the suggestion that ATX-S10(Na) is taken up by endocytosis (5), because substances taken up by endocytosis usually accumulate in lysosomes. Interestingly, ATX-S10(Na) is taken up by retinal pigment epithelial cells (RPE) more slowly than by endothelial cells, and the amount of dye taken up seems to be less in retinal pigment epithelial cells, although quantification of dye uptake has not yet been investigated. The reduced and slower uptake of ATX-S10(Na) by RPE compared to endothelial cells might allow for selective treatment of choroidal neovascularization (CNV) *in vivo.*

CYTOCIDAL EFFECT OF ATX-S10(Na) TO HUMAN MICROVASCULAR ENDOTHELIAL CELLS AND RETINAL PIGMENT EPITHELIAL CELLS *IN VITRO*

Two different PDT protocols, early and late PDT, resulted in different effects on cell viability. In early PDT treatment, the vascular endothelial or RPE were incubated in a medium containing ATX-S10(Na) for 5 minutes and, without washing out the dye with phosphate-buffered saline, the cells were irradiated with a diode laser at 670 nm. Early PDT treatment is considered a model of laser irradiation immediately after dye injection *in vivo.* In late PDT, the cells were incubated in a medium containing ATX-S10(Na) for more than 30 minutes. After washing out the dye with phosphate-buffered saline, the cells were irradiated with a diode laser. Because ATX-S10(Na) is taken up by cells with incubation for 30 minutes or longer, this PDT protocol is considered a model of PDT performed at some time interval after dye injection *in vivo.* Cell viability was determined by MTS assay using Cell Titer 96 (Promega, Madison, WI).

The results showed that in early PDT, more than 90% of endothelial cell death was achieved with media containing ATX-S10(Na) at concentration of 6.3 µg/mL and 50 J/cm^2 radiance. Retinal pigment epithelial cells, however, were not injured under such conditions. Endothelial cells are thought to be more sensitive than RPE to ATX-S10(Na)-induced membrane photodamage; therefore, early PDT treatment–induced selective damage to vascular endothelial cells. In contrast, the rate of cell death with late PDT increased depending on dye concentration and incubation time for both cells. More than 90% of endothelial cell death was achieved with 1 hour incubation in the medium containing 50 µg/mL ATX-S10(Na) and for 100 J/cm^2 radiance, or 2 hours incubation and 50 J/cm^2 radiance. Under these conditions, the rate of retinal pigment epithelial cell death was 87% and 97%, respectively. Selectivity, therefore, seemed poorer in late PDT than early PDT. It should be noted, however, that in this experiment the RPE were exposed ATX-S10(Na) at their apical side directly, whereas *in vivo* the dye leaks from the choriocapillaris and exists in Bruch's membrane at the basal side of retinal pigment epithelial cells. Therefore, the *in vitro* results have to be interpreted with caution.

MODE OF CELL DEATH BY PHOTODYNAMIC THERAPY USING ATX-S10(Na)

Mode of endothelial cell death was investigated using both PDT protocols that induced greater than 90% cell death. After staining the nuclei with propidium iodide, the number of apoptotic cells was counted using a laser scanning cytometer.

The results showed that early PDT predominantly induced necrosis, whereas late PDT resulted in apoptosis. In early PDT, ATX-S10(Na) was present mainly around the cells and on the cell membrane. The extracellular photosensitizer appeared to induce necrosis following direct photochemical damage to the cell membrane. In contrast, using the late PDT protocol, the dye was taken up by cells and localized in lysosomes, inducing apoptosis. This result is consistent with previous reports that dyes localized in the cell membrane, such as hematoporphyrin derivatives, induce necrosis, and dyes localized in mitochondria and lysosomes induce apoptosis (9,10).

From these *in vitro* studies of endothelial and retinal pigment epithelial cells, early PDT is superior to late PDT from the standpoint of induced cell death; that is, there is a possibility that the endothelial cells can be selectively destroyed. However, apoptosis was predominantly induced by late PDT. It is still unclear which mode is appropriate for the therapy of ocular new vessels. Our *in vivo* studies described in the following suggest that inflammation after PDT might induce regrowth of new vessels. If this suggestion is true, apoptotic cell death of vascular endothelial cells may be more suitable than necrosis, because apoptosis minimizes inflammation.

TIME COURSE ANALYSIS OF THE DISTRIBUTION OF ATX-S10(Na) IN NEOVASCULARIZED EYES

Photodynamic effects are closely related to the biodistribution of the dye in the tissue; therefore, accumulation of ATX-S10(Na) to neovascular tissue was investigated.

Nitrogen-Pulsed Laser Spectrofluorometry

Gohto and associates (4) measured the amount of ATX-S10(Na) in corneal neovascularization in rabbits semi-quantitatively, using nitrogen-pulsed laser spectrofluorometry, and showed that ATX-S10(Na) gradually accumulated in corneal neovascularization and reached maximal levels at 2 to 4 hours after dye administration (Fig. 6.5). In contrast, plasma ATX-S10(Na) concentration decreased rapidly after injection, as shown in Figure 6.3. ATX-S10(Na) is excreted promptly from the body (a few hours after administration), but is retained in neovascular tissue.

Fluorescence Microscopy

Selective accumulation of ATX-S10 in CNV lesions was observed in rats (11). Choroidal neovascularization was induced by intense argon laser photocoagulation. After injection of ATX-S10, the eyes were enucleated at various time intervals and frozen sections were observed by fluorescence microscope coupled with a cooled Charge-Coupled Device (CCD) camera and image processing system (ARGUS-50.C-CCD, Hamamatsu Photonics, Hamamatsu, Japan).

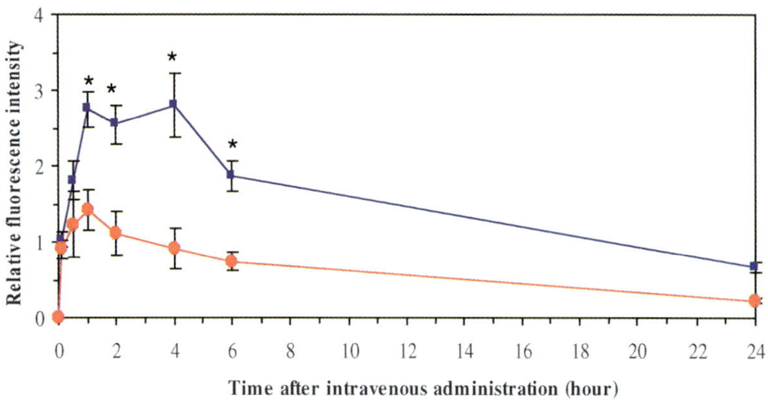

FIGURE 6.5. Time course of relative fluorescence intensity of ATX-S10(Na) on rabbit cornea. *Square:* ATX-S10(Na) fluorescence detected at site of corneal neovascularization. *Circle:* ATX-S10(Na) fluorescence detected at a nonvascularized portion of cornea. Mean ± SEM. *$p < .01$. (From: Gohto Y, Obana A, Kaneda K, et al. Accumulation of a photosensitizer ATX-S10(Na) to experimental corneal neovascularization. *J Jpn Ophthalmol Soc* 1998;102: 724–730, with permission.)

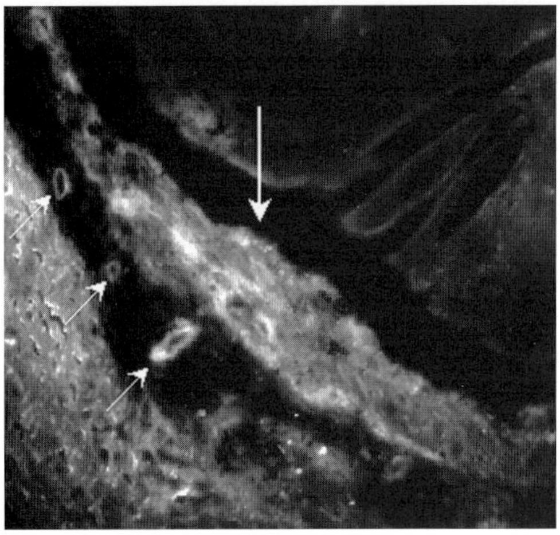

FIGURE 6.6. Fluorescence microscopy of experimentally induced CNV in rat eye. One hour after administration of ATX-S10 (16 mg/kg). Bright fluorescence is observed in CNV *(large arrow)* and choroidal artery walls *(arrows)*. (From: Obana A, Gohto Y, Kaneda K, et al. Selective occlusion of choroidal neovascularization by photodynamic therapy with a water-soluble photosensitizer, ATX- S10. *Lasers Surg Med* 1999;24:209–222, with permission.)

At 5 minutes after dye injection, the dye exists in the CNV and in the lumen of choroidal vessels. Choroidal artery wall and the sclera were also heavily stained, whereas dye accumulation in the RPE was very weak. Fluorescence intensity in CNV increased gradually after that, and selective accumulation of ATX-S10 in CNV was obtained from 2 to 4 hours after administration (Fig. 6.6).

ATX-S10(Na) Angiography

The localization of ATX-S10(Na) was analyzed *in vivo* in primate eyes using ATX-S10(Na) angiography (12). Choroidal neovascularization was induced in the posterior pole of the monkey eyes with a krypton laser. After intravenous injection of ATX-S10(Na), the fluorescence of the dye from the fundus was detected by a modified fundus camera (TRC-50IA, Topcon, Tokyo, Japan), which included a 670-nm wavelength diode laser (Hamamatsu Photonics, Hamamatsu, Japan) as the stimulation source and a cooled CCD camera (KP-160, Hitachi, Ibaragi, Japan) as a detector.

In ATX-S10(Na) angiography, dye appeared in the retinal arteries and in the venous return within 10 seconds, and hyperfluorescence representative of CNV was observed (Fig. 6.7A). At 10 to 20 minutes, ATX-S10(Na) fluorescence in the retinal capillaries faded away, whereas that in the retinal arteries/veins persisted. At 30 minutes, CNV lesions showed an increase in fluorescence intensity and mild dye leakage was noted (Fig. 6.7B), although the leakage was less obvious than that by fluorescein angiography. In the next few hours, fluorescence from CNV persisted, whereas that in the retinal arteries/veins decreased. By 24 hours, ATX-S10(Na) fluorescence was entirely gone from all structures. Figure 6.8 shows the change of fluorescence intensity from CNV and retinal artery measured by National Institutes of Health imaging software. Between 1 and 3 hours after injection, the intensity from CNV was significantly higher than that from the retinal artery. The property of less leakage of ATX-S10(Na) from CNV is related to the higher affinity of this dye to the plasma pro-

A

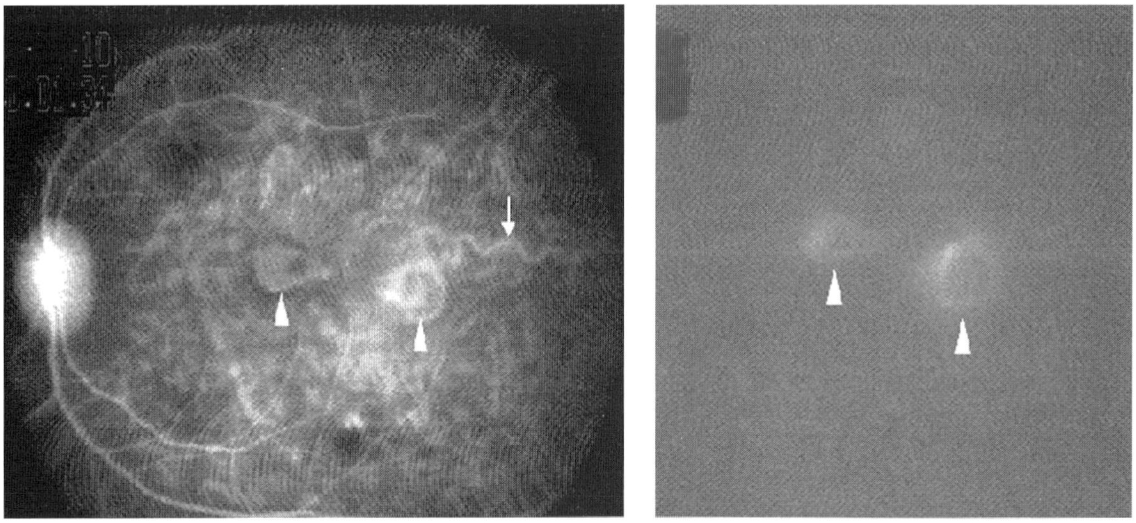

B

FIGURE 6.7. A: ATX-S10(Na) angiogram at 90 seconds after dye injection. *Arrow:* posterior ciliary artery. *Arrowheads:* choroidal neovascularization (CNV). **B:** Angiogram at 40 minutes after dye injection. Fluorescence persisted in CNV with mild dye leakage *(arrowheads)*. (From: Obana A, Gohto Y, Kaneda K, et al. PDT to monkey CNV with ATX-S10(Na): Inappropriateness of early laser irradiation for selective occlusion. *Invest Ophthalmol Vis Sci* 2001;42:2639–2645, with permission.)

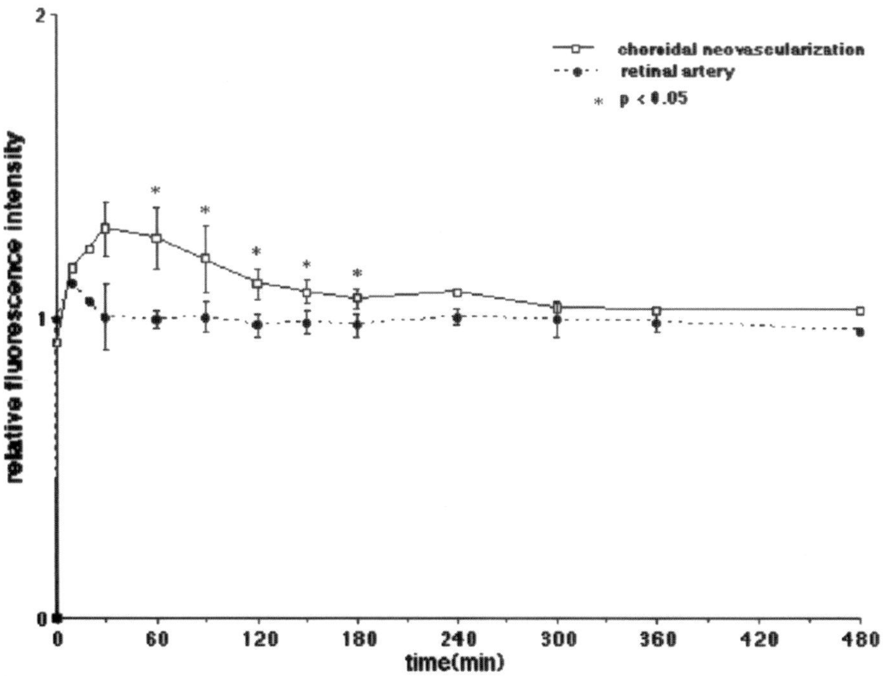

FIGURE 6.8. Time course of fluorescence intensity in ATX-S10(Na) angiography with a dye dose of 8 mg/kg body weight. Relative intensity was calculated as follows: fluorescence intensity of choroidal neovascularization (CNV) or retinal artery divided fluorescence intensity of the background. *Square:* CNV. *Circle:* retinal artery.

teins, and it decreases the adverse effect of PDT on the sensory retina.

PHOTODYNAMIC THERAPY OF EXPERIMENTAL CHOROIDAL NEOVASCULARIZATION

Treatment Parameters of Photodynamic Therapy

For CNV treatment, occlusion of CNV without damage to the surrounding normal tissue, especially the neurosensory retina, is important. Such a selective occlusion of CNV by PDT depends on three treatment parameters: dose of dye administered, dose of laser irradiation, and the time interval between dye injection and irradiation. Concerning the time interval, it is still controversial whether laser irradiation, immediately or some interval after dye injection, gives a selective injuring effect on CNV (13–21). The proposal of immediate irradiation comes from the interpretation that high concentrations of blood-borne dye at an early time give the maximal photodynamic effect on vascular endothelial cells by generating a large amount of radical species even with low doses of photosensitizer and irradiation. In contrast, PDT performed after some time interval results from photoactivation of the dye taken up into the target cells. Therefore, the optimal treatment parameters for selective occlusion of CNV were evaluated in rat and monkey CNV models induced by intense laser photocoagulation. In these experiments, CNV occlusion was evaluated using fluorescein angiography and histology.

Photodynamic Therapy on Choroidal Neovascularization in Rat Eyes

After intravenous injection of ATX-S10, CNV lesions were irradiated with a 670-nm diode laser at various time intervals. There were no apparent color changes in any treated areas immediately after PDT. One day after PDT, different extents of deep retinal whitening appeared, depending on the intensity of irradiation. The area of whitening usually corresponded to the size of the laser irradiation spot, but in the lesions treated with high exposure, it was larger than the size of the laser irradiation spot. Choroidal neovascularization closure was achieved without closure of retinal capillaries and choroidal large vessels when PDT was performed immediately after dye injection of 16 mg/kg body weight with irradiation at 7.4 J/cm^2 (exposure of 30.8 mW/cm^2 for 4 minutes) and at 2 or 4 hours after dye injection with irradiation at 22.0 J/cm^2 (exposure of 91.7 mW/cm^2 for 4 minutes) (11). The irradiance used was too low to induce thermal effects. Timing of 2 or 4 hours after dye injection was considered optimal because the difference between the amount of dye in the CNV and in the retinal and choroidal vessels during this period was large. The reason for selectivity immediately after dye injection was not considered to result from differences in dye accumulation, but differences in sensitivity between CNV and retinal and large choroidal vessels. Light microscopy revealed CNV closure with thrombus, and electron microscopy showed disruption of the endothelial cells of CNV lesions, which were filled with platelets, erythrocytes, and fibrin. The basement membrane was preserved.

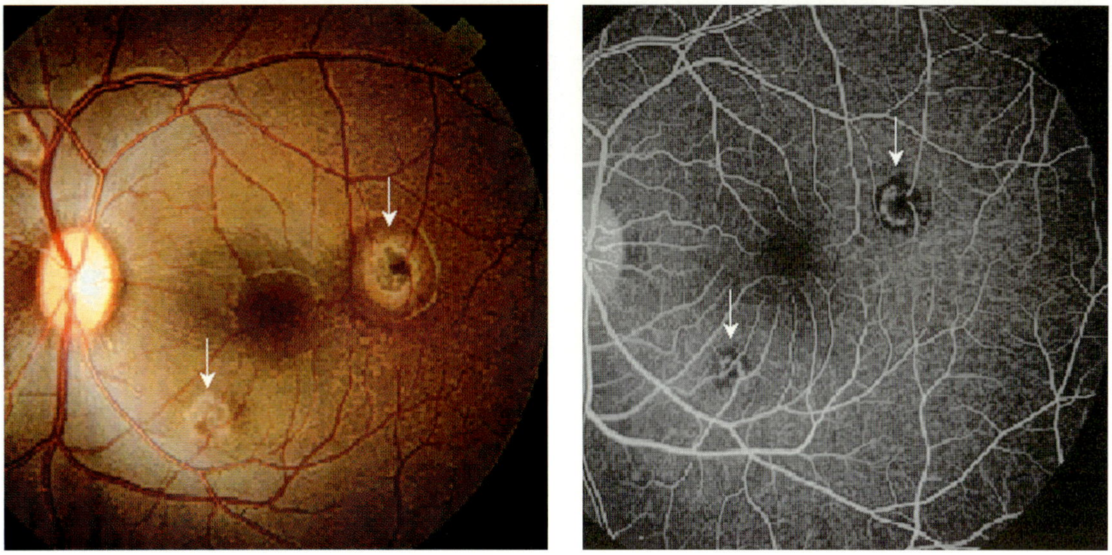

A B

FIGURE 6.9. CNV before photodynamic therapy. **A:** Choroidal neovascularization revealed as yellowish gray subretinal proliferative tissue with serous detachment of sensory retina by ophthalmoscopy *(arrows)*. **B:** Fluorescein angiography shows ring hyperfluorescence *(arrows)* with late fluorescein leakage. (From: Obana A, Gohto Y, Kanai M, et al. Selective photodynamic effects of the new photosensitizer ATX-S10(Na) on choroidal neovascularization in monkeys. *Arch Ophthalmol* 2000;118:650–658, with permission.)

Photodynamic Therapy on Choroidal Neovascularization in Monkey Eyes

Figure 6.9 shows CNV before PDT. One day after PDT (Fig. 6.10), occlusion of CNV was represented by hypofluorescence with no ring hyperfluorescence in fluorescein and little dye leakage in late-phase fluorescein angiography. Choriocapillary occlusion, as indicated by hypofluorescence in fluorescein angiography, was concurrently detected. Destruction of the blood–retinal barrier in the retinal pigment epithelium was assumed from the fluorescein leakage in the boundary of irradiated areas. It was determined that CNV was occluded selectively in the lesions where retinal vessels were well perfused. Light

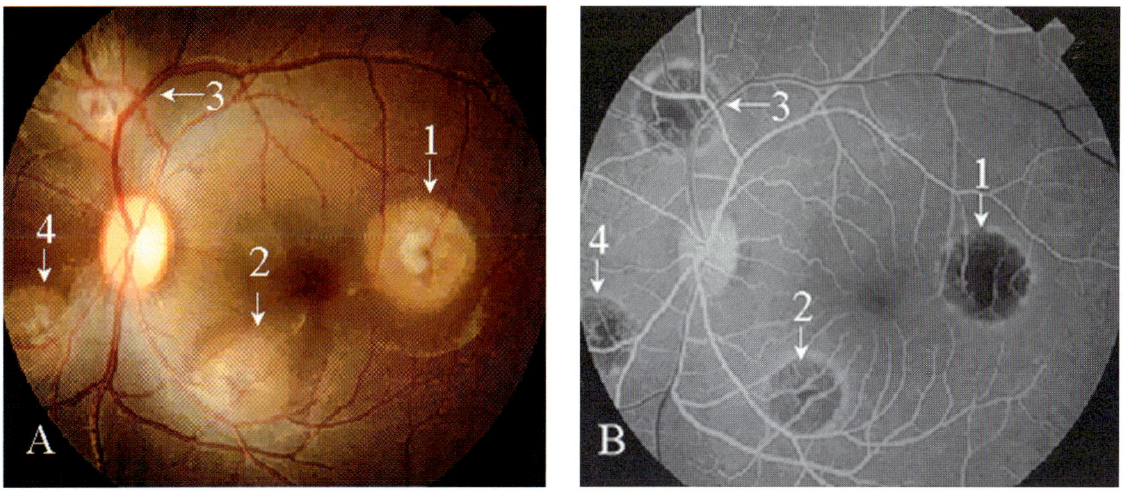

FIGURE 6.10. CNV 1 day after photodynamic therapy. Four lesions of CNV were irradiated in different conditions: lesion 1, 89.5 J/cm^2 at 70 minutes after dye injection; lesion 2, 21.1 J/cm^2 at 40 minutes; lesion 3, 10.6 J/cm^2 at 15 minutes; and lesion 4, 52.8 J/cm^2 at 63 minutes. Dye dose is 8 mg/kg body weight. **A:** Fundus photography shows a color change into mild gray in all lesions. **B:** Fluorescein angiogram shows hypofluorescence indicative of CNV closure in all lesions. Retinal arterioles and venules exhibit normal features in all lesions except lesion 3. (From: Obana A, Gohto Y, Kanai M, et al. Selective photodynamic effects of the new photosensitizer ATX-S10(Na) on choroidal neovascularization in monkeys. *Arch Ophthalmol* 2000;118:650–658, with permission.)

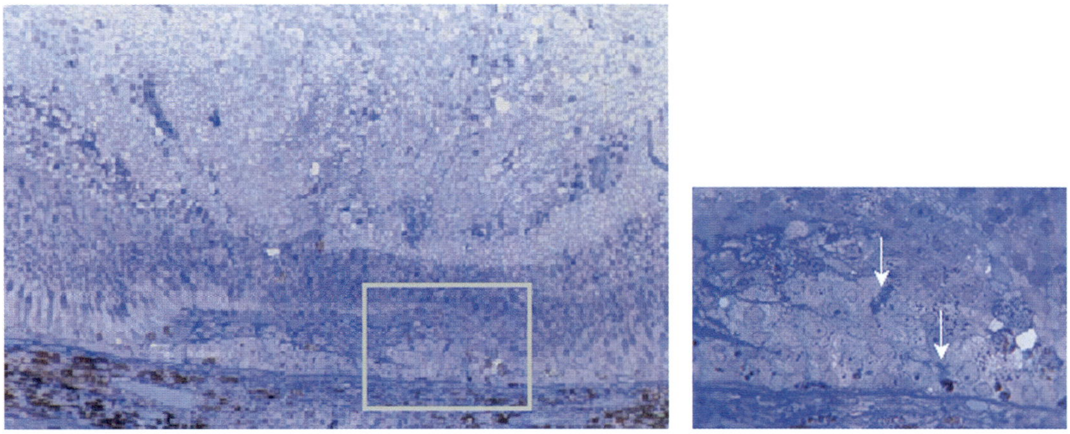

FIGURE 6.11. Light micrograph at 1 week after photodynamic therapy. CNV is occluded *(arrows in inset)*. Toluidine blue-staining. (Original magnification, ×250)

microscopy analysis demonstrated that CNV was occluded by thrombi.

At later than 1 week, the retinal opacity decreased and detachment of the sensory retina recovered in most of the CNV-occluded lesions, although pigment irregularity remained to some extent (Fig. 6.11). However, at 1 to 4 weeks, ring-shaped hyperfluorescence with late dye leakage, which represented recurrent CNV, appeared in some lesions in fluorescein angiography (Fig. 6.12). Histologic analysis revealed new vessels surrounded by many macrophages and double-layered RPE cells. Occluded retinal arterioles and venules after intensive PDT usually underwent recanalization.

In our experiments (12,22), optimal treatment parameters for achieving selective occlusion of CNV were investigated with dye doses of 2, 4, 8, and 12 mg/kg body weight. Selective occlusion of CNV was achieved with the following conditions: (a) 50 to 70 J/cm^2 irradiation at 30 to 40 minutes after 4 mg/kg body weight dye injection; (b) 30 to 74 J/cm^2 irradiation at 30 to 74 minutes after 8 mg/kg dye injection; and (c) 1 to 29 J/cm^2 at 30 to 74 minutes or 30 to 74 J/cm^2 irradiation at 75 to 150 minutes after 12 mg/kg dye injection. Irradiation within 20 minutes at a dye dose of 2 mg/kg body weight failed to achieve selective CNV occlusion without neovascular recurrence. Recurrence of CNV was noted particularly in those lesions that received excessive PDT and retinal vessel occlusion.

As described, ATX-S10(Na) accumulated to a greater extent in CNV between 30 and 120 minutes. This time interval is compatible with that of laser irradiation for selective CNV occlusion. The nonselectivity of the injuring effect of PDT performed within 20 minutes after dye injection is believed to result from lack of preferential accumulation of dye in CNV lesions during this time period.

The optimal conditions for selective PDT in human age-related macular degeneration (AMD) may differ from those

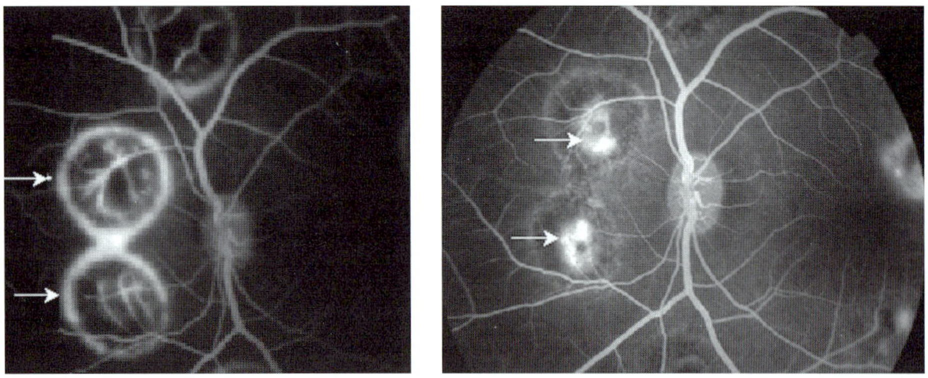

FIGURE 6.12. A: Fluorescein angiography at 1 day after PDT. CNV is closed *(arrows)*. **B:** Fluorescein angiography at 2 weeks after PDT. Ring-shaped hyperfluorescence that represents CNV recurrence is observed *(arrows)*. (From: Obana A, Gohto Y, Kaneda K, et al. PDT to monkey CNV with ATX-S10(Na): Inappropriateness of early laser irradiation for selective occlusion. *Invest Ophthalmol Vis Sci* 2001;42:2639–2645, with permission.)

observed in our experimental studies, because the pathogenesis of experimental CNV is not identical to that of CNV associated with AMD. Further study is necessary for a future clinical trial.

PHOTODYNAMIC THERAPY TO NORMAL RETINA AND CHOROID

Previous studies have shown that PDT, under conditions needed to treat experimental CNV, leads to changes in normal retina and choroid (23,24). The collateral effects to retina and choroid under conditions that induced selective occlusion of CNV with ATX-S10(Na), therefore, was investigated in normal eyes (12,22). The results confirmed that ATX-S10(Na) PDT did lead to occlusion of the choriocapillaris and damage to the retinal pigment epithelial cells, but that large choroidal vessels and retinal vessels, including capillaries, were spared. At 1 day after PDT, damage to the barrier function of RPE leads to edema of the outer layer of the retina and a color change from grayish to whitish in the deep retina by ophthalmoscopy. At 1 week, choriocapillary occlusion partly persisted, but blood–brain barrier function was reestablished, as shown by cessation of dye leakage in fluorescein angiography. At 2 to 3 weeks, PDT-treated lesions showed pigment mottling by ophthalmoscopy. Histology demonstrated that RPE preserved its original structure of a single-cell layer, and that many macrophages accumulated on the apical side of RPE (Fig. 6.13). The choroid showed the normal architecture with patent choriocapillaries. Outer segments of photoreceptors became shortened or were absent in parts. Most of the nuclei in the outer nuclear layer were weakly stained with toluidine blue, and some showed pyknotic changes. Nerve fibers and ganglion cell layers were normal in appearance. In general, the choriocapillaris and RPE are directly injured by PDT, which is followed by secondary damage to the photoreceptor cells to some extent. However, such injury is significantly less than that caused by thermal coagulation.

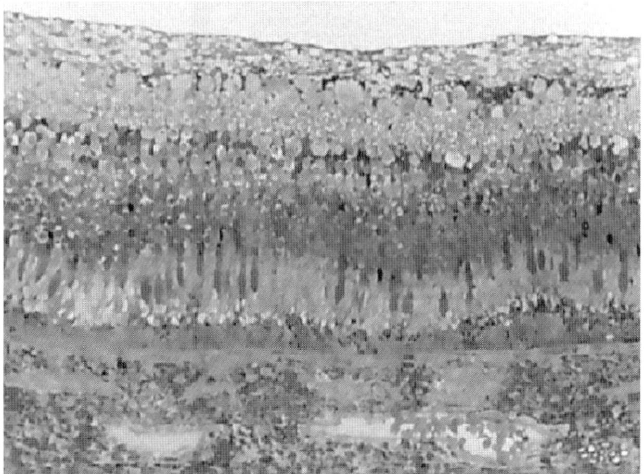

FIGURE 6.13. Light micrograph at 1 week after photodynamic therapy to normal retina and choroid. Toluidine blue-staining. (Original magnification, ×250) (From: Obana A, Gohto Y, Kanai M, et al. Selective photodynamic effects of the new photosensitizer ATX-S10(Na) on choroidal neovascularization in monkeys. *Arch Ophthalmol* 2000;118:650–658, with permission.)

SPECULATION FOR THE MECHANISM OF RECURRENCE OF CHOROIDAL NEOVASCULARIZATION

Recurrence of CNV is one of the major shortcomings of PDT in the clinic (25,26). Although the mechanism of recurrence is not known, it is assumed that feeder vessels of CNV, surviving after PDT, may be responsible (27). From our experiments (12,22), the possibility of recurrence from residual CNV after insufficient PDT is excluded because recurrence frequently occurred after excessive irradiation. Furthermore, recurrence usually was observed when retinal vessels were damaged. From these observations, three causes are postulated: (a) inflammation evoked by excessive PDT; (b) ischemia of the sensory retina following retinal vessel occlusion; and (c) destruction of RPE covering CNV. Photodynamic therapy–induced damage of the retina and choroid induces infiltration of macrophages, which may produce vascular endothelial growth factor (VEGF) (28) and contribute to induction of CNV. It has also been reported that RPE release VEGF under hypoxic conditions (29). On the other hand, RPE may be responsible for preventing the proliferation of endothelial cells of underlying CNV probably by secreting inhibitory factors such as transforming growth factor-β and promoting the maturation of neovascularization (30). Although the mechanism of CNV development may differ between AMD and this experimental model, the present findings strongly suggest that excessive PDT could promote the recurrence of CNV.

In order to avoid undesirable photodynamic damage, we propose that PDT should be performed when the dye diminishes from the normal tissue and selectively accumulates in CNV, and that laser irradiation should be focused strictly to CNV. If the apoptotic mode of cell death minimizes inflammatory elements, this suggests that there may be no advantage to supralethal PDT.

DEVELOPMENT OF A NEW DEVICE FOR PHOTODYNAMIC THERAPY

Photodynamic therapy currently is performed using a slit-lamp system, with which laser light is delivered as a single circular spot and CNV is illuminated as a circle through a hand-held contact lens. However, the shape of CNV is not always circular, and photosensitizers retained in the normal

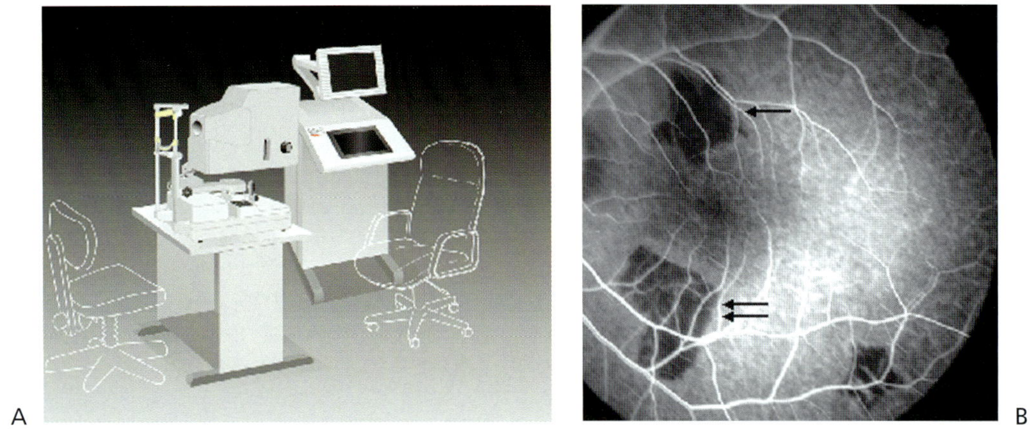

FIGURE 6.14. A: Scanning laser ophthalmoscope for PDT (Hamamatsu Photonics, Hamamatsu, Japan). **B:** Fluorescein angiogram at 1 day after PDT using the scanning laser ophthalmoscope. Choriocapillary occlusion of star *(arrow)* and square *(double arrow)* shapes is achieved.

tissue may induce unnecessary injury in the tissue surrounding CNV. Therefore, we are currently developing a scanning laser ophthalmoscope specially designed for PDT for focal irradiation strictly fitted to CNV (Fig. 6.14A, Hamamatsu Photonics, Hamamatsu, Japan) (31). With this device, we can irradiate the eye fundus in any shape, as shown in Figure 6.14B, and avoid unnecessary irradiation of normal tissue. There are still some problems with the present prototype device, such as necessity of long exposure time and management of eye movement during long-time treatment, and further improvements are necessary. However if these problems are solved, the scanning system will be a potent device for PDT.

CONCLUSION

ATX-S10(Na) is an amphiphilic photosensitizer that accumulates in CNV. Photodynamic therapy using ATX-S10(Na) and diode laser effectively and selectively occlude CNV in rat and monkey eyes. A clinical trial of PDT using this agent is warranted.

AKNOWLEDGMENTS

The author thanks Susumu Nakajima (Health Care Administration Center, Obihiro University of Agriculture and Veterinary Medicine), Kenji Kaneda (Department of Anatomy, Osaka City University Graduate School of Medicine), and Yuko Gohto (Department of Ophthalmology and Visual Sciences, Osaka City University Graduate School of Medicine) for their collaboration for the present study; Isao Sakata (Photochemical Co., Ltd.) for providing ATX-S10(Na); Sueo Miyaki and Shinichi Fujisaka (Hamamatsu Photonics Co., Ltd.); Toru Hirano (Hamamatsu University School of Medicine); Kouji Kobayashi (Kowa Co., Ltd.) for providing the diode laser and scanning laser system; and Gerald W. De Vries (Allergan Co., Ltd.) for kind suggestions. Thanks are also owing to Reginal Birngruber (Luebeck Laser Institute) and Ursula Schmidt-Erfurth (University Eye Hospital, Luebeck) for their useful discussion on our PDT project.

The present PDT study was supported by Health Science Research Grants of the Ministry of Health and Welfare (H10-018), a Science Research Grant of the Ministry of Education (CO9671812) (C13671849), the Fund of the Osaka Eye Bank, and the Fund for Medical Research of Osaka City University Medical Research Foundation.

REFERENCES

1. Nakajima S, Sakata I, Takemura T, et al. Tumor-localizing and photosensitization of photo-chlorin ATX-S10. In: Spinelli P, Dal Fante M, Marchesini R, eds. *Photodynamic therapy and biomedical lasers.* Amsterdam: Elsevier Science, 1992:531–534.
2. Sakata I, Inui Y, Maruyama I, et al. Synthesis and properties of ATX-S10 analogues. *Proc Conf Jpn Soc Laser Med* 1996;16: 161–168.
3. Nakajima S, Sakata I, Hirano T, et al. Therapeutic effect of interstitial photodynamic therapy using ATX-S10(Na) and a diode laser on radio-resistant SCCVII tumors of C3H/He mice. *Anti-Cancer Drugs* 1998;9:539–543.
4. Gohto Y, Obana A, Kaneda K, et al. Accumulation of a photosensitizer ATX-S10(Na) to experimental corneal neovascularization. *J Jpn Ophthalmol Soc* 1998;102:724–730.
5. Mori M, Kuroda T, Obana A, et al. In vitro plasma protein binding and cellular uptake of ATX-S10(Na), a hydrophilic chlorin photosensitizer. *Jpn J Cancer Res* 2000;91:845–852.
6. Nakajima S, Moriyama T, Hayashi H, et al. Hemopexin as a carrier protein of tumor-localizing Ga-metalloporphyrin-ATN-2. *Cancer Lett* 2000;149:221–226.
7. Roberts WG, Berns MW. In vitro photosensitization 1. Cellular uptake and subcellular localization of mono-l-aspartyl chlorin e6, chloro-aluminum sulfonated phthalocyanine, and photofrin II. *Lasers Surg Med* 1989;9:90–101.

8. Moan J, Berg K. The photodegradation of porphyrins in cells can be used to estimate the lifetime of singlet oxygen. *Photochem Photobiol* 1991;53:549–553.
9. Luo Y, Kessel D. Initiation of apoptosis versus necrosis by photodynamic therapy with chloroaluminum phthalocyanine. *Photochem Photobiol* 1997;66:479–483.
10. Kessel D, Luo Y, Mathieu P, Reiners Jr JJ. Determinants of the apoptosis response to lysosomal photodamage. *Photochem Photobiol* 2000;71:196–200.
11. Obana A, Gohto Y, Kaneda K, et al. Selective occlusion of choroidal neovascularization by photodynamic therapy with a water-soluble photosensitizer, ATX-S10. *Lasers Surg Med* 1999;24:209–222.
12. Obana A, Gohto Y, Kaneda K, et al. PDT to monkey CNV with ATX-S10(Na): Inappropriateness of early laser irradiation for selective occlusion. *Invest Ophthalmol Vis Sci* 2001;42:2639–2645.
13. Kliman GH, Puliafito CA, Stern D, et al. Phthalocyanine photodynamic therapy: new strategy for closure of choroidal neovascularization. *Laser Surg Med* 1994;15:2–10.
14. Lin SC, Lin CP, Feld JR, et al. The photodynamic occlusion of choroidal vessels using benzoporphyrin derivaive. *Curr Eye Res* 1994;13:513–522.
15. Peyman GA, Moshfeghi DM, Moshfegbi A, et al. Photodynamic therapy for choriocapillaris using tin ethyl etiopurpurin (SnET2). *Ophthalmic Surg Lasers* 1997;28:409–417.
16. Mori K, Yoneya S, Ohta M, et al. Angiographic and histologic effects of fundus photodynamic therapy with a hydrophilic sensitizer (mono-L-aspartyl chlorin e6). *Ophthalmology* 1999;106: 1384–1391.
17. Gohto Y, Obana A, Kaneda K, et al. Photodynamic effect of a new photosensitizer ATX-S10 on corneal neovascularization. *Exp Eye Res* 1998;67:313–322.
18. Haimovici R, Kramer M, Miller JW, et al. Localization of lipoprotein-delivered benzoporphyrin derivative in the rabbit eye. *Curr Eye Res* 1996;16:83–90.
19. Kim RY, Hu LK, Flotte TJ, et al. Digital angiography of experimental choroidal melanomas using benzoporphyrin derivative. *Am J Ophthalmol* 1997;123:810–816.
20. Kanai M, Obana A, Gohto Y, et al. Long-term occlusion of photodynamic therapy by using a hydrophilic photosensitizer ATX-S10(Na) against experimental choroidal neovascularization in rats. *Lasers Surg Med* 2000;26:48–57.
21. Gohto Y, Obana A, Kanai M, et al. Treatment parameters for selective occlusion of experimental corneal neovascularization by photodynamic therapy using a water soluble photosensitizer, ATX-S10(Na). *Exp Eye Res* 2001;72:13–22.
22. Obana A, Gohto Y, Kanai M, et al. Selective photodynamic effects of the new photosensitizer ATX-S10(Na) on choroidal neovascularization in monkeys. *Arch Ophthalmol* 2000;118: 650–658.
23. Husain D, Miller JW, Michaud N, et al. Intravenous infusion of liposomal benzoporphyrin derivative for photodynamic therapy of experimental choroidal neovascularization. *Arch Ophthalmol* 1996;114:978–985.
24. Husain D, Kramer M, Kenny AG, et al. Effects of photodynamic therapy using verteporfin on experimental choroidal neovascularization and normal retina and choroid up to 7 weeks after treatment. *Invest Ophthalmol Vis Sci* 1999;40:2322–2311.
25. Schmidt-Erfurth U, Miller JW, Sickenberg M, et al. Photodynamic therapy with verteporfin for choroidal neovascularization caused by age-related macular degeneration. Results of a retreatments in a phase 1 and 2 study. *Arch Ophthalmol* 1999;117: 1177–1187.
26. Treatment of Age-related Macular Degeneration with Photodynamic Therapy (TAP) Study Group. Photodynamic therapy of subfoveal choroidal neovascularization in age-related macular degeneration with verteporfin. One-year results of 2 randomized clinical trials. *Arch Ophthalmol* 1999;117:1329–1345.
27. Schmidt-Erfurth U, Michels S, Hager A, et al. ICG-angiographic analysis of the photodynamic mechanism in treatment of choroidal neovascularization. *Invest Ophthalmol Vis Sci* 1998;39: S242.
28. Sunderkoetter C, Steinbrink K, Goebeler M, et al. Macrophages and angiogenesis. *J Leukoc Biol* 1994;55:410–422.
29. Adams AP, Shima DT, Yeo KT, et al. Synthesis and secretion of vascular endothelial growth factor by human retinal pigment endothelial cells. *Biochem Biophys Res Commun* 1993;193:631–638.
30. Miller H, Miller B, Ryan SJ. The role of retinal pigment epithelium in the involution of subretinal neovascularization. *Invest Ophthalmol Vis Sci* 1986;27:1644–1652.
31. Obana A, Gohto Y. Scanning laser system for photodynamic therapy of choroidal neovascularization. *Lasers Surg Med* 2002; 30:370–375.

7

PHOTODYNAMIC THERAPY FOR EXPERIMENTAL CHOROIDAL NEOVASCULARIZATION USING PURLYTIN

DARIUS M. MOSHFEGHI
GHOLAM A. PEYMAN

Tin ethyl etiopurpurin (SnET2) is a metallopurpurin synthetic chlorin second-generation photosensitizer (Fig. 7.1). It is formulated for human use under the trade name Purlytin (Miravant Medical Technologies, Santa Barbara, CA) in a hydrophobic, isotonic, isoosmotic lipid emulsion that can be administered by intravenous (iv) infusion. Like most photosensitizers, it has several absorption peaks (Fig. 7.2) (1). The 664-nm excitation peak is used in ophthalmology for its superior penetrance through biologic tissues (1,2). It has been demonstrated *in vitro* that the action spectrum for phototoxicity of SnET2 occurs at 655 and 670 nm (1).

Early work in evaluating SnET2 photodynamic therapy in rats provided the broad parameters for treatment: 1 mg/kg, treatment initiated 24 hours after iv infusion, and excitation with red light (>590 nm) (1–4). These studies demonstrated that at concentrations of SnET2 of 10 mg/kg or higher, serious cutaneous photosensitivity reactions occurred (1–3). The carrier (lipid, emulsion, or cyclodextrin) for SnET2 was also noted to be a significant factor in the efficacy of SnET2 (5,6).

Because SnET2 was originally studied in transplantable tumor models (1–4), its efficacy was judged by the amount of tumor death and, subsequently, its mechanism of action was inferred to occur by disruption of the tumor blood supply. Selman and associates demonstrated a decrease in blood flow to a tumor model in rats following SnET2 photodynamic therapy, but were unable to localize the level at which the damage was occurring: endothelial or subendothelial (7). Further work showed that following SnET2 photodynamic therapy, singlet oxygen species were generated that resulted in lipid peroxidation with subsequent cellular membrane and mitochondrial damage (8,9). These investigators provided data indicating that SnET2 damages the endothelial cells lining the rat aorta directly following application of red light, even after the SnET2 is no longer circulating in the blood (10). These studies seemed to indicate that, similar to the proposed mechanism for other photosensitizers (11), SnET2 is activated to a triplet state following activation by laser light of a specific wavelength, generating singlet and reactive oxygen species that cause damage to the endothelial cells of the vasculature, releasing subendothelial clotting factors, with subsequent occlusion of the vessel. Flower and Snyder recently proposed that the SnET2 photodynamic effect is mediated by direct damage to erythrocyte membranes, which then release hemoglobin (12). Hemoglobin acts as a vasoconstrictor *in vivo*

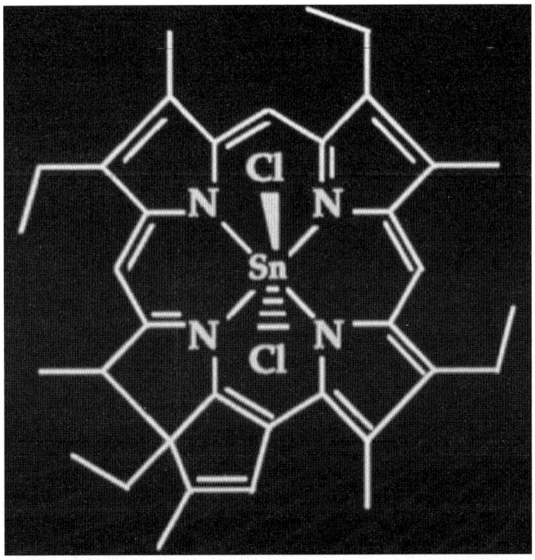

FIGURE 7.1. SnET2 chemical structure demonstrating a metallopurpurin based on tin.

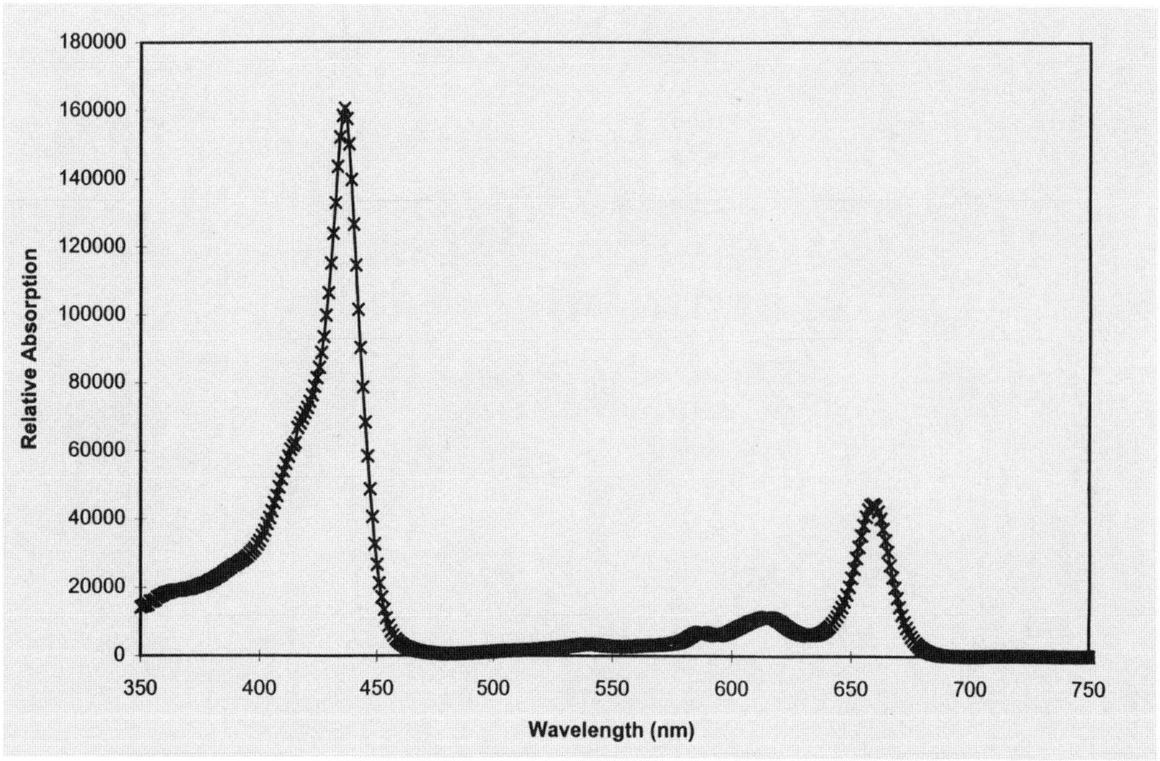

FIGURE 7.2. The absorption spectra of SnET2 demonstrating the 664-nm peak used for treatment of normal choriocapillaris. (From: Moshfeghi DM, Peyman GA, Moshfeghi AA, et al. Ocular vascular thrombosis following tin ethyl etiopurpurin (SnET2) photodynamic therapy: time dependencies. *Ophthalmic Surg Lasers* 1998;29:664, with permission.)

and it is this action that leads to the appearance of vascular occlusion on fluorescein angiography (12). Although this effect may be occurring, it is demonstrated in the following that vascular occlusion, however short-lived, definitely occurs in the choriocapillaris.

CHORIOCAPILLARIS CLOSURE IN RABBITS

SnET2 offered another choice of photosensitizing agent for the treatment of choroidal neovascularization (CNV) in addition to verteporfin, mono-L-aspartyl chlorin, and the phthalocyanines. It was a desirable agent in that it was readily available, already in clinical testing for cutaneous lesions, and active in the red wavelength. However, SnET2 is hydrophobic, as is verteporfin, and necessitated iv infusion. Unlike verteporfin and mono-L-aspartyl chlorin, it was associated with prolonged cutaneous photosensitivity in nonhuman models (1–3).

Crean and associates (13) showed that in rabbits, SnET2 reached peak concentrations in the vascular structures of the eye and in the blood within 1 hour of iv infusion and persisted for up to 28 days, possibly contributing to its prolonged cutaneous sensitivity. The investigations of Peyman

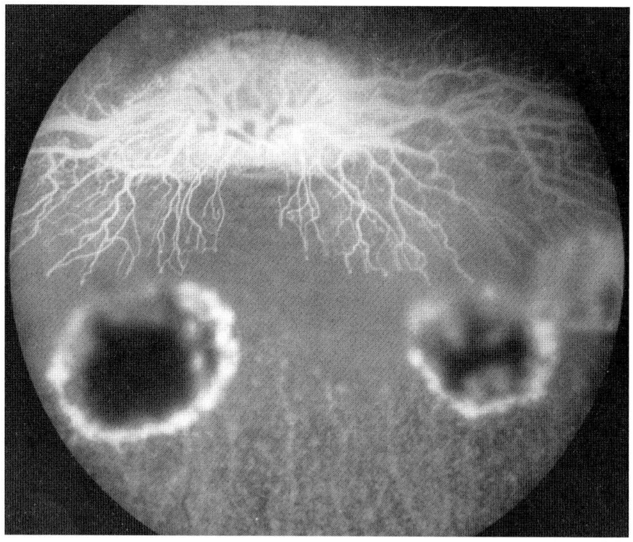

FIGURE 7.3. Fluorescein angiogram of a pigmented rabbit following SnET2 photodynamic therapy. There is central hypofluorescence, indicating vascular nonperfusion, with surrounding hyperfluorescence. (From: Peyman GA, Moshfeghi DM, Moshfeghi A, et al. Photodynamic therapy for choriocapillaris using tin ethyl etiopurpurin (SnET2). *Ophthalmic Surg Lasers* 1997;28: 414, with permission.)

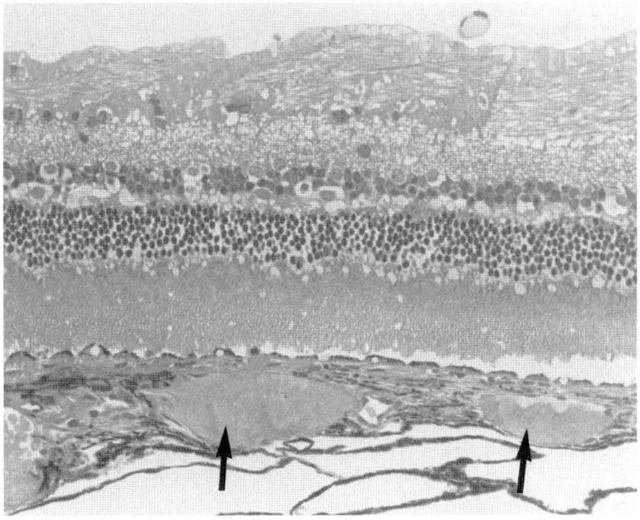

FIGURE 7.4. Histopathologic specimen obtained from a pigmented rabbit 24 hours following SnET2 photodynamic therapy, demonstrating thrombus formation in the large choroidal vessels (*arrows*). There is occlusion of the normal choriocapillaris with relative preservation of the overlying neurosensory retina. (From: Moshfeghi DM, Peyman GA, Moshfeghi AA, et al. Ocular vascular thrombosis following tin ethyl etiopurpurin (SnET2) photodynamic therapy: time dependencies. *Ophthalmic Surg Lasers* 1998;29:667, with permission.)

and colleagues into the viability of SnET2 as a potential ophthalmological therapeutic agent for CNV focused on its ability to close normal choriocapillaris vessels in pigmented rabbits (14,15). They demonstrated that vascular occlusion was observable both angiographically (Fig. 7.3) and histologically (Fig. 7.4) following photodynamic therapy with SnET2 (dose 0.5 to 1.0 mg/kg, 664-nm laser irradiation beginning 15 to 45 minutes after infusion, 5 to 20 J/cm^2) (15,16).

Baumal and coworkers found PDT with SnET2 and a 665-nm diode laser effective at producing selective closure of CNV in a primate model (16). Moshfeghi and associates subsequently demonstrated that the optimal time for laser irradiation was between 5 and 20 minutes after iv infusion for a concentration of 0.5 mg/kg of SnET2 (17). Using these parameters, vascular occlusion was determined to occur between 70 and 120 minutes and 40 and 90 minutes after SnET2 PDT in the albino and pigmented rabbits, respectively. Apparently, these studies sufficed to allow human Phase I/II open-label studies using SnET2 PDT for the treatment of subfoveal CNV (18).

CONCLUSION

Tin ethyl etiopurpurin is a hydrophobic second-generation photosensitizer that is effective following irradiation with 664-nm light at 5 to 20 minutes after iv infusion. It has been demonstrated to work *in vivo* by vascular occlusion, and there is some *in vitro* evidence suggesting that the release of hemoglobin following damage to erythrocytes may result in a vascular constriction of treated vessels. The concentrations used preclinically for treatment of normal rabbit choriocapillaris were 0.5 and 1.0 mg/kg. Cutaneous photosensitivity was noted at higher doses in other animal species. To our knowledge, no published data exist on the efficacy of SnET2 for treatment of experimental CNV in nonhuman primates.

REFERENCES

1. Morgan AR, Garbo GM, Keck RW, et al. Tin (IV) etiopurpurin dichloride: an alternative to DHE? New directions in photodynamic therapy. *SPIE Proc* 1988;847:172–179.
2. Morgan AR, Garbo GM, Keck RW, et al. New photosensitizers for photodynamic therapy: combined effect of metallopurpurin derivatives and light on transplantable bladder tumors. *Cancer Res* 1988;48:194–198.
3. Morgan AR, Garbo GM, Keck RW, et al. Metallopurpurins and light: effect on transplantable rat bladder tumors and murine skin. *Photochem Photobiol* 1990;51:589–592.
4. Morgan AR, Garbo GM, Mastroianni M, et al. New photosensitizers for PDT. In: Optical methods for tumor treatment and early diagnosis: mechanisms and techniques. *SPIE Proc* 1991; 1426:350–355.
5. Garbo GM. The use of liposomes, emulsion or inclusion complexes may potentiate in vivo effects of SnET2. Photodynamic therapy: mechanisms II. *SPIE Proc* 1990;1203:118–125.
6. Kessel D, Garbo GM, Hampton J. The role of lipoproteins in the distribution of tin etiopurpurin (SnET2) in the tumor-bearing rat. *Photochem Photobiol* 1993;57:298–301.
7. Selman SH, Qin B, James HR, et al. Hemodynamic effect of the metallopurpurin SnET2 and light on transplantable FANFT induced bladder tumor. *J Urol* 1990;143:630–633.
8. Morgan AR, Cheng LS, Skalkos D, et al. Tin etiopurpurin dichloride-sensitized lipid photooxidation of erythrocyte membranes. *Photochem Photobiol* 1990;52:987–991.
9. Kessel D, Morgan A, Garbo GM. Sites and efficacy of photodamage by tin etiopurpurin in vitro using different delivery systems. *Photochem Photobiol* 1991;54:193–196.
10. He DP, Hampton JA, Keck R, et al. Photodynamic therapy: effect on the endothelial cell of the rat aorta. *Photochem Photobiol* 1991;54:801–804.
11. Schmidt-Erfurth U, Hasan T. Mechanisms of action of photodynamic therapy with verteporfin for the treatment of age-related macular degeneration. *Surv Ophthalmol* 2000;45: 195–214.
12. Flower RW, Snyder WJ. Expanded hypothesis on the mechanism of photodynamic therapy action on choroidal neovascularization. *Retina* 1999;19:365–369.
13. Crean DH, Gebhardt BM, Falco V, et al. Distribution of a photosensitizer within ocular tissues and blood. *Invest Ophthalmol Vis Sci* 1997;38(Suppl):S140.
14. Peyman GA, Moshfeghi DM, Moshfeghi A, et al. The effect of light-activating tin ethyl etiopurpurin (SnET2) on normal rabbit choriocapillaries. *SPIE Proc* 1996;2673:174–181.
15. Peyman GA, Moshfeghi DM, Moshfeghi A, et al. Photodynamic therapy for choriocapillaris using tin ethyl etiopurpurin (SnET2). *Ophthal Surg Lasers* 1997;28:409–417.

16. Baumal CR, Puliafito CA, Peiroth L, et al. Photodynamic therapy (PDT) of experimental choroidal neovascularization with tin ethyl etiopurpurin. *Invest Ophthalmol Vis Sci* 1996;37(Suppl): S122.
17. Moshfeghi DM, Peyman GA, Moshfeghi AA, et al. Ocular vascular thrombosis following tin ethyl etiopurpurin (SnET2)-photodynamic therapy: time dependencies. *Ophthalmic Surg Lasers* 1998;29:663–668.
18. Thomas EL, Rosen R, Murphy R, et al. Purlytin (SnET2)-photodynamic therapy produces closure of subfoveal choroidal neovascularization in humans. *Invest Ophthalmol Vis Sci* 1998;39 (Suppl):S242.

8

PHOTODYNAMIC THERAPY FOR EXPERIMENTAL CHOROIDAL NEOVASCULARIZATION USING LU-TEX

J. DANIEL ARBOUR
DANNY GAUTHIER

Photodynamic therapy (PDT) has recently emerged as a new form of treatment for a significant number of patients affected by choroidal neovascularization (CNV) involving the macula (1–4). A photosensitizer is administered intravenously and activated by nonthermal light irradiation at a specific wavelength according to its absorption profile. Energy absorbed by the photosensitizer is transferred in its immediate environment, leading to thrombosis of the neovascular vessels. The exact mechanisms are described in detail in the preceding chapters. Several major classes of photosensitizers have been used *in vitro* and *in vivo* (Table 8.1), including tetrapyrrole derivatives, phthalocyanine, chlorins, and xanthene derivatives. Several have been used in preclinical investigation, including DHE/photofrin5, RB6, CASPc 7, 8, tin ethyl etiopurpurin/purlytin 9, and BPD/verteporfin. Verteporfin, a second-generation porphyrin, also known as benzoporphyrin derivative (BPD) monoacid was the first and still is the only photosensitizer to receive approval from the US Food and Drug Administration (FDA) and other health agencies around the world for the treatment of subfoveal CNV secondary to age-related macular degeneration (AMD) (1,10–12). This chapter reviews the biochemical characteristics of another photosensitizer, motexafin lutetium (Lu-Tex), and the results of experimentation to determine dosimetry and efficacy of this photosensitizer in the treatment of CNV in a nonhuman primate model, making Lu-Tex a potential photodynamic agent for the treatment of neovascular AMD and other causes of CNV. The potential clinical applications of Lu-Tex as an imaging dye are reviewed as well.

BIOCHEMICAL PROPERTIES

Motexafin lutetium (Lu-Tex/PCI 0123) is a photosensitizing dye that belongs to the family of metallo-motexafins. They represent a second generation of expanded porphyrin compounds applied as photosensitizers (13). Lu-Tex is water soluble and fully aromatic, with a molecular weight of 1,165.4 g/mol. It appears as a green solution. Motexafins are characterized by the presence of central metallic ions. The Lu-Tex molecule contains a heavy lutetium atom that allows for long-lived singlet oxygen production with a quantum yield between 10% and 70% when activated at its lowest energy maximum (732 nm) (14). The large molecular central core of Lu-Tex is responsible for its ability to form a stable complex with metal cations, and therefore a strong barrier against dissociation (15). The Lu-Tex spectrum of absorption is in the near-infrared, with an absorption peak at 732 nm (Fig. 8.1), which theoretically allows for its activation through blood and retinal tissues. The Lu-Tex fluorescence emission band is centered at 740 nm (16). Graham and coworkers (17) took advantage of these characteristics to perform digital angiography using Lu-Tex in a

TABLE 8.1. CLASSIFICATION OF THERAPEUTIC PHOTOSENSITIZERS USED FOR THE TREATMENT OF OCULAR NEOVASCULARIZATION

Chlorins
Chlorin e6
Bacteriochlorin a
Phtalocyanines
Chloroaluminum sulfonated phthalocyanine
Zinc phthalocyanine
Tetrapyrrole derivatives
Hematoporphyrin derivative
Photofrin (porfimer sodium/dihematoporphyrin ether)
Benzoporphyrin derivative
Tin ethyl etiopurpurin
Motexafin lutetium
Xanthene derivatives
Rose Bengal

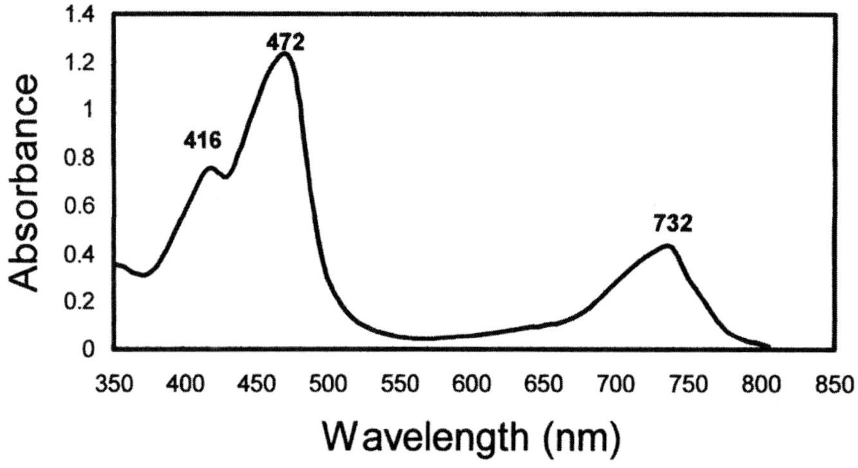

FIGURE 8.1. Absorption spectrum of motexafin lutetium.

monkey model of choroidal neovascularization. They observed an accumulation of the agent in the CNV with rapid clearance of the compound from the retinal vessels. Blumenkranz and associates obtained similar results with a definite enhancement of experimental CNV (18). They also found rapid clearance of the photosensitizer from the plasma with a 39.7% fraction bound to high-density lipoprotein, whereas 15.8% was bound to the low-density lipoproteins.

Lipid-based formulations are known to accumulate in tissues for a long period of time. Photofrin has a measurable plasma concentration up to 1 year after injection, whereas Lu-Tex has a plasma half-life of about 7 hours (19). When used for solid malignancies, Lu-Tex was not associated with significant systemic skin phototoxicity (20), whereas confocal laser scanning microscopy identified the lysosome as the intracellular localizing site (21).

CLINICAL APPLICATIONS OF LU-TEX

The successful clinical application of a photosensitizer depends on its ability to selectively concentrate in the target tissue and maintain good agent retention for PDT. It should be easily activated with low levels of energy and associated with minimal side effects. Lu-Tex is an attractive dye because of its water solubility and its stability as a solution. Investigators involved in the field of oncology have been using the affinity of Lu-Tex for tumor tissues in order to destroy cancer cells (22–24).

Proliferating tumor cells may preferentially take up the newly formed complex of Lu-Tex combined to lipoproteins. It also may result from the fact that tumor cells have a higher mitotic activity combined with a high expression of low-density lipoprotein (LDL) receptors. Hammer-Wilson and coworkers (23) looked at the efficacy of PCI-0123 (motexafin lutetium) as a PDT agent. They evaluated the response of the SMT-F tumor model to PDT. Lu-Tex was found to be more effective than photofrin with a 100% response rate and a 55% cure rate (40 mg/kg dose) compared to animals treated with photofrin (16% cure rate). No toxic effects were reported with a dose regimen below 40 mg/kg in this mouse model. The SMT-F mouse mammary tumor model demonstrated a selective uptake (15 times higher than plasma) of Lu-Tex drug at the site of the tumor 24 hours postinjection. Its tumor selectivity also has been demonstrated by magnetic resonance imaging (25). The mechanism of its selectivity for these tissues remains unclear but it may be related to its interaction with LDLs (23).

Photodynamic therapy is generally known to be minimally successful for the treatment of pigmented melanoma (22). Low light penetration in pigmented tumors is responsible for this poor response. Motexafin lutetium PDT in the highly pigmented B16F10 murine melanoma model showed promising results. Coagulative necrosis was observed histologically, and was surrounded by noncoagulative necrosis (apoptosis, pyknosis, and karyorrhexis). PCI-0123 also was associated with increased survival and significant tumor growth delay. Woodburn and colleagues (26) postulated that the higher responsiveness compared to previously studied agents might be related to the higher affinity of PCI-0123 for tumor tissues. Apo-E deficient mice in this study (lipoprotein profile similar to humans) also had favorable results. The high tumor concentration of this agent can initiate highly oxidative attacks for which melanoma cells seem to be very susceptible. The 732-nm wavelength also may achieve deeper penetration in pigmented tissues.

Photodynamic therapy effectiveness with Lu-Tex, therefore, may be attributed to its lower tissue attenuation. Higher local concentrations can be obtained and its optical absorption in the near infrared range has been associated with tissue penetration of at least 6 mm (27).

Photodynamic therapy has also expanded its applications to the field of cardiovascular diseases. Photoangioplasty for atherosclerosis (photoatherolysis) using cylindrical light-emitting fiberoptic catheters is a novel therapeutic approach. A photosensitizing agent is injected and then light activation is used to remove endovascular atherotic plaques. The therapeutic agent must have the ability to be activated in the presence of blood. The near infrared absorption spectrum of the molecule represents a real advantage for this purpose. The safety of Antrin (motexafin lutetium) was demonstrated in a Phase I study (28,29). A balloon injury model of iliac arteries demonstrated a high concentration of Lu-Tex in atheromatous plaques and a small decrease in the amount of atheroma following treatment. Normal vessel walls were not injured and there was an absence of endothelial cell damage (30).

Finally, Renno and associates examined the effect of combining angiostatin with photodynamic therapy using Lu-Tex as the photosensitizing agent (described more fully in Chapter 4). They observed a synergistic cytotoxicity on bovine retinal capillary endothelial cells (BRCE) at all fluences when angiostatin was administered prior to the PDT. Retinal pigment epithelial cells did not present so much damage. This interesting combination may provide an increased selectivity of PDT using Lu-Tex (31).

EXPERIMENTAL PHOTODYNAMIC THERAPY WITH LU-TEX IN THE ANIMAL MODEL

Experiments were conducted to determine the efficacy and the dosimetry of PDT using Motexafin lutetium (Lu-Tex/PCI-0123) in the photodynamic treatment of experimental choroidal neovascularization (CNV) in a monkey model.

Cynomolgus monkeys weighing from 2.5 to 6.5 kg were anesthetized using intramuscular injections of ketamine hydrochloride (20 mg/kg), acepromazine maleate (0.125 mg/kg), and atropine sulfate (0.125 mg/kg). The animals were then placed in a comfortable restraint device to maintain an adequate head position during photography, angiography, and PDT. Choroidal neovascularization was induced in each eye studied by placing seven to nine photocoagulation spots between the major retinal arcades using an argon green laser with a power of 350 to 450 mW, a spot size of 50 μm, and a duration of 0.1 second. A digital angiography system (Topcon 50-VT fundus camera and IMAGEnet 1024 digital imaging system) was used for fundus photography and fluorescein angiography (FA) performed before CNV induction (Fig. 8.2A) and weekly thereafter to assess development of CNV characterized by early hyperfluorescence with leakage in the later frames of the angiogram (Figs. 8.2C and 8.2D). Lu-Tex/PCI-0123, a sterile, pyrogen-free, dark green aqueous solution was administered intravenously over 30 seconds at doses of 1.0, 1.5, 2.0, or 6.0 mg/kg followed by an intravenous flush of saline or mannitol. Photodynamic therapy was performed after calibration of spot size and light irradiation intensity using an argon/dye laser with a wavelength of 732 nm, at fluences of 50, 100, 150, or 300 J/cm^2 at a constant irradiance of 600 mW/cm^2. Timing of laser irradiation was predetermined and monitored from 5 minutes to a maximum of 3 hours after the start of the dye injection. Treatment spots measuring 1,000, 1,250, 3,000, or 4,000 μm were placed directly over CNVs and normal choroid to serve as control spots to each CNV treated. After PDT, color fundus pictures were obtained (Fig. 8.2B) and the animal was kept in the dark for 24 hours. The animals were then enucleated under deep anesthesia and euthanized immediately after enucleation except for one animal followed for 1 month after PDT. Enucleated eyes were fixed for 20 minutes using a modified Karnovsky fixative (pH 7.4) then bisected 2 mm posterior to the limbus and replaced in the fixative for 24 hours at 4°C. After fixation the eyes were placed in 0.1 M cacodylate buffer (pH 7.4) and cut into block size, then postfixed in 2% osmium tetroxide. Specimens were dehydrated in ethanol and embedded in Epon, then sectioned at 1 μm for light microscopy. For electron microscopy, thin sections were stained using uranyl acetate in methanol and Sato lead stains.

ANGIOGRAPHY RESULTS

The first goal of PDT is to effectively close the CNV. Successful CNV closure is characterized by an absence of leakage on FA at 24 hours after the treatment, with hypofluorescence seen in the early frames of the angiogram and leakage of dye from the rim of the treated spot in the later frames of the angiogram (Figs. 8.2E and 8.2F). Failure of treatment was defined as early hyperfluorescence in the area of the CNV, with leakage of dye in the later frames.

Seventy-one CNV were treated with Lu-Tex PDT with irradiation at 5 minutes to 3 hours after the start of the drug injection (Fig. 8.3). Using 2 mg/kg body weight of Lu-Tex with a fluence of 50 and 100 J/cm^2, effective closure was seen in all cases when light was applied within 20 minutes after the start of the drug infusion (Fig. 8.4). Efficiency rates decreased to 50% at 50 J/cm^2 and 89% at 100 J/cm^2 when light was applied between 20 and 40 minutes after the start of the injection, and with irradiation more than 40 minutes after the start of the Lu-Tex injection PDT at 2 mg/kg body weight failed to close the CNV in more than 50% of the cases (Fig. 8.4). The time window for effective closure of CNV was longer at 2 mg/kg than at 1 or 1.5 mg/kg, suggesting a dye dose response. Fluence dose

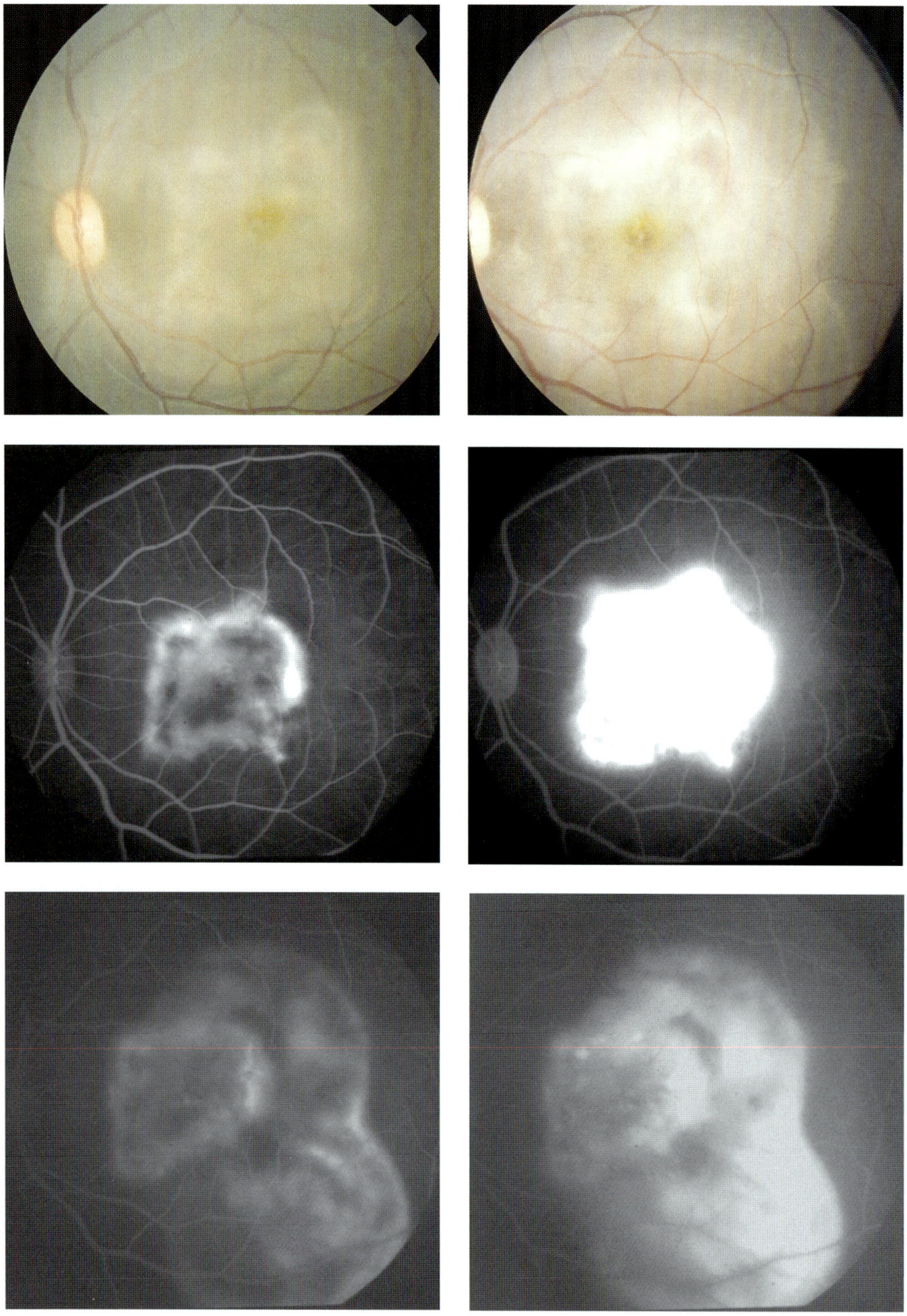

A B C D E F

FIGURE 8.2. **A:** Color photos of a fundus, before photodynamic therapy (PDT). **B:** Color photos of the same fundus, 24 hours after PDT using Lu-Tex, 2 mg/kg and 50J/cm^2. **C:** Fluorescein angiography before PDT showing early hyperfluorescence in the area of choroidal neovascularization (CNV) (42 seconds). **D:** Fluorescein angiography before PDT showing late leakage of fluorescein from the CNV (8 minutes). **E:** Fluorescein angiography 24 hours after PDT using Lu-Tex at 2 mg/kg and a fluence of 50 J/cm^2. Early frames show early hypofluorescence in the area corresponding to CNV (11 seconds). **F:** Fluorescein angiography 24 hours after PDT using Lu-Tex at 2 mg/kg and a fluence of 50 J/cm^2. Later frames show hyperfluorescence starting at the rim of the treatment spot with staining of the fibrosis within the CNV but with no leakage from the CNV (5 minutes 27 seconds).

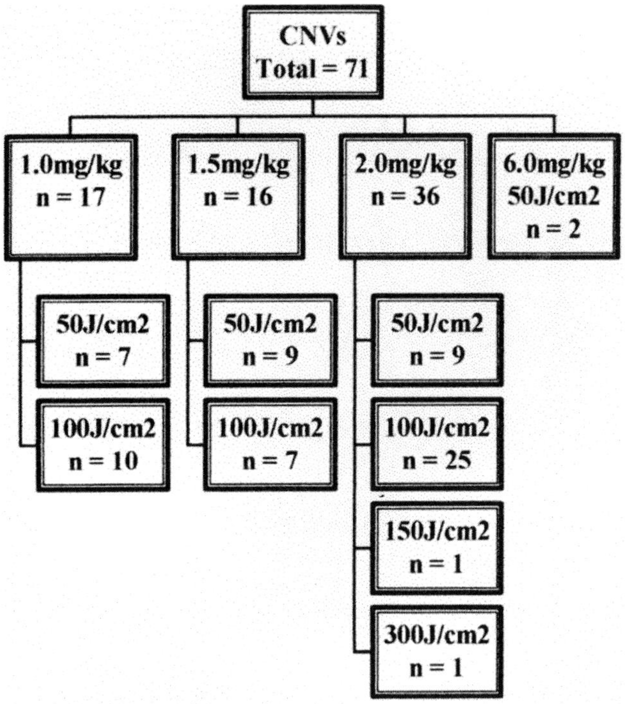

FIGURE 8.3. Distribution of eyes treated with photodynamic therapy using Lu-Tex according to dose and fluence.

response was also demonstrated: using the same dose, at 2 mg/kg, a higher fluence also produced higher rates of success at CNV closure (Fig. 8.4).

A 6 mg/kg dose of Lu-Tex was tested in one animal at a fluence of 50 J/cm^2 with irradiation performed at 15 minutes and 3 hours after the start of the infusion. Successful closure of CNV was observed at 15 minutes; however, retinal damage was also apparent. At 3 hours after Lu-Tex injection, partial closure was demonstrated with some angiographic leakage.

One animal was treated with 2 mg/kg Lu-Tex at 50 and 100 J/cm^2 and sacrificed 1 month after PDT to evaluate long-term effects. Closure of CNV was seen after 1 week at 50 J/cm^2 with irradiation done at 12 minutes after Lu-Tex injection. Fluorescein leakage reappeared at 2 weeks after PDT. At 100 J/cm^2 and irradiation performed 15 minutes after Lu-Tex injection, the treated CNV was closed for 2 weeks on FA and showed fluorescein leakage at 3 weeks after PDT.

HISTOLOGIC FINDINGS

Both treated CNV and normal retina control spots were examined histopathologically. Treated CNV showed damage to endothelial cells with extravasation of erythrocytes and fibrin. Damaged erythrocytes, fibrin, and platelets

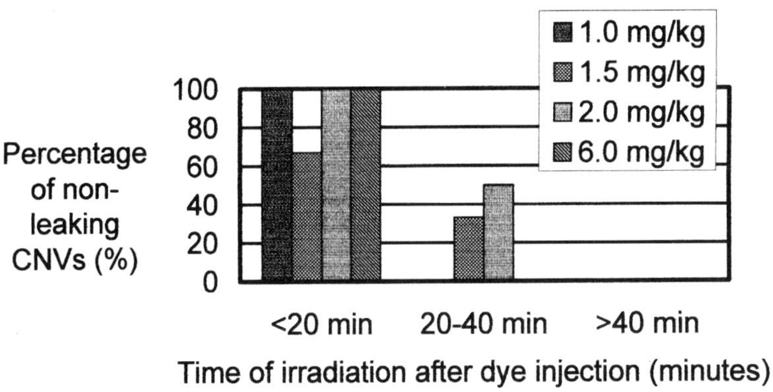

A

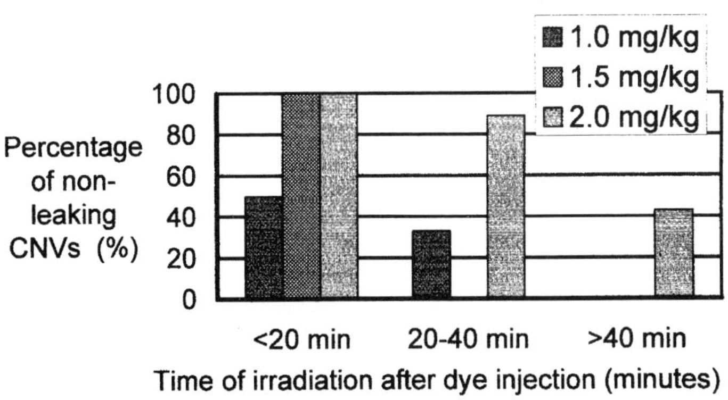

B

FIGURE 8.4. A: Bar graph of the percentage of choroidal neovascularization (CNV) closure at 1, 1.5, 2, and 6 mg/kg, and 50 J/cm^2 according to the time of irradiation after Lu-Tex injection. **B:** Bar graph of the percentage of CNV closure at 1, 1.5, and 2 mg/kg, and 100 J/cm^2 according to the time of irradiation after Lu-Tex injection.

A 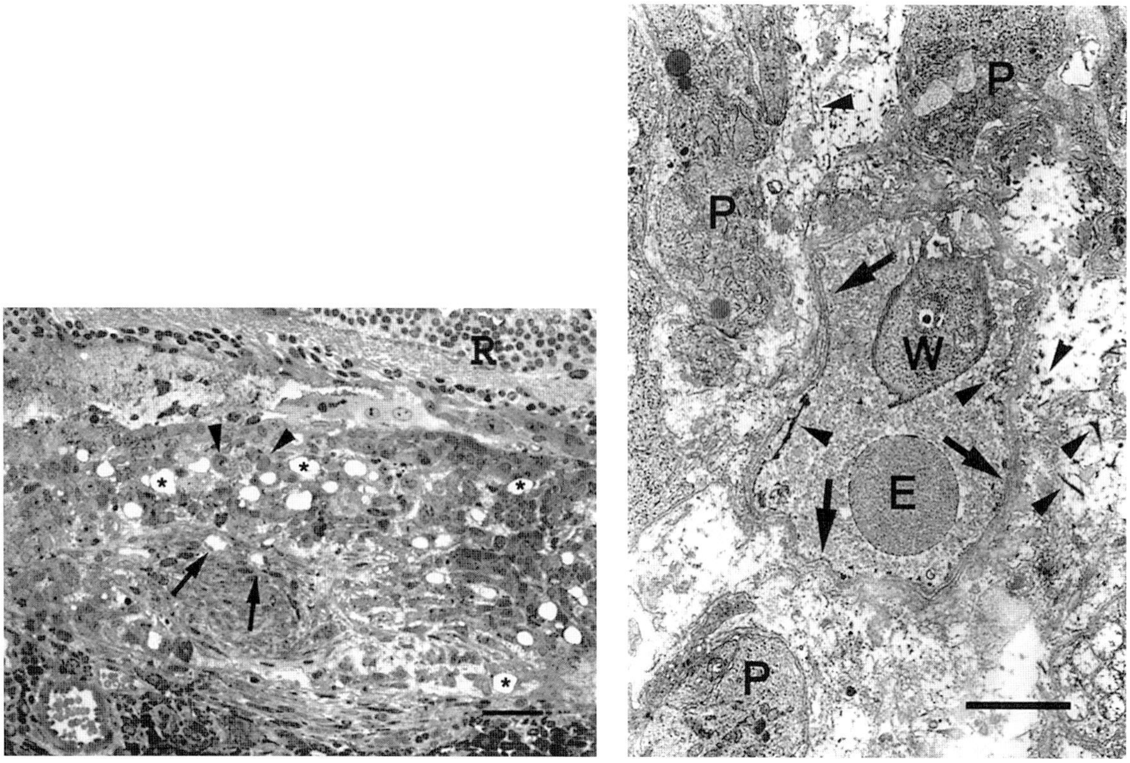 B

FIGURE 8.5. A: Light micrograph of choroidal neovascularization (CNV) 24 hours after photodynamic therapy treatment using Lu-Tex, 2 mg/kg and 50 J/cm^2. The retina *(R)* is in disarray above a CNV showing both open *(arrows)* and closed *(arrowheads)* vessels as well as retinal pigment epithelial cells (RPE) vacuoles *(asterisks)* (bar = 50 microns). **B:** Transmission electron micrograph of a capillary from the lesion shown in **(A).** The luminal surface is denuded of endothelium *(arrow)* and fibrin deposits *(arrowheads)* are seen within and outside of the capillary. The capillary is between groups of proliferating RPE cells *(P)* and contains a probable damaged erythrocyte *(E)* and white blood cell *(W)* (bar = 3 υm).

filled the lumen of capillaries within the CNV (Fig. 8.5). Similar to the findings with verteporfin 11 the retinal pigmented epithelium (RPE) was necrotic and the choriocapillaris was mostly occluded.

In the monkey model of CNV the induction of subretinal neovascularization in itself damages the outer retinal layers. In order to assess and categorize the effects of PDT on normal retina and choroid we used a grading scheme modified from a previously published version 11. According to this system (Table 8.2), grade 1 was the lowest damage observed and grade 5 the most severe. Acceptable damages (grades 1 to 3) included disruption of the RPE, closure of choriocapillaris, mild disorganization of the inner and outer segments of photoreceptors, and up to 50% pyknosis in the outer nuclear layer (ONL). Unacceptable damage (grades 4 and 5) included more than 50% pyknosis in the ONL, damage to the medium and large choroidal vessels or retinal vessels, or damage to the inner retina (Fig. 8.6). Over a total number of 79 treated lesions, 72 were found on pathological sections. The vast majority of the lesions were grade 1

TABLE 8.2. GRADING SCHEME OF PHOTODYNAMIC THERAPY EFFECT ON NORMAL RETINA/CHOROID

Grade	Damaged Retinal/Choroidal Layers
1	Retinal pigment epithelial cells (RPE) only; or RPE + slight photoreceptor changes + <10% pyknosis in the outer nuclear layer (ONL); with or without choriocapillaris closure
2	Choriocapillaris closure + RPE + photoreceptors + 10–20% pyknosis in the ONL
3	Choriocapillaris closure + RPE + photoreceptors + ONL pyknosis ≤50%
4	Choriocapillaris closure + RPE + photoreceptors + ONL pyknosis >50%
5	Choriocapillaris closure + RPE + photoreceptors + ONL pyknosis >50%, or choroidal vessel damage (medium and large), or retinal vessel or inner retinal damage

From Kramer M, Miller JW, Michaud N, et al. Liposomal benzoporphryn derivative verteporfin photodynamic therapy. Selective treatment of choroidal neovascularization in monkeys. *Ophthalmology* 1996;103:427–438, with permission.

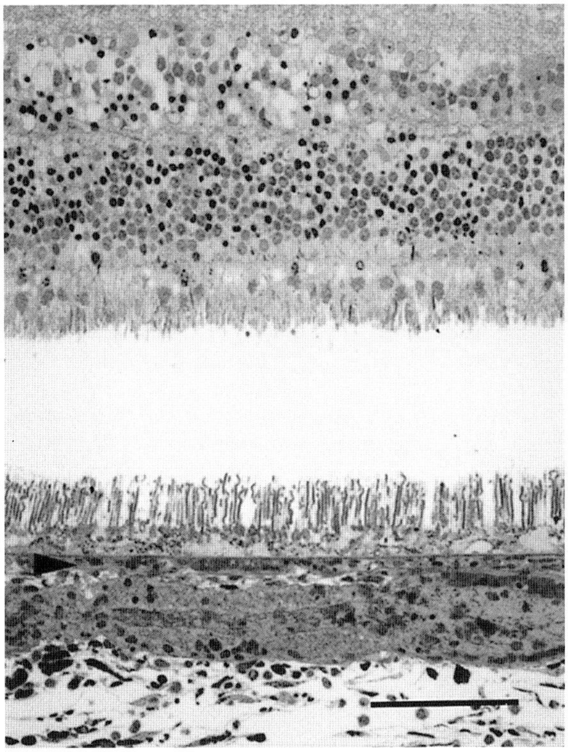

FIGURE 8.6. Light micrograph of a normal retina/choroid spot 24 hours after photodynamic therapy using Lu-Tex, 2 mg/kg and 50 J/cm² with very early irradiation time showing grade 5 damage. There is pyknosis in the inner and outer nuclear layers, closure of large choroidal vessels, as well as choriocapillaris *(arrowhead).* Retinal pigment epithelial cells (RPE) are also necrotic. Separation of retina and RPE is an artifact of preparation. Not shown are the closed inner blood vessels (bar = 100 μm).

(n = 58 or 80.5%), four were grade 2 (5.5%), one was grade 4 (1.4%), and nine were grade 5 (12.5%). At 2 mg/kg grades and 100 J/cm² grades 4 and 5 were seen at 68 minutes after injection (unacceptable pyknosis) and when irradiation was delivered early from 5 to 17 minutes (retinal vessel staining on FA) with histological damage seen at 5 minutes only. Higher fluences of 150 J/cm² and 300 J/cm² were tested in one animal irradiated at 11 and 28 minutes, respectively, with a dose of 2 mg/kg and both lesions were graded 5 because of important pyknosis in the ONL and retinal vessel closure (Fig. 8.6). A higher dose of 6 mg/kg applied at 15 minutes after the dye injection with a fluence of 50 J/cm² produced damage to the retinal vessel that was not found on the control spot classified as grade 1.

One animal was sacrificed 1 month after PDT with Lu-Tex at 2 mg/kg and a fluence of 50 or 100 J/cm² to study long-term effects of PDT. Histopathological examination showed reopened choriocapillaris, and repopulated multilayered RPE (Fig. 8.7). Occasional pyknosis of the ONL was the only change seen in the neurosensory retina.

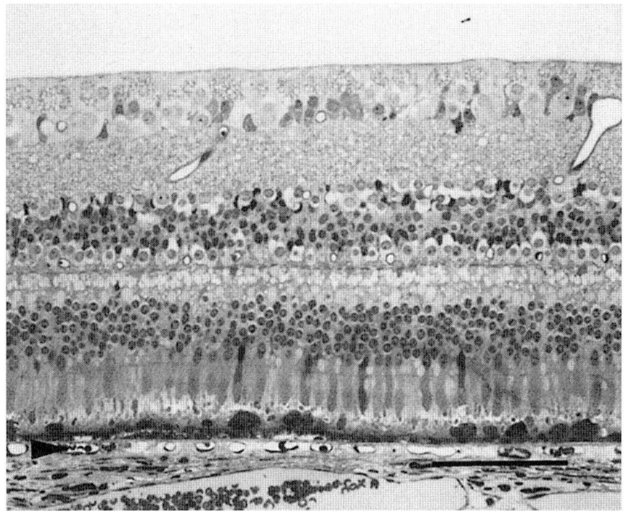

FIGURE 8.7. Light micrograph of a normal retina/choroid spot 4 weeks after photodynamic therapy using Lu-Tex, 2 mg/kg and 50 J/cm². Retina shows normal organization, although there is occasional pyknosis in the outer nuclear layer. There also is minimal fragmentation of the outer segments and large pigment-containing cells overlying the recovered retinal pigment epithelial cells and choriocapillaris *(arrowhead)* (bar = 100 μm).

CONCLUSIONS

Photodynamic therapy has revolutionized the treatment of subfoveal CNV. Because the approval of verteporfin PDT for the treatment of subfoveal CNV secondary to the exudative form of AMD, the previous standard of care guidelines established by the macular photocoagulation study (MPS) no longer apply. However, the results of PDT treatment with the only FDA-approved photosensitizer (verteporfin) are not ideal because not all the patients are eligible for treatment, only a few patients show an improvement in their vision, and the vast majority of treated patients still encounter further loss of vision. The quest for the perfect photosensitizer or treatment regimen probably is not yet over. Ideally, this photosensitizer would be chemically stable, nontoxic, with a rapid clearance from the body but persistence in the CNV, therefore allowing for specific treatment of the abnormal vessels with no harm to the surrounding normal tissues (32). Its absorption profile should be maximal in the deep penetrating wavelengths of higher than 600 nanometers to allow activation through blood and fibrous tissues; also, its triplet state quantum yield should be high to maximize the phototoxic effect (33). Motexafin lutetium is a third-generation hydrophilic photosensitizer that corresponds to these criteria. Angiographic studies performed with Lu-Tex in the monkey model of neovascularization (described elsewhere in this text) demonstrated fluorescence from the retinal vessels, choroid, and CNV starting as early as 1 minute after iv injection with rapid clearance from the retinal vessels and persistence in the

CNV for up to 50 minutes after the dye injection. This sufficient time-window allowed for experimentation of PDT with Lu-Tex in the same animal model of CNV, demonstrating angiographic closure of the CNV at 24 hours after PDT under several parameters with relative sparing of the surrounding neuroretina and underlying choroidal medium and large vessels, makes Lu-Tex an effective and selective photosensitizer for this purpose. Nonselective effects were noted if irradiation was carried out within 10 minutes after an injection of Lu-Tex at a dose of 2 mg/kg, or at 15 minutes at a dose of 6 mg/kg of Lu-Tex. Higher fluences of 150 or 300 J/cm^2 with irradiation at 11 or 28 minutes, respectively, produced retinal and large choroidal vessel damage. Effects of PDT with Lu-Tex were established histopathologically with examination of control choroidal spots. Unlike the results obtained with verteporfin Lu-Tex PDT rarely led to pyknosis in the ONL. Effective closure of CNV was achieved at a dose of 2 mg/kg, with an irradiance of 600 mW/cm^2 at fluences of both 50 and 100 J/cm^2, when irradiation was performed between 10 and 40 minutes after the start of the dye injection. Earlier irradiation might lead to retinal vessel damage and irradiation performed later than 20 minutes after the start of the Lu-Tex injection was not as efficient, especially with a fluence of 50 J/cm^2 at a dose of 2 mg/kg. Longer-term evaluation of up to 1 month after PDT with Lu-Tex demonstrated a good recovery of both the RPE and the choriocapillaris with preservation of a normal neurosensory retina histopathologically. These preclinical results provided a safe and apparently effective dosimetry for clinical experimentation in the human that are described elsewhere in this text.

REFERENCES

1. Bressler NM. Photodynamic therapy of subfoveal choroidal neovascularization in age-related macular degeneration with verteporfin: two-year results of 2 randomized clinical trials. *Arch Ophthalmol* 2001;119:198–207.
2. Bressler NM. Verteporfin therapy of subfoveal choroidal neovascularization in age-related macular degeneration: two-year results of a randomized clinical trial including lesions with occult with no classic choroidal neovascularization-verteporfin in photodynamic therapy report 2. *Am J Ophthalmol* 2002;133:168–169.
3. Sharma S, Hollands H, Brown GC, et al. Improvement in quality of life from photodynamic therapy: a Canadian perspective. *Can J Ophthalmol* 2001;36:332–338.
4. Miller JW, Schmidt-Erfurth U, Sickenberg M, et al. Photodynamic therapy with verteporfin for choroidal neovascularization caused by age-related macular degeneration: results of a single treatment in a phase 1 and 2 study. *Arch Ophthalmol* 1999;117: 1161–1173.
5. Thomas EL, Langhofer M. Closure of experimental subretinal neovessels with dihematoporphyrin ether augmented argon green laser photocoagulation. *Photochem Photobiol* 1987;46: 5881–5886.
6. Miller H, Miller B. Photodynamic therapy of subretinal neovascularization in the monkey eye. *Arch Ophthalmol* 1993;111: 855–860.
7. Kliman GH, Puliafito CA, Stern D, et al. Phthalocyanine photodynamic therapy: new strategy for closure of choroidal neovascularization. *Lasers Surg Med* 1994;15:2–10.
8. Iliaki OE, Naoumidi II, Tsilimbaris MK, et al. Photothrombosis of retinal and choroidal vessels in rabbit eyes using chloroaluminum sulfonated phthalocyanine and a diode laser. *Lasers Surg Med* 1996;19:311–323.
9. Kreimer-Birnbaum M. Modified porphyrins, chlorins, phthalocyanines, and purpurins: second-generation photosensitizers for photodynamic therapy. *Semin Hematol* 1989;26:157–173.
10. Husain D, Kramer M, Kenny AG, et al. Effects of photodynamic therapy using verteporfin on experimental choroidal neovascularization and normal retina and choroid up to 7 weeks after treatment. *Invest Ophthalmol Vis Sci* 1999;40:2322–2331.
11. Kramer M, Miller JW, Michaud N, et al. Liposomal benzoporphyrin derivative verteporfin photodynamic therapy. Selective treatment of choroidal neovascularization in monkeys. *Ophthalmology* 1996;103:427–438.
12. Miller JW, Walsh AW, Kramer M, et al. Photodynamic therapy of experimental choroidal neovascularization using lipoprotein-delivered benzoporphyrin. *Arch Ophthalmol* 1995;113: 810–818.
13. Sessler JL, Miller RA. Texaphyrins: new drugs with diverse clinical applications in radiation and photodynamic therapy. *Biochem Pharmacol* 2000;59:733–739.
14. Harriman A, Maiya BG, Murai T, et al. Metallotexaphryns: a new family of photosensitizers for efficient generation of singlet oxygen. *J Chem Soc Chem Commun* 1989;5:314–316.
15. Sessler JL, Hemmi G, Mody TD, et al. Texaphrins: synthesis and applications. *Am Chem Soc Accounts Chem Res* 1994;27:43–50.
16. Zellweger M, Radu A, Monnier P, et al. Fluorescence pharmacokinetics of Lutetium Texaphyrin (PCI-0123, Lu-Tex) in the skin and in healthy and tumoral hamster cheek-pouch mucosa. *J Photochem Photobiol B* 2000;55:56–62.
17. Graham K, Arbour JD, Connolly E, et al. Digital angiography using lutetium motexafin in a monkey model of choroidal neovascularization. *Arvo Abs* 1999;40:402.
18. Blumenkranz MS, Woodburn KW, Qing F, et al. Lutetium texaphyrin (Lu-Tex): a potential new agent for ocular fundus angiography and photodynamic therapy. *Am J Ophthalmol* 2000;129: 353–362.
19. Bellnier DA, Dougherty TJ. A preliminary pharmacokinetic study of intravenous Photofrin in patients. *Med Phys* 1996;26:1552–1558.
20. Young LH, Howard MA, Hu LK, et al. Photodynamic therapy of pigmented choroidal melanomas using a liposomal preparation of benzoporphyrin derivative. *Arch Ophthalmol* 1996;114: 186–192.
21. Woodburn K, Fan Q, Miles D, et al. Localization and efficacy analysis of the phototherapeutic lutetium Texaphyrin (PCI-0123) in the murine EMT6 sarcoma model. *Photochem Photobiol* 1997;65:410–415.
22. Pass HI. Photodynamic therapy in oncology: mechanisms and clinical use. *J Natl Cancer Inst* 1993;85:443–456.
23. Hammer-Wilson MJ, Ghahramanlou M, Berns MW. Photodynamic activity of lutetium-texaphyrin in a mouse tumor system. *Lasers Surg Med* 1999;24:276–284.
24. Grossweiner L. Photodynamic therapy. *J Laser Appl* 1995;7: 51–57.
25. Young SW, Woodburn KW, Wright M, et al. Lutetium texaphyrin (PCI-0123): a near-infrared, water-soluble photosensitizer. *Photochem Photobiol* 1996;63:892–897.
26. Woodburn KW, Fan Q, Kessel D, et al. Photodynamic therapy of B16F10 murine melanoma with lutetium texaphyrin. *J Invest Dermatol* 1998;110:746–751.
27. Wilson BC. Photodynamic therapy: light delivery and dosage for

second generation photosensitizers. Photosensitizing compounds: their chemistry, biology, and clinical use. In: Bock G, Hartnett S, eds. *Ciba Foundation Symposium 146.* New York: Wiley, 1989: 60–77.

28. Rockson SG. Lutetium texaphyrin: a new therapeutic tool for human atherosclerosis. *Curr Treat Options Cardiovasc Med* 1999; 1:199–202.
29. Rockson SG, Kramer P, Razavi M, et al. Photoangioplasty for human peripheral atherosclerosis: results of a phase I trial of photodynamic therapy with motexafin lutetium (Antrin). *Circulation* 2000;102:2322–2324.
30. Hayase M, Woodbum KW, Perlroth J, et al. Photoangioplasty with local motexafin lutetium delivery reduces macrophages in a rabbit post-balloon injury model. *Cardiovasc Res* 2001;49: 449–455.
31. Renno RZ, Delori FC, Holzer RA, et al. Photodynamic therapy using Lu-Tex induces apoptosis in vitro, and its effect is potentiated by angiostatin in retinal capillary endothelial cells. *Invest Ophthalmol Vis Sci* 2000;41:3963–3971.
32. Lui H, Anderson RR. Photodynamic therapy in dermatology: recent developments. *Dermatol Clin* 1993;11:1–13.
33. Takemura T, Ohta N, Nakajima S, et al. Critical importance of the triplet lifetime of photosensitizer in photodynamic therapy of tumor. *Photochem Photobiol* 1989;50:339–344.

9

PHOTODYNAMIC THERAPY FOR IRIS NEOVASCULARIZATION

DEEBA HUSAIN
JOAN W. MILLER
EVANGELOS S. GRAGOUDAS

Growth of new blood vessels on the iris is a devastating complication of ocular ischemia, and often leads to neovascular glaucoma and optic atrophy with loss of vision and pain that frequently necessitates enucleation. Iris neovascularization is thought to occur when ischemic tissue releases angiogenic factors, such as vascular endothelial growth factor (VEGF) that lead to new blood vessel growth on the iris (1,2). The conditions that lead to iris neovascularization (rubeosis) include diabetic eye disease, retinal vein occlusion, ocular tumors, longstanding retinal detachment, and carotid artery disease (3). These new vessels can lead to hyphema and iritis, and can cause closure of the angle, leading to intractable glaucoma. The current treatment for iris neovascularization and neovascular glaucoma is retinal ablation by panretinal photocoagulation or cryotherapy (4). Goniophotocoagulation is occasionally used to stabilize the angle. Topical steroids, mydriatics, topical and oral glaucoma medications, and even filtration or shunt procedures may be required to treat the neovascular glaucoma. However, retinal ablation takes 4 to 6 weeks to take effect and angle closure can occur in the interim. Photodynamic therapy (PDT) has been shown to close experimental iris neovascularization within 24 hours after treatment (5–7), and may offer an adjunctive therapy to the existing treatment modalities.

Photodynamic therapy using the photosensitizer verteporfin is a new treatment for choroidal neovascularization (CNV) in macular degeneration and other disorders approved by health authorities in the United States and abroad. It is a localized treatment that relies on chemical effects of photosensitized tissues exposed to light of a specific wavelength. The treatment involves injection of a photosensitizer dye that accumulates in proliferating tissues such as tumors and new vessels. This photosensitized tissue is then exposed to light at an absorption maximum of the dye, leading to formation of singlet oxygen and reactive intermediates, which can cause autoxidation and direct damage to cell membranes, nucleus, lysosomes, and mitochondria (8,9). Tumor studies have suggested two mechanisms for PDT effect; a direct cytotoxic effect on tumor cells and occlusion of tumor vessels (9–12).

Photodynamic therapy has not been used clinically in iris neovascularization but has been tested in experimental model. Three photosensitizers have been studied, namely, hematoporphyrin (HpD) (5), phthalocyanine (CASPc) (6), and benzoporphyrin derivative or verteporfin (7). All three studies created iris neovascularization in the monkey eye using the model described by Virdi and Hayreh (13) or its modification by Miller and associates (6). This model involves occlusion of three or all of the major branches of the retinal vein using argon laser or yellow dye laser, leading to widespread ischemia of the retina. Iris neovascularization developed in almost all eyes within 7 to 10 days of the laser induction. A grading scheme has been developed based on the fluoroangiographic appearance of the iris vessels (Table 9.1). This grading scheme has been used in studies of photodynamic therapy of iris neovascularization.

TABLE 9.1. GRADING SCHEME FOR IRIS NEOVASCULARIZATION

Grade	Description
0	Vessels may or may not be visible; no leakage on fluorescein (FA) (normal iris)
1	Prominent, tortuous, and discontinuous vessels; do not leak on FA
2	Prominent, nonradial vessels that leak on FA; less than standard photograph 2A
3	Prominent nonradial vessels that leak early on FA (20–30 s); greater than standard photograph 2A
4	Individual vessels cannot be delineated on early frames (20–30 s) of FA; iris appears as a diffuse opaque fluorescent sheet
5	Identical to grade 4, associated with glaucoma, hyphema, or ectropion uvea

ANGIOGRAPHY OF IRIS NEOVASCULARIZATION

Iris vessels are visualized and documented with fluorescein angiography (5–7) (Figs. 9.1 and 9.2). The normal iris in the early phase of the angiogram shows radial hyperfluorescent vessels that do not leak or stain in the late phase. In contrast, iris neovascularization is seen in the early phase as tortuous radial or nonradial vessels or a sheet of hyperfluorescence that leaks in the late phase of the angiogram. Angiography of the iris also has been performed using indocyanine green (7), which showed deeper iris vessels that are tortuous but do not leak in the late phase of the angiogram. In contrast, iris neovascularization was seen as tortuous hyperfluorescent vessels that leaked in the late phase. Liposomal benzoporphyrin derivative (BPD) or verteporfin, has been used to perform iris angiography as well (7). Normal iris showed radial hyperfluorescent vessels in the early phase of the angiogram with no leakage of the dye in the late phase. Iris neovascularization appeared as tortuous dilated hyperfluorescent vessels in the early phase of the angiogram and showed staining of the vessel wall in the late phase.

CLINICAL COURSE OF IRIS NEOVASCULARIZATION

Iris neovascularization is always secondary to an ocular or systemic disorder (1,2). The exact pathogenesis is not known, but it is postulated that retinal ischemia leads to the release of angiogenic factors, such as vascular endothelial growth factors. These vasoproliferative factors gain access to the iris and anterior chamber and lead to the formation of new vessels (14).

The clinical course of iris neovascularization has been divided into three stages. The first stage is the appearance of small individual vessels at the pupillary border and the angle of the anterior chamber. This may be difficult to diagnose by slit-lamp biomicroscopy, but fluorescein angiography shows leakage of dye from areas of neovascularization (15). The second stage of this disease involves clinically

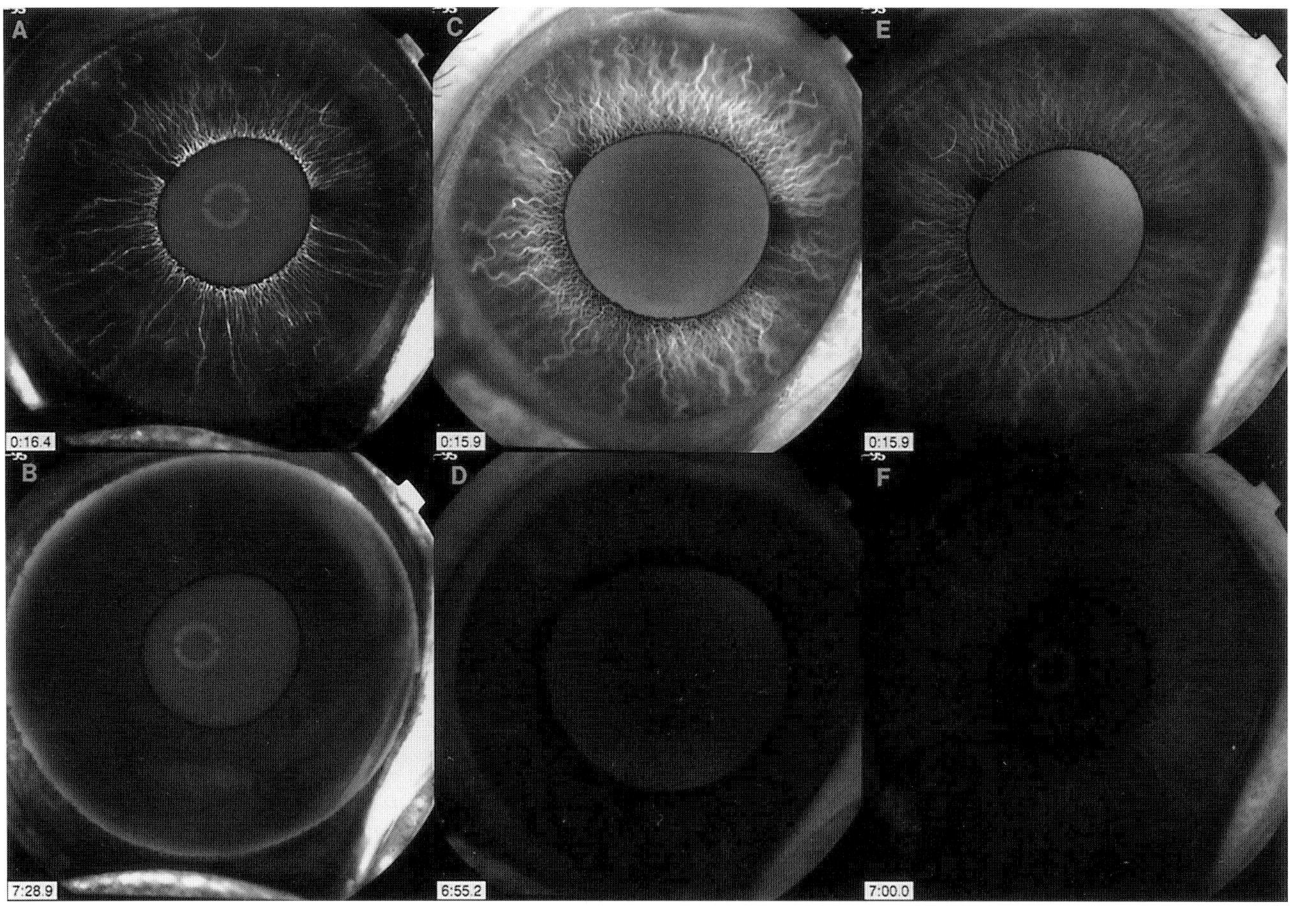

FIGURE 9.1. Angiography of normal cynomolgus monkey iris. **A,B:** Fluorescein angiography of normal iris shows fine radial vessels with no leakage in the late phase *(B)*. **C,D:** Indocyanine green angiography of normal iris demonstrates higher density of larger and tortuous vessels with no leakage or staining in the late phase *(D)*. **E,F:** Liposomal benzoporphyrin derivative angiography of normal iris demonstrates radial and tortuous vessels and no staining in the late phase.

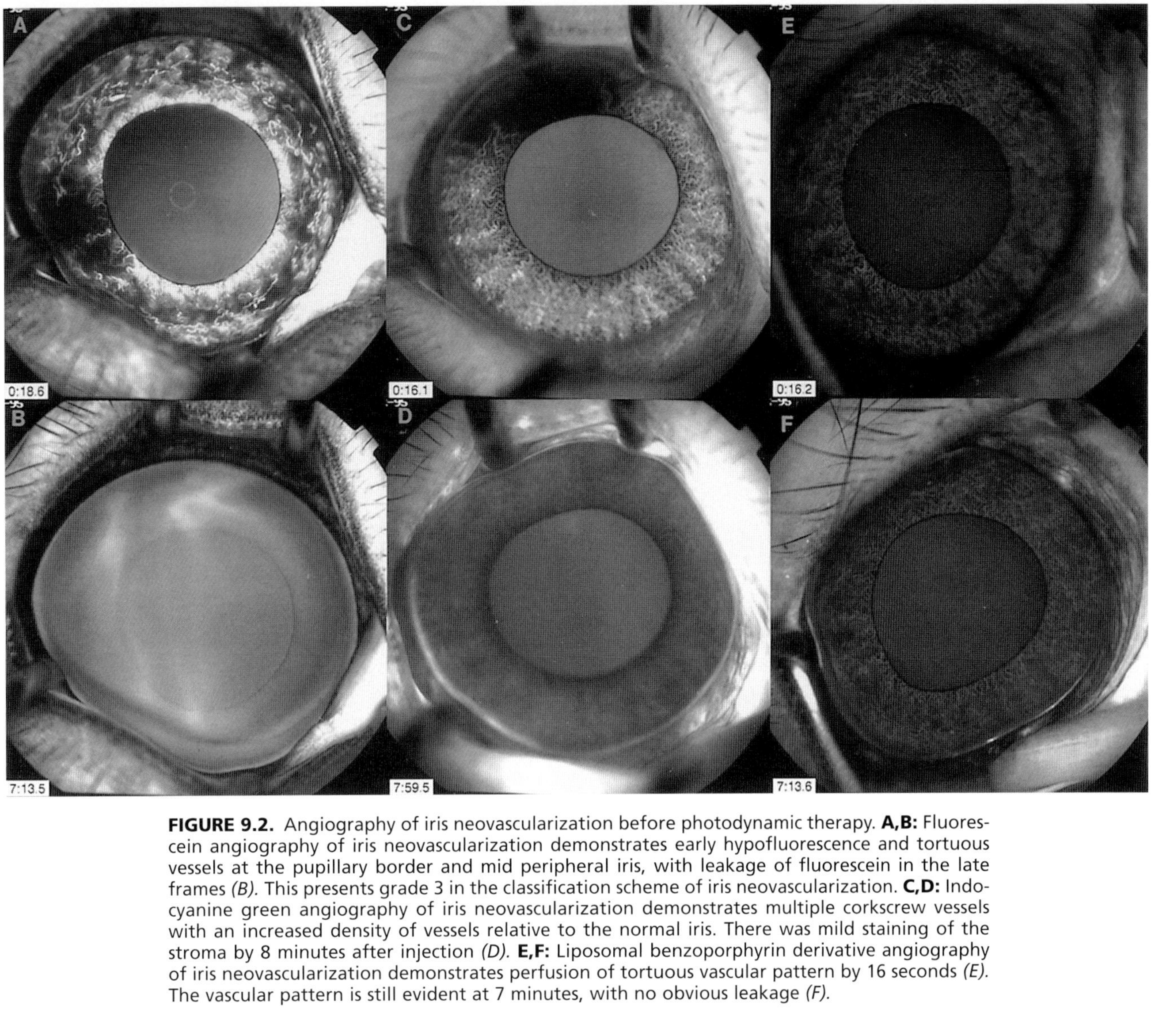

FIGURE 9.2. Angiography of iris neovascularization before photodynamic therapy. **A,B:** Fluorescein angiography of iris neovascularization demonstrates early hypofluorescence and tortuous vessels at the pupillary border and mid peripheral iris, with leakage of fluorescein in the late frames *(B)*. This presents grade 3 in the classification scheme of iris neovascularization. **C,D:** Indocyanine green angiography of iris neovascularization demonstrates multiple corkscrew vessels with an increased density of vessels relative to the normal iris. There was mild staining of the stroma by 8 minutes after injection *(D)*. **E,F:** Liposomal benzoporphyrin derivative angiography of iris neovascularization demonstrates perfusion of tortuous vascular pattern by 16 seconds *(E)*. The vascular pattern is still evident at 7 minutes, with no obvious leakage *(F)*.

apparent new vessels, which cover the iris surface and branch into the angle of anterior chamber. The eye pressure may be high at this stage but the angles are open (16). The third stage of the disease involves new vessels on the iris surface and angle with the formation of peripheral anterior synechiae and neovascular glaucoma.

PHOTODYNAMIC THERAPY USING HEMATOPORPHYRIN

Hematoporphyrin derivative is a photosensitizer that is activated by a light at 630 nm. Hematoporphyrin derivative localizes to rapidly proliferating tissues such as neoplastic tissues, proliferating new vessels and regenerative tissues (17). Packer and colleagues (5) used a dose of 3 mg/kg of intravenous (iv) hematoporphyrin derivative to treat four eyes of cynomolgus monkeys with experimental iris neovascularization. Irradiations were performed at 3½ to 8¾ hours after administration of the photosensitizer, with light at 630 nm from an argon dye laser. The total light dose delivered to the iris was 538 to 540 J/cm^2. In two eyes the whole iris was irradiated, in one eye the nasal iris was treated, and in one eye the inferior iris was treated. All treated irides showed angiographic closure of neovascularization at 24 hours after the treatment. Anterior chamber inflammation was seen in all eyes, and one eye developed very high intraocular pressure (70 mm Hg) that resolved in one day. Additionally, one eye showed a small hemorrhage over the iris in the treated area. Two eyes that were followed for 2 weeks after treatment developed leaky new vessels at 6 to 7 days after PDT. These vessels were successfully treated a second time with PDT using the same parameters.

Hematoporphyrin derivative (18) has several disadvantages because is it is not a pure compound but a mixture of porphyrins, and it absorbs poorly at longer wavelengths; thus, tissue penetration of the treatment may be limited. Hematoporphyrin derivative is retained in the skin as well and causes photosensitization for several weeks.

PHOTODYNAMIC THERAPY USING PHTHALOCYANINE

Chloroaluminum sulfonated phthalocyanine (CASPc) is a relatively pure compound that is stable at room temperature. Plasma levels of CASPc peak at 6 minutes after iv injection in animal models (19). It is retained by skin, but does not seem to cause photosensitivity. It absorbs light maximally at 675 nm, with good tissue penetration (8). Phthalocyanines are hydrophilic and lipophilic, depending on the degree of sulfonation, and have been shown to localize in lysosomes. Miller and associates (6) studied the effect of CASPc photodynamic therapy in experimental iris neovascularization. Chloroaluminum sulfonated phthalocyanine was used at a dose of 0.5 to 1 mg/kg of body weight, and irradiation was performed at 5 minutes after dye injection. Laser light of 675 nm was applied using an argon dye laser delivered as a 10-mm diameter beam. Sectors of iris were shielded using different shaped apertures. The light doses used were 34, 68, and 102 J/cm^2, at 200 mW with treatment times of 133 to 399 seconds. Effective closure of iris neovascularization was seen by fluorescein angiography (FA) and confirmed by histopathology using light doses of 68 and 102 J/cm^2. The vessels remained closed for 7 days and neovascularization recurred at 13 days after PDT.

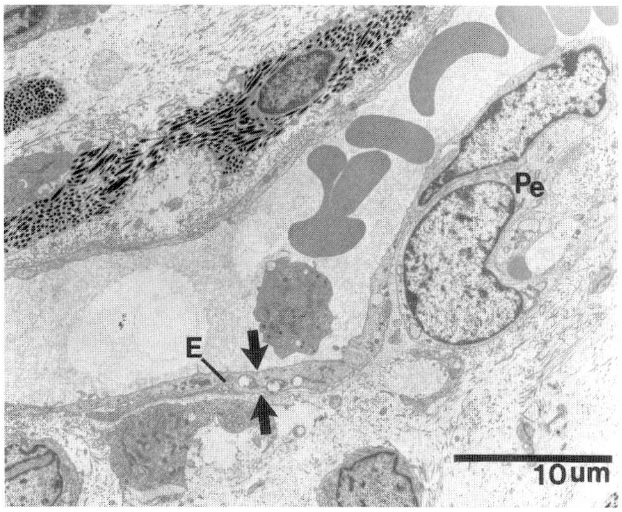

FIGURE 9.3. Electron micrograph of iris 1 hour after treatment demonstrating endothelial damage in a patent vessel. There is swelling of the nuclei and vacuolization of the cytoplasm *(between arrows)* of both endothelial cells (E) and pericytes (Pe). Cells adjacent to the vessels appear undamaged. (Original magnification, ×1,900)

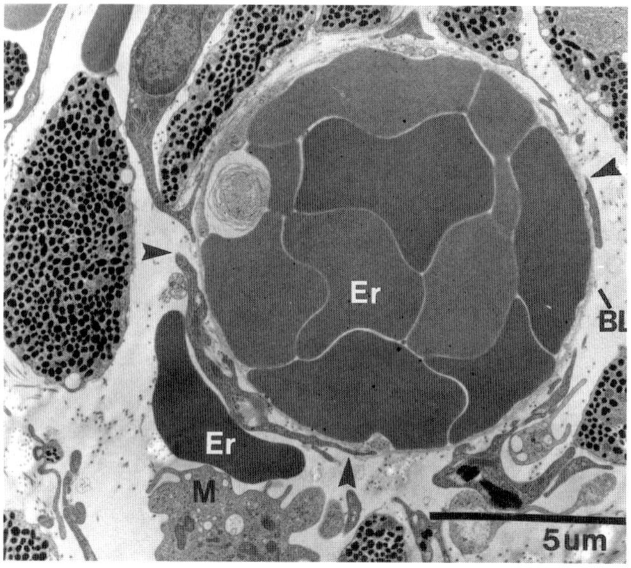

FIGURE 9.4. Electron micrograph of iris 3 days after treatment. Packed erythrocytes (Er) are surrounded by disintegrating endothelium. The basal lamina (BL) is relatively well preserved. Macrophage processes *(arrowheads)* are wrapped around the basal lamina. M = macrophages. (Original magnification, ×5,200)

Light microscopy at 1 hour after PDT showed vascular occlusion by thrombus with aggregated platelets and trapped red cells. Electron microscopy (Fig. 9.3) at this stage showed vacuolization in endothelial cells and pericytes. Platelets and erythrocytes were adherent to basal lamina where endothelium was disrupted. At 2 to 3 days after PDT, fluorescein angiography showed no perfusion of iris new vessels. Light and electron microscopy showed clumps of RBCs surrounded by disintegrating endothelial cells, and macrophages were seen around these occluded vessels, a picture consistent with partially resorbed occluded vessels (Fig. 9.4). At 5 days after PDT, angiography still showed no perfusion in iris vessels. Electron microscopy showed only vessel remnants with basal lamina outlining empty lumens surrounded by macrophages, indicating complete resorption of vessels (Fig. 9.5). At day 13 after PDT, the iris vessels perfused and showed leakage on angiography. Histopathology showed new vessels on the surface of iris and in the stroma, indicating recurrence of neovascularization. Rare whorls of fibrous such as cells that were consistent with remnants of occluded vessels were seen (Fig. 9.6).

The side effects of CASPc PDT were minimal; one eye showed an acute rise of intraocular pressure up to 23 mm Hg at 1 hour after treatment, which resolved within 48 hours. Mild lid swelling and conjunctival chemosis was seen as well as minimal anterior chamber inflammation (1 + cells/flare), all of which resolved by 48 hours. However, the long-term systemic side effects of CASPc are not well known.

The authors suggested that the most likely mechanism of phthalocyanine PDT using these parameters was vascular damage based on this study. This could be explained by membrane damage both to intracellular and extracellular

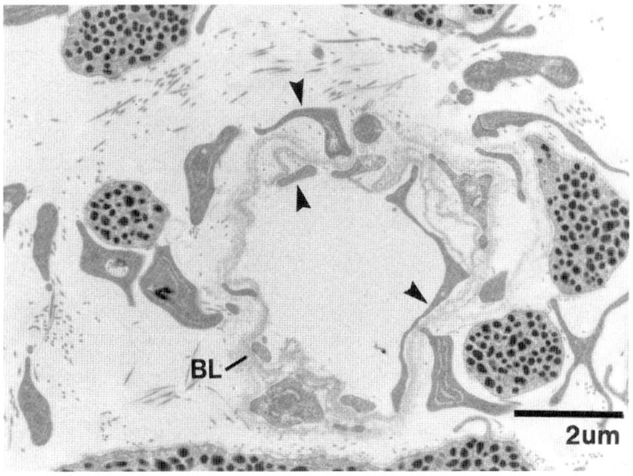

FIGURE 9.5. Electron micrograph of iris 5 days after treatment. Basal lamina (BL) outlines an empty lumen, associated with macrophage processes *(arrowheads).* No endothelial cells or pericytes are seen. (Original magnification, ×5,200)

organelles. Following PDT the endothelial cells lost their normal junctions, leading to exposure of basal lamina and aggregation of platelets and RBC, which resulted in vascular occlusion. The damage seemed to be limited to endothelial cells and pericytes with sparing of stromal cells.

PHOTODYNAMIC THERAPY USING LIPOSOMAL BENZOPORPHYRIN DERIVATIVE (VERTEPORFIN)

Liposomal benzoporphyrin derivative (BPD) or verteporfin has been used extensively in patients for the treatment of choroidal neovascularization, as well as some limited use in dermatology clinical trials and is safe for human use (20). It has been found to be effective *in vitro* and *in vivo* (21). It is rapidly cleared from the body, with a half-life of 30 minutes, thus reducing the risk of systemic photosensitivity (22). It absorbs light at 580 and 690 nm, although PDT is done with 690 nm light to achieve better tissue penetration (21).

The effect of verteporfin PDT on iris neovascularization was studied at our institution, in experimental iris neovascularization in four cynomolgus monkeys. Intravenous infusion of 0.375 to 0.75 mg/kg body weight of verteporfin was given over 10 minutes. Irradiation was performed 10 to 50 minutes after drug administration. Light was generated at 689 nm using a photoactivation diode laser and slit-lamp delivery system. Treatment parameters included a fluence of 150 J/cm^2, irradiance of 600 mW/cm^2 with a treatment time of 4 minutes and 9 seconds. Light was delivered as a 4-mm spot, using either three to four spots placed on each iris with untreated areas in between or seven confluent spots to cover the entire iris surface.

Verteporfin PDT at a dose of 0.75 mg/kg with light parameters given in the preceding, was effective in acute closure (24 hours) of iris neovascularization (Fig. 9.7). Light microscopy showed vascular occlusion with white cells, RBC, and platelets in the neovascularization of the anterior border of iris extending into the anterior stroma. Damage to the iris was more severe to the iris root than the pupillary margin. The ciliary body also showed vascular occlusion and epithelial damage. Electron microscopy of occluded vessels showed loss of endothelial cells or vacuolization. Deeper iris stromal vessels were closed at higher drug doses with irradiation at earlier time points after the start of drug infusion. Follow up of the treated eyes showed loss of the neovascular tissue over the iris at 3, 6, and 9 days after PDT, indicating atrophy of the neovascularization

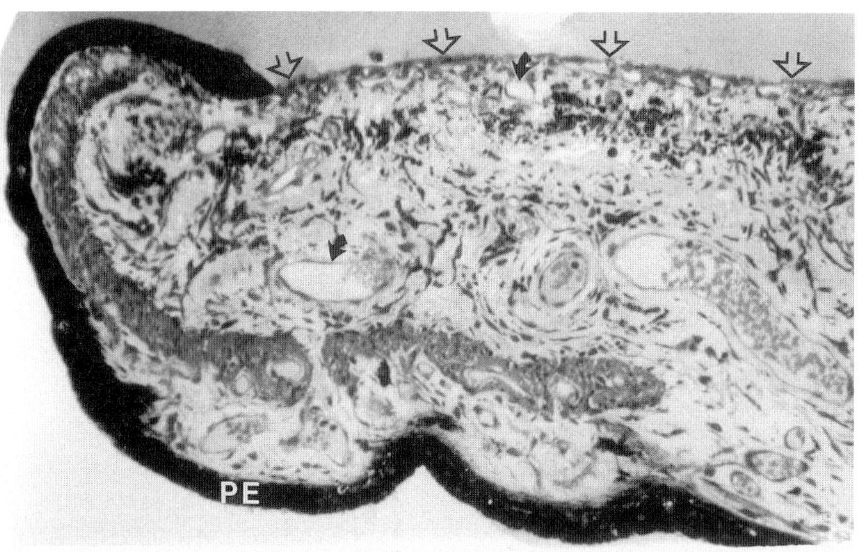

FIGURE 9.6. Light micrograph of iris 13 days after treatment. Open vessels are apparent on the surface of the iris and in the stroma *(arrows).* A fibrovascular membrane is evident over the surface of the iris *(open arrows),* causing ectropion uveae. PE, pigment epithelium. (Original magnification, ×100)

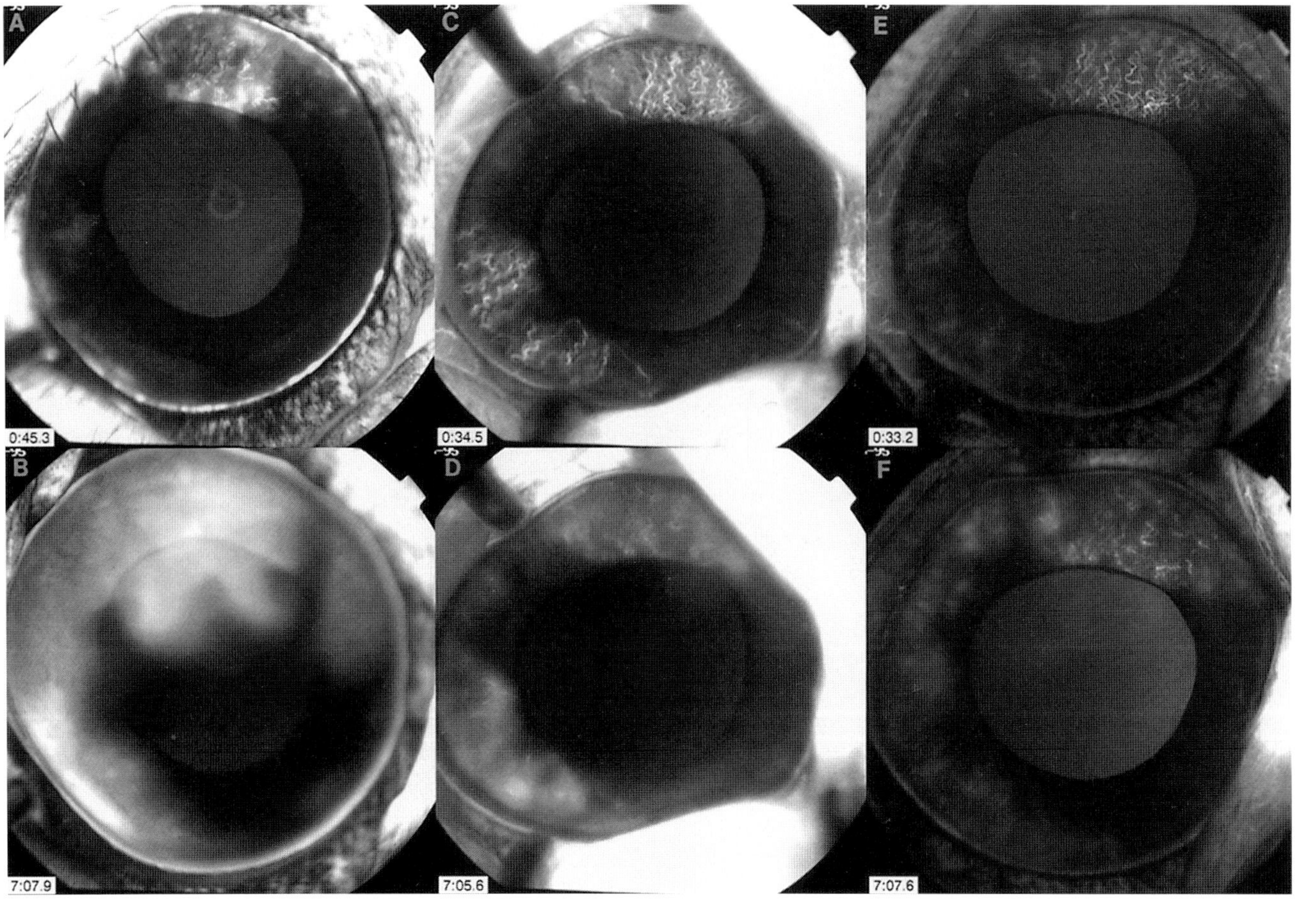

FIGURE 9.7. Iris angiography at 24 hours after PDT of the eyes in Figure 9.2, with seven contiguous spots starting at the 1 o'clock position. **A,B:** Fluorescein angiography at 24 hours after PDT shows hypofluorescence of the iris from 1 to 11 o'clock in early frames, with perfusion of vessels at the 12 o'clock position corresponding to the area irradiated latest (41 minutes) after the start of dye infusion. Leakage is evident in the later frames primarily originating from the 12 o'clock area. **C,D:** Indocyanine green angiography 24 hours after PDT demonstrates hypofluorescence throughout most of the iris except for some perfusion of vessels at the 11 to 1 o'clock and 7 to 8 o'clock positions. The vascular pattern between the 7 and 8 o'clock positions appears less dense than prior to PDT. A later frame shows staining and leakage from the same area. **E,F:** Liposomal benzoporphyrin derivative angiography 24 hours after PDT demonstrates hypofluorescence from the 1 to 11 o'clock positions. There is some faint fluorescence between the 7 and 8 o'clock positions. Some staining of vessels is seen in the later frames, with patchy staining in the stroma.

after successful PDT. Few open capillaries with plump nuclei were seen, which may represent recanalization or growth of new vessels owing to continued retinal ischemic stimulus.

No significant side effects were observed after verteporfin PDT. No significant inflammation was seen. The angle structures did not show any abnormality on histopathology after PDT and intraocular pressures did not show a significant rise. There was no evidence of neovascular glaucoma, and histopathology showed damage to ciliary vasculature and ciliary epithelium. This may indicate that PDT using verteporfin may be successful as a cyclodestructive method for reducing aqueous production in causes of severe neovascular glaucoma.

SUMMARY

Iris neovascularization and neovascular glaucoma are rare but dreaded complications of ocular ischemia, which presumably result from release of factors such as vascular endothelial growth factor in several ocular disorders. The accepted treatment is retinal ablation, but it requires several weeks to take effect. In the interim the angle can close, leading to intractable glaucoma, severe pain, and loss of vision. Photodynamic therapy of iris neovascularization offers an adjunctive therapy to retinal ablation. Photodynamic therapy of iris neovascularization in the primate model, using various photosensitizers (hematoporphyrin, phthalocyanine, and verteporfin) has shown acute closure of the iris new vessels within 24 to 48 hours of treatment. The effect of treatment is damage to the endothelial cells, causing thrombosis and closure of vessels that is demonstrated on fluorescein angiography as lack of perfusion. Verteporfin PDT also showed damage to ciliary epithelium, which may reduce aqueous production and help control intraocular pressure. Reparative process and recanalization or new vessel growth was observed 1 to 2 weeks after treatment with all photosensitizers. Therefore, repeat treatments may be needed until the retinal ablation takes effect or photodynamic therapy may be combined with antiangiogenic drugs.

REFERENCES

1. Schultze RR. Rubeosis iridis. *Am J Ophthalmol* 1967;63:487–495.
2. Glaser BM, D'Amore PA, Michels RG, et al. The demonstration of angiogenic activity from ocular tissues. Preliminary report. *Ophthalmology* 1980;87:440–446.
3. Gartner S, Henkind P. Neovascularization of the iris (rubeosis iridis). *Surv Ophthalmol* 1978:22:291–312.
4. Wand M, Dueker DK, Aiello LM, et al. Effects of panretinal photocoagulation on rubeosis iridis, angle neovascularization, and neovascular glaucoma. *Am J Ophthalmol* 1978;86:332–339.
5. Packer AJ, Tse DT, Gu XG, et al. Hematoporphyrin photoradiation for iris neovascularization. *Arch Ophthalmol* 1984;102:1193–1197.
6. Miller JW, Stinson WG, Gregory WA, et al. Phthalocyanine photodynamic therapy of experimental iris neovascularization. *Ophthalmology* 1991;98:1711–1719.
7. Husain D, Miller JW, Kenney AG, et al. Photodynamic therapy and digital angiography of experimental iris neovascularization using liposomal benzoporphyrin derivative. *Ophthalmology* 1997;104:1242–1250.
8. Manyak MJ, Russo A, Smith PD, et al. Photodynamic therapy. *J Clin Oncol* 1988;6:380–391.
9. Nelson JS, Liaw LH, Orenstein A, et al. Mechanism of tumor destruction following photodynamic therapy with hematoporphyrin derivative, chlorin, and phthalocyanine. *J Natl Cancer Inst* 1988;80:1599–1605.
10. Zhou CN. Mechanism of tumor necrosis induced by photodynamic therapy. *J Photochem Photobiol* 1989;3:299–318.
11. Weiman TJ, Mang TS, Fingar VH, et al. Effects of photodynamic therapy on blood flow in normal and tumor vessels. *Surgery* 1988;104:512–517.
12. Milanesi C, Biolo R, Reddi E, et al. Ultrastructural studies on the mechanism of the photodynamic therapy of tumors. *Photochem Photobiol* 1987;46:675–681.
13. Virdi PS, Hayreh SS. Ocular neovascularization with retinal vein occlusion. *Arch Ophthalmol* 1982;100:331–341.
14. Glaser BM, D'Amore PA, Michels RG, et al. Demonstration of vasoproliferative activity from mammalian retina. *J Cell Biol* 1980;84:298–304.
15. Mitsui Y, Matsubara M, Kanagawa M. Fluorescence irido corneal photography. *Br J Ophthalmol* 1969;53:505–512.
16. Grant WM. Management of neovascular glaucoma. In: Leopold IH (ed). Symposium on ocular therapy. St. Louis, MO: Mosby, 1974:36–61.
17. Dougherty TJ, Kaufman JE, Goldfarb A, et al. Photoradiation therapy for treatment of malignant tumors. *Cancer Res* 1978;38:2628–2635.
18. Kreimer-Birnbaum M. Modified porphyrins, chlorins, phthalocyanines and purpurins: second generation photosensitizers for photodynamic therapy. *Semin Hematol* 1989;26:157–173.
19. Chan WS, Marshall JF, Lam GYF, et al. Tissue uptake, distribution and potency of photoactivable dye chloroaluminum sulfonated phthalocyanine in mice bearing transplantable tumors. *Cancer Res* 1988;48:3040–3044.
20. Lui J, Hruza L, Kollias N, et al. Photodynamic therapy of malignant tumors with Benzoporphyrin derivative monoacid ring A (BPD-MA): preliminary investigations. In Anderson RR, Shapshay SM, White JV, eds. Lasers in otolaryngology, dermatology, and tissue welding. *SPEI* 1993;1876:147–151.
21. Aveline B, Hasan T, Redmond RW. Photophysical and photosensitizing properties of benzoporphyrin derivative monoacid ring A (BPD-MA). *J Photochem Photobiol* 1994;59:328–335.
22. Richter AM, Cerruti-Sola S, Sternberg ED, et al. Biodistribution of tritiated benzoporphyrin derivative(3H-BPD-MA), a new potent photosensitizer, in normal and tumor bearing mice. *J Photochem Photobiol B* 1990;5:231–244.

10

RECOVERY AFTER REPEATED PHOTODYNAMIC THERAPY TREATMENTS FOR NORMAL RETINA AND CHOROID

MARTIN H. REINKE
EVANGELOS S. GRAGOUDAS
JOAN W. MILLER

Several ocular conditions—including age-related macular degeneration (AMD), high myopia, ocular histoplasmosis syndrome, and angioid streaks—can lead to the formation of subfoveal choroidal neovascularization (CNV). Few great treatment options exist in the management of CNV in these diseases (1,2). Much attention is paid to treatment of CNV secondary to AMD because this condition poses the largest health risk in the general population and accounts for the majority of CNV cases in the United States (2,3).

Although conventional laser photocoagulation has been shown to be successful in limiting long-term vision loss owing to subfoveal CNV in many diseases, the treatment requires destruction of normal overlying retina in order to achieve control of neovascularization. Recurrence or persistence of lesions in nearly one-half of AMD patients often requires further laser photocoagulation and produces accompanying damage to overlying and adjacent normal retinal structures (4–9).

Photodynamic therapy (PDT) for use in ophthalmology originated from earlier dermatology and oncology studies where tumors were selectively treated while minimizing damage to surrounding normal structures. This concept is now being applied toward management of subfoveal CNV caused by AMD, high myopia, ocular histoplasmosis, and other inflammatory diseases (10–15). Photodynamic therapy aims to destroy CNV while preserving normal retina and choroid.

Several activating agents used for PDT are being studied, although most attention has been directed toward the use of verteporfin (Visudyne, Novartis Pharmaceuticals, Basel, Switzerland) because the drug is Food and Drug Administration–approved for treatment of CNV secondary to AMD, pathologic myopia, and ocular histoplasmosis (16–19). Other agents in clinical trials include tin ethyl etiopurpurin (Purlytin, Miravant Medical Technologies, Santa Barbara, CA) (20,21) and lutetium taxaphyrin (Lu-Tex, Pharmacyclics, Inc., Sunnyvale, CA). Also, preclinical studies are proceeding using mono-L-aspartyl chlorin e6 PDT to treat experimental CNV in primates (22–25).

Trials with verteporfin PDT and Purlytin have shown that multiple treatments using these photosensitizing chemicals are needed in varying frequencies in order to control neovascularization. Evidence of leakage or reperfusion within 1 to 3 months after PDT is expected in most treated eyes. Current protocol using verteporfin in the Treatment of Age-Related Macular Degeneration with Photodynamic Therapy (TAP) and Verteporfin in Photodynamic Therapy (VIP) studies dictates that retreatments are to be completed in 3-month intervals.

This chapter addresses retreatment issues. First, the effects of PDT laser treatments and retreatments on normal retina and choroid in preclinical trials are described. Second, available information on cumulative effects owing to multiple treatments in clinical trials is summarized. Finally, future directions and concepts concerning PDT retreatment are addressed.

EFFECTS OF PHOTODYNAMIC THERAPY ON NORMAL RETINA

Photodynamic therapy affects the retina by production of a photochemical reaction leading to the production of free radicals and singlet oxygen that damage surrounding cells and cell membranes. Initially, a chemical agent is localized to a neovascular membrane and then activated by a long-pulse low-irradiance light at an absorption peak of the photosensitizer. Intracellular oxidation leads to free radical production and subsequent damage to proteins followed by platelet activation and thrombosis of neovascular tissues. Histopathologic studies by Ghazi, Jabbour, de la Cruz, and others appear to verify this mechanism (26). The applied light is described as nonthermal because maximum temperature rise is estimated to be only 2°C (27). This photochemical mechanism is in contrast to conventional photocoagulation, where short-pulse laser produces photothermal reactions caused by absorption of energy by pigmented structures such as the retinal pigment epithelium. The expected maximal retinal temperature rise using conventional photocoagulation is approximately 42°C.

Multiple chemical agents have been evaluated for use in PDT treatment of CNV. Selective localization of the chemical in the abnormal neovascular tissue with minimal concentration in normal retinal structures is needed prior to application of laser light. It has been shown that normal retinal tissues retain at least some concentration of chemical throughout the time frame for which CNV treatment is ideal.

Several preclinical studies described the effects of PDT treatment of normal retina and choroid. Most published work concerns benzoporphyrin derivative monoacid (BPD-MA, verteporfin) and its effects when used as the active chemical in PDT treatments to rabbit and monkey eyes (28–34). Photographic, angiographic, and histologic descriptions have been made in order to understand effects on normal retinal structures.

The use of photodynamic therapy in the posterior segment of the rabbit eye showed that verteporfin-induced effects led to closure of normal choroidal vessels with damage to overlying neural retina (29). Other rabbit work included evaluating the localization properties of BPD-MA (28) (see Chapter 11).

Subsequent studies evaluated the potential role for verteporfin in controlling experimental CNV in primates (29–34). The effects of PDT on normal retina and choroid were included in these studies. Multiple factors can be altered in any PDT treatment. These include: medication dose (listed either in mg/kg or mg/m^2), infusion time duration, light parameters such as irradiance (mW/cm^2), fluence (J/cm^2) and treatment duration, and onset of irradiation relative to infusion onset. Each of these factors plays a role in affecting change in the neovascular membrane being treated and the overlying and underlying normal retinal and choroidal tissues. Appropriate dosing and timing result in selective closure of CNV while minimizing damage to adjacent neurosensory retina and choroid. Photodynamic therapy effects on normal retina and choroid were evaluated in many preclinical trials.

Miller, Walsh, Kramer, and others narrowed the useful ranges of the above parameters in an early study demonstrating closure of CNV in cynomolgus monkeys (30). Irradiance, dye dose, and fluence were varied. Intravenous lipoprotein-delivered BPD dye doses of 1 to 2 mg/kg were used and showed that the 2 mg/kg dose resulted in RPE necrosis and photoreceptor damage with pyknosis of the outer nuclear layer. The lower drug dose (1 mg/kg) led to less normal tissue damage. Later studies using a newer liposomal BPD dye formulation showed that a liposomal BPD dye dose of 0.25 mg/kg was the low threshold dose for closing choriocapillaris and 0.375 mg/kg appeared optimal (31).

Information concerning the timing of irradiation as it relates to damage to normal tissues has been evaluated in preclinical studies (30,31). Placement of irradiation soon after dye injection—within 20 minutes and especially within 5 minutes—showed that some larger choroidal vessels were closed and some retinal vessels were affected. One explanation for this observation was that plasma levels of BPD in the larger choroidal and retinal vessels were high soon after dye injection and activation of this dye too early led to nonselective damages.

An irradiance of 150 mW/cm^2 was used initially to show closure of CNV. Miller, Walsh, Kramer, and others found higher irradiances of 300 mW/cm^2 and 600 mW/cm^2 to be helpful because treatment times could be shortened to less than 10 minutes. At these higher irradiances, neither additional damage to normal retinal tissues nor thermal damage was identified (30).

A 1999 paper by Husain, Kramer, Kenney, and others described the effects of single PDT spots on normal primate retina and choroid using liposomal BPD. These lesions were followed for 4 to 7 weeks (33). Laser light at 689 or 692 nm was applied with an irradiance of 600 mW/cm^2 and fluence of 150 J/cm^2. Intravenous liposomal BPD (0.375 mg/kg or approximately 6 mg/m^2) was infused as a bolus, slow infusion, or fast infusion. The onset of subsequent laser light application varied from 10 to 71 minutes after the start of infusion.

In all groups fundus photography demonstrated mild graying of treatment areas at 24 hours that transformed into mild pigmentary change by 1 week. Pigment mottling eventually diminished at 4 weeks and was no longer present at the 7-week examination. Fluorescein angiography at 24 hours showed early hypofluorescence at the treatment site with late hyperfluorescence. Overlying retinal vasculature grossly appeared intact. Indocyanine green angiography at 24 hours after PDT showed early and late hypofluorescence of the treatment area but confirmed perfusion of the retinal and large choroidal vessels. Fluorescein angiography at 7 weeks showed no early changes but minimal hypofluorescence and hyperfluorescence persisted. At the 5-week stage, ICG angiography still showed late hypofluorescence to be present in the treatment areas. One can postulate that the hypofluorescence at 24 hours noted by fluorescein and ICG angiography may result from choriocapillaris occlusion or blockage from retinal pigment epithelium swelling.

Light microscopy at 4 weeks showed occasional pyknosis in the inner retina, mild disarray of outer segments, and normal retinal vessels. Presumably, phagocytic pigment-laden cells were overlying a single-layered RPE. Transmission electron microscopic evaluation of the treatment sites at 4 weeks showed the RPE to be intact but photoreceptor outer segments were still disorganized. The RPE, however, had varied pigmentation, rudimentary basal infolding, elongated microvilli, and contained lysosomes with outer segment material. The choriocapillaris and underlying choroid were patent and appeared recovered although areas of reduplicated basement membrane were present.

This study by Husain and others confirmed retinal recovery after initial choriocapillaris closure, RPE cell necrosis, and outer nuclear layer pyknosis. Retinal pigment epithelium repopulation and reestablishment of normal function appeared to occur by 4 to 7 weeks after a single PDT treatment to normal retina and choroid. Also, the choriocapillaris appeared to be well perfused by the 4- to 7-week period. This recovery by the retinal pigment epithelium is consistent with prior work evaluating RPE response after conventional laser photocoagulation (35–39).

In summary, normal segments of the fundus are affected by single PDT treatments. Overall, choriocapillaris closure and minimal damage to the outer neurosensory retina resulted from successful treatment of CNV in the primate model. Initial mild disruption of the RPE, minimal pyknosis of the outer retina, and swelling of the outer segments were followed in time by recovery of the RPE and choriocapillaris.

VERTEPORFIN PHOTODYNAMIC THERAPY RETREATMENT EFFECTS ON NORMAL RETINA AND CHOROID IN PRIMATES

Liposomal BPD is very effective in closing neovascular membranes. However, reperfusion usually arises between 1 week and 3 months. As a result, retreatment issues were evaluated in preclinical studies in primates.

Reinke and others studied verteporfin PDT retreatment of normal monkey retina and choroid (34). Analysis by fundus photography, fluorescein angiography, and light and electron microscopy led to a better understanding of retreatment effects. The verteporfin dose was varied from 6 mg/m^2 to 12 mg/m^2 to 18 mg/m^2. All dye concentrations were injected over a 10-minute interval and laser irradiation was initiated 20 minutes after the start of dye infusion. Light dosimetry was kept constant at an irradiance of 600 mW/cm^2 and a fluence of 100 J/cm^2, which was felt to be the maximal tolerated fluence for treatment of CNV. A 4-mm diameter spot size was used as the light was applied for 166.6 seconds. In this study either the fovea or optic nerve in one eye was treated every 2 weeks for a total of three treatment sessions. Follow-up times ranged from 2 to 7 weeks after the last treatment.

Fundus photography documented retinal whitening at 24 hours after the initial treatment (Fig. 10.1). Severe whitening leading to retinal vessel obscuration was present in the higher verteporfin dose groups (12 mg/m^2 and 18 mg/m^2). After the second and third applications, whitening was not found at the central macula. Pigmentary change developed in all eyes within weeks of the initial treatments but remained very apparent over the course of the study in the 12 mg/m^2 and 18 mg/m^2 groups. In the 6 mg/m^2 group, mild foveal granularity decreased by 6 weeks after the third treatment and the treatment zone border became inapparent (Fig. 10.2). These fundus findings appear to represent RPE reaction and recovery in the 6 mg/m^2 monkeys.

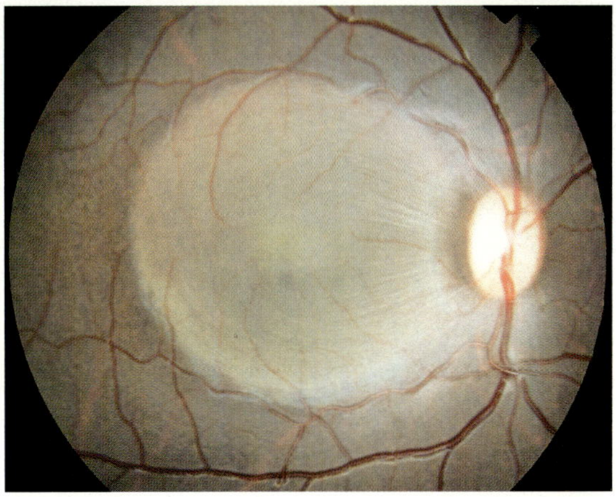

FIGURE 10.1. Fundus photograph 24 hours after first photodynamic therapy application to fovea with verteporfin dose of 6 mg/m^2. Color photograph shows typical deep retinal whitening seen after initial application in all animals. (From: Reinke M, Canakis C, Husain D, et al. Verteporfin photodynamic therapy retreatment of normal retina and choroid in the cynomolgus monkey. *Ophthalmology* 1999;106:1915–1923, with permission.)

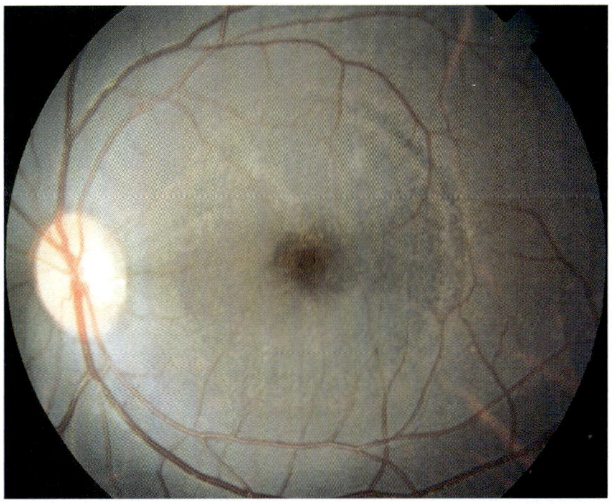

FIGURE 10.2. Fundus photograph 6 weeks after third PDT application to fovea with verteporfin dose of 6 mg/m^2. Relative recovery of retinal pigment epithelium is present with mild pigment mottling. (From: Reinke M, Canakis C, Husain D, et al. Verteporfin photodynamic therapy retreatment of normal retina and choroid in the cynomolgus monkey. *Ophthalmology* 1999; 106:1915–1923, with permission.)

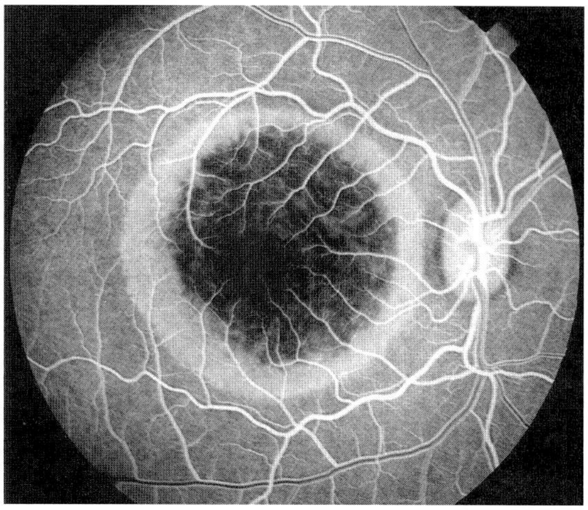

FIGURE 10.3. Early-frame fluorescein angiograph 24 hours after first PDT application to fovea with verteporfin dose of 6 mg/m^2. Early central hyperfluorescence is seen at the treatment site. (From: Reinke M, Canakis C, Husain D, et al. Verteporfin photodynamic therapy retreatment of normal retina and choroid in the cynomolgus monkey. *Ophthalmology* 1999;106: 1915–1923, with permission.)

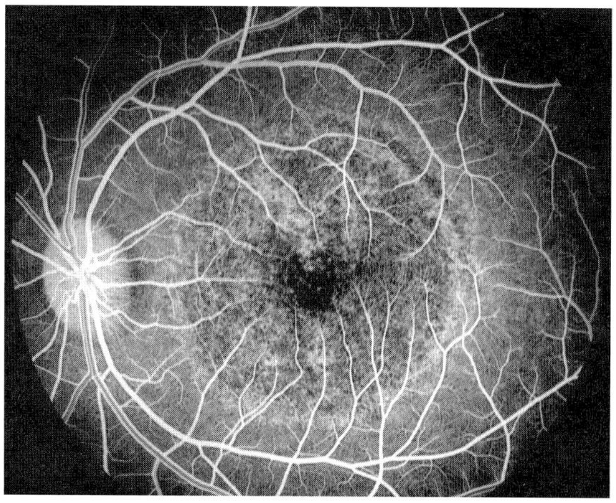

FIGURE 10.5. Early-frame fluorescein angiograph 6 weeks after third PDT application to fovea with verteporfin dose of 6 mg/m^2. Early scattered punctate hyperfluorescence is present. (From: Reinke M, Canakis C, Husain D, et al. Verteporfin photodynamic therapy retreatment of normal retina and choroid in the cynomolgus monkey. *Ophthalmology* 1999;106:1915–1923, with permission.)

Fluorescein angiography at 24 hours after the initial treatment showed early hypofluorescence with late staining at the foveal treatment site (Figs. 10.3 and 10.4). Subsequent angiograms in the 6 mg/m^2 group demonstrated late leakage up to 1 week after the initial treatment but only 24 hours after the second and third treatments. Figures 10.5 and 10.6 show punctate hyperfluorescence with no late leakage or staining at 6 weeks. Late fluorescein leakage was noted at all time points in the two higher verteporfin dose groups.

Histopathology confirmed that retreated retinal tissues were recovering much more in the 6 mg/m^2 group than in the 12 mg/m^2 and 18 mg/m^2 groups. At 3 weeks after the third PDT treatment in the 6 mg/m^2 group, light microscopy showed mild outer nuclear layer (ONL) disruption with outer segment shortening, RPE multilayering, and presence of overlying pigment-laden cells. The inner retina, choriocapillaris, and deep choroid appeared normal (Fig. 10.7). At 7 weeks after the third PDT treatment to the macula in this 6 mg/m^2 group, the RPE cells had repopulated and few pigment-laden

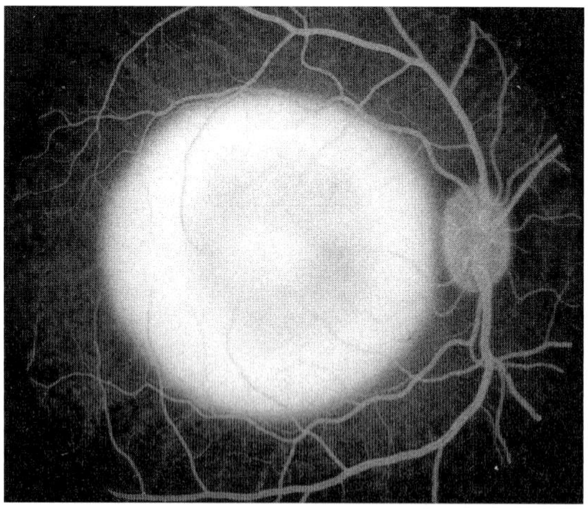

FIGURE 10.4. Late-frame fluorescein angiograph 24 hours after first PDT application to fovea with verteporfin dose of 6 mg/m^2. Progressive late staining of treatment site originates from the treatment border. (From: Reinke M, Canakis C, Husain D, et al. Verteporfin photodynamic therapy retreatment of normal retina and choroid in the cynomolgus monkey. *Ophthalmology* 1999; 106:1915–1923, with permission.)

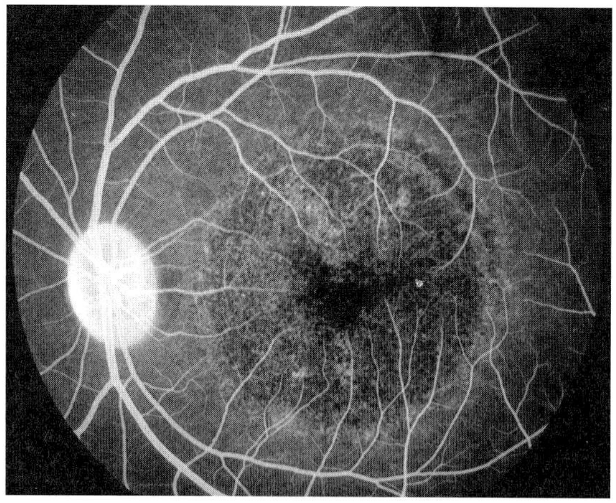

FIGURE 10.6. Late-frame fluorescein angiograph 6 weeks after third PDT application to fovea with verteporfin dose of 6 mg/m^2. Punctate hyperfluorescence is present in a zone of relative hypofluorescence. No significant leakage or staining is present. (From: Reinke M, Canakis C, Husain D, et al. Verteporfin photodynamic therapy retreatment of normal retina and choroid in the cynomolgus monkey. *Ophthalmology* 1999;106:1915–1923, with permission.)

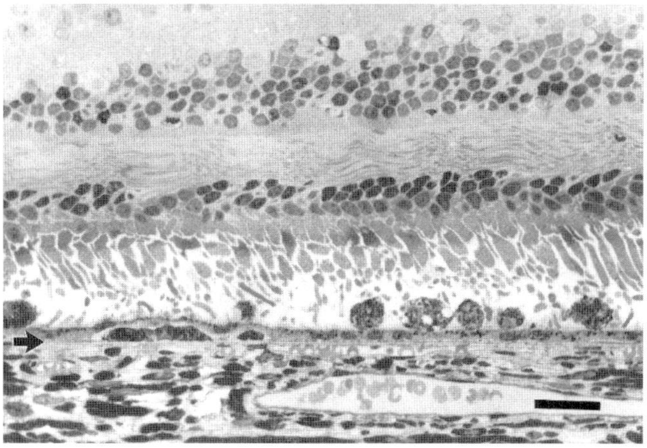

FIGURE 10.7. Light micrograph of macula 3 weeks after the third PDT application with verteporfin dose of 6 mg/m^2. At the edge of the fovea, there are shortened inner and outer segments and pigment-laden cells that overlie renewed retinal pigment epithelium (*arrow,* Bruch's membrane). The choriocapillaris is patent, and the outer nuclear layer and inner retina appear normal (stain, toluidine blue; bar, 25 μm). (From: Reinke M, Canakis C, Husain D, et al. Verteporfin photodynamic therapy retreatment of normal retina and choroid in the cynomolgus monkey. *Ophthalmology* 1999;106:1915–1923, with permission.)

cells were found. Again, the inner retina, choriocapillaris, and deep choroid appeared normal (Fig. 10.8).

Good retinal recovery was not achieved in the 12 mg/m^2 and 18 mg/m^2 verteporfin groups. In monkeys from these treatment groups, the ONL, RPE, and choriocapillaris all were absent at 6 and 7 weeks after three treatments to the fovea. In addition, there was loss of perifoveal inner retinal vessels in the 18 mg/m^2 group.

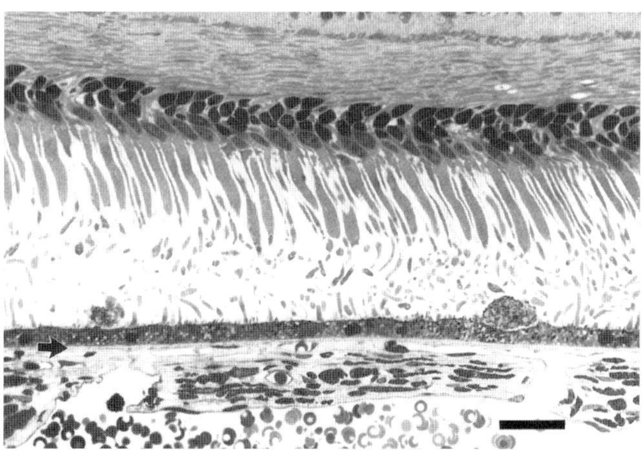

FIGURE 10.8. Light micrograph of macula 7 weeks after the third PDT application with verteporfin dose of 6 mg/m^2. The retinal pigment epithelium (RPE) is cuboidal with some microvilli and a few pigment-laden cells remaining. The outer and inner segments are long but distorted by a probable artifactual separation of the retina and RPE. The choriocapillaris remains patent, and the inner retina appears normal (*arrow,* Bruch's membrane; stain, toluidine blue; bar, 25 μm). (From: Reinke M, Canakis C, Husain D, et al. Verteporfin photodynamic therapy retreatment of normal retina and choroid in the cynomolgus monkey. *Ophthalmology* 1999;106:1915–1923, with permission.)

This preclinical study showed that the primate retina can recover from verteporfin retreatments to normal retina and choroid. Also, a dye dose threshold was found. Retinal pigment epithelium recovery appeared to be present in the 6 mg/m^2 treatment group. By the seventh week after three PDT applications, these cells, choriocapillaris, deep choroid, and inner neurosensory retina all appeared largely to have recovered.

PHASE I AND II CLINICAL TRIALS

Phase I and II clinical trials studied early short-term effects of verteporfin treatments and retreatments in human eyes (10,11) and are described in more detail in Chapter 14, Part 5 by Miller. The study parameters were based on data from prior preclinical work. Retreatment intervals of 2 or 4 weeks were evaluated using a 6 mg/m^2 dye dose, irradiance of 600 mW/cm^2, and fluence of 50 J/cm^2 to 100 J/cm^2.

Results of a single PDT treatment with verteporfin in a phase I and II study provided initial clinical data showing selective closure of CNV with preservation of normal retina and choroid. These studies involving 128 patients were designed to identify the most ideal dose regimens needed to achieve CNV control with minimal surrounding damage. A series of five general treatment protocols based on preclinical data was evaluated. The verteporfin dose was 6 mg/m^2 or 12 mg/m^2 and the duration of infusion was always 10 minutes. The light doses (fluence in J/cm^2) were increased sequentially from as low as 12.5 J/cm^2 to 150 J/cm^2. The time of light application after start of infusion varied between 10 and 30 minutes. The irradiance was kept constant at 600 mW/cm^2 in all treatments.

There were several conclusions concerning light doses and damage to normal retina. The minimum effective light doses were 12.5 J/cm^2 and 25 J/cm^2. The 100 J/cm^2 dose was felt to be the maximum tolerated light dose in clinical trial data. The 150 J/cm^2 light dose was too high because neurosensory retinal vessel closure was noted in four of eight patients receiving this dose. Other adverse ocular events that may have been related to natural disease progression or treatments included: increased subretinal hemorrhage (8.6%), increased fibrosis associated with CNV (8.6%), increased RPE atrophy (3.9%), subretinal hemorrhage (3.1%), choroidal vessel staining (1.6%), and vitreous hemorrhage (1.6%).

Overall the phase I and II single treatment studies showed that fluorescein dye leakage from CNV could be stopped or slowed in most patients without significant associated loss of visual acuity owing to collateral damage. Stabilization or improvement of vision could be achieved by the 12-week visit.

Progressive increased angiographic leakage was noted through weeks 4 through 12, however. The most desirable

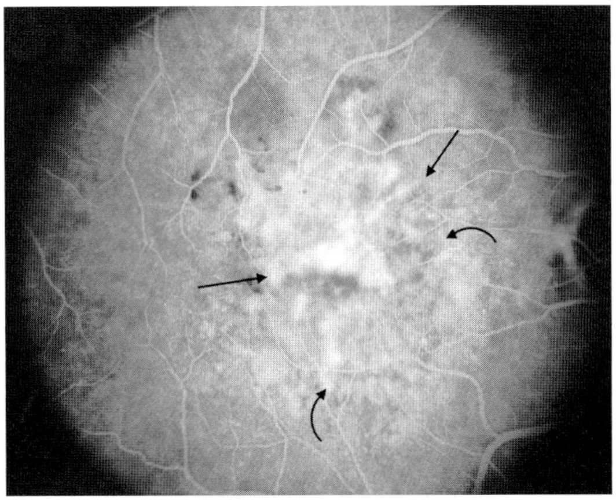

FIGURE 10.9. Baseline and follow-up of multiple verteporfin treatments using a light dose of 100 J/cm^2. Baseline fluorescein angiogram (visual acuity 20/40) showing early-phase classic CNV *(straight arrows)* and occult CNV *(curved arrows).* (From: Schmidt-Erfurth U, Miller JW, Sickenberg M, et al. Photodynamic therapy with verteporfin for choroidal neovascularization caused by age-related macular degeneration. Results of retreatments in a phase 1 and 2 study. *Arch Ophthalmol* 1999;117: 1177–1187, with permission.)

treatment regimen—verteporfin dose 6 mg/m^2, 10 minute infusion, light dose 50 J/cm^2 begun 15 minutes after infusion—still led to progression or moderate leakage in nearly 50% of patients by week 4 and 70% to 80% of patients by week 12. Some fluorescein leakage was noted to reappear in most patients between 1 and 4 weeks. Clearly, retreatments were indicated.

Retreatment regimens were evaluated in the phase I and II study. Thirty-one eyes from the single treatment study were given up to two retreatments at 2- or 4-week intervals and five additional patients received retreatments at or after

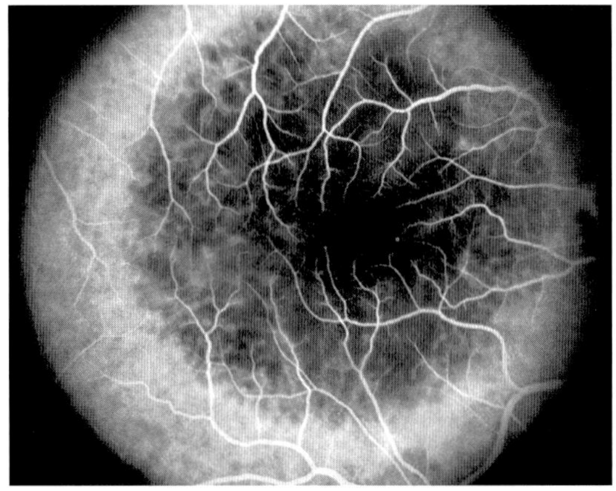

FIGURE 10.11. One week after PDT early-phase angiography shows central hypofluorescence (visual acuity 20/40). (From: Schmidt-Erfurth U, Miller JW, Sickenberg M, et al. Photodynamic therapy with verteporfin for choroidal neovascularization caused by age-related macular degeneration. Results of retreatments in a phase 1 and 2 study. *Arch Ophthalmol* 1999;117: 1177–1187, with permission.)

12 weeks. Based on data from the single treatment phase I and II trials, all retreatment regimens involved a verteporfin dose of 6 mg/m^2 infused over 10 minutes with an irradiance of 600 mW/cm^2.

One retreatment study protocol used a light dose of 100 J/cm^2 given 20 minutes after the start of infusion with retreatment intervals at 2 to 4 weeks. Among the 16 patients treated in this manner, the mean visual acuity was unchanged when measured 3 months after the last retreatment. An additional five patients had two retreatments at a frequency of every 2 weeks. Three months after these sessions, the average visual acuity had changed by +0.4 lines. Figures 10.9 through 10.18

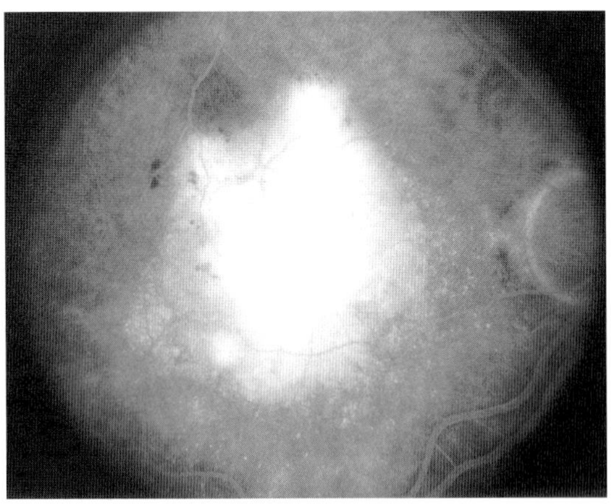

FIGURE 10.10. Baseline late-phase fluorescein angiogram showing leakage. (From: Schmidt-Erfurth U, Miller JW, Sickenberg M, et al. Photodynamic therapy with verteporfin for choroidal neovascularization caused by age-related macular degeneration. Results of retreatments in a phase 1 and 2 study. *Arch Ophthalmol* 1999;117:1177–1187, with permission.)

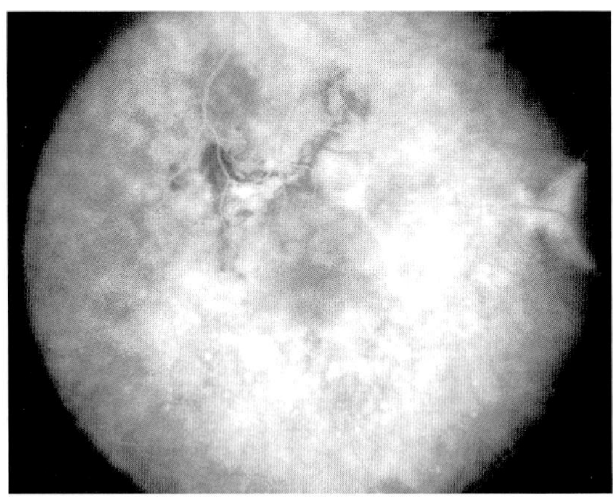

FIGURE 10.12. Late-phase angiogram at 1 week shows absence of central fluorescence but pericentral staining or leakage. (From: Schmidt-Erfurth U, Miller JW, Sickenberg M, et al. Photodynamic therapy with verteporfin for choroidal neovascularization caused by age-related macular degeneration. Results of retreatments in a phase 1 and 2 study. *Arch Ophthalmol* 1999;117:1177–1187, with permission.)

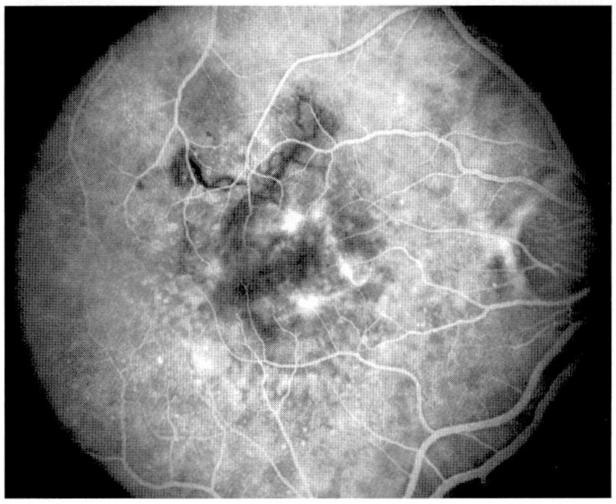

FIGURE 10.13. Four weeks after the initial treatment (visual acuity 20/50) an early-phase angiogram shows several areas of hyperfluorescence corresponding to classic choroidal neovascularization. (From: Schmidt-Erfurth U, Miller JW, Sickenberg M, et al. Photodynamic therapy with verteporfin for choroidal neovascularization caused by age-related macular degeneration. Results of retreatments in a phase 1 and 2 study. *Arch Ophthalmol* 1999;117:1177–1187, with permission.)

show fluorescein angiogram changes associated with multiple treatments in a patient receiving a light dose of 100 J/cm^2.

Another retreatment protocol varied the light dose from 50 to 75 to 100 J/cm^2. Irradiation in this group was applied 15 minutes after the start of infusion. Ten patients in this group received retreatments at 2- to 4-week intervals. Visual acuity was stable or improved by one line at 1 and 4 weeks after each treatment and by 12 weeks after the last retreatment, the average visual acuity decreased one line.

Fluorescein evaluation in these patients showed absence of leakage from CNV at 1 week after each treatment and retreatment. Recurrence was noted by week 4 in most eyes.

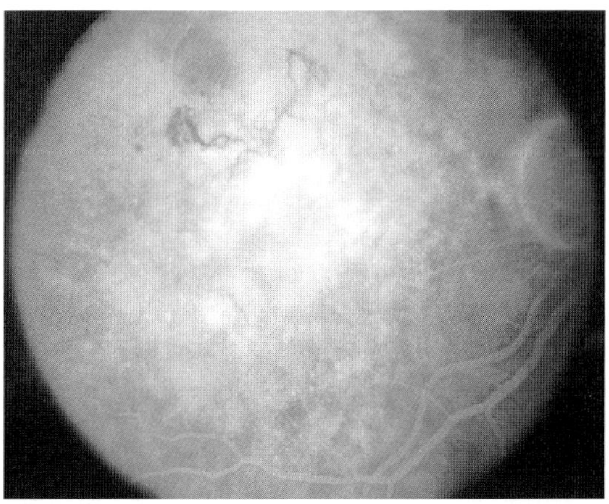

FIGURE 10.14. Late-phase angiogram at 4 weeks demonstrates leakage. (From: Schmidt-Erfurth U, Miller JW, Sickenberg M, et al. Photodynamic therapy with verteporfin for choroidal neovascularization caused by age-related macular degeneration. Results of retreatments in a phase 1 and 2 study. *Arch Ophthalmol* 1999;117:1177–1187, with permission.)

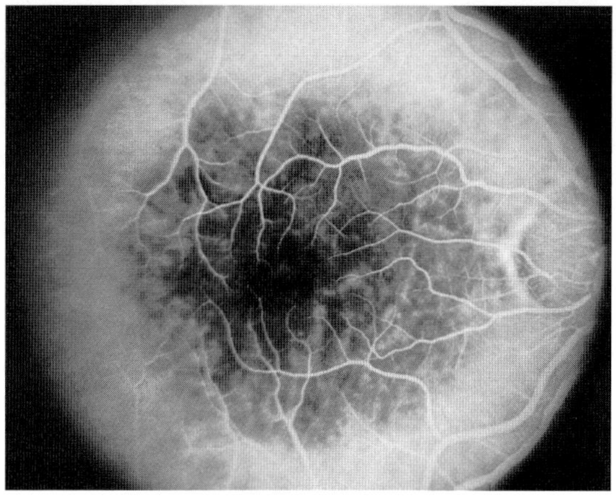

FIGURE 10.15. One week after PDT retreatment (visual acuity 20/26) early hypofluorescence is present. (From: Schmidt-Erfurth U, Miller JW, Sickenberg M, et al. Photodynamic therapy with verteporfin for choroidal neovascularization caused by age-related macular degeneration. Results of retreatments in a phase 1 and 2 study. *Arch Ophthalmol* 1999;117:1177–1187, with permission.)

In general, however, leakage at the last visit was typically less than at the angiographic baseline.

Relative stability of vision in the study groups using retreatments at 2- to 4-week intervals showed that the PDT protocols did not lead to significant adverse effects in normal retina and choroid at least over short time intervals. No individuals lost more than six lines of vision from the time of retreatment. Retinal pigment epithelium atrophy, however, increased in 11 patients (39%) but involved only a small segment of the treated retina. No correlation between the number of retreatments and RPE atrophy was noted. In addition, the published data did not specify whether the RPE atrophy developed primarily in the eyes

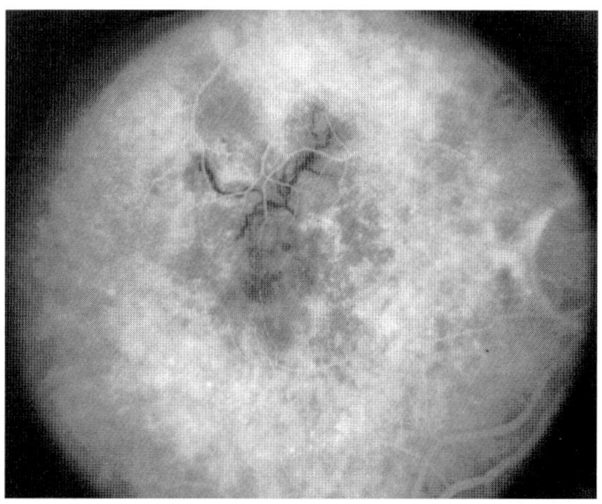

FIGURE 10.16. Late-phase angiogram 1 week after PDT retreatment shows slight staining. (From: Schmidt-Erfurth U, Miller JW, Sickenberg M, et al. Photodynamic therapy with verteporfin for choroidal neovascularization caused by age-related macular degeneration. Results of retreatments in a phase 1 and 2 study. *Arch Ophthalmol* 1999;117:1177–1187, with permission.)

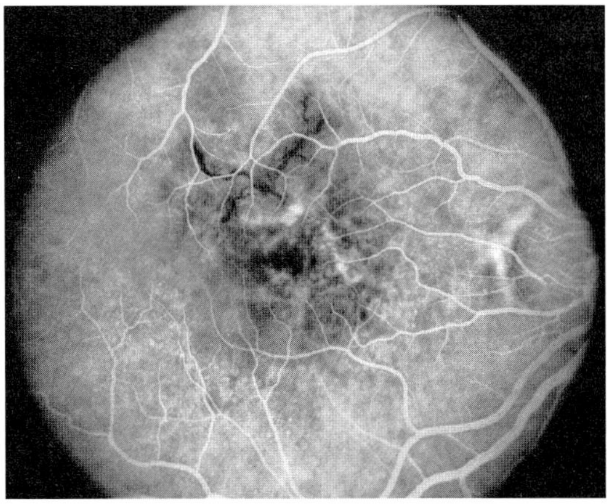

FIGURE 10.17. Angiography four weeks after retreatment (visual acuity 20/64) shows some early hyperfluorescence owing to classic choroidal neovascularization. (From: Schmidt-Erfurth U, Miller JW, Sickenberg M, et al. Photodynamic therapy with verteporfin for choroidal neovascularization caused by age-related macular degeneration. Results of retreatments in a phase 1 and 2 study. *Arch Ophthalmol* 1999;117:1177–1187, with permission.)

receiving 50 J/cm^2 or 100 J/cm^2 light doses. Other retinal changes included retinal capillary nonperfusion in four patients (14%) and retinal vascular leakage in three patients (10%). The nonperfusion cases affected less than 30% of the treated lesion area and involved only one or two tiny capillaries.

Several conclusions concerning retreatment intervals were made. First, it was noted that the visual acuity was maintained for as long as 3 months after the last retreatment session. Second, concerns about long-term induction

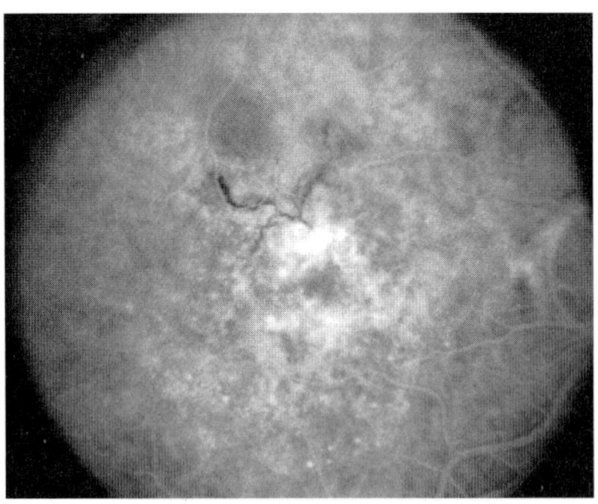

FIGURE 10.18. Late leakage on angiography 4 weeks after retreatment is less than at 4 weeks after the initial treatment. (From: Schmidt-Erfurth U, Miller JW, Sickenberg M, et al. Photodynamic therapy with verteporfin for choroidal neovascularization caused by age-related macular degeneration. Results of retreatments in a phase 1 and 2 study. *Arch Ophthalmol* 1999; 117:1177–1187, with permission.)

of retinal pigment epithelium atrophy were noted, especially with respect to the 100 J/cm^2 light dose. Cumulative RPE damage could limit the preservation of neurosensory retina function. The goal of therapy was to avoid too many retreatments in order to allow RPE recovery and repopulation between applications. This was balanced by the need to stop progression of neovascularization.

PHASE III CLINICAL TRIALS

The Treatment of Age-Related Macular Degeneration with Photodynamic Therapy (TAP) study and the Verteporfin in Photodynamic Therapy (VIP) study demonstrate significant safety using photodynamic therapy (12,14,15). The parameters for the phase III trials were identified with the goal of minimizing damage to normal retinal structures. The best parameters from the phase I and II studies were: verteporfin dose of 6 mg/m^2 with a 10-minute infusion, fluence 50 J/cm^2, irradiance 600 mW/cm^2, onset of irradiation 15 minutes after start of infusion. Retreatments were to be placed every 3 months if fluorescein leakage was found.

The TAP study group published Report 1 in October 1999 (12). Six hundred nine eyes were assigned to receive either verteporfin (402 eyes) or placebo (207 eyes) treatment. This study is discussed in greater detail by Arnold in Chapter 14, Part 6. Overall, multiple measures of vision were better in the verteporfin group and therefore confirmed the safety of this procedure. Safety data showed limited effects of PDT treatment and retreatment on normal retina and choroid. Development of RPE atrophy attributable to verteporfin PDT was not found in this phase III clinical trial. Also, problems related to retinal arteriolar or venular nonperfusion were not found using the 50 J/cm^2 light dose and retreatments at 3-month intervals.

Safety profiles with treatments and retreatments were evaluated. Visual disturbances were noted in 89 (22.1%) eyes receiving verteporfin compared to 32 (15.5%) eyes receiving placebo. Most of these problems were considered mild and transient. The visual disturbances encompassed reports of abnormal vision in 41 verteporfin-treated patients (10.2%) versus 13 placebo-treated patients (6.3%), decreased vision in 58 verteporfin-treated patients (14.4%) versus 24 placebo-treated patients (11.6%), and visual field defects in 24 verteporfin-treated patients (6.0%) versus seven placebo-treated patients (3.4%). Four episodes of severe vision loss—defined as loss of at least four lines of vision within 7 days of treatment—were reported in three patients receiving verteporfin PDT.

The 24-month data confirmed good safety outcomes. The average number of verteporfin treatments in the first year of the TAP study was 3.4 and in the second year 2.2. No striking loss of vision or atrophy of RPE was identified in the TAP study. Importantly, the TAP authors noted that

> the distribution of the size of the lesion plus any surrounding atrophy was not significantly different from the distribution of the size of the lesion without the inclusion of surrounding atrophy, suggesting that by the month 24 examination, verteporfin-treated eyes had developed no additional surrounding atrophy compared with placebo-treated eyes. (14)

In summary, TAP Reports 1 and 2 verified the safety of the treatment regimen using a verteporfin dose of 6 mg/m^2, light dose of 50 J/cm^2, irradiance of 600 mW/cm^2, and treatment 15 minutes after the onset of a 10-minute dye infusion. When retreatments were completed at 3-month intervals, the normal retina and choroid in patients appeared to tolerate the multiple treatments. Minimal visual acuity loss and stabilization of contrast sensitivity and fluorescein leakage suggest that PDT selectively treats CNV while minimizing damage to photoreceptors, retinal pigment epithelium, and choroidal tissues.

The VIP study was established to determine if verteporfin PDT could reduce the risk of moderate visual acuity loss (at least 15 letters) among patients with occult but no classic CNV, patients with classic CNV and initial visual acuity better than 20/40, and patients with CNV caused by pathologic myopia. VIP Report 2 again confirmed relative safety using verteporfin for treatment in these first two subgroups over the course of 24 months (15). This study is described in further detail by Arnold in Chapter 14, Part 6.

Safety issues among the VIP study patients showed that no subgroups were identified in which eyes receiving placebo fared better than eyes treated with verteporfin. Ten of 225 verteporfin-treated patients (4.4%), however, were noted to have a severe visual acuity decrease of at least 20 letters. Nine events occurred after the initial treatment and one occurred after the second treatment. Five of these patients had recovery of vision to less than 20 letters lost. The causes included: extensive subretinal fluid development (one case), sub-RPE hemorrhage (three cases), and no obvious etiology (six cases).

Subjective visual disturbances were reported in 94 verteporfin-treated cases (42%) compared to 26 placebo-treated cases (23%). The disturbances at 12 months were categorized as abnormal vision in 39 verteporfin-treated patients (17.3%) versus 11 placebo-treated patients (9.6%), decreased vision in 62 verteporfin-treated eyes (27.6%) versus 13 placebo-treated eyes (11.4%), and visual field defects in 32 verteporfin-treated eyes (14.2%) versus six placebo-treated eyes (5.3%). At the 24-month stage, the visual disturbances were listed as abnormal vision in 46 verteporfin-treated patients (20%) versus 14 placebo-treated patients (12%), decreased vision in 67 verteporfin-treated patients (30%) versus 15 placebo-treated patients (13%), and visual field defects in 34 verteporfin-treated patients (15%) versus eight placebo-treated patients (7%). These events were mild to moderate and usually were transient.

Overall the VIP trial has shown that multiple verteporfin treatments are safe and effective in patients with occult but no classic CNV. A positive treatment benefit was confirmed at the 24-month stage after initiation of treatment. Ten patients were noted to have severe vision loss in this report. Nine of the episodes, however, happened after the first treatment; therefore, they could not be attributed to cumulative retreatment damage to normal retina and choroid. Neither progressive RPE atrophy nor cumulative retinal damage was described in VIP Report 2.

Additionally, verteporfin PDT has been shown to benefit patients with CNV caused by pathologic myopia, ocular histoplasmosis syndrome, angioid streaks, and idiopathic causes (13). A phase I and II study of 13 patients published in 2000 demonstrated a benefit using verteporfin for treatment of CNV. Effects of verteporfin treatment on normal retina and choroid were minimal in these subgroups.

Eight patients were treated once, two patients were treated twice, one patient was treated three times, and two patients were treated four times. The retreatment intervals varied from 4 to 21 weeks with final follow-up completed 12 weeks after the last PDT treatment. At the end of the trial, no patients experienced a decrease in visual acuity. Among the patients receiving multiple treatments, two of five patients had no change in visual acuity and three of five had improved visual acuity. This safety study showed no adverse effects on the retina, RPE, or choroid owing to single treatments or retreatments using intervals as frequent as every 4 weeks.

The preceding studies have shown that multiple treatments to control neovascularization over several years can be placed without significant damage to adjacent normal retina, choriocapillaris, and choroid in patients with AMD.

CONCLUSIONS

Photodynamic therapy retreatment using verteporfin has been shown to be safe in numerous clinical studies. The approved protocol was based on initial phase I and II trials and prior preclinical studies involving cynomolgus monkeys. The TAP and VIP studies have shown that although nearly all membranes in AMD patients are closed after one PDT treatment, the neovascularization may leak again by 4 to 6 weeks. As such, many lesions are active yet not treated—according to the TAP protocol established several years ago—until 3 months after the initial or subsequent treatment.

There are little data regarding the best and safest times for retreatment. However, some specialists retreat at 1 to 2 months based on angiographic leakage, increased size of CNV, and worsening visual acuity with exudative signs present on clinical examination. Some argue that treating at intervals earlier than 3 months may lead to better visual acuity outcomes and decrease the total number of retreatments.

Based on the present existing data, however, there is no scientific evidence available demonstrating a definite vision benefit utilizing a protocol other than that from the TAP study. One probably should be careful in basing retreatment decisions on fluorescein angiogram interpretation alone. Angiographic benefit from PDT is not always equivalent to visual acuity benefit.

The issue of retreatment and recovery of normal tissues is important because if the fundus is treated too frequently, the normal retinal structures may receive too many "hits" too frequently from which they cannot recover. We know at present that after several years the human retina can withstand and recover from a series of treatments 3 months apart with an average of 5.6 total treatments.

In order to help answer the uncertainties surrounding time of retreatment, the Verteporfin in Early Retreatment (VER) Trial was established. This 2-year trial will determine whether early retreatment with verteporfin at 6 weeks safely reduces the risk of moderate vision loss compared with the standard approved TAP retreatment protocol where retreatments occur every 3 months.

The rationale for the VER study is based on 2-year TAP data showing that 75% of vision lost by patients with predominantly classic CNV occurred within the first 6 months of the initial verteporfin treatment. The protocol being studied will randomize AMD patients to receive verteporfin PDT as often as every 6 weeks for the first 6 months compared to the presently approved regimen of retreatment every 3 months. Safety using retreatment intervals of 2 to 4 weeks was shown in the phase I and II clinical trials (11). It is hoped that the VER trial will reconfirm the safety of shorter retreatment intervals and demonstrate sustained benefit using verteporfin PDT.

Future studies concerning retreatment intervals may very well alter the frequency of PDT applications in AMD patients. In addition, retreatment intervals may vary according to the etiology of the CNV. Neovascular progression or persistence in patients with AMD is different than in other diseases such as myopia, ocular histoplasmosis, angioid streaks, or in idiopathic cases. When one considers the inherent baseline health of the involved treated tissues, it is expected that younger patients will respond to PDT insults more effectively than older patients.

In conclusion, verteporfin PDT treatment and retreatment for CNV can be applied safely. Preclinical studies evaluating photographic, angiographic, and histological data showed good recovery of normal retinal and choroidal tissues. Clinical trials over the past several years have confirmed that visual acuity is stabilized after multiple PDT treatments. Preclinical and clinical data show that PDT retreatment can remain safe when applied judiciously.

REFERENCES

1. Bressler NM, Bressler SB, Gragoudas ES. Clinical characteristics of choroidal neovascular membranes. *Arch Ophthalmol* 1987; 105:209–213.
2. Ferris FL III, Fine SL, Hyman L. Age-related macular degeneration and blindness due to neovascular maculopathy. *Arch Ophthalmol* 1984;102:1640–1642.
3. Klein R, Klein BEK, Linton KLP. Prevalence of age-related maculopathy. The Beaver Dam Eye Study. *Ophthalmology* 1992;99: 933–943.
4. Macular Photocoagulation Study Group. Recurrent choroidal neovascularization after argon laser photocoagulation for neovascular maculopathy. *Arch Ophthalmol* 1986;104:503–512.
5. Macular Photocoagulation Study Group. Argon laser photocoagulation for neovascular maculopathy. Three year results from randomized clinical trials. *Arch Ophthalmol* 1986;104:694–701.
6. Macular Photocoagulation Study Group. Argon laser photocoagulation for neovascular lesions of age-related macular degeneration. Five-year results from randomized clinical trials. *Arch Ophthalmol* 1991;109:1109–1114.
7. Macular Photocoagulation Study Group. Laser photocoagulation of subfoveal neovascular lesions in age-related macular degeneration. Results of a randomized clinical trial. *Arch Ophthalmol* 1991;109:1220–1231.
8. Macular Photocoagulation Study Group. Laser photocoagulation of subfoveal neovascular lesions of age-related macular degeneration. Updated findings from two clinical trials. *Arch Ophthalmol* 1993;111:1200–1209.
9. Macular Photocoagulation Study Group. Persistent and recurrent neovascularization after laser photocoagulation for subfoveal choroidal neovascularization of age-related macular degeneration. *Arch Ophthalmol* 1994;112:497–499.
10. Miller JW, Schmidt-Erfurth U, Sickenberg M, et al. Photodynamic therapy with verteporfin for choroidal neovascularization caused by age-related macular degeneration. Results of a single treatment in a phase 1 and 2 study. *Arch Ophthalmol* 1999;117: 1161–1173.
11. Schmidt-Erfurth U, Miller JW, Sickenberg M, et al. Photodynamic therapy with verteporfin for choroidal neovascularization caused by age-related macular degeneration. Results of retreatments in a phase 1 and 2 study. *Arch Ophthalmol* 1999;117: 1177–1187.
12. Treatment of Age-Related Macular Degeneration with Photodynamic Therapy (TAP) Study Group. Photodynamic therapy of subfoveal choroidal neovascularization in age-related macular degeneration with verteporfin. One-year results of 2 randomized clinical trials. *Arch Ophthalmol* 1999;117:1329–1345.
13. Sickenberg M, Schmidt-Erfurth U, Miller JW, et al. A preliminary study of photodynamic therapy for choroidal neovascularization in pathologic myopia, ocular histoplasmosis syndrome, angioid streaks, and idiopathic causes. *Arch Ophthalmol* 2000; 117:327–336.
14. Treatment of Age-Related Macular Degeneration with Photodynamic Therapy (TAP) Study Group. Photodynamic therapy of subfoveal choroidal neovascularization in age-related macular degeneration with verteporfin. Two-year results of 2 randomized clinical trials. *Arch Ophthalmol* 2001;119:198–207.
15. Verteporfin in Photodynamic Therapy Study Group. Verteporfin therapy of subfoveal choroidal neovascularization in age-related macular degeneration: two-year results of a randomized clinical trial including lesions with occult with no classic choroidal neovascularization. *Am J Ophthalmol* 2001;131:541–560.
16. Soubrane G, Bressler N. Treatment of subfoveal choroidal neovascularisation in age related macular degeneration: focus on

clinical application of verteporfin photodynamic therapy. *Br J Ophthalmol* 2001;85:483–495.

17. Donati D, Kapetanios AD, Pournaras CJ. Principles of treatment of choroidal neovascularization with photodynamic therapy in age-related macular degeneration. *Semin Ophthalmol* 1999;14: 2–10.
18. Husain D, Miller JW. Photodynamic therapy for macular degeneration. *Semin Ophthalmol* 1997;12:14–25.
19. Schmidt-Erfurth U, Miller J, Sickenberg M, et al. Photodynamic therapy of subfoveal choroidal neovascularization: clinical and angiographic examples. *Graefes Arch Clin Exp Ophthalmol* 1998; 236:365–374.
20. Peyman GA, Moshfeghi DM, Moshfeghi A, et al. Photodynamic therapy of choriocapillaris using tin ethyl etiopurpurpin (SnET2). *Ophthalmic Surg Lasers* 1997;28:409–417.
21. Moshfeghi DM, Peyman GA, Moshfeghi A, et al. Ocular vascular thrombosis following tin ethyl etiopurpurin (SnET2) photodynamic therapy: time dependencies. *Ophthalmic Surg Lasers* 1998;29:663–668.
22. Peyman GA, Kazi AA, Moshfeghi D, et al. Threshold and retreatment parameters of NPe6 photodynamic therapy in retinal and choroidal vessels. *Ophthalmic Surg Lasers* 2000;31:323–327.
23. Peyman GA, Kazi AA, Unal M, et al. Problems with and pitfalls of photodynamic therapy. *Ophthalmology* 2000;107:29-35.
24. Nakashizuka T, Mori K, Hayashi N, et al. Retreatment effect of NPe6 photodynamic therapy on the normal primate macula. *Retina* 2001;21:493–498.
25. Photodynamic therapy of experimental choroidal neovascularization with a hydrophilic photosensitizer mono-L-aspartyl chlorin e6. *Retina* 2001;21:499–508.
26. Ghazi NG, Jabbour NM, De la Cruz ZC, et al. Clinicopathologic studies of age-related macular degeneration with classic subfoveal choroidal neovascularization treated with photodynamic therapy. *Retina* 2001;21:478–486.
27. Mainster MA, Reichel E. Transpupillary thermotherapy for age-related macular degeneration: long-pulse photocoagulation, apoptosis, and heat shock proteins. *Ophthalmic Surg Lasers* 2000; 31:359–373.
28. Haimovici R, Kramer M, Miller JW, et al. Localization of lipoprotein-delivered benzoporphyrin derivative in the rabbit eye. *Curr Eye Res* 1997;16:83-90.
29. Schmidt-Erfurth U, Hasan T, Gragoudas E, et al. Vascular targeting in photodynamic occlusion of subretinal vessels. *Ophthalmology* 1994;101:1953–1961.
30. Miller JW, Walsh AW, Kramer M, et al. Photodynamic therapy of experimental choroidal neovascularization using lipoprotein-delivered benzoporphyrin. *Arch Ophthalmol* 1995;113:810–818.
31. Kramer M, Miller JW, Michaud N, et al. Liposomal benzoporphyrin derivative verteporfin photodynamic therapy. Selective treatment of choroidal neovascularization in monkeys. *Ophthalmology* 1996;103:427–438.
32. Husain D, Miller JW, Michaud N, et al. Intravenous infusion of liposomal benzoporphyrin derivative for photodynamic therapy of experimental choroidal neovascularization. *Arch Ophthalmol* 1996;114:978–985.
33. Husain D, Kramer M, Kenney AG, et al. Effects of photodynamic therapy using verteporfin on experimental choroidal neovascularization and normal retina and choroid up to seven weeks after treatment. *Invest Ophthalmol Vis Sci* 1999;40:2322–2331.
34. Reinke M, Canakis C, Husain D, et al. Verteporfin photodynamic therapy retreatment of normal retina and choroid in the cynomolgus monkey. *Ophthalmology* 1999;106:1915–1923.
35. Wallow IHL, Tso MOM. Repair after xenon arc photocoagulation. 3. An electron microscopic study of the evolution of retinal lesions in rhesus monkeys. *Am J Ophthalmol* 1973;75:957–972.
36. Marshall J. Interactions between sensory cells, glial cells and the retinal pigment epithelium and their response to photocoagulation. *Dev Ophthalmol* 1981;2:308-317.
37. Smiddy WE, Fine SL, Quigley HA, et al. Cell proliferation after laser photocoagulation in primate retina. An autoradiographic study. *Arch Ophthalmol* 1986;104:1065–1069.
38. Heriot WJ, Machemer R. Pigment epithelial repair. *Graefes Arch Clin Exp Ophthalmol* 1992;230:91–100.
39. Valentino TL, Kaplan HJ, Del Priore LV, et al. Retinal pigment epithelial repopulation in monkeys after submacular surgery. *Arch Ophthalmol* 1995;113:932–938.

11

THE OCULAR LOCALIZATION OF PHOTOSENSITIZERS

SEAN KOH
ROBERT HAIMOVICI

Photodynamic therapy (PDT) depends on the interaction among a photosensitizer, light, and molecular oxygen. As discussed in Chapter 2, the photosensitizer is excited to its singlet state by light of the appropriate wavelength. The excited photosensitizer can react with oxygen via energy transfer processes, generating reactive oxygen species such as singlet oxygen ($^1O_2$) and free radicals such as $\cdot OH$, $HO\cdot_2$ and $\cdot O_2^-$ that are able to damage cellular structures (1). These reactive oxygen species travel fewer than several tens of nanometers before reacting with biomolecules. This suggests that the intracellular action of photosensitizers may be restricted to the site of their subcellular location and the surrounding radius of not more than 40 nm (2). Photosensitizers differ in their subcellular localization, suggesting that the choice of photosensitizer may influence the outcome of PDT. Few of the very many known candidate PDT agents have been investigated for their ocular localization. In this chapter, we review the available data on the ocular localization of these photosensitizers and discuss the potential factors that may influence photosensitizer localization.

PRINCIPLES OF PHOTOSENSITIZER LOCALIZATION

Classification of Photosensitizers

Several classes of photosensitizers have been used *in vitro* and in animal models for the study of the mechanisms of photodynamic injury and to develop an optimal agent for PDT for human malignancies and the treatment of ocular neovascularization. They are listed in Table 11.1. The absorption spectra as a function of wavelength for these agents differ markedly. Composite normalized absorption spectra for some of these photosensitizers are presented in Figures 11.1 and 11.2. Among these agents, only verteporfin (benzoporphyrin derivative monoacid) (Visudyne, Novartis Pharmaceuticals, Basel, Switzerland) has been approved by health authorities including the US Food and Drug Administration (FDA) for the treatment of various types of choroidal neovascularization (CNV). The purpurin tin ethyl etiopurpurin (SnET2) is currently in human trials for similar indications.

Xanthene Derivatives

Rose Bengal is a halogenated fluorescein derivative with increased singlet oxygen yields and photosensitizing ability that has been used to produce vascular damage of ocular vessels (3,4). It has an absorption peak at about 550 nm and is quite hydrophilic. Because of its high absorption coefficient (5) and high singlet oxygen quantum yield, it is widely used to generate singlet oxygen in biological systems (3,5,6). It is not currently under investigation for PDT in humans because of systemic toxicity.

Porphyrin and Benzoporphyrin Derivatives

Most early clinical PDT experience came from using the porphyrin derivatives, hematoporphyrin derivative (HPD), and dihematoporphyrin ether (DHE). Hematoporphyrin derivative contains several porphyrins including monomers, dimers, and oligomers. Hematoporphyrin derivative was partially purified to form DHE (Photofrin, QLT Therapeutics, Vancouver, BC, Canada), the earliest widely used photosensitizer in clinical PDT (1). Other, later-generation photosensitizers have been introduced into clinical trials and practice because of the long-lasting skin phototoxicity induced by Photofrin, a complex chemical composition, as well as its small absorption peak at tissue-penetrating longer wavelengths (7).

Benzoporphyrin derivative (BPD or verteporfin) is one of the newer generation photosensitizers with more rapid plasma and tissue clearance, enhanced tumor to normal tissue selectivity, and superior light absorption of visible red and near infrared light (8). It has an absorption maximum of about 690 nm and is rapidly inactivated or

TABLE 11.1. MAJOR CLASSES OF PHOTOSENSITIZERS

Xanthene derivatives (ex) Rose Bengal Hematoporphyrins (ex) Hematoporphyrin derivative (HPD), dihematoporphyrin ether (DHE) Benzoporphyrins (ex) Verteporfin (benzoporphyrin derivative monoacid) Chlorins and bacteriochlorins (ex) Chlorin e6, mono-L-aspartyl chlorin e6 (NPe6), Bacteriochlorin a, Lysyl chlorin p6	Phthalocyanines and naphthalocyanines (ex) Chloroaluminum sulfonated phthalocyanine (CASPc), zinc phthalocyanine (ZnPc), silicon naphthalocyanine (SINc) Texaphyrins (ex) Lutetium texaphyrin (Lu-Tex) Purpurins (ex) Tin ethyl etiopurpurin (SnET2) Benzochlorins (ex) Tinoctaethylbenzochlorin (BNZ-203) Others (ex) ATX-S10 (13,17-bis [1-carboxy-priopionyl] carbamoylethyl-8-ethenyl-2-hydroxy-3-hydroxyiminoethylidene-2,7,12,18-tetramethyl porphyrin sodium)

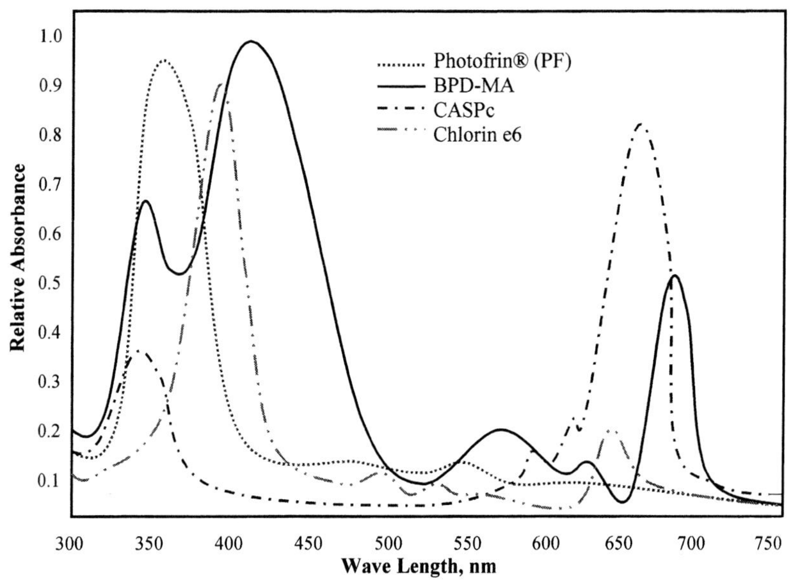

FIGURE 11.1. The relative absorbance versus wavelength for Photofrin, BPD-MA, CASPc, and Chlorin e6. (From: Liu H, Anderson RR. Photodynamic therapy in dermatology: recent developments. *Dermatol Clin* 1993;11:1–13, with permission.)

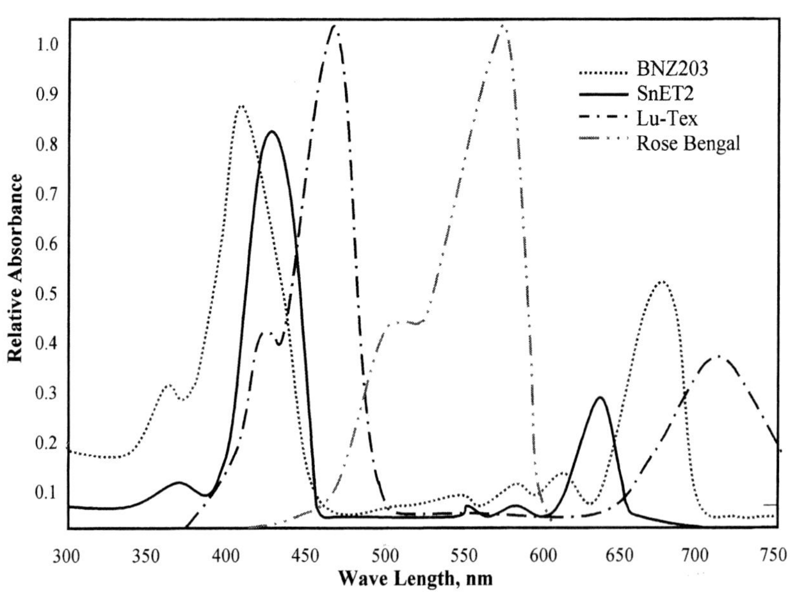

FIGURE 11.2. The relative absorbance versus wavelength for BNZ 203, SnET2, Lu-tex, and Rose Bengal. (From: Hill RA, Crean DH, Doiron DR, et al. Photodynamic therapy of the ciliary body with tin ethyl etiopurpurin and tin octaethyl benzochlorin in pigmented rabbits. *Ophthalmic Surg Lasers* 1997;28:948–953; Blumenkranz MS, Woodburn KW, Qing F, et al. Lutetium texaphyrin: a potential new agent for ocular fundus angiography and photodynamic therapy. *Am J Ophthalmol* 2000;129:353–362; Luttrull DK, Valdes-Aguilera O, Linden SM, et al. Rose Bengal aggregation in rationally synthesized dimeric systems. *Photochem Photobiol* 1988;47:551–557, with permission.)

cleared from the body with no significant phototoxicity after 24 hours (8).

Chlorins and Bacteriochlorins

Chlorins are derived either by modifying a porphyrin (reducing one of the pyrrolic rings of the porphyrin macrocycle) or from chlorophyll as the starting material for synthesis (9). Chlorin e6 is a hydrophobic chlorin derivative that has a strong absorption band at 654 nm in the red part of the spectrum (10). Mono-L-aspartyl chlorin e6 (NPe6) is a water-soluble chlorin derivative that has an absorption peak at 664 nm (11). Bacteriochlorin is a chlorin derivative that has a maximum light absorption at 760 nm (12).

Phthalocyanines and Naphthalocyanines

Phthalocyanines are another class of photosensitizers with a strong absorption band at 675 nm (13). Central metals such as zinc and aluminum are incorporated into their structure to increase the triplet state and singlet oxygen yields. Their solubility and cellular localization are at least partially determined by the number and charge of their side chains (13). CASPc is a hydrophilic dye that effectively generates singlet oxygen, absorbs in the red part of spectrum at 675 nm, and has been studied for potential ocular applications (14). Naphthalocyanines (maximum absorption at 770 nm) have red-shifted absorption spectra compared with phthalocyanines. However, unlike zinc and aluminum phthalocyanines, zinc and aluminum naphthalocyanines are unstable and tend to aggregate *in vitro*, making them relatively inactive photochemically (15).

Texaphyrins

The texaphyrins are synthetic water-soluble tripyrrolic pentaaza-expanded porphyrins, which have the capacity to bind large metal cations and exhibit strong, low-energy optical absorption in the 700 to 780 nm range (16). Lu-Tex, a specific member of this class of compounds, exhibits broad absorption peaks in the Soret-like band at 474 nm and the Q-like absorption band of 732 nm (17). Because of its polyether and hydroxyl peripheral functional groups, Lu-Tex is an amphipathic molecule and possesses a broad characteristic fluorescence emission band centered at 750 nm.

Purpurins

Purpurins are formally chlorins, because they have one reduced pyrrole group as well as a fused six-member isocyclic ring (18). Tin ethyl etiopurpurin (SnET2) is a hydrophobic molecule that is formulated in an isotonic, isoosmotic lipid emulsion that is suitable for intravenous (iv) use. It is currently in phase III trials as a photosensitizing agent for the treatment of CNV and glaucoma (19,20).

Benzochlorins

Benzochlorins are synthesized from meso-substituted porphyrins and consist of a benzene ring fused to the tetrapyrrolic structure (21). Tin octaethyl benzochlorin (BNZ 203) is a member of this group that has been tested for efficacy by *in vitro* and *in vivo* methods (22). BNZ 203 has a maximum red absorption at 689 nm. It is a lipophilic compound that requires formulation in a lipid-rich environment such as a liposome.

ATX-S10

ATX-S10 [13,17-bis (1-carboxy-propionyl)carbamoylethyl-8-ethenyl-2-hydroxy-3-hydroxyiminoethylidene-2,7,12,18-tetramethyl porphyrin sodium] is a water-soluble modified porphyrin compound that has a half-life in plasma of only 30 minutes (23). It has a major absorption peak at 401 nm with minor peaks at 510, 557, 611, and 670 nm. Recently, the accumulation of this photosensitizer has been investigated in experimental CNV (see the following discussion) (24,25).

Cellular Localization of Photosensitizers

Responses to PDT are dependent on the concentration of the photosensitizer used, the solvent, the route of administration, the illumination conditions, the oxygenation status of the tissue, the cell type under study, and the use, if any, of carrier molecules (26). The distribution of a photosensitizer also depends on intrinsic physicochemical and biochemical properties of the photosensitizer. Many of these potential factors are listed in Table 11.2. For example, hydrophilic photosensitizers are likely to be taken up by pinocytosis or endocytosis and become localized in lysosomes or endosomes, whereas many hydrophobic photosensitizers such as hematoporphyrin derivative and verteporfin localize to the mitochondrial membranes and exert their actions there. ATX-S10(Na), an amphiphilic photosensitizer, localizes to a variety of subcellular organelles (27). Porphyrins have been shown to have a high affinity for the peripheral benzodiazepine receptor (28), a protein localized in the outer mitochondrial membrane. Peng and coworkers (29) used confocal laser scanning microscopy to determine the intracellular distribution of aluminum phthalocyanine with various degrees of sulfonation in an *in vitro* human melanoma cell line. Tetrasulfonated and trisulfonated phthalocyanines ($AlPcS_4$ and $AlPcS_3$) localized in the lysosomes, whereas the monosulfonated and disulfonated phthalocyanines ($AlPcS_2$ and $AlPcS_1$) showed a diffuse distribution throughout the cytoplasm. The distribution of these anionic dyes suggests a relationship between the number of negatively charged groups attached to the photosensitizing core and its mode of entry into the cell, which in turn, determines the intracellular distribution pattern. Boyle and Dolphin (30) inves-

TABLE 11.2. PHYSICOCHEMICAL AND BIOCHEMICAL PROPERTIES OF PHOTOSENSITIZERS THAT AFFECT CELLULAR LOCALIZATION

Hydrophobicity/hydrophilicity
Type, number, and arrangement of charged groups
Nature of and presence of central atom in the tetrapyrrole structure
Aggregation state
Charge: mass ratio
Partitioning within serum
Affinity for particular subcellular organelles

From Moor A. Invited review: signaling pathways in cell death and survival after photodynamic therapy. *J Photochem Photobiol, B: Biol* 2000;57:1–13, with permission.

tigated the uptake of two cationic *meso*-tetra-pyridyl porphyrins, quaternized with methyl and hexyl residues, in human dermal fibroblasts. Important differences were found, with the methyl derivative being taken up faster and localizing in the nucleus, whereas the hexyl analog entered the cells much more slowly and was distributed in the cytoplasm. These results illustrate the importance of charge-to-mass ratio in determining intracellular distribution.

The subcellular localization patterns of the photosensitizer may also help to determine the nature and extent of tissue injury. In general, mitochondria localized photosensitizers are able to induce apoptosis rapidly, whereas photosensitizers that bind to the plasma membrane or lysosomes, but not to mitochondria, kill cells less efficiently and by necrosis rather than apoptosis (31). Examples of selected photosensitizers with their primary subcellular localization sites are shown on Table 11.3. Photodynamic therapy may also lead to lipid peroxidation of membrane-bound organelles leading to release and redistribution of the photosensitizer. For example, anionic tetrasulfonated Zn(II) phthalocyanines and tetraglycine Zn(II) phthalocyanine have been shown to migrate from lysosomes to the region of the nucleus after low-level light irradiation (32). To date, the relationship between subcellular photosensitizer localization and photodynamic injury has not been investigated in ocular tissues.

TABLE 11.3. PRIMARY SUBCELLULAR LOCALIZATION SITES OF SELECTED PHOTOSENSITIZERS

Plasma membrane
Chlorin e6
Lysyl chlorin e6 imide
Mitochondria
Lysyl chlorin e6 imide
Silicon phthalocyanine
Dihematoporphyrin ether (DHE)
Verteporfin (BPD-MA)
Lysosomes
Mono-L-aspartyl chlorin e6 (NPe6)
Lysyl chlorin p6 ester
Tetrasulfonated and trisulfonated phthalocyanines (Al PcS_3, Al PcS_4, $ZnPcS_4$)
Tin octaethyl benzochlorin (BNZ203)
Tin ethyl etiopurpurin (SnET2)
Lutetium texaphyrin (Lu-Tex)
Cytoplasm
Monosulfonated and disulfonated aluminum phthalocyanines (Al PcS_1, Al PcS_2)
Zinc phthalocyanine (ZnPc)
Widely distributed within the cell
ATX-S10

From Mori M, Kuroda T, Obana A, et al. In vitro plasma protein binding and cellular uptake of ATX-S10(Na), a hydrophilic chlorin photosensitizer. *Jpn J Cancer Res* 2000;91:845–852; Boyle RW, Dolphin D. Structures and biodistribution relationships of photodynamic sensitizers. *Photochem Photobiol* 1996;64:469–485; Rosenkranz AA, Jans DA, Sobolev AS. Targeted intracellular delivery of photosensitizers to enhance photodynamic efficiency. *Immunol Cell Biol* 2000;78:452–464; Pogue BW, Ortel B, Chen N, et al. A photobiological and photophysical-based study of two chlorins. *Cancer Res* 2001;61:717–724, with permission.

Systems for Photosensitizer Delivery into Cells

A variety of approaches have been used to try to enhance PDT efficacy and selectivity. The most popular and promising approach has been to use various carriers (33) such as monoclonal antibodies, microspheres, liposomes, folate-liposomes, immunoliposomes, lipoproteins, oil emulsions, and ligands to deliver the photosensitizer into the cell (Table 11.4). Lipid-based delivery vehicles were used for delivering porphyrin-type photosensitizers to tumors after

TABLE 11.4. EXAMPLES OF CARRIERS FOR PHOTOSENSITIZER DELIVERY

Monoclonal antibodies
Microspheres
Liposomes
Folate-liposomes
Immunoliposomes
Lipoproteins
Oil emulsions
Ligands

From Rosenkranz AA, Jans DA, Sobolev AS. Targeted intracellular delivery of photosensitizers to enhance photodynamic efficiency. *Immunol Cell Biol* 2000;78:452–464, with permission.

it was recognized that coupling them to a hydrophobic vehicle increased their affinity for neoplastic tissues (34). For example, the selective biodistribution of porphyrin-type photosensitizers is enhanced by their incorporation into amphiphilic systems such as oil emulsions, which are stable in an aqueous milieu yet possess apolar compartments where hydrophobic substrates are embedded (35). Similarly, liposome-associated photosensitizers exhibited greater efficiency and selectivity of tumor targeting as compared with the same photosensitizer administered in a homogeneous aqueous solution (36).

The association of the photosensitizers to lipoproteins, in particular to LDL, could result in selective or preferential uptake to neoplastic cells probably owing to relative abundance of the LDL receptors in tumor plasma membrane (37). These receptors promote the internalization of the LDL-bound photosensitizers by endocytosis (38). Porphyrin-type photosensitizers largely localize in membranous domains, including the plasma membrane and mitochondrial membrane (38). The conjugation of CASPc, a water-soluble sensitizer to diplasmenylchlorine-folate liposomes has been shown to enhance its tumor selectivity and phototoxicity compared to folate-free counterpart (39). These results imply that high concentrations of a water-soluble photosensitizer could be delivered to target cells using the folate receptor-mediated pathway.

Microspheres are another type of carrier that has been shown to enable the intracellular delivery of photosensitizers to phagolysosomes. For example, the covalent attachment of chlorin e6 to polystyrene microspheres results in its entry into MGH-U1 human transitional cell bladder carcinoma via phagocytosis (40). The specificity of PDT can be also improved by conjugating photosensitizers to monoclonal antibodies (mAb) or ligands specific for receptors or antigens on the tumor cell surface. For instance, immunoconjugates of chlorin e6 monoethylene diamine monamide with a mAb specific for uveal melanoma cells produce fourfold greater damage than the free photosensitizers at the same concentration (41).

Immunoliposomes have been shown to improve the efficacy of antibody conjugated photosensitizer therapy by facilitating penetration into the target cells (42). Comparison of conjugates of the photosensitizer CASPc with antibodies alone or in combination with monolayer immunoliposomes has revealed that the photodynamic activity of immunoliposomes on bladder carcinoma cells *in vitro* is 13-fold higher than that of the photosensitizer-antibody conjugates alone (42). In summary, preclinical studies in nonocular, mostly tumor, models have illustrated numerous ways in which photosensitizer localization patterns can be altered resulting in increased photodynamic efficacy. As research in ocular PDT expands it is likely that these and other refinements in photosensitizer delivery will be investigated for increasing the efficacy and specificity of ocular PDT.

LOCALIZATION OF PHOTOSENSITIZERS TO OCULAR STRUCTURES

The short distance over which photosensitizers exert their effect after light excitation suggests that the results of ocular PDT depends in part on photosensitizer localization to the eye. Theoretical advantages of the eye as a target organ for PDT include the high transmission characteristics of the ocular media that allow for light to interact directly with vascular structures such as the choroid or CNV after iv administration of the photosensitizer. Contiguous structures such as the retina and RPE could be at risk of PDT-mediated injury, although at least in the case of verteporfin, photosensitizer–light combinations with acceptably reduced collateral damage have been demonstrated in clinical trials. Over the past two decades, a number of investigators have evaluated the ocular localization of photosensitizers. Methods that have been used include postmortem techniques such as fluorescence microscopy and spectrofluorometry (43,44) as well as *in vivo* fluorescence angiography (FA) using the candidate photosensitizer. Unfortunately, for most of the photosensitizers studied with fluorescence microscopy (with the exception of HPD, verteporfin, and ATX-S10), only ciliary body distribution data is available (45–47). Qualitative assessments of photosensitizer accumulation in the posterior segment have been made with a number of photosensitizers using *in vivo* FA (11,24,48–50), but quantitative data as provided by spectrofluorometric evaluation of postmortem tissue are lacking for all but verteporfin. The variety of agents studied and the nonuniform evaluation of these agents make it difficult to generalize the findings. In the following we summarize the available information regarding the ocular localization of widely studied photosensitizers.

Hematoporphyrin Derivative and Dihematoporphyrin Ether

Gomer and coworkers (43) used pigmented rabbits with an amelanotic melanoma heterotransplanted to the iris to obtain quantitative tissue levels of HPD by scanning spectrofluorometry as well as to document HPD localization by fluorescence microscopy. HPD was administered iv at a dose of 5 mg/kg for spectrofluorometry and 10 mg/kg for fluorescence microscopy. Vascular structures such as the iris, choroid, retina, and tumor all demonstrated rapid uptake of HPD. In addition, the aqueous in eyes with anterior chamber tumors also accumulated significant levels of HPD within 30 minutes after HPD administration. The sclera and aqueous from eyes without tumors had extremely low concentrations of HPD at all time intervals after drug administration. The drug was not detected in avascular structures such as the lens or cornea. Hematoporphyrin derivative was cleared from all ocular structures except the tumor and choroid-retina by 24 hours following injection (43).

Hill and coworkers (45) investigated the localization of DHE using fluorescence microscopy in a pigmented rabbit model. Dihematoporphyrin ether (10 mg/kg) in a 0.9% saline solution was injected and biodistribution studies were performed using fluorescence microscopy at 1 and 24 hours after the dye injection. The studies showed that DHE was seen primarily in the intravascular space of the ciliary body at 1 hour. At 24 hours, DHE exhibited good localization to the ciliary body epithelium. Posterior segment localization studies of DHE were not performed.

Verteporfin (BPD-MA)

Verteporfin, a liposomal preparation of BPD monoacid, is currently the only FDA-approved drug for PDT of CNV. Kim and coworkers (50) investigated the localization of BPD-MA using digital BPD FA in experimental choroidal melanomas. Ten albino rabbits with experimental choroidal melanomas were administered 1 mg/kg BPD-MA iv while images of tumor, normal choroid, or iris were obtained. Follow-up images were obtained during the first 3 and at 24 hours after injection. The time of peak dye accumulation ranged between 15 and 45 minutes for the tumors. A small amount of dye was still present within the tumors 3 hours after injection, and decreased to only trace amounts at 24 hours. However, in the surrounding retina and choroid, the amount of dye decreased steadily within the first 10 minutes and was not detectable by 3 hours. These data may suggest selective accumulation of BPD-MA into the experimental choroidal melanomas.

Haimovici and coworkers (44) also investigated the localization of this photosensitizer using fluorescence microscopy and quantified its presence in ocular tissues after porphyrin extraction using fluorescence spectroscopy. Albino rabbits were administered 2 mg/kg BPD-MA precomplexed with low-density lipoprotein (LDL) iv. The eyes were enucleated at intervals between 5 minutes and 24 hours after dye injection and were studied with light and fluorescence microscopy, or dissected for porphyrin extraction. At 5 minutes after dye injection, there was bright fluorescence from the choroid and RPE with trace retinal outer segment fluorescence. After 20 minutes, there was increased photoreceptor outer segment and RPE fluorescence but decreased choroidal fluorescence. By 2 hours no fluorescence remained in either the choroid or the photoreceptors and there was diminished fluorescence of the RPE. Trace RPE fluorescence was still visible at 24 hours. Using fluorescence spectroscopy, the highest BPD-MA levels from the eye were measured in the retina/RPE/uvea complex with lower levels measured from the sclera and cornea. It is believed that the rapid accumulation of BPD in the RPE and retina is at least in part owing to the high lipid content of these structures. The authors also suggest that the presence of LDL receptors on the RPE may contribute to BPD localization via a receptor-mediated mechanism (51).

Silicon Naphthalocyanine (SINc)

Hill and coworkers (46) studied the localization of SINc in rabbit eyes using fluorescence microscopy. SINc (0.5 mg/kg) dissolved in canola oil was administered iv. The localization studies were performed in frozen sections by fluorescence microscopy using a charged-coupled device (CCD) camera-based, low light detection system with digital image processing. The studies showed a primarily intravascular distribution of SINc in the ciliary body at 1 hour. After 24 hours, the SINc underwent redistribution into the substantia propria of the rabbit ciliary body. Posterior segment localization studies of SINc were not performed.

Tin Octaethyl Benzochlorin (BNZ 203)

Hill and coworkers (47) investigated the biodistribution of iv BNZ 203 (0.5 mg/kg) by fluorescence microscopy in pigmented rabbit eyes. The pharmacokinetics of BNZ 203 was examined in frozen sections by fluorescence microscopy using a CCD-based low-light detection system at 1 and 24 hours after injection. Localization studies of BNZ 203 showed spotty intravascular distribution in the ciliary body within 1 hour after administration. Selective retention of BNZ 203 in the ciliary processes was further diminished at 24 hours. No posterior segment localization studies were performed.

Tin Ethyl Etiopurpurin (SnET2)

Hill and coworkers (47) also investigated the localization of SnET2 by fluorescence microscopy in rabbits. SnET2 was administered iv at a dose of 1.0 mg/kg. The pharmacokinetics of SnET2 was determined in frozen sections by fluorescence microscopy using CCD camera system with digital image processing at 1 and 24 hours. The studies showed that SnET2 was distributed intravascularly within the ciliary processes by 1 hour after the injection. At 24 hours, SnET2 was found primarily within the nonpigmented epithelium of the ciliary processes. The authors concluded that this localization pattern suggests the possibility of developing a selective nonpigmented epithelium cyclodestructive surgery. No posterior segment localization studies of SnET2 were performed.

Lutetium Texaphyrin (Lu-Tex)

Blumenkranz and associates (49) investigated the suitability of Lu-Tex as a fluorescence imaging agent in the delineation of retinal vascular and choroidal vascular diseases. Fundus FA using Lu-Tex was compared with conventional FA and indocyanine green (ICG) angiography in normal and laser-injured New Zealand white rabbits. Lu-Tex imaging was performed by exciting the photosensitizer at around 500 nm and collecting the resultant emission signal using a 10-nm bandwidth, 750-nm interference filter. Normal retinal and choroidal vasculature was well delineated by Lu-Tex angiography, which also accurately illustrated the site and the severity of laser-induced vasculitis of the medullary ray. Whereas FA showed profound early leakage and late indistinct fluorescence, Lu-Tex angiography better defined the extent of vascular injury, presumably secondary to its higher molecular weight and protein binding.

Plasma pharmacokinetic data and plasma protein binding were also assessed after Lu-Tex (10 μm/kg) was administered iv. In the rabbits administered Lu-Tex, plasma protein binding analysis showed that 15.8% of the Lu-Tex was associated with LDL, 39.7% with high-density lipoprotein (HDL), and 44.5% with other serum proteins, including albumin and globulin. Because albumin and globulin account for most of the total rabbit plasma protein, the authors concluded that HDL and LDL have a great affinity for Lu-Tex and that the plasma protein binding of this photosensitizer to lipoprotein receptors could contribute to their accumulation in both neoplastic and non-neoplastic–associated neovascularization (17).

ATX-S10

Obana and coworkers (25) investigated the localization of iv ATX-S10 (16 mg/kg) in rats with experimental CNV using fluorescence microscopy. Retinal vascular fluorescence was greatest at the 5-minute time point, whereas retinal outer segment and RPE/Bruch's membrane fluorescence was greatest at the 30-minute time point. Fluorescence intensity of the photosensitizer within the CNV peaked somewhat later and was greatest at the 30-minute and 2-hour time points. Hikichi and coworkers (24) investigated the selective accumulation of ATX-S10 in experimental CNV in rats using FA. ATX-S10 (16 mg/kg) was injected iv, the retinas were excited with 405 to 435 nm light, and the emitted light was passed through a 680-nm bandpass filter before being detected by CCD camera. Immediately after the injection, fluorescence appeared within the retinal vessels and then throughout the entire retina. Thirty minutes postinjection, the intensity of the fluorescence was still strong from the whole retina and the CNV was not discernible. One hour after injection, retinal fluorescence was weak but still observable. At 1.5 hours postinjection, retinal fluorescence was undetectable but fluorescence from the CNV was strong. After 2 hours postinjection, there was no residual fluorescence from the CNV. Based on these results, the authors suggested that ATX-S10 might accumulate somewhat preferentially within experimental CNV. Recently, Obana and coworkers (52) performed ATX-S10(Na) angiography in monkeys with experimental laser-induced CNV. After iv injection of ATX-S10(Na) (4 mg/kg or 8 mg/kg), a 670-nm diode laser was used to stimulate the photosensitizer and ATX-S10(Na) fluorescence was detected by a cooled CCD camera as a detector using a barrier filter appropriate for this photosensitizer. ATX-S10(Na) fluorescence persisted in retinal arteries and veins during the first 10 to 20 minutes but began to diminish after 30 minutes. Hyperfluorescence from the choroidal neovascular membranes persisted until 90 minutes for the 4 mg/kg dose and 120 minutes for the 8 mg/kg dose. The authors conclude that ATX-S10(Na) accumulates preferentially within experimental CNV in monkeys between 30 and 120 minutes.

Rose Bengal, Chlorin e6, and Aluminum Phthalocyanine Tetrasulfonate

Recently, Haimovici and coworkers (53) studied the ocular distribution of Rose Bengal, chlorin e6, and aluminum phthalocyanine tetrasulfonate (CASPc) in rabbits using fluorescence microscopy and digital angiography to determine if these structurally different photosensitizers also localized differently. Albino rabbits were administered Rose Bengal (40 mg/kg), CASPc (5 mg/kg), and chlorin e6 (2 mg/kg). The eyes were enucleated and examined at intervals from 5 minutes to 24 hours after dye injection using fluorescence microscopy. By 5 minutes after dye injection, all three dyes studied showed prominent fluorescence from the ciliary epithelium and less extensive fluorescence form the ciliary body stroma. (It is presumed that the dyes initially localized to the vascular ciliary body stroma after iv injection.) The extent of ciliary epithelial fluorescence declined over the first 2 hours and trace residual fluorescence was detected at 24 hours with all three photosensitizers. In the posterior segment, all three photosensitizers demonstrated bright fluorescence from the choroid and retinal pigment epithelium (RPE) with trace retinal outer segment fluorescence at 5 minutes. Initial RPE fluorescence was slightly less with CASPc than with Rose Bengal and chlorin e6. Choroidal, RPE, and outer retinal fluorescence slowly declined over time. Some intermediate time points (60 minutes to 2 hours) showed corneal endothelial and inner retinal fluorescence possibly owing to anterior chamber or vitreous transport from the ciliary body. Scleral fluorescence was less than choroidal and RPE fluorescence at the early time points (5 and 20 minutes) for all three photosensitizers. Generally, scleral fluorescence was least for chlorin e6, intermediate for Rose Bengal, and most for CASPc.

Fundus angiography was also performed with Rose Bengal, chlorin e6, and CASPc. Good quality FA could be performed that delineated the retinal vessels in pigmented rabbits and retinal and choroidal vessels during the transit phase in albino rabbits (Fig. 11.3A). Choroidal vascular detail was better visualized in both pigmented and albino rabbits with CASPc and chlorin e6 angiography because of their longer excitation and emission wavelengths compared to Rose Bengal (Figs. 11.1 and 11.2). Retinal vascular fluorescence persisted for less than 10 minutes for Rose Bengal, 1 hour for

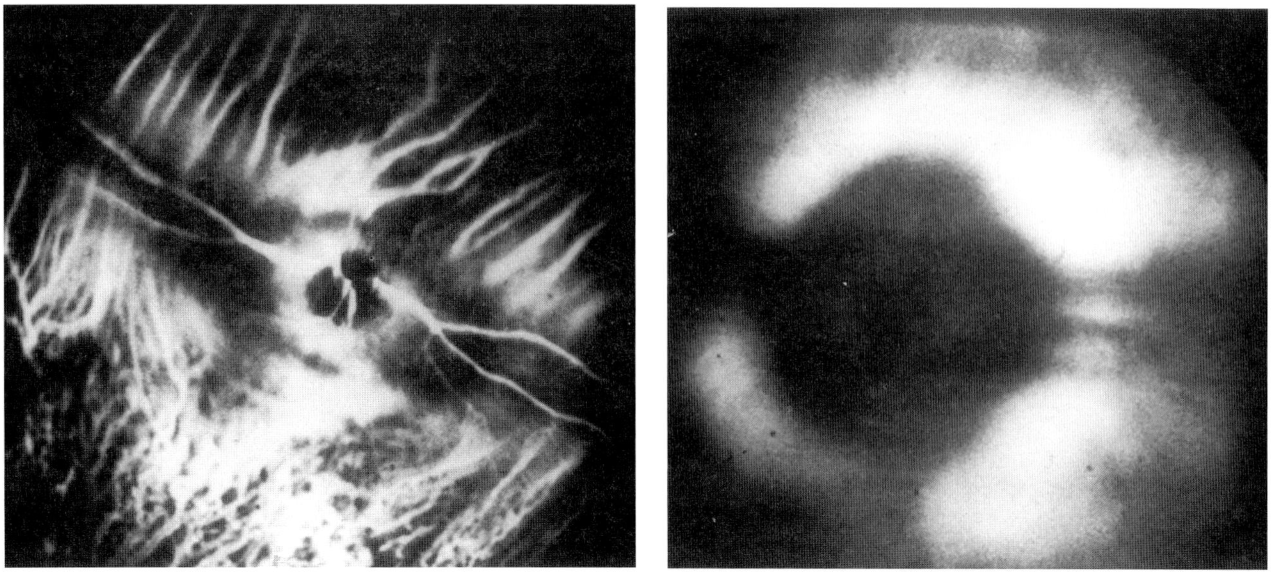

A B

FIGURE 11.3. CASPc (2 mg/kg) fluorescence angiogram. Albino rabbit. **A:** Transit phase. The retinal and choroidal arteries are brightly fluorescent and there is some choroidal venous filling. **B:** Twenty-four hours after dye injection, there is persistent marked fundus fluorescence. Fluorescence microscopy studies performed on other eyes after the same dose of CASPc suggest that the fluorescence visible at 24 hours is localized to the sclera. (From: Haimovici R, Ciulla TA, Miller JW, et al. Localization of Rose Bengal, CASPc, and chlorin e6 in the rabbit eye. *Retina* 2002;22:65–74, with permission.)

chlorin e6, and up to 2 hours for CASPc. Scleral fluorescence was particularly strong for CASPc, persisting for 24 hours (Fig. 11.3B). The authors suggested that the increased scleral fluorescence of CASPc was caused by its high water solubility. The authors also concluded that although differences in localization were demonstrated, the localization patterns of these photosensitizers to the posterior segment were somewhat similar. The relative permeability of the choroidal vasculature to the photosensitizers was ascribed to the large size of endothelial fenestrations in rabbits (54) and possibly osmotic opening of the blood–retinal barrier (55). The significance of these findings to potential PDT therapy with these agents requires further investigation.

Kliman and associates (48) investigated the localization of CASPc in experimental CNV in monkeys using CASPc angiography. Three cynomolgus monkeys were administered CASPc 3 mg/kg iv. The dye was visualized within normal retinal and choroidal vessels 30 seconds after injection. Hyperfluorescence also was seen in an area of CNV. At 1 hour after injection, the dye had largely cleared from normal retina and choroidal vessels, but the area of CNV remained intensely hyperfluorescent. The authors concluded that CASPc selectively accumulates within CNV in monkeys.

Mono-L-aspartyl Chlorin e6 (NPe6)

Moshfeghi and coworkers (11) evaluated the localization of NPe6 using FA. Four pigmented rabbits, four pigmented rats and two African green monkeys were administered NPe6 (2mg/kg) iv. The photosensitizer (peak excitation 664 nm) was excited by the Helium-Neon laser (He-Ne; 633 nm) and a 665-nm barrier filter was placed between the He-Ne laser and the scanning laser ophthalmoscope (SLO). In a pattern similar to FA, NPe6 was initially observed within the choroid followed by the retinal vasculature. NPe6 fundus fluorescence disappeared most quickly in the monkey, intermediate in the rabbit, and slowest in the rat.

CONCLUSIONS AND FUTURE DIRECTIONS

In this chapter we have attempted to summarize the theoretical factors that may influence ocular localization of photosensitizers as well as review the results of previous studies of the ocular localization of photosensitizers. It is difficult to generalize the results of these investigations because many different photosensitizers have been studied using different techniques in a variety of species. Many photosensitizers administered iv have been imaged successfully within the choroid and retinal vessels, and in some cases experimental CNV, using a variety of imaging modalities. Subtle differences in localization were demonstrated by one study (53) that compared different agents simultaneously. In general, however, localization studies have not to date identified a more ideal photosensitizer for PDT of the posterior segment than verteporfin, which is currently in clinical use. The few fluorescence microscopic studies (25,44,53) performed suggest that the RPE (and to a lesser extent, retina) are potential sites of photosensitizer accumulation after iv administration of photosensitizers, a finding that is not evident from FA studies. The possibility that retinal, RPE, and choroidal vascular cells differ in their susceptibility to or ability to recover from photodynamically mediated injury is starting to be investigated (56) and might explain how verteporfin/light combinations that occlude CNV in humans while minimizing RPE and retinal damage could be developed despite the presence of low levels of photosensitizer within these structures (57,58). Future research may evaluate whether initial PDT disrupts the permeability characteristics of the RPE (thereby altering photosensitizer localization patterns) or renders the RPE and retina more susceptible to further photodynamic injury. Such changes could explain why repeated PDT especially with higher doses of photosensitizers increases the risk of RPE and retina damage (59,60).

The study of photosensitizer localization as it pertains to ocular photodynamic therapy remains in its infancy. New photosensitizers continue to be developed and will need to be evaluated for ocular indications. With the exception of liposomes, more selective targeting systems being studied in other investigational PDT models have yet to be applied to ocular photodynamic therapy. Many questions remain unanswered. Can photosensitizers such as verteporfin be more selectively localized to choroidal neovascular membranes or ocular tumors? Will more selective targeting of choroidal neovascular membranes improve the therapeutic index of PDT, expand its indications, or reduce the rate of recurrence of these membranes? Is there a more rational approach to developing candidate photosensitizers tailored to ocular indications (61)? If so, what is the role of *in vitro* and animal biodistribution studies in their development? We expect that future studies will address these and other questions and lead to further refinement in the understanding of photosensitizer localization and the increasing role of photodynamic therapy in the treatment of ocular disorders.

REFERENCES

1. Dougherty TJ. Photodynamic therapy. *Photochem Photobiol* 1993;58:895–900.
2. Takemura T, Ohta N, Nakajima S, et al. Critical importance of the triplet lifetime of the photosensitizer in photodynamic therapy of tumors. *Photochem Photobiol* 1989;50:339–344.
3. Gandin E, Lion Y, van de Vorst A. Quantum yield of singlet oxygen production by xanthene derivatives. *Photochem Photobiol* 1983;37:271–278.
4. Royster AJ, Nanda SK, Hatchell DL, et al. Photochemical initiation of thrombosis. *Arch Ophthalmol* 1988;106:1608–1614.
5. Linden S, Neckers D. Type I and type II sensitizers based on rose bengal onium salts. *Photochem Photobiol* 1988;47:543–550.
6. Gottfried C, Peled D, Winkelman J, et al. Photosensitizers in organized media: singlet oxygen production and spectral properties. *Photochem Photobiol* 1988;48:157–163.
7. Gomer CJ. Preclinical examination of first and second generation photosensitizers used in PDT. *Photochem Photobiol* 1991;54: 1093–1097.
8. Richter AM, Kelly B, Chow J, et al. Preliminary studies on a more effective phototoxic agent than hematoporphyrin. *JNCI* 1987;79:1327–1332.
9. Fisher AM, Murphree AL, Gomer CJ. Clinical and preclinical photodynamic therapy. [Review] *Lasers Surg Med* 1995;17:2–31.
10. Spikes J. New trends in photobiology (invited review) chlorins as photosensitizers in biology and medicine. *J Photochem Photobiol B, Biology* 1990;6:259–274.
11. Moshfeghi D, Peyman GA, Kazi AA, et al. Fluorescence properties of a hydrophilic sensitizer in pigmented rats, rabbits, and monkeys. *Ophthal Surg Lasers* 1999;30:750–753.
12. Schuitmaker JJ, van Best JA, van Delft JL, et al. Bacteriochlorin a, a new photosensitizer in PDT. *Invest Ophthalmol Vis Sci* 1990; 31:1444–1450.
13. Morgan AR, Skalkos D. Second generation sensitizers: where are we and where should we be going? *SPIE* 1990;6:87–106.
14. Kreimer-Birnbaum M. Modified porphyrins, chlorins, phthalocyanines and purpurins: second generation photosensitizers for photodynamic therapy. *Semin Hematol* 1989;26:157–173.
15. van Lier JE, Spikes JD. The chemistry, photophysics and photosensitizing properties of phthalocyanines. *Ciba Found Symp* 1989;146:17–26.
16. Sessler JL, Hemmi G, Mody TD, et al. Texaphyrins: synthesis and applications. *Am Chem Soc Accounts Chem Res* 1994;27: 43–50.
17. Young S, Woodburn K, Wright M, et al. Lutetium texaphyrin (PCI-0123): a near-infrared water-soluble photosensitizer. *Photochem Photobiol* 1996;63:892–897.
18. Morgan AR. Reduced porphyrins as photosensitizers: synthesis and biological effects. In: Henderson BW, Dougherty TJ, eds. *Photodynamic therapy, basic principles and clinical applications.* New York: Marcel Dekker, 1992:157–172.
19. Baumal CR, Puliafito CA, Pieroth L, et al. Photodynamic therapy of experimental choroidal neovascularization with tin ethyl etiopurpurin. *Invest Ophthalmol Vis Sci* 1996;37:122.
20. Hill RA, Crean DH, Doiron DR, et al. Photodynamic therapy for antifibrosis in a rabbit model of filtration surgery. *Invest Ophthalmol Vis Sci* 1995;36:877.
21. Garbo GM. Purpurins and benzochlorins as sensitizers for photodynamic therapy. *J Photochem Photobiol B, Biol* 1996;34: 109–116.
22. Kessel D, Morgan A. Photosensitization with etiobenzochlorins and octaethyl benzochlorins. *Photochem Photobiol* 1993;58:521–526.
23. Nakajima S, Sakata I, Takemura T, et al. Tumor-localizing and photosensitization of photochlorin ATX-S10. In: Spinelli P, Fante Dal M, Marchesini R, eds. *Photodynamic therapy and biomedical lasers.* Amsterdam: Elsevier Science, 1992.531–534.
24. Hikichi T, Mori F, Nakajima S, et al. Dynamic observation of selective accumulation of a photosensitizer and its photodynamic effects in rat experimental choroidal neovascularization. *Retina* 2001;21:126–131.
25. Obana A, Gohto Y, Kaneda K, et al. Selective occlusion of choroidal neovascularization by photodynamic therapy with a water-soluble photosensitizer, ATX-S10. *Lasers Surg Med* 1999;24: 209–222.
26. Moor A. Invited review: signaling pathways in cell death and survival after photodynamic therapy. *J Photochem Photobiol B, Biol* 2000;57:1–13.
27. Mori M, Kuroda T, Obana A, et al. In vitro plasma protein binding and cellular uptake of ATX-S10(Na), a hydrophilic chlorin photosensitizer. *Jpn J Cancer Res* 2000;91:845–852.
28. Verma A, Facchina SL, Hirsch DJ, et al. Photodynamic tumor therapy: mitochondrial benzodiazepine receptors as a therapeutic target. *Mol Med* 1998;4:40–45.

29. Peng Q, Farrants GW, Madslien K, et al. Subcellular localization, redistribution and photobleaching of sulfonated aluminum phthalocyanines in a human melanoma cell line. *Int J Cancer* 1991;49:290–295.
30. Boyle RW, Dolphin D. Structures and biodistribution relationships of photodynamic sensitizers. *Photochem Photobiol* 1996;64: 469–485.
31. Kessel D, Luo Y. Mitochondrial photodamage and PDT-induced apoptosis. *J Photochem Photobiol B, Biol* 1998;42:89–95.
32. Wood SR, Holroyd JA, Brown SB. The subcellular localization of Zn (II) phthalocyanines and their redistribution on exposure to light. *Photochem Photobiol* 1997;65:397–402.
33. Rosenkranz AA, Jans DA, Sobolev AS. Targeted intracellular delivery of photosensitizers to enhance photodynamic efficiency. *Immunol Cell Biol* 2000;78:452–464.
34. Berg K, Anholt H, Moan J, et al. Photobiological properties of haematoporphyrin diesters: evaluation of possible applications in photochemotherapy. *J Photochem Photobiol B, Biol* 1993;20: 37–45.
35. Ricchelli F, Gobbo S, Jori G, et al. Photosensitization of mitochondria by liposome-bound porphyrins. *Photochem Photobiol* 1993;58:53–58.
36. Jori G. Tumour photosensitizers: approaches to enhance the selectivity and efficiency of photodynamic therapy. *J Photochem Photobiol B, Biol* 1996;36:87–93.
37. Allison BA, Pritchard PH, Levy JG, et al. Evidence for low-density lipoprotein receptor-mediated uptake of benzoporphyrin derivative. *Br J Cancer* 1994;69:833–839.
38. Soncin M, Polo L, Reddi E, et al. Effect of axial ligation and delivery system on the tumor-localising and -photosensitising properties of Ge(IV)-octabutoxy-phthalocyanines. *Br J Cancer* 1995;71:727–732.
39. Qualls MM, Thompson DH. Chloroaluminum phthalocyanine tetra sulfate delivered via acid-labile diplasmenylcholine-folate liposomes: intracellular localization and synergistic phototoxicity. *Int J Cancer* 2001;93:384–392.
40. Bachor R, Shea CR, Gillies R, et al. Photosensitized destruction of human bladder carcinoma cells treated with chlorin e6-conjugated microspheres. *Proc Natl Acad Sci USA* 1991;88:1580–1584.
41. Hu LK, Hasan T, Gragoudas ES, et al. Photoimmunotherapy of human uveal melanoma cells. *Exp Eye Res* 1995;6:385–391.
42. Morgan J, Lottman H, Abbou CC, et al. A comparison of direct and liposomal antibody conjugates of sulfonated aluminum phthalocyanines for selective photoimmunotherapy of human bladder carcinoma. *Photochem Photobiol* 1994;60:486–496.
43. Gomer CJ, Jester JV, Razum NJ, et al. Photodynamic therapy of intraocular tumors: examination of hematoporphyrin derivative distribution and long-term damage in rabbit ocular tissue. *Cancer Res* 1985;45:3718–3725.
44. Haimovici R, Kramer M, Miller JW, et al. Localization of lipoprotein-delivered benzoporphyrin derivative in the rabbit eye. *Current Eye Res* 1997;16:83–90.
45. Hill RA, Esterowitz T, Ryan J, et al. Photodynamic laser cyclodestruction with chloroaluminum sulfonated phthalocyanine (CASPc) or Photofrin (PII) vs. Nd:YAG laser cyclodestruction in a pigmented rabbit model. *Lasers Surg Med* 1995;17:166–171.
46. Hill RA, Garret J, Reddi S, et al. Photodynamic therapy (PDT) of the ciliary body with silicon naphthalocyanine (SINc) in rabbits. *Lasers Surg Med* 1996;18:86–91.
47. Hill RA, Crean DH, Doiron DR, et al. Photodynamic therapy of the ciliary body with tin ethyl ethyl purpurin and tin octaethyl benzochlorin in pigmented rabbits. *Ophthal Surg Lasers* 1997;28: 948–953.
48. Kliman GH, Puliafito CA, Stern D, et al. Phthalocyanine photodynamic therapy: new strategy for closure of choroidal neovascularization. *Lasers Surg Med* 1994;15:2–10.
49. Blumenkranz MS, Woodburn KW, Qing F, et al. Lutetium texaphyrin: a potential new agent for ocular fundus angiography and photodynamic therapy. *Am J Ophthalmol* 2000;129:353–362.
50. Kim RY, Hu LK, Flotte TJ, et al. Digital angiography of experimental choroidal melanomas using benzoporphyrin derivative. *Am J Ophthalmol* 1997;123:810–816.
51. Hayes KC, Lindsey S, Stephan ZF, et al. Retinal pigment epithelium possesses both LDL and scavenger receptor activity. *Invest Ophthalmol Vis Sci* 1989;30:225–232.
52. Obana A, Gohto Y, Kaneda K, et al. PDT to monkey CNV with ATX-S10(Na): inappropriateness of early laser irradiation for selective occlusion. *Invest Ophthalmol Vis Sci* 2001;42: 2639–2645.
53. Haimovici R, Ciulla TA, Miller JW, et al. Localization of Rose Bengal, CASPc, and chlorin e6 in the rabbit eye. *Retina* 2002; 22:65–74.
54. Melamed S, Ben-Sira I, Sen-Shaul Y. Ultrastructure of fenestrations in endothelial choriocapillaris of the rabbit. *Br J Ophthalmol* 1980;64:537–543.
55. Rapoport S. Osmotic opening of the blood-brain and blood-ocular barriers. *Exp Eye Res* 1977;(Suppl):499–509.
56. Renno RZ, Delori FC, Holzer RA, et al. Photodynamic therapy using Lu-tex induces apoptosis in vitro, and its effect is potentiated by angiostatin in retinal capillary endothelial cells. *Invest Ophthalmol Vis Sci* 2000;41:3963–3971.
57. Verteporfin in Photodynamic Therapy Study Group. Verteporfin therapy of subfoveal choroidal neovascularization in age-related macular degeneration: two-year results of a randomized clinical trial including lesions with occult with no classic choroidal neovascularization—verteporfin in photodynamic therapy report 2. *Am J Ophthal* 2001;131:541–560.
58. TAP study group. Photodynamic therapy of subfoveal choroidal neovascularization in age-related macular degeneration with verteporfin. *Arch Ophthalmol* 2001;119:198–207.
59. Reinke MH, Canakis C, Husain D. Verteporfin photodynamic therapy retreatments of normal retina and choroid in the cynomolgus monkey. *Ophthalmology* 1999;106:1915–1923.
60. Peyman GA, Kazi AA, Unal M, et al. Problems with and pitfalls of photodynamic therapy. *Ophthalmology* 2000;107:29–35.
61. Lange N, Ballini JP, Wagnieres G, van den Bergh H. A new drug-screening procedure for photosensitizing agents used in photodynamic therapy for CNV. *Invest Ophthalmol Vis Sci* 2001;42: 38–46.
62. Pogue BW, Ortel B, Chen N, et al. A photobiological and photophysical-based study of two chlorins. *Cancer Res* 2001;61: 717–724.

12

PHOTODYNAMIC THERAPY OF EXPERIMENTAL CHOROIDAL NEOVASCULARIZATION USING NPE6

SHIN YONEYA
DARIUS M. MOSHFEGHI
GHOLAM A. PEYMAN

Mono-L-aspartyl chlorin e6 (NPe6), a second-generation photosensitizer (Meiji Seika Kaisha, Ltd., Tokyo, Japan), differs from the benzoporphyrins and metallopurpurins in its hydrophilicity and availability as an aqueous preparation (1–4). NPe6 has a molecular weight of 711 (Fig. 12.1) and absorption peaks at 202, 284, 400, 502, and 664 nm (1); the 664-nm peak has been used for photodynamic therapy (PDT) because of the superior transmittance through biologic tissues (1).

The original description of NPe6 PDT was for treatment of BALB/c tumors in mice (1). This study demonstrated the lack of cutaneous photosensitivity as evaluated by the presence of skin erythema at concentrations of 10 mg/kg and fluence of 1000 J/cm^2, using 664-nm light (1). Following intravenous (iv) injection, NPe6 appeared to localize specifically and preferentially within lysosomes as demonstrated by acridine orange staining of PTK_2 cells (2).

In vitro studies evaluated the effective photosensitizing ability of NPe6 over a range of irradiances (630 to 664 nm) as well as its low phototoxicity (8% loss of Chinese hamster ovary [CHO] cells when exposed to 15 µg/mL of NPe6 alone, 2% loss of CHO cells when exposed to light alone). Further studies by Roberts and Berns demonstrated that NPe6 localized to lysosomes through the process of endocytosis (pinocytosis) (3). *In vitro* studies with CHO cells showed that when the cell line was cooled to 2°C, a process that is known to inhibit endocytosis while permitting diffusion, there was minimal fluorescence within the cell. At a dose of 15 µg/mL, which is normally 100% phototoxic, cooling to 2°C resulted in a phototoxicity of only 35% (3). Using PTK_2 cells (which localize NPe6 identically to CHO cells) (2), transmission electron microscopy demonstrated lysosomal disruption following NPe6 PDT (4). This disruption was characterized by swelling of the lysosomes and vacuoles, breaks in the lysosomal membrane, and the presence of intralysosomal debris. Mitochondria were relatively unaffected.

In another study using a chick chorioallantoic membrane/embryo model, NPe6 was shown to localize within proliferating microvascular cells as opposed to rapidly dividing embryo cells (5). In a mouse model, peak concentrations of NPe6 were seen 2 to 60 minutes following administration (6). There is evidence that NPe6 PDT is mediated by a type-II photosensitization, involving the generation of singlet oxygen species (6). Mori and coworkers demonstrated that NPe6 PDT with 664-nm irradiation generates 2.3-fold more singlet oxygen than hematoporphyrin derivative (7). Similarly, Grossweiner reported that NPe6 results in greater singlet oxygen yields than hematoporphyrin derivative, phthalocyanines, and purpurins (6). All of these properties of NPe6—its hydrophilic nature, rapid biodistribution, low cutaneous photosensitivity, high photosensitizing ability, endocytotic uptake—suggested that it would be a useful agent for the treatment of choroidal neovascularization (CNV).

FLUORESCENCE PROPERTIES OF NPE6

Moshfeghi and coworkers investigated the fluorescence properties of NPe6 in pigmented rabbits, rats, and nonhuman primates (African green monkeys) (8) (Fig. 12.2). Following iv injection of NPe6 (2 mg/kg), a helium-neon (HeNe) laser mounted within a Rodenstock scanning laser ophthalmoscope (SLO) 101 system (Rodenstock, Danbury, CT) delivered 633-nm light to the fundus of the animals. A barrier filter of 665 nm mounted between the HeNe laser and the SLO allowed optimal fluorescence while minimizing any photodynamic effect. Results were continuously recorded on super-VHS videotape. NPe6 fluorescence was found to persist for 5 hours in the rat, 3 hours in the rabbit, and 1.5 hours in the nonhuman primate, indicating the possibility of using NPe6 for angiography followed by PDT, and eliminating the need for fluorescein angiography.

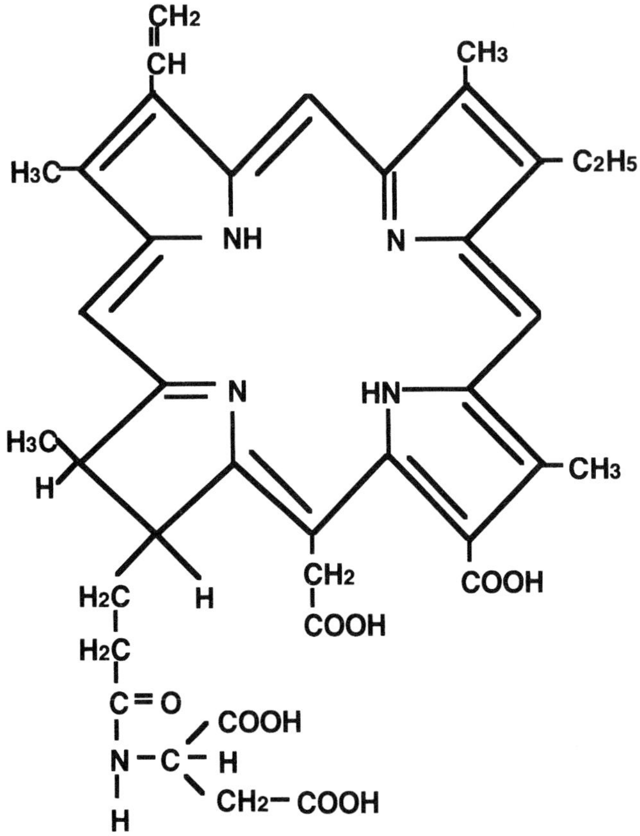

FIGURE 12.1. Chemical structure of mono-L-aspartyl chlorin e6 (MW, 711). (From: Mori K, Yoneya S, Ohta M, et al. Angiographic and histologic effects of fundus photodynamic therapy with a hydrophilic sensitizer (mono-L-aspartyl chlorin e6). *Ophthalmology* 1999;106:1384–1391, with permission.)

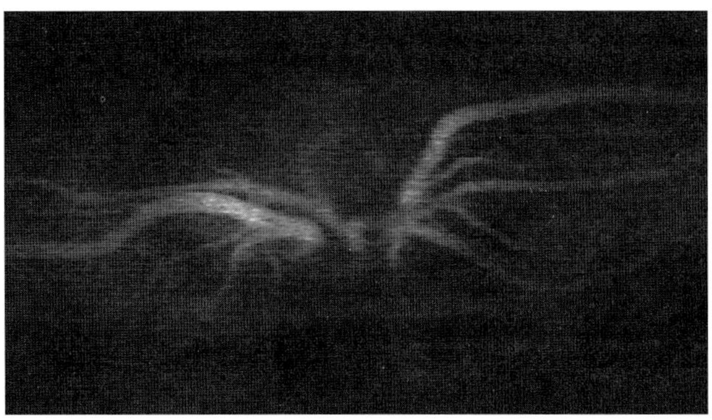

FIGURE 12.2. Middle-phase retinal angiogram in rabbit. This photograph shows the retinal vasculature moments after intravenous injection of NPe6. (From: Moshfeghi D, Peyman GA, Kazi AA, et al. Fluorescence properties of a hydrophilic sensitizer in pigmented rats, rabbits, and monkeys. *Ophthalmic Surg Lasers* 1999;30:750–753, with permission.)

NPE6 RETINAL TOXICITY

El-Dessouky and associates evaluated the retinal toxicity of NPe6 following direct intravitreal injection (9). These experiments involved 12 pigmented rabbits divided into five experimental groups receiving intravitreal injections in each eye of NPe6 (6.25, 12.5, 25, 50, or 100 μg) and one control group receiving intravitreal injection of saline in each eye. One eye of each rabbit was sutured closed following injection to test the effect of ambient lighting on NPe6 and retinal toxicity. Electroretinograms (ERG) were performed prior to intervention and at 2 days, 1 week, and 2 weeks postinjection. At the end of 2 weeks, the eyes were enucleated and prepared for histology. Fundus findings of uncovered eyes treated with PDT at 1 week postinjection revealed central vein occlusion at doses of 50 μg or more. Covered eyes developed retinal pigment epithelial (RPE) proliferation. Electroretinogram results demonstrated absent retinal responses at 100 μg and mild toxicity at 50 μg. No toxicity was noted at intravitreal doses of 25 μg or less.

NPE6 PHOTODYNAMIC THERAPY OF NORMAL PIGMENTED RABBIT AND NONHUMAN PRIMATE FUNDI

Mori and coworkers examined the efficacy of NPe6 in closing normal choroidal vessels in pigmented rabbits and nonhuman primates (*Macaca fuscata*) (10). The objectives of the study were fourfold: to determine (a) the efficacy of NPe6 in closing normal choroidal vessels; (b) the selectivity of NPe6 PDT; (c) any funduscopic and angiographic changes following NPe6 PDT; and (d) the optimal NPe6 PDT parameters for normal choroidal vascular occlusion. Laser light was delivered to the fundi of the experimental animals with a GaAlInAs diode laser (Matsushita, Osaka, Japan) tuned to 664 nm coupled to a slit-lamp biomicroscope (Topcon SL-7F, Tokyo, Japan) with a filter in front of the illuminating light to prevent inadvertent activation of NPe6.

The optimal parameters of dye concentration (testing 2, 10, 25, 50, and 100 mg/kg) and laser fluence (0.46, 0.75, 2.3, 3.75, 4.6, and 7.5 J/cm^2) were determined in the pigmented rabbits using a spot size of 1,000 μm, laser duration of 1 to 10 seconds, and power of 3.6 or 5.9 mW. Indirect ophthalmoscopy and fluorescein angiography were performed both 2 hours and 7 days following treatment, after which the eyes were enucleated under deep anesthesia. The monkeys were treated with a similar regimen using an NPe6 concentration of either 2 or 10 mg/kg.

Choroidal vascular occlusion and blood–retinal barrier breakdown on fluorescein angiography (FA) occurred at all tested doses in the pigmented rabbit study (10). At higher concentrations (10 mg/kg or more), choroidal lesions overlapped the initial treatment zone. The optimal concentration and fluence were 2 mg/kg and 0.75 J/cm^2, respectively. No adverse systemic effects were noted. No fundus changes were seen in those animals receiving only dye. Histopathology of the 2-hour post-PDT specimens in rabbits revealed endothelial cell necrosis, scattered choriocapillaris occlusion, occasional necrosis of the RPE, and preservation of the overlying neurosensory retina (Fig. 12.3).

Early hypofluorescence and intense dye leakage were observed on late-phase angiograms in most treated areas of the monkey eyes at a concentration of 2 mg/kg and a laser fluence of 2.3 to 7.5 J/cm^2, although these findings were not evident at the 2-hour post-PDT examination (10). Similarly, no funduscopic changes were noted at 2 hours post-PDT. However, by 7 days after PDT, a yellowish retinochoroidal lesion was visible. At a concentration of 10 mg/kg and fluences of 3.75 to 7.5 J/cm^2, the retinal vessels were occluded. At 7 days, a white, full-thickness retinochoroidal lesion was present in the treatment zone. Histologic analysis divided retinal damage into three grades: (a) grade 0, no reaction; (b) grade 1, choroidal vascular occlusion only; and (c) grade 2, retinochoroidal vascular occlusion. Grade 1 lesions demonstrated choriocapillaris damage, occlusion, and vacuolations of the RPE cells, with preservation of the neurosensory retina. Most grade 2 lesions demonstrated occlusion of retinal vessels. Based on these results, the optimal dye concentration was determined to be 2 mg/kg, with fluence between 2.3 and 7.5 J/cm^2.

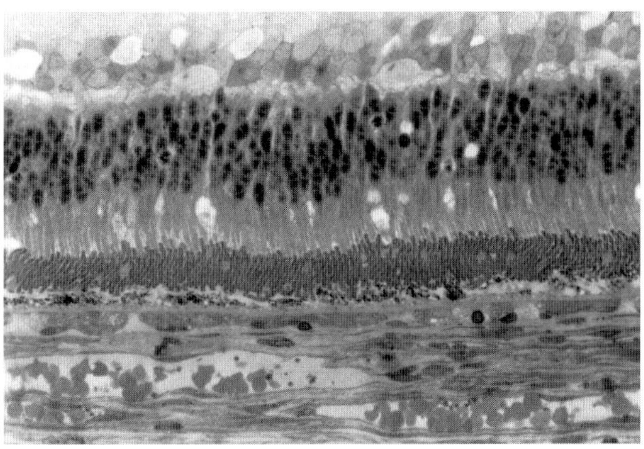

FIGURE 12.3. Light micrograph obtained 2 hours after photodynamic therapy (0.75 J/cm^2, 25 mg/kg). Note the necrosis of endothelial cells and occasional capillary occlusion on choroidal vessels. Necrotized retinal pigment epithelial cells are also evident. In contrast, the architecture of sensory retina is approximately intact except for the loss of a few visual cells. (From: Mori K, Yoneya S, Ohta M, et al. Angiographic and histologic effects of fundus photodynamic therapy with a hydrophilic sensitizer (mono-L-aspartyl chlorin e6). *Ophthalmology* 1999;106: 1384–1391, with permission.)

VARIABLES OF NPE6 PHOTODYNAMIC THERAPY

Peyman and colleagues performed a series of experiments on pigmented rabbits, nonpigmented rabbits, and nonhuman primates to determine the factors that influence successful NPe6 PDT (11). They evaluated the effect of fundus pigmentation, intraocular pressure, laser spot focus/defocus, region of fundus treated, fluence equivalency (power × time), and retreatment on NPe6 PDT. Results indicated that fundus pigmentation was a factor at only the lowest fluence (1 mW, 10 sec) in pigmented rabbits (4/12 demonstrating a lesion, compared to 12/12 nonpigmented rabbits) (Fig. 12.4). Intraocular pressure (IOP) steadily retarded the effect of NPe6 PDT, with complete lesion manifestation in 100% of treated areas at normal IOP, 40% of lesions at 30 mm Hg, and 0% at IOP sufficient to blanch the optic nerve. Laser focus/defocus had no effect on lesion development, attesting to the lack of thermal input necessary for successful PDT. Areas treated in the fovea resulted in larger lesion size than those treated in the periphery. Longer durations of PDT with lower power were associated with larger lesions compared with shorter durations with higher power (Fig. 12.5). Finally, retreatment resulted in a progressive thinning of the neurosensory retina with loss of photoreceptor outer segments and nuclei in rabbits.

THRESHOLD LEVELS FOR NPE6 PHOTODYNAMIC THERAPY

Kazi and coworkers evaluated the threshold fluence to create a choroidal vascular occlusion using NPe6 PDT in pigmented and nonpigmented rabbits (12). Group 1 rabbits were treated with fluences that varied from 0.44 to 4.42 J/cm^2, with a constant concentration of 2 mg/kg NPe6 and irradiance applied with a 664-nm laser 5 to 10 minutes postinjection. Threshold was defined as the level at which all treated lesions appeared on FA. Group 2 rabbits received NPe6 at 2 mg/kg, fluence of 8.84 J/cm^2, and irradiation beginning from 5 minutes to 3 hours postinjection. Fluorescein angiography was performed 24 hours later to determine the presence of lesions in the treatment zone.

Group 3 rabbits were the same pigmented rabbits that were used in Group 1; they underwent FA at 30 minutes to 24 hours post-PDT to determine when the treatment lesion developed. Threshold for choriocapillaris occlusion as determined by FA was 0.88 J/cm^2 for nonpigmented rabbits and 2.65 J/cm^2 for pigmented rabbits. Five minutes following injection was found to be the optimal timing of postinjection irradiation to achieve angiographic evidence

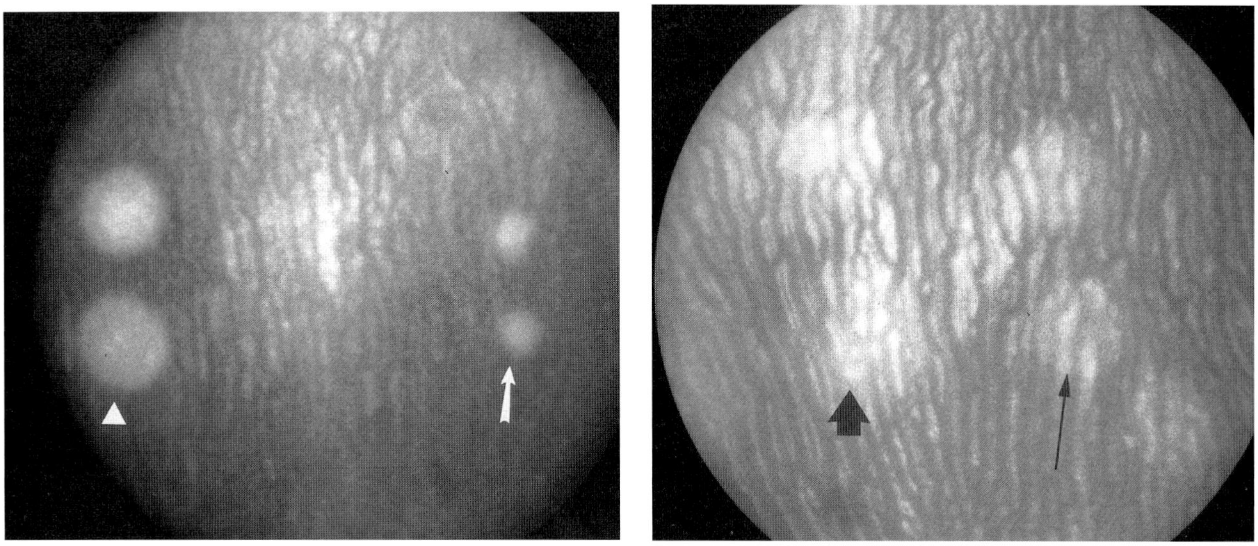

A B

FIGURE 12.4. A: Fundus photograph of a pigmented rabbit showing lesions made at a spot size of 1.2 mm at a power of 1 mW for 10 seconds *(arrow)* and at a power of 3 mW for 10 seconds *(arrowhead).* **B:** Fundus photograph of a nonpigmented rabbit showing lesions made at a spot size diameter of 1.2 mm at a power of 1 mW for 10 seconds *(thin arrow)* and at a power of 3 mW for 10 seconds *(thick arrow).* Note that the lesions placed in the nonpigmented rabbit fundus **(B)** are larger in diameter than those at the same parameters in the pigmented rabbit fundus. (From: Peyman GA, Kazi AA, Unal M, et al. Problems with and pitfalls of photodynamic therapy. *Ophthalmology* 2000;107:29–35, with permission.)

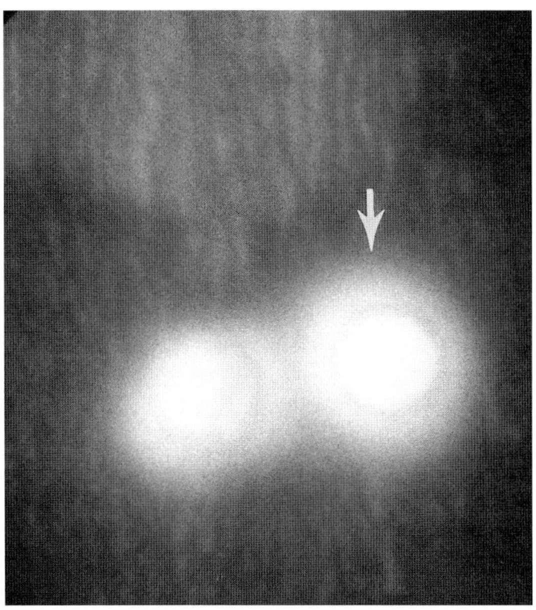

FIGURE 12.5. Fluorescein angiogram of a rabbit avascular fundus demonstrating the effect of equivalent fluence after photodynamic therapy. The lesion made with 5 mW for 10 seconds *(arrow)* on the right-hand side is larger than the lesion made with 10 mW for 5 seconds adjacent to it. (From: Peyman GA, Kazi AA, Unal M, et al. Problems with and pitfalls of photodynamic therapy. *Ophthalmology* 2000;107:29–35, with permission.)

of closure with NPe6 PDT. Photodynamic therapy applied 1 hour postinjection produced lesions significantly smaller in size than those made at 5 minutes postinjection; no angiographically evident lesions were visible after PDT applied 3 hours postinjection. Fluorescein evidence of choriocapillaris occlusion was not noted until 2 hours post-PDT application.

Peyman and colleagues continued this investigation in rats, rabbits, and nonhuman primates to investigate the existence of a threshold for retinal damage that is higher than the threshold for choroidal damage following NPe6 PDT (13). Two groups were evaluated: a primary and a retreatment group. In the primary treatment group, rats received two lesions each at fluences ranging from 5.1 to 101.9 J/cm^2. Similarly, rabbits were treated with fluences ranging from 2.7 to 17.7 J/cm^2 and monkeys received one treatment at each fluence between 2.7 to 53.1 J/cm^2. All animals were given 2 mg/kg of NPe6 iv followed by 664-nm laser irradiation 5 minutes postinjection. In the retreatment group, four rabbits received treatment with the 664-nm laser at 2.7, 4.4, 8.8, and 17.7 J/cm^2 fluences 5 minutes after being injected with 2 mg/kg of NPe6. These areas were retreated at the same parameters 1 week later and the eyes underwent subsequent FA.

In the primary treatment groups of all three species, a higher fluence was required to close retinal vessels than choroidal vessels: rats (15.3 J/cm^2 for choroid, 101.9 J/cm^2 for retina), rabbits (2.7 J/cm^2 for choroid, 17.7

J/cm² for retina), and monkeys (17.7 J/cm² for choroid, 53.1 J/cm² for retina) (13). In the retreatment group, choroidal occlusion was noted on angiography at all fluences. Retreatment did not result in retinal damage (demonstrated angiographically) until the fluence exceeded 17.7 J/cm². This study demonstrated the relative safety of NPe6 PDT retreatment as long as the retinal threshold for vascular occlusion was avoided.

REPEAT NPE6 PHOTODYNAMIC THERAPY IN NONHUMAN PRIMATES

Mori and coworkers expanded these retreatment studies by evaluating the effect of NPe6 retreatment on the normal fovea and choroid in nonhuman primates (*Macaca fuscata*) (14). NPe6 was injected iv at a concentration of 2 mg/kg; PDT irradiation was applied with a 664-nm laser 5 minutes postinjection at a fluence of 7.5 J/cm² and spot size of 1,000 μm for 10 seconds. PDT was repeated every 2 weeks for a total of three treatments to each fovea and midperipheral fundus. Following the third treatment, eyes were enucleated and prepared for histology. Histopathologic examination demonstrated proliferation (Fig. 12.6) and duplication of the RPE, fibrous tissue plaques around the RPE, and occlusion of the choriocapillaris and large choroidal vessels. The retinal vessels and overlying neurosensory retina were spared (14).

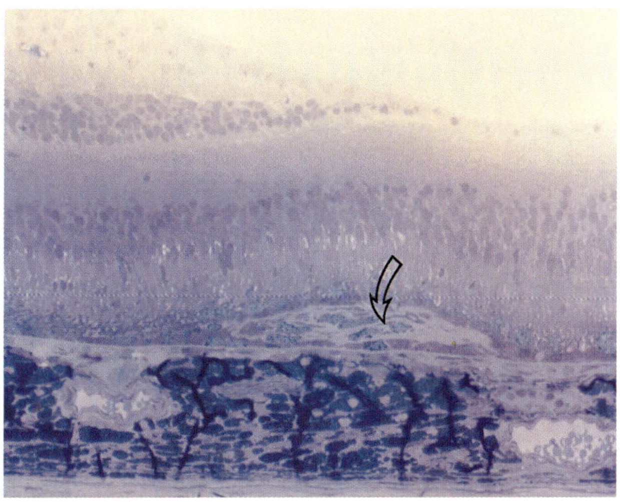

FIGURE 12.6. Light micrograph of triply treated eye demonstrates extensive proliferation of the retinal pigment epithelial layer *(arrow)* combined with near-complete occlusion of the choriocapillaris. The inner sensory retina remained intact despite some shortening of outer segments. (Toluidine blue, magnification ×150) (From: Nakashizuka T, Mori K, Hayashi N, et al. Retreatment effect of NPe6 photodynamic therapy on the normal primate macula. *Retina* 2001;21:493–498, with permission.)

NPE6 PHOTODYNAMIC THERAPY OF EXPERIMENTAL CHOROIDAL NEOVASCULARIZATION IN NONHUMAN PRIMATES

In one of the final sets of preclinical experiments, Mori and colleagues evaluated the localization of NPe6 in experimental CNV in nonhuman primates (*Macaca fuscata*) (15). Sixty-seven experimental CNV lesions were created using the modified Ryan's model. NPe6 angiography was performed in 16 lesions using suprathreshold concentrations (20 mg/kg) to ensure that if the dye localized to the CNV, it would be visible on super-VHS videotape. Blue-green light (488 nm) from a laser coupled to an SLO was used to excite one of the minor excitation peaks. Angiography, performed continuously for the first 10 minutes after injection and then every 10 minutes for the next hour, demonstrated localization of NPe6 to experimental CNV between 20 and 60 minutes, with a peak at 20 minutes after injection. At the completion of this study, the animals were euthanized and their eyes were prepared for fluorescence microscopy studies, which revealed that the magnitude of NPe6 fluorescence was greatest around experimental CNV and RPE and less around choroidal vessels (Fig. 12.7). Retinal stroma did not fluoresce.

The remaining 51 CNV lesions were entered into the NPe6 PDT arm of the study: 30 received NPe6 PDT (0.5 to 10.0 mg/kg, 7.5 to 225 J/cm², irradiation at 0 to 60 minutes postinjection, spot size 1,000 μm, and duration 10 to 300 seconds), 13 received NPe6 (0.5 to 10.0 mg/kg) alone, and eight CNV lesions were treated with laser irradiation alone. Eyes were enucleated and prepared for histopathology. Fluorescein and indocyanine angiographic studies of experimental CNV treated with NPe6 PDT demonstrated effective closure of experimental CNV at all test doses. Histopathologic studies confirmed this finding, demonstrating necrosis of experimental CNV endothelial cells with preservation of the overlying neurosensory retina. The conclusion of this study was that NPe6 PDT results in effective localization to experimental CNV with subsequent effective vascular occlusion.

SUMMARY

NPe6 is a hydrophilic photosensitizing agent available in aqueous solution. Treatment with NPe6 PDT in nonhuman primates has demonstrated separate choroidal and retinal thresholds for damage. Retreatment does not appear to affect the neurosensory retina adversely even while effectively closing normal choroidal vessels, as long as PDT parameters are below the threshold for retinal damage. NPe6 has a high degree of photosensitizing abil-

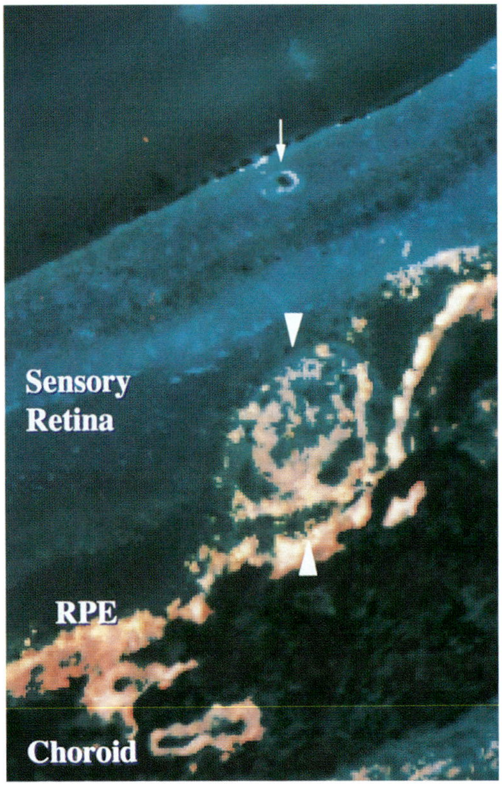

FIGURE 12.7. Fluorescence microscopy of NPe6. Fluorescence of NPe6 accumulated intensively in the choroidal neovascularizations *(arrowheads)* and retinal pigment epithelial cells. Some choroidal vascular walls also fluoresced moderately. In contrast, there was trace fluorescence in retinal vascular walls *(arrow)* and microcapillaries. There was little fluorescence of NPe6 detected in retinal stroma, vascular lumen of the retina and choroid, vitreous cavity, and subretinal space. (Original magnification, ×175) (From: Mori K, Yoneya S, Anzail K, et al. Photodynamic therapy of experimental choroidal neovascularization with a hydrophilic photosensitizer: mono-L-aspartyl chlorin e6. *Retina* 2001;21: 499–508, with permission.)

ity and effectively localizes to experimental CNV, causing the occlusion of these abnormal vessels following 664-nm irradiation at low fluences (7.5 J/cm^2) with preservation of the overlying neurosensory retina. These studies have demonstrated that NPe6 is a promising agent for clinical evaluation.

REFERENCES

1. Nelson JS, Roberts WG, Berns MW. In vivo studies on the utilization of mono-l-aspartyl chlorin (NPe6) for photodynamic therapy. *Cancer Res* 1987;47:4681–4685.
2. Roberts WG, Shiau FY, Nelson JS, et al. In vitro characterization of monoaspartyl chlorin e6 and diaspartyl chlorin e6 for photodynamic therapy. *J Natl Cancer Inst* 1988;80:330–336.
3. Roberts WG, Berns MW. In vitro photosensitization. I. Cellular uptake and subcellular localization of mono-L-aspartyl chlorin e6, chloro-aluminum sulfonated phthalocyanine, and Photofrin II. *Lasers Surg Med* 1989;9:90–101.
4. Roberts WG, Liaw LHL, Berns MW. In vitro photosensitization. II. An electron microscopy study of cellular destruction with mono-L-aspartyl chlorin e6 and Photofrin II. *Lasers Surg Med* 1989;9:102–108.
5. Roberts WG, Hasan T. Role of neovasculature and vascular permeability on the tumor retention of photodynamic agents. *Cancer Res* 1992;52:924–930.
6. Grossweiner LI. *The science of phototherapy.* Boca Raton, FL: CRC Press, 1994:27–49,139–155,175–177.
7. Mori K, Ohta M, Sano A, et al. [Potential of photodynamic therapy with a second-generation sensitizer: mono-L-aspartyl chlorin e6]. *Nippon Ganka Gakkai Zasshi. Acta Societatis Ophthalmologicae Japonicae* 1997;101:134–140.
8. Moshfeghi DM, Peyman GA, Kazi AA, et al. Fluorescence properties of a hydrophilic sensitizer in pigmented rats, rabbits, and monkeys. *Ophthal Surg Lasers* 1999;30:750–753.
9. El-Dessouky ES, Moshfeghi AA, Peyman GA, et al. Toxicity of the photosensitizer NPe6 following intravitreal injection. *Ophthal Surg Lasers* 2001;32:316–321.
10. Mori K, Yoneya S, Ohta M, et al. Angiographic and histologic effects of fundus photodynamic therapy with a hydrophilic sensitizer (mono-L-aspartyl chlorin e6). *Ophthalmology* 1999;106: 1384–1391.
11. Peyman GA, Kazi AA, Unal M, et al. Problems with and pitfalls of photodynamic therapy. *Ophthalmology* 2000;107: 29–35.
12. Kazi AA, Peyman GA, Unal M, et al. Threshold power levels for NPe6 photodynamic therapy. *Ophthalmic Surg Lasers* 2000;31: 136–142.
13. Peyman GA, Kazi AA, Moshfeghi D, et al. Threshold and retreatment parameters of NPe6 photodynamic therapy in retinal and choroidal vessels. *Ophthalmic Surg Lasers* 2000;31:323–327.
14. Nakashizuka T, Mori K, Hayashi N, et al. Retreatment effect of NPe6 photodynamic therapy on the normal primate macula. *Retina* 2001;21:493–498.
15. Mori K, Yoneya S, Anzail K, et al. Photodynamic therapy of experimental choroidal neovascularization with a hydrophilic photosensitizer: mono-L-aspartyl chlorin e6. *Retina* 2001;21: 499–508.

13

PHOTODYNAMIC THERAPY FOR EXPERIMENTAL INTRAOCULAR TUMORS

ROSA Y. KIM
LUCY H.Y. YOUNG

Photodynamic therapy (PDT) is an attractive modality for the treatment of intraocular tumors for several reasons. The clear media of the eye permit an accurate alignment of the illuminating beam of light with the intraocular tumor, thus sparing the adjacent normal tissues. In addition, the optical property of the eye permits a variety of microlenses, allowing a good visualization of intraocular structures. Finally, leaky tumor vasculature, combined with an intact blood–retina barrier in the adjacent tissue, allow the photosensitizing dye to accumulate within the tumor bed, further enhancing the efficacy of PDT.

RETINOBLASTOMA

Photodynamic therapy for retinoblastoma (RB) is at an early investigational stage. The first studies in animal models were performed using hematoporphyrin derivative (HPD) as the photosensitizer (1,2). Tumors derived from six patients with RB were implanted in the anterior chambers of the nude mice. Using HPD as the photosensitizer, four of the six RB lines demonstrated response to PDT with tumor necrosis. Tumors produced by poorly vascularized lines, including Y79, which is a well-established avascular human RB cell line, did not show regression. This study has demonstrated that a well-vascularized tumor bed is necessary to achieve the effects of PDT (1).

Few clinical studies describing PDT of retinoblastoma have been reported (3). Using HPD as the photosensitizer, seven eyes in six patients with retinoblastoma were treated. The light doses ranged from 60 to 400 J/cm^2, with a single exception of one patient, who received 1,000 J/cm^2. Whereas one patient with vitreous seeding showed absolutely no response to PDT, the others with discrete, solitary tumors responded by decrease in tumor size within the first 2 months. However, all of these patients exhibited tumor growth after 3 to 4 months. Most likely, the patient with vitreous seedings did not show any response to PDT because of a lack of blood supply to this region; the vitreous HPD level would have been subtherapeutic (4).

In another clinical study, photodynamic therapy has been used in conjunction with radiation therapy in treatment of RB (5). Four of five children who underwent PDT received radiation before PDT using HPD. Fluorescein angiograms (FA) performed following the treatment showed tumor hypofluorescence in all patients. Histologic examinations of the tumors from the patients treated only with PDT revealed tumor angionecrosis. Various side effects from PDT described in this study included vitreous hemorrhage and retinal damage to the surrounding retina following excessive irradiation (5). Ohnishi and coworkers concluded that tumors less than 4-disc diameter in size might be adequately treated by PDT alone. Despite the previously mentioned side effects of PDT in these patients, a combination of PDT and radiation might still have a role in reducing the doses of radiation in cases of larger tumors.

Photodynamic therapy for RB needs further investigation. None of the currently available animal models closely resemble RB in humans. Thus, further studies are necessary to identify a more optimal animal model system.

UVEAL MELANOMA

Because the early clinical studies were performed on very advanced diseases using HPD, which tend to have poor tissue penetration, the results have been mixed and often unsuccessful (6–9). Tse and associates treated seven patients with uveal melanoma, including three patients with choroidal melanoma, two with ciliary body tumors, one with an iris tumor, and one who developed an orbital recurrence after exenteration for a postenucleation recurrence of an iris melanoma (9). Each patient was treated with HPD and received light doses ranging from 360 to 720 J/cm^2. Unfortunately, the authors observed complications, including external skin sunburns, iritis, neovascular glaucoma in patients with iris tumors, and serous retinal detachment. Although these patients showed clinical response with reduction in tumor size, all had histological evidence of residual neoplasm.

In another study, various tumor volumes ranging from 500 mm^3 to 1,000 mm^3 were exposed to 630-nm laser light with total light doses of 300 to 3,000 J/cm^2 via transpupillary and transscleral methods (6). The treated tumors were followed for 3 months, and the authors observed that the smaller-volume tumors displayed a more dramatic response to PDT than the larger ones. In this study, high doses of light resulted in secondary thermal effects in addition to direct PDT toxicity.

Other studies have purposefully attempted to eliminate the thermal effect by maintaining the light doses below the thermal threshold (3,7). A variety of tumors were treated, including pigmented and nonpigmented choroidal melanomas, amelanotic iris melanoma, and ciliary body melanoma. Interestingly, the nonpigmented tumors responded well to PDT using HPD with no evidence of regrowth in 2 months, whereas the pigmented tumors showed only a partial reduction in tumor size.

Finally, in another study by Sery and coworkers (8), the authors also observed that pigmented tumors required much greater light doses compared to the amelanotic tumors. The pigmented iris tumors only turned gray after PDT but did not show any reduction in size even with a total light dose of approximately 7,000 J/cm^2. Increased light absorption by the pigment was a potential reason for the poor response in these tumors.

With these mixed reports from the early clinical studies, several investigational studies of PDT on experimental uveal melanomas were performed using amelanotic Greene hamster melanoma cell line (10–14). Unlike the initial clinical studies, which were performed using HPD, the subsequent studies were performed using second-generation photosensitizers, including chloroaluminum sulfonated phthalocyanine (CASPc) (12), 2, 3-Naphthalocyanine (10), and benzoporphyrin derivatives (BPD) (13,14). Early investigations with CASPc demonstrated that a successful treatment of an amelanotic iris tumor required only 10 to 30 J/cm^2, whereas an amelanotic choroidal tumor needed 22 to 60 J/cm^2. At higher light doses (57 to 60 J/cm^2), iris tumor treatment suffered complications of hyphema and severe inflammatory responses. For the choroidal tumors, a light dose higher than 43 J/cm^2 resulted in intraretinal and subretinal hemorrhages and exudative retinal detachments (12).

Later studies by Hill and associates (10) showed fewer complications using the 2,3-Naphthalocyanine. The authors reported that only 20 J/cm^2 was necessary to achieve tumor destruction of more than 3.5 mm in depth. Histopathologic examination displayed a sharp demarcation between the treated and nontreated areas. Unlike other reports (15,16), exudative retinal detachments were not noted.

Although these data with second-generation photosensitizers were encouraging with their improved tissue penetration and reduced side effects, the preceding studies performed on amelanotic melanoma were not clinically applicable because the pigmented tumors represented more than 90% of human ocular melanomas. An animal model of pigmented choroidal melanoma was developed in our laboratory (17). We performed multiple studies using CASPc and BPD as photosensitizers with this model. Our initial studies were performed using CASPc (15). Fluences ranging from 25 to 70 J/cm^2 were used to treat 20 tumor-bearing rabbits with heights ranging from 2.0 to 4.8 mm. These animals were followed for 4.5 to 8 weeks. All tumors treated with 40 J/cm^2 or more resulted in tumor regression with histologic examination demonstrating vascular occlusions within the tumor.

Although our initial results with CASPc were very optimistic, this dye was not clinically practical, because PDT had to be performed 24 hours after the dye injection. Our next studies were performed with liposomal preparation of BPD with the pigmented experimental choroidal melanomas. First, biodistribution studies were performed using digital angiography and fluorescence microscopy to determine the time of the maximum dye accumulation in the experimental choroidal melanoma with minimal fluorescence in the surrounding normal tissue (18). Filters designed specifically for BPD were used with peak absorption at 580 nm and peak emission at 695 nm. Benzoporphyrin derivative at concentration of 1 mg/kg was injected via ear vein, and digital images of tumor, normal choroidal, and iris were obtained at various time points until 24 hours. Fluorescence microscopy was performed using the same time points, and the two sets of the data were compared for maximum dye accumulation. Both studies demonstrated that maximal intratumoral BPD fluorescence occurred 15 to 45 minutes after BPD administration.

Using this information, we performed PDT on 18 tumor-bearing rabbits with intravenous BPD (2 mg/kg) (19). Argon-pumped dye laser (692 nm) delivered fluences of 40 to 150 J/cm^2 15 minutes after the dye injection. Tumor regression was evident in all eyes treated with 60 J/cm^2 or greater (Fig. 13.1); however, with light dose of 40 J/cm^2, tumor regrowth was observed within 10 days after the treatment. Histological studies on eyes enucleated immediately after the treatment with both photosensitizer and light showed prominent vascular occlusion throughout the full thickness of the tumor.

Following this study, we performed PDT on the same experimental choroidal melanoma with only half the previous BPD dose at 1 mg/kg. In addition, we allowed the tumors to reach a higher thickness prior to PDT (3.1 to 4.6 mm). Total fluences ranging from 60 to 120 J/cm^2 were

A 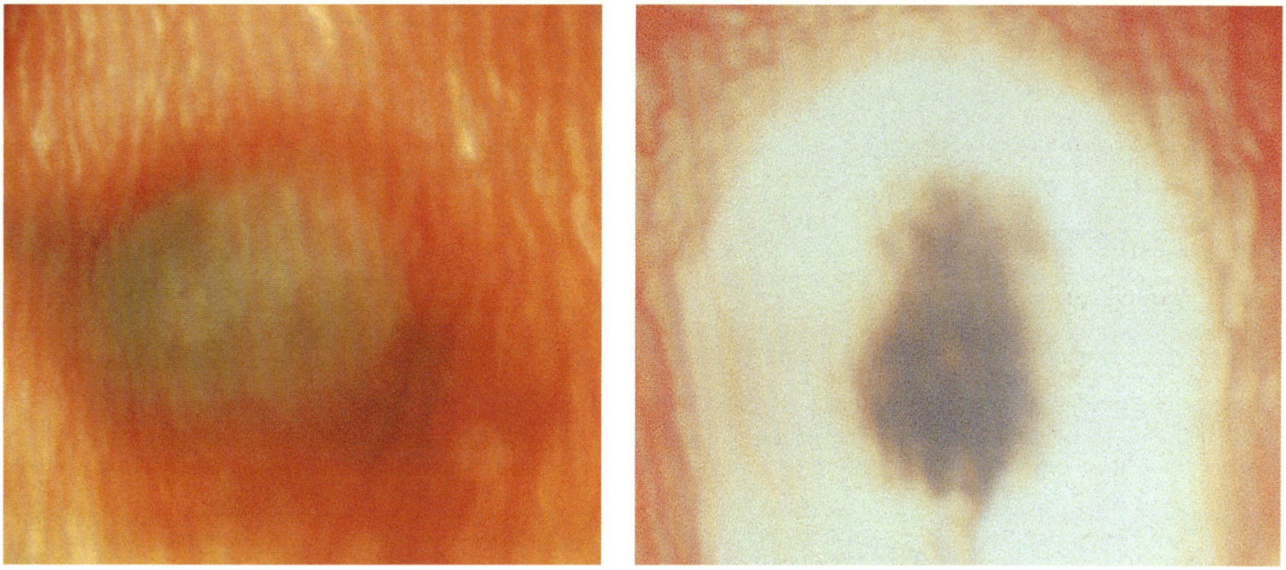 B

FIGURE 13.1. **A:** Pretreatment color fundus photograph of a pigmented choroidal melanoma. **B:** Post-treatment fundus photograph of the same tumor 6 weeks after PDT using benzoporphyrin derivative and light at 80 J/cm^2.

used to execute PDT. All animals treated with 80 J/cm^2 or greater exhibited tumor arrest. Clinically, immediately after the treatment, these tumors demonstrated blanching of the surface vessels and closure of surrounding choroidal vessels. Fluorescein angiography confirmed these findings with hypofluorescence of the tumor and surrounding tissues, suggesting vascular occlusion. One consistent side effect included serous retinal detachment overlying the treated tumors. This exudative process peaked within several hours of the treatment but unfailingly reabsorbed within 14 days after the treatment. As the exudative retinal detachment spontaneously resolved, the tumors were reduced in size and less pigmented. In some cases, tumors became almost completely flat. The adjacent choroid became avascular and fibrotic, leading to chorioretinal scars with a surrounding ring of atrophy. Two control groups, one treated with the light only and the other with BPD only, displayed continuous tumor growth, which filled most of the vitreous cavity within 3 weeks. No vascular changes were noted in the control eyes treated with either light or dye alone. Histological studies of the regressed tumors showed tumor necrosis and extensive infiltration of mononuclear cells and pigment-laden macrophages at the tumor site.

More recently, our laboratory has performed PDT without the external photosensitizer. The theory behind this new modality is at the molecular level involving free radicals. Efficacy of PDT is believed to be secondary to the free radical species that are produced when the photosensitizers react with a substrate such as molecular oxygen, which subsequently cause irreversible damage to cellular components (20–22). Hence, if endogenous free radicals could be produced by a laser capable of producing such free radical species, theoretically one could perform PDT without the external photosensitizers. This approach would eliminate any drug toxicity and skin photosensitivity associated even with the second-generation photosensitizers. In addition, as previous studies have shown (3,8), the dark pigmentation of the choroidal melanoma is a further complicating factor with PDT, because this optical density of melanin limits the light delivery to the full thickness of the tumor (23).

Our most recent studies have shown that melanin-containing tumors may be destroyed by a combination of thermal and photodynamic effects in the absence of external photosensitizers using ultrafast lasers (24,25). A single treatment with a highly focused, raster-scanned laser beam at 1,047 nm was effective in the destruction of experimental choroidal melanomas. These results warrant further studies to differentiate the thermal and photodynamic effects in attaining tumor regression.

SUMMARY

Photodynamic therapy on experimental intraocular tumor has made significant progress in recent years. Many investigators have achieved tumor destruction with the surge of second-generation photosensitizers and the development of clinically applicable animal models of choroidal melanoma. The new modality in the horizon involves PDT without the external photosensitizers. With its combination of thermal and photodynamic effects, we have observed single-treatment tumor regression. Additional studies are necessary to further understand and elucidate the mechanisms of this new ultrafast laser in PDT of ocular tumors.

REFERENCES

1. Benedict WF, Lingua RW, Doiron DR, et al. Tumor regression of human retinoblastoma in the nude mouse following photoradiation therapy: a preliminary report. *Med Pediatr Oncol* 1980;8: 397–401.
2. Winther J. Porphyrin photodynamic therapy in an experimental retinoblastoma model. *Ophthal Paediatr Genet* 1987;8:49–52.
3. Murphree AL, Cote M, Gomer CJ. The evolution of photodynamic therapy techniques in the treatment of intraocular tumors. *Photochem Photobiol* 1987;46:919–923.
4. Gomer CJ, Jester JV, Razum NJ, et al. Photodynamic therapy of intraocular tumors: examination of hematoporphyrin derivative distribution and long-term damage in rabbit ocular tissue. *Cancer Res* 1985;45:3718–3725.
5. Ohnishi Y, Yamana Y, Minei M. Photoradiation therapy using argon laser and a hematoporphyrin derivative for retinoblastoma—a preliminary report. *Jpn J Ophthalmol* 1986;30: 409–419.
6. Bruce RA Jr. Evaluation of hematoporphyrin photoradiation therapy to treat choroidal melanomas. *Lasers Surg Med* 1984;4: 59–64.
7. Davidorf J, Davidorf F. Treatment of iris melanoma with photodynamic therapy. *Ophthalmic Surg* 1992;23:522–527.
8. Sery TW, Shields JA, Augsburger J, et al. Photodynamic therapy of human ocular cancer. *Ophthalmic Surg* 1987;18:413–418.
9. Tse DT, Dutton JJ, Weingeist YA, et al. Hematoporphyrin photoradiation therapy for intraocular and orbital malignant melanoma. *Arch Ophthalmol* 1984;102:833–838.
10. Hill RA, Reddi S, Kenny ME, et al. Photodynamic therapy of ocular melanoma with bis silicon 2,3-naphthalocyanine in a rabbit model. *Invest Ophthalmol Vis Sci* 1995;36:2476–2481.
11. Ozler SA, Nelson JS, Liggett PE, et al. Photodynamic therapy of experimental subchoroidal melanoma using chloroaluminum sulfonated phthalocyanine. *Arch Ophthalmol* 1992;110: 555–561.
12. Panagopoulos JA, Svitra PP, Puliafito CA, et al. Photodynamic therapy for experimental intraocular melanoma using chloroaluminum sulfonated phthalocyanine. *Arch Ophthalmol* 1989;107: 886–890.
13. Schmidt-Erfurth U, Bauman W, Gragoudas ES, et al. Photodynamic therapy of experimental choroidal melanoma using lipoprotein-delivered benzoporphyrin. *Ophthalmology* 1994;101: 89–99.
14. Schmidt-Erfurth U, Flotte TJ, Gragoudas ES, et al. Benzoporphyrin-lipoprotein mediated photodestruction of intraocular tumors. *Exp Eye Res* 1996;62:1–10.
15. Gonzalez VH, Hu LK, Theodossiadis P, et al. Photodynamic therapy of pigmented choroidal melanomas. *Invest Ophthalmol Vis Sci* 1995;36:871–878.
16. Kim RY, Hu LK, Foster BS, et al. Photodynamic therapy of pigmented choroidal melanomas of greater than 3-mm thickness. *Ophthalmology* 1996;103:2029–2036.
17. Hu LK, Huh K, Gragoudas ES, et al. Establishment of pigmented choroidal melanomas in a rabbit model. *Retina* 1994;14: 264–269.
18. Kim RY, Hu LK, Flotte TJ, et al. Digital angiography of experimental choroidal melanomas using benzoporphyrin derivative. *Am J Ophthalmol* 1997;123:810–816.
19. Young LH, Howard MA, Hu LK, et al. Photodynamic therapy of pigmented choroidal melanomas using a liposomal preparation of benzoporphyrin derivative. *Arch Ophthalmol* 1996;114: 186–192.
20. Dougherty TJ. Photosensitizers: therapy and detection of malignant tumors. *Photochem Photobiol* 1987;45:879–889.
21. Gibson SL, Hilf R. Photosensitization of mitochondrial cytochrome c oxidase by hematoporphyrin derivative and related porphyrin in vitro and in vivo. *Cancer Res* 1983;43:4191–4197.
22. Foote CS. Photosensitized oxidation and singlet oxygen: consequences in biological systems. In: Pryor WA, ed. *Free radicals in biology.* Orlando, FL: Academic Press, 1985:1976.
23. Busetti A, Soncin M, Jori G, et al. Treatment of malignant melanoma by high peak-power 1064 nm irradiation followed by photodynamic therapy. *Photochem Photobiol* 1998;68:377–381.
24. Krause M, Xiong J, Gragoudas ES, et al. Photodynamic therapy of experimental choroidal melanoma by multiphoton excitation of melanin precursors. *Invest Ophthal Vis Sci* 2001;41(suppl): S386.
25. Krause M, Xiong J, Gragoudas ES, et al. Treatment of experimental choroidal melanoma with a Nd:YLF laser at 1047 nm. *Invest Ophthal Vis Sci* 2001;42(suppl):S338.

14

VERTEPORFIN PHOTODYNAMIC THERAPY FOR AGE-RELATED MACULAR DEGENERATION

Part 1: Verteporfin Photodynamic Therapy for Age-Related Macular Degeneration: How To Do It

RENÉ-PIERRE COPT
LEONIDAS ZOGRAFOS

Verteporfin photodynamic therapy (PDT) for subfoveal choroidal neovascularization (CNV) is a two-step procedure. The first step involves preparation and infusion of the photosensitizing dye; the second step involves application of nonthermal laser light to activate the photosensitizing dye.

Once the appropriate indications for PDT are met (1–4), you need to:

1. Prepare the dye.
2. Inject the dye.
3. Apply laser light.
4. Explain the effects of the treatment to the patient.

Each of the different photosensitizing dyes has unique physical properties and pharmacokinetic characteristics. The following discussion pertains to photodynamic therapy with the photosensitizing dye known as verteporfin (Visudyne, Novartis Pharmaceuticals, Basel, Switzerland) (5).

PREPARATION OF THE DYE

Verteporfin is supplied in single-use 15-mg vials as a sterile, lipid-based, lyophilized green powder that requires reconstitution with sterile water and dilution with 5% dextrose solution before administration. Avoid exposure of the drug to direct bright light.

Storage

Verteporfin should be stored at room temperature between 20°C and 25°C (68°F to 77°F) and must be protected from light.

Reconstitution

For a total volume of 7.5 mL of reconstituted drug, 7 mL sterile water is injected into the verteporfin vial, which should then be gently agitated until the verteporfin powder is completely dissolved. The reconstituted solution must be protected from light and used within 4 hours. The use of saline solution is contraindicated because verteporfin precipitates in saline.

Dilution

Prior to injection, further dilution with 5% dextrose is required to achieve a drug dose of 6 mg/m^2 of body surface area and a total infusion volume of 30 mL. The body surface area is calculated from a standard nomogram using the patient's height and weight measurements (Fig. 14.1.1).

ADMINISTRATION OF THE DRUG

Infusion of the Dye

The solution is infused intravenously (iv) at a rate of 3 mL per minute over 10 minutes. Routine precautions must be taken to ensure sterility and exclusion of air, and to prevent extravasation.

Standard precautions to prevent extravasation include, but are not limited to, the following:

1. A free-flowing iv line should be established before starting verteporfin infusion, and the line should be monitored carefully.
2. It is strongly recommended that the largest possible vein in the arm, preferably antecubital, be used for the infu-

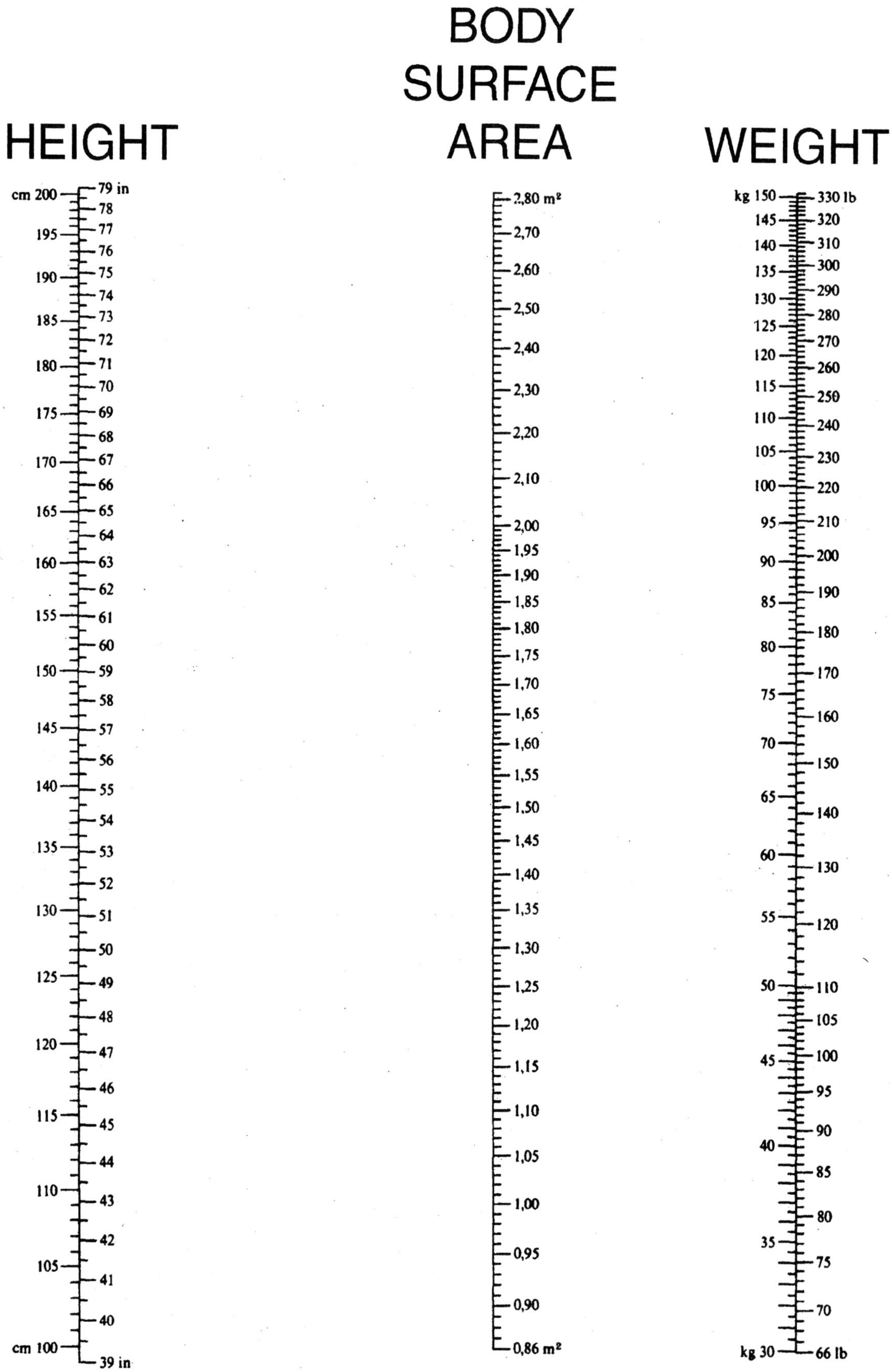

FIGURE 14.1.1. A nomogram to determine body surface area based on patient's weight and height. (Dose in mL, 3* BSA.)

sion because of possible fragility of vein walls in some elderly patients.
3. Small veins in the back of the hand should be avoided, because even long sleeves may not completely cover the site after treatment, which will be extremely light sensitive.

Extravasation of the Dye

Verteporfin extravasation can cause severe pain, inflammation, swelling, and discoloration at the injection site; an analgesic may be necessary to relieve the pain. The infusion must be stopped immediately if the patient indicates discomfort or pain at or near the infusion site, or if extravasation occurs.

1. Obtain better venous access as soon as possible and restart the infusion if less than half of the solution is estimated to have been administrated iv. Light application should be carried out 15 minutes after the second start of the infusion. If venous access cannot be obtained after several attempts, the patient can be retreated not less than 24 hours later.
2. Discontinue the infusion if more than half of the solution is estimated to have been administrated iv. Light application can be carried out 15 minutes after the start of the reinfusion, even if the duration of the infusion is less than 10 minutes.
3. Discontinue the infusion if extravasation has occurred. Immediate application of a cold compress or ice is recommended and the patient's arm should be elevated for 1 day if possible. Warm compress can be used 24 hours after the event. The site of extravasation must be protected from direct light for a minimum of 2 days after the infusion or for as long as swelling and discoloration of the skin is visible.
4. The patient should be retreated after 7 days if venous access has not been obtained and treatment has not been given. The patient should return for the regularly scheduled examination after 3 months if venous access has been achieved and the treatment has been given.

THE LIGHT APPLICATION

Determination of Spot Size and Location

Fluorescein angiography (FA) is used to visualize the CNV and the angiogram is then used to calculate the greatest linear dimension (GLD) of the CNV. The spot size of the laser is determined by measuring the GLD of the entire lesion, including all classic and occult CNV, blood, and all blocked fluorescence. This measurement is estimated using a transparent millimeter rule placed on the FA obtained with the fundus camera (Fig. 14.1.2). The GLD is divided by the camera lens magnification to obtain the actual diameter of the lesion in the fundus in microns (μm). Table 14.1.1 identifies some of the more commonly used film-based camera systems and the magnification of the film image. If the magnification of the camera system is unknown, the GLD of the CNV can be estimated by using a standard

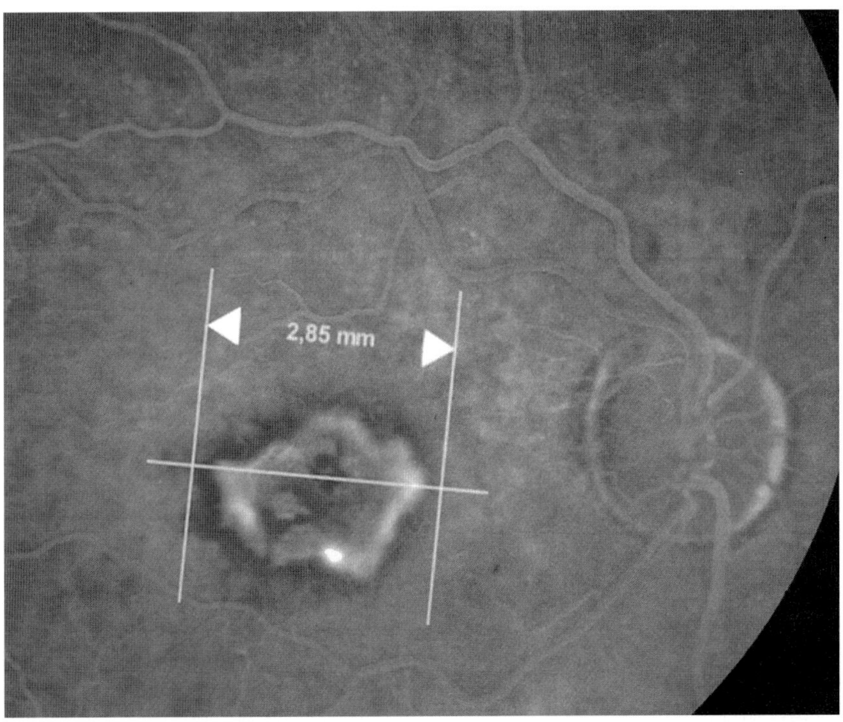

FIGURE 14.1.2. Transparent millimeter rule placed on the FA obtained with the fundus camera.

TABLE 14.1.1. RETINAL MAGNIFICATION OF SELECTED FILM-BASED FUNDUS CAMERAS

	Angles of View						
Camera Model	20	30	35	40	45	50	60
Zeiss FF450	4.33x	2.6x				2.0x	
Zeiss FF4/3/2		2.5x					
Topcon 50F/X/EX/IA	3.7x		2.5x			1.8x	
Nikon NFC 50/505	3.66x	2.41x				1.45x	
Kowa Pro 1/2/3	4.3x		7.5x			1.7x	
Kowa RC-XV	3.7x	2.5x			1.7x		
Kowa fx500			2.6x			2.0x	
Canon 60U				2.5x			1.7x

Fundus camera magnification reference guide provided courtesy of Zeiss Humphrey Systems.

optic disc diameter of 1.5 mm and then calculating the GLD using the optic disc as an internal standard.

Using a digital-based camera, the size of the lesion can be immediately read on the screen.

Figure 14.1.2 depicts an FA image of a subfoveal CNV photographed with a Canon digitalized system. In this example, the GLD of the CNV measures 2.85 mm.

Early- to mid-phase angiographic images are typically the most useful frames for measuring the GLD of the classic lesion. If some occult component needs to be included, the late-phase angiogram will yield the size to be treated. An additional 1,000 μm is added to the GLD to allow a 500-μm margin, ensure full coverage of the lesion, and allow for small movements of the eye. It is recommended that the FA used to calculate the GLD be obtained within 1 week prior to PDT.

Irradiation of the Optic Disc

The light spot covering the lesion must come no closer than 200 μm to the temporal edge of the optic disc, even if the lesion is located closer the disc. It is considered appropriate to leave this portion of the lesion untreated if the lesion or calculated treatment area extends closer to the optic disc than 200 μm.

Application of Light

The fundus is visualized with one of several available fundus contact lenses at the time of treatment. Each contact lens has a different magnification; therefore, the spot size of the laser light has to be adjusted according to the lens. Table 14.1.2 lists some of the more commonly used contact lenses and their respective magnifications.

Zeiss, Coherent, and Quantel Medical manufacture laser delivery systems suitable for verteporfin PDT. The software package in each system requires that the ophthalmologist enter the GLD of the CNV and the magnification of the fundus contact lens. The spot size of the aiming beam and power output of the laser are then determined automatically.

The spot size of the aiming beam is the same as the spot size of the laser light used for treatment. The green light or the filtered white light from the slit-lamp can be used if additional fundus illumination is necessary. The aiming beam is positioned using retinal landmarks so that the CNV is illuminated. The laser treatment consists of a light wavelength of 689 nm and a power density of 600 mW/cm^2 for a duration of 83 seconds to deliver a total light dose of 50 J/cm^2. Brief interruptions are permitted if the patient cannot maintain the eye in a steady position. There is no noticeable change in the CNV during the 83-second treatment.

Concurrent Bilateral Treatment

To treat both eyes with one infusion, the first eye is treated as described in the preceding, with light application 15 minutes after beginning the infusion. At completion of light application to the first eye, the laser setting should be adjusted immediately to introduce treatment parameters for the second eye, with the same light dose and intensity as for the first eye. Light application to the second eye should begin no more than 20 minutes after the start of the infusion.

TABLE 14.1.2. RETINAL MAGNIFICATION OF SELECTED CONTACT LENSES

Fundus Contact Lens	Magnification
Volk, Area Centralis	1.04x
Haig-Streit 901 Fundus Lens	1.04x
Ocular, Mainster Standard	1.05x
Ocular 3, Mirror Universal Long (direct)	1.08x
Ocular 3, Mirror Universal Long (direct)	1.08x
Ocular, Fundus Laser	1.08x
Yannuzzi Fundus Laser Lens	1.10x
Volk, Trans Equator	1.44x
Ocular, Mainster Wide Field	1.50x
Ocular, Mainster Ultra Field PRP	1.90x
Volk, SuperQuad 160	1.92x
Volk, Quadra-Aspheric	2.01x

Retreatment

Patients should return for follow-up examination 3 months after treatment. Patients who have not experienced any serious adverse event likely to be associated with the laser therapy can be retreated if there is evidence on an FA of leakage from any classical or occult CNV. Further follow-up examinations are scheduled at 3-month intervals.

Patients who experience severe vision loss of four or more lines within 1 week of treatment should not be retreated, at least until their vision has returned to pretreatment levels. The potential benefits and risks of subsequent treatment must be carefully considered by the treating physician.

PATIENT INFORMATION

Photosensitivity

Patients are advised to avoid exposure of unprotected skin or eyes to direct sunlight or bright indoor light, especially halogen lighting, for 48 hours after treatment.

Dark sunglasses, long sleeves, and slacks need to be worn by patients who must go outdoors during the first 48 hours after treatment.

Patients must be advised that use of sunscreen provides no protection against a photosensitivity reaction, but they can be assured that watching television does not cause photosensitivity reactions. Exposure to low levels of normal indoor light should be encouraged, because this helps inactivate the drug through photobleaching.

Routine visits to a dentist and any elective surgery should be rescheduled, because powerful examination operating lights may cause tissue necrosis, especially during abdominal surgery.

Patients are advised to wear a wristband indicating their potential photosensitivity in the event of emergency surgery. During the first 48 hours after the treatment of an accident entails hospitalization, the patient must be handled with extreme care and, if at all possible, under low light. All parts of the body not involved in any necessary surgery should be covered, and the procedure kept as short as possible.

REFERENCES

1. Bressler NM. Photodynamic therapy of subfoveal choroidal neovascularization in age-related macular degeneration with verteporfin: two-year results of 2 randomized clinical trials. *Arch Ophthalmol* 2001;119:198–207.
2. Verteporfin in Photodynamic Therapy Study Group. Photodynamic therapy of subfoveal choroidal neovascularization in pathologic myopia with verteporfin: 1-year results of a randomized clinical trial. *Ophthalmology* 2001;108:841–852.
3. Verteporfin in Photodynamic Therapy Study Group. Verteporfin therapy of subfoveal choroidal neovascularization in age-related macular degeneration: 2-year results of a randomized clinical trial including lesions with occult with no classic choroidal neovascularization. *Am J Ophthalmol* 2001;131:541–560.
4. Bressler NM. Verteporfin therapy of subfoveal choroidal neovascularization in age-related macular degeneration: two-year results of a randomized clinical trial including lesions with occult with no classic choroidal neovascularization. *Am J Ophthalmol* 2002;133:168–169.
5. Schmidt-Erfurth U, Michels S, Barbazetto I, et al. Photodynamic effects on choroidal neovascularization and physiological choroid. *Invest Ophthalmol Vis Sci* 2002;43:830–841.

Part 2: Fluorescein Angiography and Optical Coherence Tomography in Photodynamic Therapy for Choroidal Neovascularization Caused by Age-Related Macular Degeneration

GISÈLE SOUBRANE
GABRIEL COSCAS

Fluorescein angiography (FA), the gold standard for assessment of lesions at all stages in the management of choroidal neovascularization (CNV) caused by age-related macular degeneration (AMD), is essential in diagnosis, classification of lesions, management, therapeutic decision making, and follow up. Therapeutic options include laser photocoagulation and photodynamic therapy (PDT) with verteporfin (Visudyne, Novartis Pharmaceuticals, Basel, Switzerland) as well as surgical procedures and several investigational treatment modalities (1). Fluorescein angiographic patterns were key to determining eligibility criteria in randomized trials of PDT with verteporfin (2), in which leakage of the fluorescein dye also was used to determine the need to retreat at follow up.

Optical coherence tomography (OCT) has the potential to provide additional information to aid characterization of lesions. In particular, OCT enables pseudohistologic *in vivo* imaging of the subretinal space and can show (and even quantify) fluid accumulation within or underneath the neurosensory retina (3). This additional information potentially can help in making decisions on the need for retreatment using PDT with verteporfin.

This chapter reviews the principles of FA and OCT and discusses their use to characterize the natural history of CNV and their application in PDT with verteporfin within clinical trials and routine clinical practice.

IMAGING TECHNIQUES

The assessment of CNV due to AMD using FA is well established. Fluorescein angiograms are used to identify the foveal avascular zone, locate its center, and outline the area of neovascularization before treatment (4). Indocyanine green (ICG) angiography also has been used to evaluate CNV. Although ICG angiography is less well established than FA, it may provide useful additional information in some cases (5).

Optical coherence tomography provides a cross-sectional image of the posterior pole with a maximum longitudinal resolution of approximately 10 μm (3). Images are produced by measuring the time delays of reflected diode light at a wavelength of 830 nm. Different tissue reflections are represented in false colors; bright colors (red and white) correspond to highly reflective tissues such as the RPE-Bruch's-membrane-choriocapillaris (RPE-BM-CC) complex, and dark colors (blue and black) represent regions with low reflectivity, such as fluid accumulation. In addition, retinal mapping can provide an accurate measurement of changes in the thickness of the neurosensory retina by comparing scans taken during follow up with those from the initial examination.

CLASSIFICATION OF CHOROIDAL NEOVASCULARIZATION

Fluorescein Angiography

Classification of CNV has been established based on its appearance on the early-, mid-, and late-phase frames of FAs (4) and its location relative to the fovea. Two major types have been identified: well-defined and occult CNV (6).

Well-defined CNV was first described in the landmark paper by Gass (7) and subsequently refined by the MPS Group (and is now known as "classic" CNV) (8). An area of localized choroidal hyperfluorescence or a neovascular network with well-demarcated boundaries appears during or immediately after the filling of the choriocapillaris. The sharply outlined neovascular net typically presents a central feeder vessel branching into a radiating pattern that resolves in an intensely leaking anastomotic peripheral neovascular arcade. This typical pattern may be limited to a seafan form or even to only an early hyperfluorescent spot. A surrounding hypofluorescent rim contrasts with and enhances the neovascular area. The hallmark of neovascularization is profuse leakage in the late phase of the FA. This leakage extends, resulting in an enlargement of the initial lesion and usually obscures its boundaries. Progressive pooling of dye occurs in the overlying subsensory retinal space (Fig. 14.2.1).

Occult CNV was identified in 1987 (9,10) as a poorly defined area of hyperfluorescence with late pinpoints (11). According to the MPS classification, it can be separated into fibrovascular pigment epithelial detachment (PED) (type I) or leakage of undetermined source (type II) (8). Fibrovascular PED is an area of irregular elevation of the retinal pigment epithelium (RPE) with stippled fluorescence in the mid-phase of the FA. Fluorescein staining and leakage occurs in the late phase. MPS type II occult CNV is characterized by an area of progressive and late leakage at the level of the RPE associated with pinpoints without well-demarcated early hyperfluorescence (Fig. 14.2.2).

The lack of visibility of a neovascular net on FA in MPS type II occult CNV may be overcome by Scanning Laser Ophthalmoscope (SLO)-ICG angiography (12,13). However, MPS type I occult CNV is even more challenging to identify and localize. SLO-ICG angiography is helpful because type I occult CNV may be "hidden" or "masked" by the overlying elevated RPE or the associated turbid fluid. The characterization of the lesions included in type I occult CNV is currently under profound recasting (14,15).

Classification of CNV has been further refined as a result of the Treatment of AMD with Photodynamic Therapy (TAP) study (2). As well as classifying CNV as either classic or occult, lesions can be categorized according to the proportion of each type of CNV. Predominantly classic lesions are defined as consisting of at least 50% classic CNV (Fig. 14.2.3 A and B) and minimally classic lesions as less than 50% but greater than 0% classic CNV (Fig. 14.2.3 C and D). Thus, some lesions with minimally classic CNV may have a larger area of classic than occult CNV if another component, such as blood, occupies a significant area (e.g., a lesion in which 30% of the area is blood, 40% classic, and 30% occult CNV).

The location of the CNV in relation to the fovea is an important determinant of the indication for different treatment modalities, including those with proven efficacy (e.g., laser photocoagulation and PDT with verteporfin) and those that are still under evaluation (e.g., surgery, antiangiogenic therapies, etc.). Lesions can be categorized as either extrafoveal (200 μm from the fovea), juxtafoveal (1 to 199 μm from the fovea), or subfoveal (underlying the fovea)

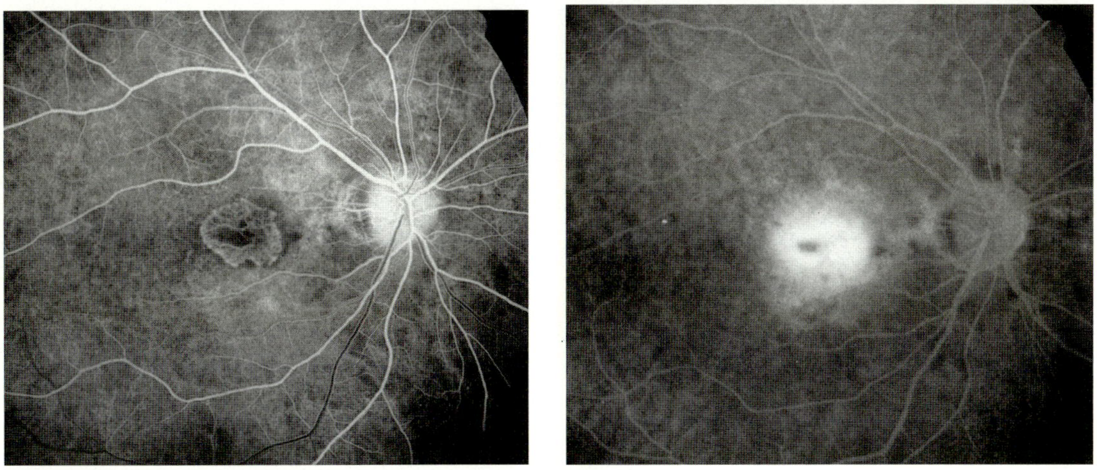

A B

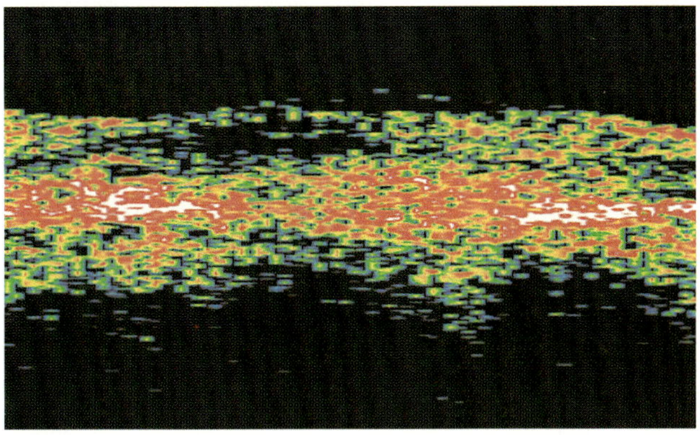

C

FIGURE 14.2.1. A: Early phase of FA: localized hyperfluorescence of a neovascular net with well-demarcated boundaries, contrasting with a limited hypofluorescent rim. **B:** Late phase of FA: profuse leakage of the dye resulting in enlargement of the initial lesion and obscuring its boundaries. **C:** Optical coherence tomography examination: fusiform thickening and disruption of the RPE-BM-CC complex, anterior to the retinal pigment epithelium but in contact with it.

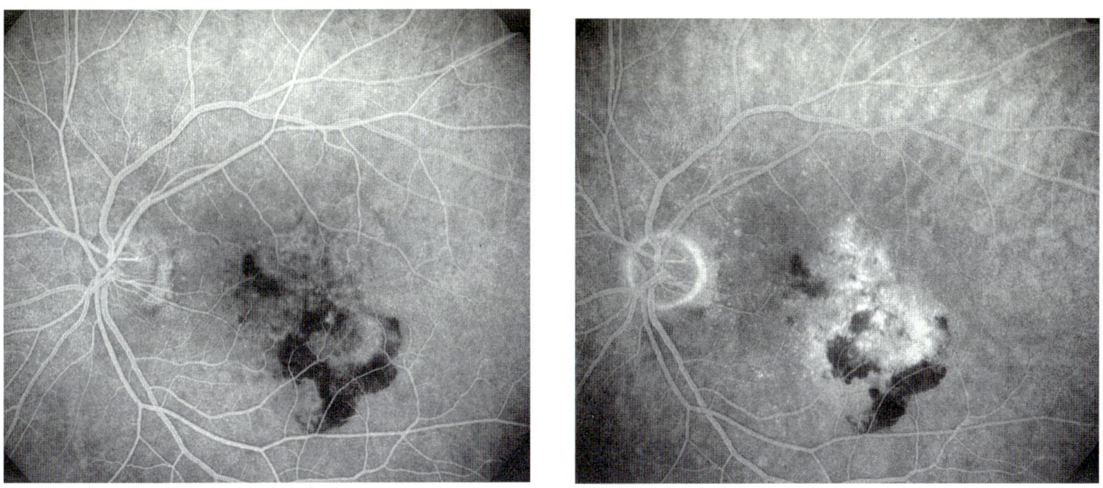

A B

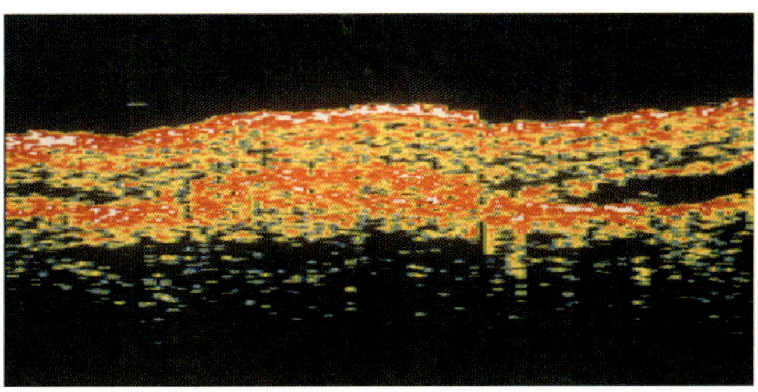

C

FIGURE 14.2.2. Occult choroidal new vessels (CNV). **A:** Early phase of FA: ill-defined area of subfoveal hyperfluorescence, irregular and not homogenous, with a rim of recent hemorrhage. **B:** Late phase of FA: progressive leakage of undetermined source and a few late pinpoints. **C:** Optical coherence tomography examination: fusiform thickening of the RPE-BM-CC complex. The focal and poorly defined hyperreflectivity extends from above to below the retinal pigment epithelium band with no separation line.

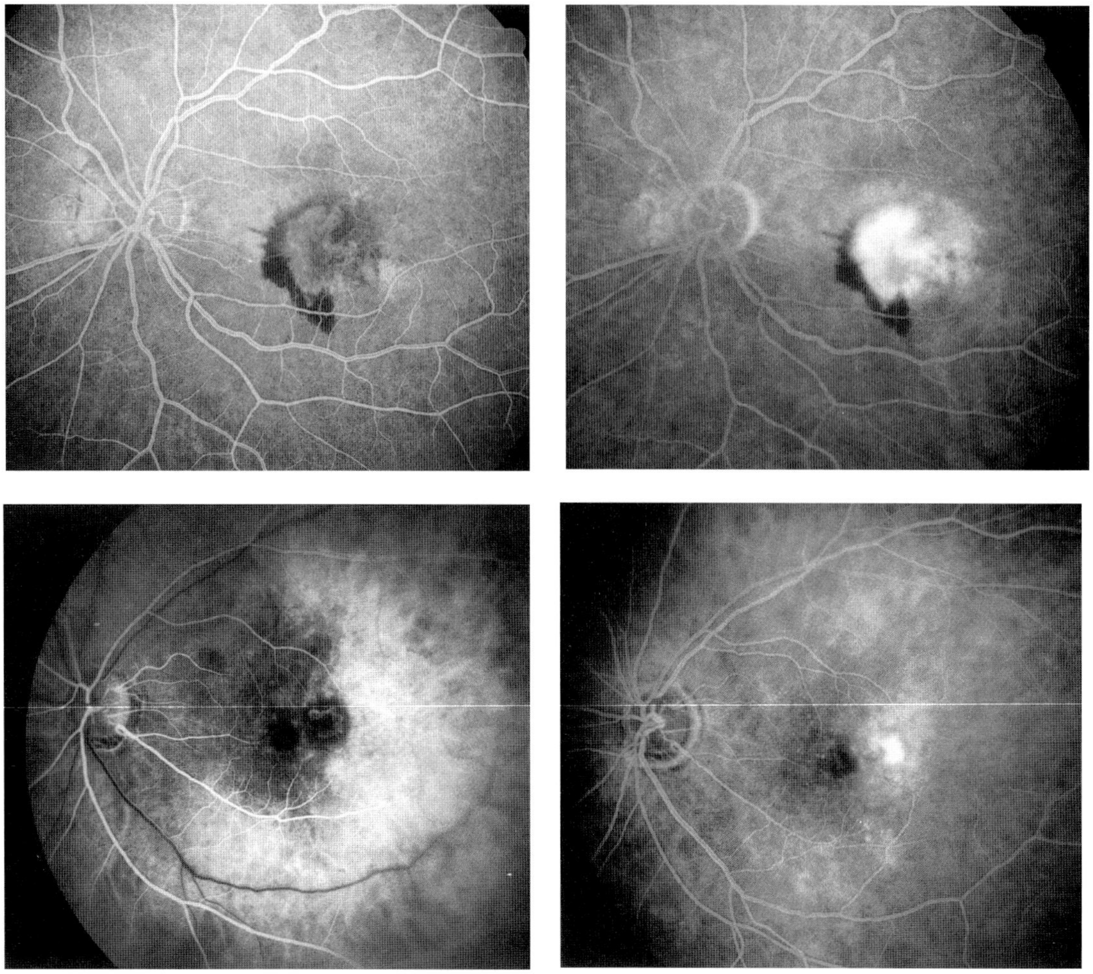

A B C D

FIGURE 14.2.3. CNV classification for PDT. Predominantly classic CNV: **A:** Early phase of FA with well-defined CNV. **B:** Late phase of FA with active and diffuse leakage from classic CNV but also from occult CNV in the temporal area. Minimally classic CNV: **C:** Early phase with extrafoveal classic CNV; **D:** Mid-phase of FA: progressive leakage from neovascular network surrounded by occult CNV.

based on the early-phase frames of the FA. Laser photocoagulation may be considered for extrafoveal or juxtafoveal lesions, whereas PDT with verteporfin may be considered for subfoveal lesions (possibly juxtafoveal).

Optical Coherence Tomography

Few reports have been published on attempts to classify CNV on OCT sections. Choroidal neovascularization appears as a hyperreflective area above or within the RPE band, with or without demarcation, because RPE and CNV have similar reflectivities (16). This interpretation has been confirmed by its disappearance after surgical ablation (17). A correlation between OCT aspects and the classification of FA has not been established yet.

Classic CNV usually presents on OCT as fusiform thickening and disruption of the RPE-BM-CC complex (Figs. 14.2.1 and 14.2.2 C). Some CNV is anterior to the RPE, but in contact with it, whereas some is separated from the RPE by a less reflective zone (yellow-green in color), suggesting an analogy with type II CNV, according to the biomicroscopic and histologic classification by Gass (18). MPS type II occult CNV appears to be characterized on OCT by a focal, irregular, poorly defined, enhanced reflectivity anterior to the choroid. The hyper-reflectivity extends from above to below the RPE with no separation line (16). Both classic and occult CNV may be associated with an elevated RPE detachment. Accumulation of intraretinal or subretinal fluid or cyst formation is necessary to visualize the presence of leakage from CNV on OCT.

A NATURAL HISTORY OF CHOROIDAL NEOVASCULARIZATION

Fluorescein angiography has helped to characterize the natural course of CNV in eyes with AMD. In addition, several studies have used FA to evaluate the natural history of AMD in untreated patient groups.

The natural history of CNV is well documented, irrespective of its initial location and extent. Choroidal neovascularization can progress rapidly; lesions have been shown to grow at a mean rate of 18 μm per day (19). Late-stage classic CNV is characterized by a macular disciform scar of variable size, sometimes limited to the posterior pole, which, in rare cases, may also take the form of a pseudotumoral pattern or profuse hemorrhaging. The goal of both evidence-based therapies (laser photocoagulation and PDT with verteporfin) is to halt or slow the growth in order to preserve residual central vision.

The natural history of occult CNV is less well documented than that of classic CNV, although occult CNV occurs more frequently. The poor visual prognosis of eyes with certain types of occult CNV underlines the importance of accurate assessment of FA to categorize the lesions and determine the most appropriate course of action.

In a retrospective study of eyes with occult CNV and poorly defined leakage on FA, 63% of 84 eyes lost three or more lines of visual acuity over 6 to 53 months (10).

Symptomatic MPS type II occult CNV is usually subfoveal in location. In another retrospective study, 16% of 82 eyes with neovascular AMD owing to occult CNV and a visual acuity of 20/100 or better at presentation lost three to six lines and 40% lost six lines or more over 12 to 84 months (11). A decrease of at least two lines over 9 to 12 months was seen in 57% of 21 eyes in a prospective study (20). Similarly, in a randomized trial of eyes presenting with juxtafoveal CNV there were decreases of at least six lines in 13% of 26 eyes during a 12-month period and in 70% of eyes over a 5-year period (21). Lesions composed of occult CNV can double in size in a 1-year period; this growth is best evaluated using ICG-angiography (22). Similarly, growth of subfoveal occult with no classic CNV was documented in the Verteporfin in Photodynamic Therapy (VIP) trial: 98% of placebo-recipients had lesions that were nine MPS disc areas or smaller at baseline, whereas at the month 24 examination, 38% of eyes had lesions that were nine MPS disc areas or larger (23). In addition, over 9 to 12 months, occult CNV may lead to the development of classic CNV in 34% to 52% of eyes (11,20,21), giving rise to minimally classic rather than predominantly classic lesions. During the development of occult CNV, a PED can occur, linking MPS types I and II occult CNV. Acute extensive sub-RPE and subretinal hemorrhages or hematomas are mainly due to MPS-type II occult CNV or RPE tears (24). Disciform scars with fibrous tissue or geographic atrophy represent the end stages of both types of CNV.

Longitudinal studies have not yet been performed to characterize the natural history of either type of CNV using OCT.

FLUORESCEIN ANGIOGRAPHY IN CLINICAL TRIALS OF PHOTODYNAMIC THERAPY WITH VERTEPORFIN

In clinical trials of treatments for CNV, the pattern of lesions on FA has laid the basis of trial design and eligibility, and is an important outcome measure. Animal studies demonstrated the potential for PDT with verteporfin to achieve closure of experimental CNV. Cessation of fluorescein leakage on angiography was associated with histological evidence of CNV closure (25).

The phase I/II study of PDT with verteporfin based on the outcomes of these animal studies was designed to assess if PDT with verteporfin could stop fluorescein dye perfusion and leakage from CNV without vision loss (26,27). Fluorescein angiography was central in determining the eligibility of patients for inclusion in this study as well as for up to 12 weeks of follow up. One week after PDT with verteporfin, the entire site of light exposure appeared deeply hyperfluorescent in FA (26) (Fig. 14.2.4). Cessation of fluorescein perfusion and leakage from classic CNV was observed in almost all eyes. No background fluorescence or visibility of the large choroidal vessels was observed in the PDT-treated area.

Nevertheless, repermeabilization, regrowth, and leakage associated with CNV recurred after temporary occlusion of CNV in at least a portion of either classic or occult CNV, sometimes with early progression. Thus, retreatment was performed in a subgroup of eyes (27). Despite the temporary nature of leakage cessation and the significant rate of recurrent leakage, FA showed that PDT with verteporfin could safely stabilize leakage from CNV for up to 3 months. The cessation of fluorescein leakage from CNV on FA appeared to correlate with visual acuity outcomes (26,27).

The FA findings in the phase I/II study were integral to the rationale for the regimen selected for further study in the phase III TAP investigation (2) and the phase IIIb VIP trial (23). Fluorescein angiography was of primary importance in determining eligibility for inclusion in the trials. In addition, the FA was used to measure the greatest linear dimension of the lesion, which was then used to select the appropriate laser treatment spot size. Early and late frames were reviewed to ensure that both the classic and occult CNV were visualized and included in the assessment of the lesion size. The size of the area to be treated is determined on FA, including features that may obscure the identification of classic and occult CNV, such as blood, hypofluorescence not from visible blood, or a serious detachment of the RPE. Retreatment was applied if any fluorescein leakage

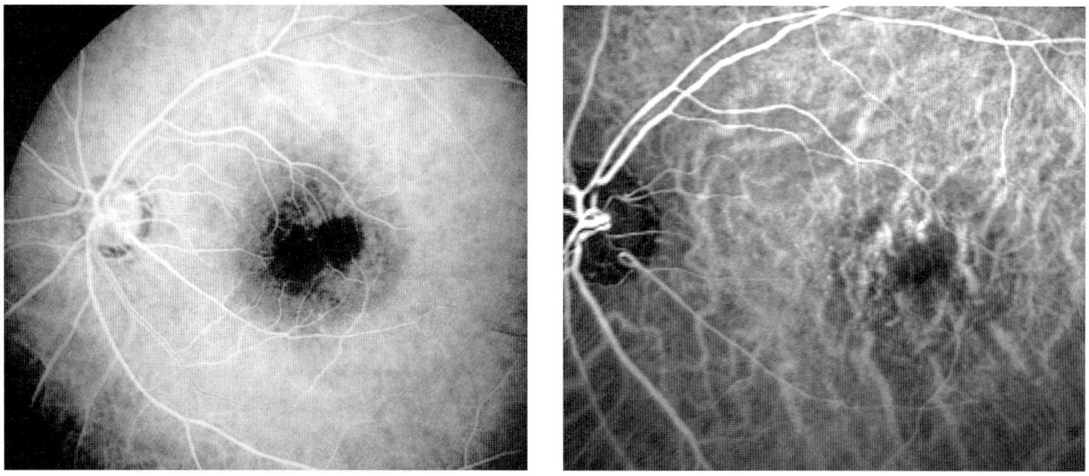

A B

FIGURE 14.2.4. Post-treatment hypofluorescent area (1 week after the first session of PDT). **A:** The classic component of the neovascular net is not perfused. **B:** The limits of the treated area can be identified on fluorescein angiography and even better on indocyanine green-angiography.

from any CNV was noted on FA performed at 3-month intervals after the initial or subsequent examination in the absence of previous serious adverse events. Repeated applications of PDT with verteporfin safely and significantly reduced the risk of vision loss in eyes with classic with no occult CNV, predominantly classic CNV, and occult with no classic CNV at 24 months.

Fluorescein angiographic criteria were correlated to functional results of PDT with verteporfin in clinical trials. Fluorescein angiographic outcomes were consistent with the visual acuity outcomes at the 24-month examinations in the eyes with predominantly classic CNV in the TAP investigation and the eyes with occult with no classic CNV in the VIP trial. These FA outcomes included progression of classic CNV beyond the boundaries of the entire lesion identified at baseline, degree of fluorescein leakage, and lesion size (measured in disc areas).

In eyes with predominantly classic CNV at baseline, the proportion of eyes with absence of leakage from classic CNV either within or beyond the area of the lesion identified at baseline increased from 19% at the 12-month examination to 51% at the 24-month examination (28). In parallel, the progression of leakage from classic CNV decreased from 46% to 23% between the 12- and 24-month examinations. Similarly, in eyes with occult with no classic CNV, progression of leakage from occult CNV occurred in 55% of eyes at 12 months and 46% at 24 months. Leakage was absent in 19% and 42% of eyes, respectively (23). However, positive FA outcomes in eyes with minimally classic lesions at baseline were not accompanied by significant reduction in the risk of losing at least three or six lines of visual acuity at the 12- or 24-month examinations (28). This finding suggests that angiographic outcomes cannot be used as the only surrogate for the benefit of PDT with verteporfin for CNV in AMD. A prospective study is in progress to determine whether eyes with minimally classic CNV benefit from either standard PDT with verteporfin or from a regimen with a reduced laser fluence (29).

The benefit of PDT with verteporfin thus is closely related to the initial pattern of CNV on the FA. In the TAP investigation, only lesion components at baseline affected the magnitude of the treatment benefit to a statistically significant degree (28). However, in eyes with occult with no classic CNV and presumed recent disease progression included in the VIP trial, both baseline lesion size and visual acuity had a significant effect on treatment outcomes (23). Eyes with small lesions (four disc areas) composed of either predominantly classic CNV (28) or occult with no classic CNV (regardless of visual acuity) (23) had better treatment outcomes (in terms of visual acuity) than eyes with larger lesions.

In the TAP investigation, 75% of vision loss in PDT with verteporfin-treated eyes with predominantly classic CNV occurred in the first 6 months. This finding provided the rationale for a new randomized controlled clinical trial, the Verteporfin in Early Retreatment (VER) study, which is evaluating the efficacy of retreatment at 6-week intervals during the first 6 months (30). As in previous trials, FA will be a key determinant of eligibility and of the need for retreatment as well as providing an important outcome measure.

Although (early or delayed) leakage is the major feature evaluated in clinical practice, many other characteristics could be analyzed, including perfusion of CNV (delayed, partial, or absent), morphology of the membrane (progression, stabilization, fragmentation, or involution), topography of CNV (within or outside of the baseline area; subfoveal or extrafoveal location), and development of RPE atrophy.

INDICATIONS FOR PHOTODYNAMIC THERAPY

Indications for PDT with verteporfin in neovascular AMD currently include most of the subfoveal lesions analyzed on FA and composed of classic CNV, predominantly classic CNV, and occult with no classic CNV (with presumed recent disease progression, visual or angiographic deterioration within the previous 3 months), or evidence of hemorrhage from CNV (23,28).

These recommendations do not apply at present to some specific patterns of AMD—minimally classic CNV, RPE tears, and late fibrous lesions.

ASSESSMENT OF PHOTODYNAMIC THERAPY OUTCOMES

Immediately after treatment, OCT examinations performed outside the trials have provided additional information to that obtained with FA. Comparison with pretreatment examinations showed that the thickness of the neurosensory retina had increased and there was accumulation of intraretinal and subretinal fluid (Fig. 14.2.5 A and B). The fluid increase suggests a breakdown of the outer retinal barrier or choriocapillaris and CNV permeability alterations (shown on ICG angiography) without damage to the retinal vascular bed, particularly with respect to the perifoveal capillary net. These changes resolved at 1 week. In animal models, the use of PDT with the same therapeutic parameters acutely damaged the RPE, followed by repopulation of the RPE cells in the treated area by 4 to 7 weeks (25).

One week after PDT, the entire site of light exposure appeared deeply hypofluorescent on FA performed in phase I/II studies (26) (Fig. 14.2.4). Cessation of fluorescein perfusion and leakage from classic CNV was observed. Absence of leakage from occult CNV was particularly difficult to assess. No background fluorescence or visibility of the large choroidal vessels was observed in the treated area. The hypofluorescent disc related to the treated area progressively merged with the normal choroidal background and its size decreased in the late phase, which suggested delayed perfusion of adjacent normal choroid. An alteration of choriocapillary perfusion is a possible correlate for angiographic hypofluorescence and was seen in the animal model when normal retina and choroid were exposed to PDT (25). The angiographic appearance followed the same pattern after subsequent treatments (27). The hypofluorescent area on FA and the accumulation of fluid on OCT progressively resolved in 4 to 6 weeks.

At the 3-month follow up, fluorescein angiogram can be used to categorize subsequent development into three groups: responders, nonresponders, and intermediate.

The responder group demonstrates the absence of progression, cessation of leakage, absence of leakage from CNV of any type, and stability of the lesion size (Fig. 14.2.6 A, B, E, and F). These characteristics indicate that retreatment is not needed, but are rarely seen in AMD after the first session of PDT with verteporfin. However, in the clinical trials there was a reduction in the likelihood that retreatment would be required subsequent to each PDT treatment, with patients receiving a mean of five to six treatments (out of a maximum of eight) during the first 2 years (23,28). This is supported by an open-label, uncontrolled extension to the TAP investigation in which the total population of PDT with verteporfin-treated patients received a mean of 1.4 treatments (out of a maximum of four) during the third year (31). The area of leakage typically decreases during follow up. The initial exudative lesion is progressively replaced by scar tissue

A 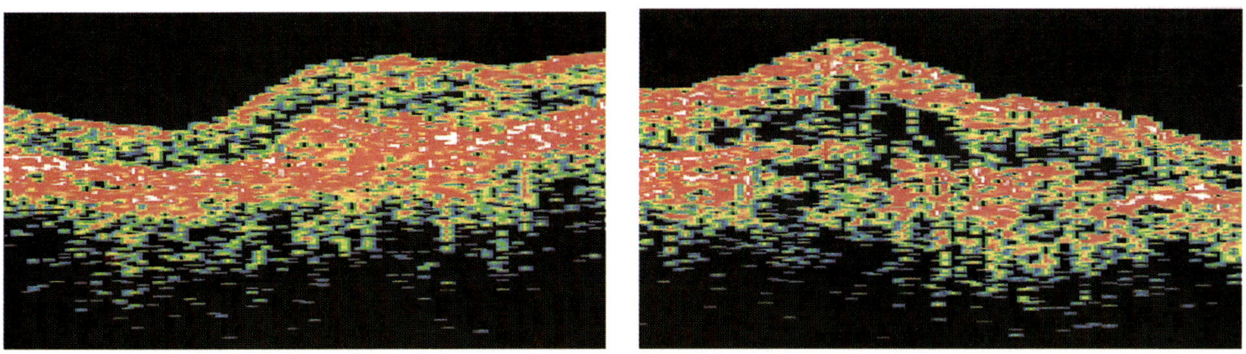 B

FIGURE 14.2.5. Optical coherence tomography examination **(A)** before and **(B)** 1 hour after the first PDT session. Increase in thickness of the neurosensory retina with accumulation of intraretinal and subretinal fluid in comparison with pretreatment examination.

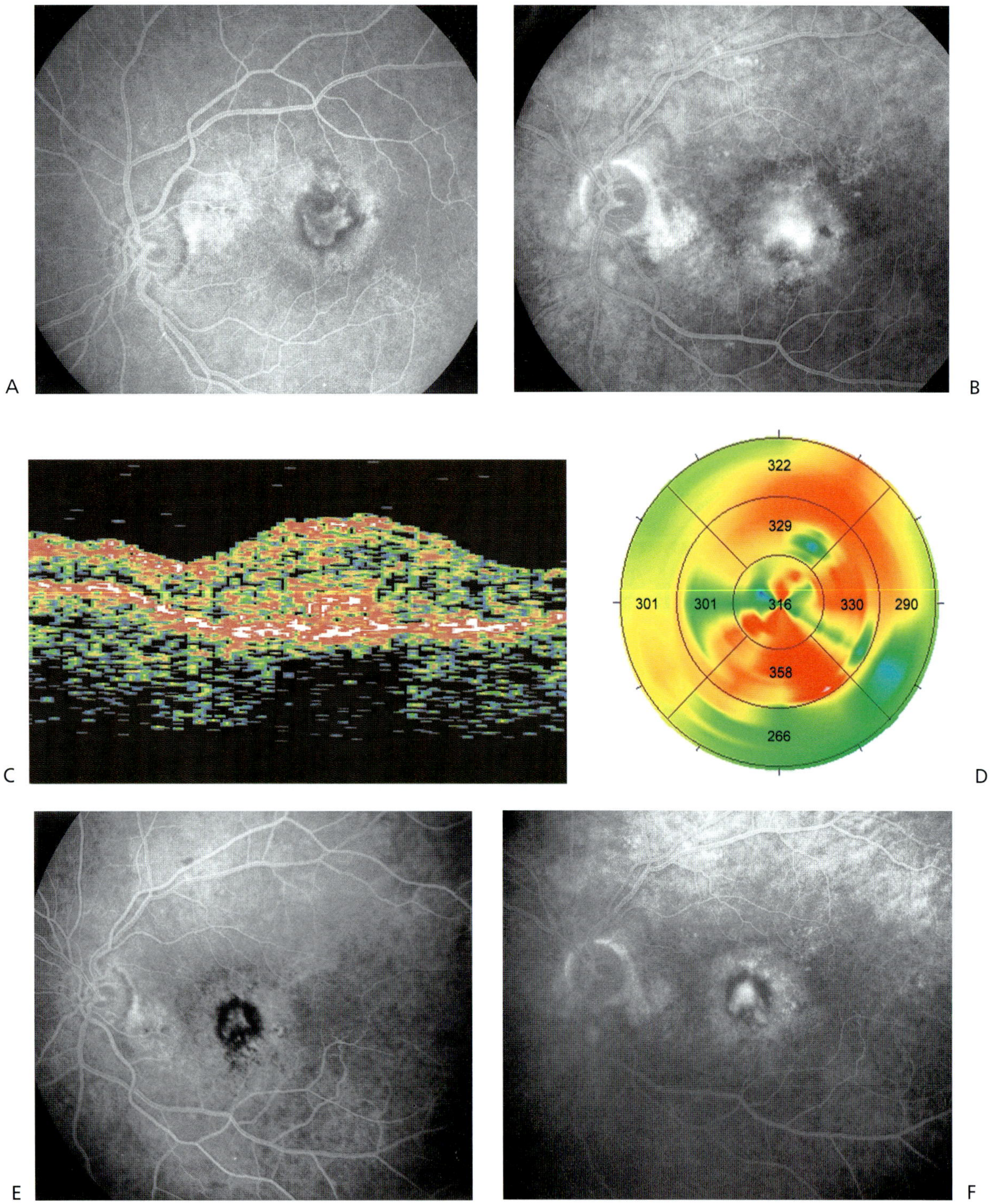

FIGURE 14.2.6. Responder group. Before treatment; visual acuity: 20/63. **A:** Mid-phase of FA: well-defined subfoveal CNV of approximately 60% of the lesion, well delimited and surrounded by a hypofluorescent rim. **B:** Late phase of FA: diffuse leakage from classic CNV and pinpoints from occult CNV at the periphery. **C:** Optical coherence tomography scan: fusiform thickening and disruption of RPE-BM-CC complex, anterior and in contact with the hyperreflective retinal pigment epithelium band; accumulation of intraretinal fluid with thickening of neurosensory retina. **D:** Optical coherence tomography mapping resulting from six radial scans: diffuse thickening of the macular retina (depicted by the yellow-reddish colors) and confirmed by the measurement of heights. Three months after the second PDT session: visual acuity 20/50. **E:** Venous phase of FA: absence of progression of the classic component with delayed hyperfluorescence. **F:** Late phase of FA: the initial exudative lesion has been replaced by staining of fibrous tissue.

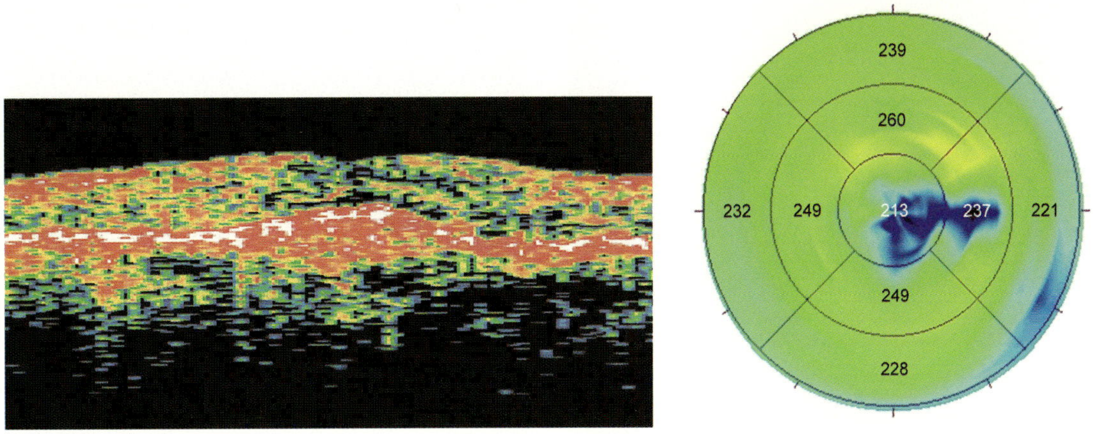

G H

FIGURE 14.2.6 *(continued).* **G:** Optical coherence tomography scan shows a localized increase in thickness and hyperreflectivity at the level of retinal pigment epithelium band corresponding to the fibrous tissue; absence of fluid accumulation in the neurosensory retina. **H:** Optical coherence tomography mapping confirms the decrease of retinal thickness.

containing various amounts of fibrotic tissue. Optical coherence tomography examination confirms the disappearance of fluid accumulation within or under the neurosensory retina and hyperreflectivity at the level of the RPE-BM-CC complex may increase in thickness (Fig. 14.2.6 C, D, G, and H).

The nonresponder group demonstrates persistent leakage and progression of CNV within or beyond the initial borders, or increase in the size of the lesion from baseline (Fig. 14.2.7 A and B). Eyes in this group need retreatment and further follow up. Optical coherence tomography examination should be considered to confirm the presence of fluid. However, discontinuation of treatment might be considered if a relatively large lesion is associated with very low visual acuity or if further treatment is unlikely to prevent further deterioration and to have a positive impact on the patient's quality of life.

The intermediate group is the most difficult and any additional information on the characteristics of the lesion, such as that obtained from OCT, are useful. On FA, perfusion of a portion of the initial CNV or regrowth (or reproliferation) gives rise to late leakage. The persistence of the

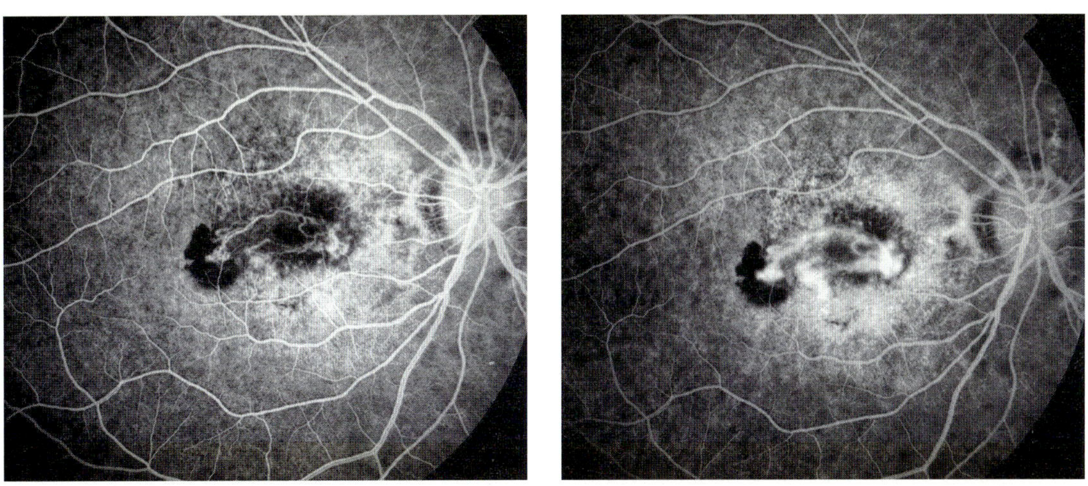

A B

FIGURE 14.2.7. Nonresponder group (same case as Fig. 14.2.1). **A:** Three months after the first session of PDT: localized persistent perfusion and leakage in the inferior nasal part of the treated area, with active temporal progression beyond the limits of the initial lesion. **B:** Late phase of FA with diffuse leakage.

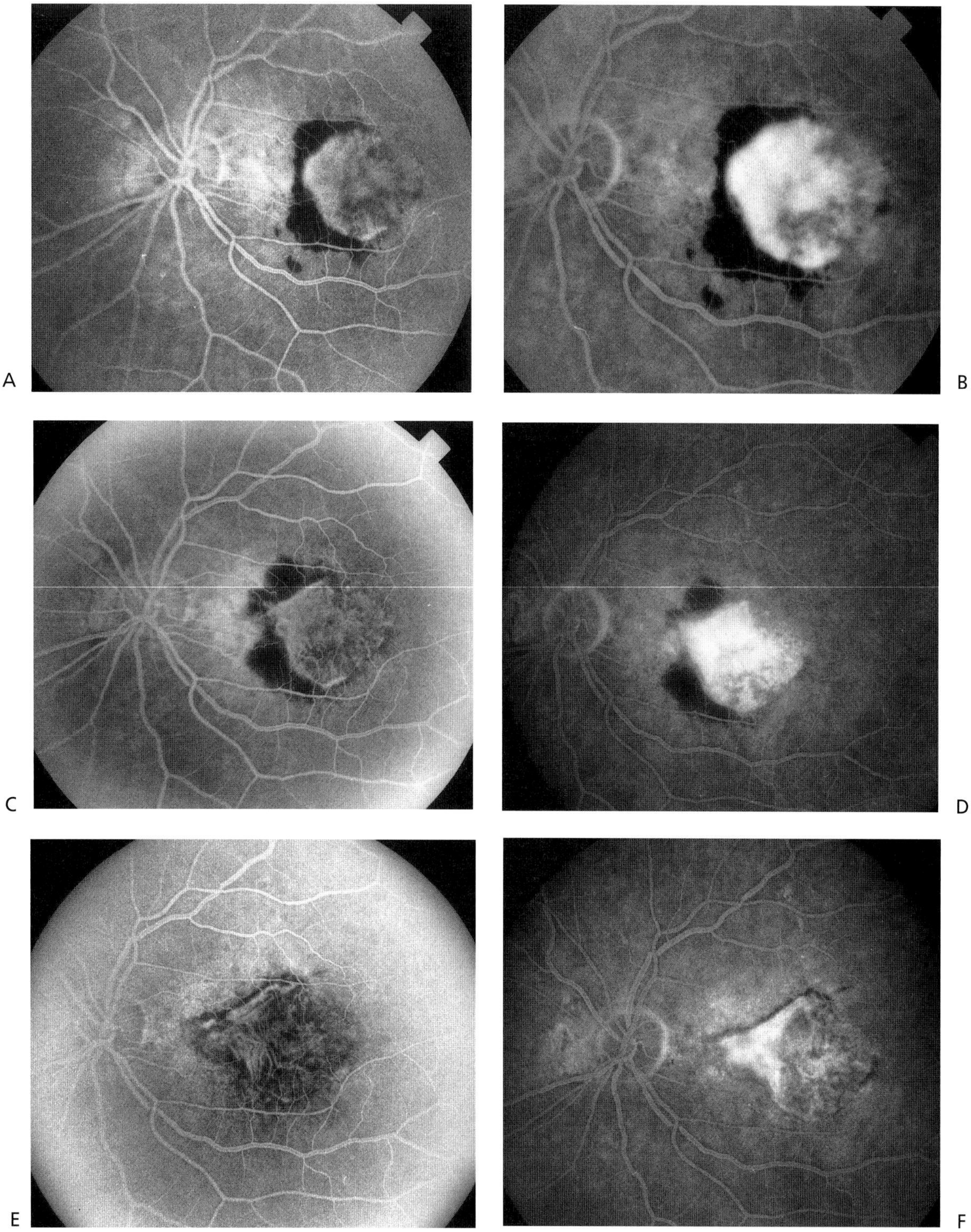

FIGURE 14.2.8. Intermediate response post-PDT (same case as Fig. 14.2.3 A and B). One month after PDT **(A)** moderate enlargement of the classic CNV, especially upward and nasally **(B)** with late leakage. Three months after PDT **(C)** moderate enlargement, only in the temporal part; progressive fibrosis in the upper and inferior region **(D)** with very limited leakage. Three months after the second course of PDT **(E)** early perfusion of persistent abnormal vessels. **F:** There is intense staining of the nasal fibrous tissue, the temporal part is atrophic, and there is no leakage.

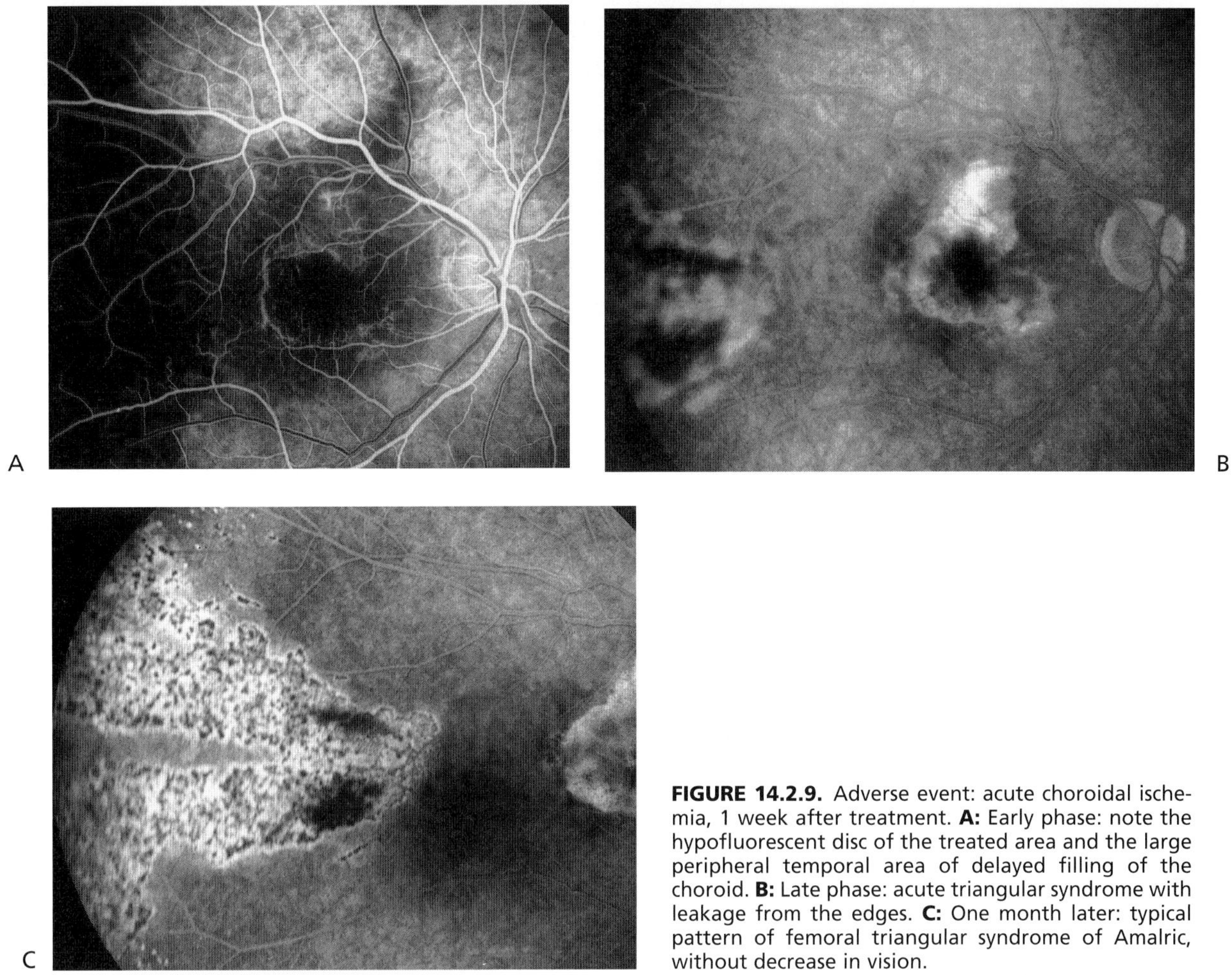

FIGURE 14.2.9. Adverse event: acute choroidal ischemia, 1 week after treatment. **A:** Early phase: note the hypofluorescent disc of the treated area and the large peripheral temporal area of delayed filling of the choroid. **B:** Late phase: acute triangular syndrome with leakage from the edges. **C:** One month later: typical pattern of femoral triangular syndrome of Amalric, without decrease in vision.

feeder vessels or rapid recanalization of transitory occluded vessels may occur if there is persistent angiogenic stimulation (32,33). Retreatment can be postponed when the biomicroscopic and FA appearance of the lesion is unchanged or decreased and visual acuity is stable. However, postponement should only be considered if there is minimal fluorescein leakage from CNV, no progression beyond the area seen at baseline, and minimal or no subretinal fluid on biomicroscopy and OCT. In the intermediate group, the major challenge is to distinguish between the localized area of minimal leakage with an overlying shallow retinal detachment and progressive and intense staining of a thick fibrotic scar, particularly in occult with no classic CNV. Accurate comparisons with previous FA might provide some clues in addition to biomicroscopic examination (Fig. 14.2.8 A through F). Similarly, the availability of OCT sections or retinal mapping can be of instrumental importance, particularly if compared with OCT examination performed before the first session of PDT (Fig. 14.2.6 C, D, G, and H). Retreatment had to be performed in the clinical trials if leakage was suspected. In clinical routine, the addition of OCT examinations to the assessment of the lesion might provide information that could prove decisive in determining the most appropriate course of action. Repeated short-term clinical and FA examinations also can provide an alternative approach to this decision-making process.

Some adverse events that result in severe vision decrease are best identified on FA that can also provide information on the underlying causes. Acute severe visual decrease may be due to choroidal ischemia occurring in the first week after PDT that appears as a triangular area of deep hypoperfusion, resulting in extensive serous retinal detachment (measurable in OCT) that resolves spontaneously. Diagnosis is challenging when the detachment occurs at the pos-

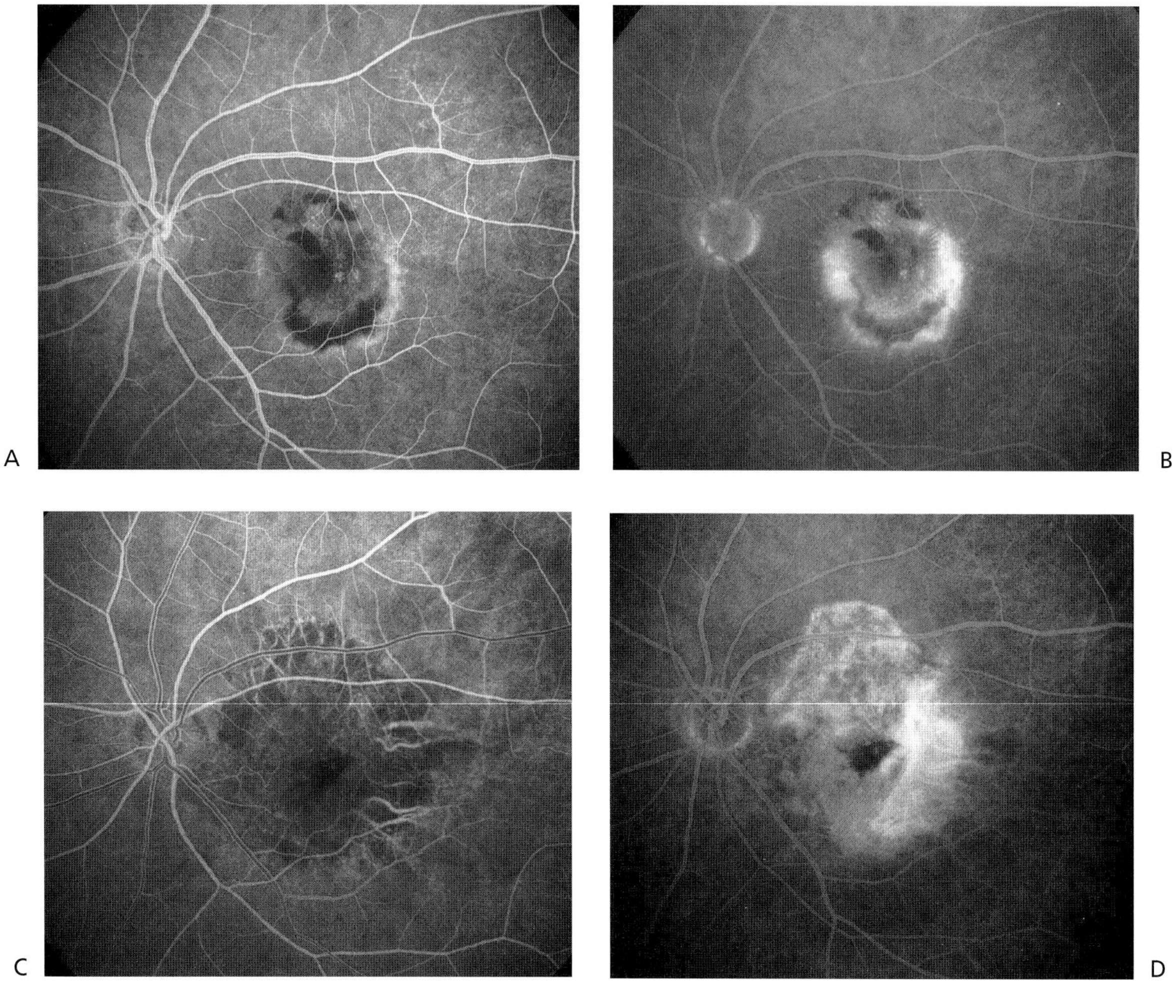

FIGURE 14.2.10. Adverse event: retinal pigment epithelium tear. **A and B:** Fibrovascular pigment epithelial detachment, irregular in shape with nonhomogenous fluorescence, with progressive leakage and a small rim of hemorrhages. **C and D:** Extensive retinal pigment epithelium tear (270°) with severe decrease in vision and fibrovascular scar (1 year later).

terior pole because an increase in the retinal detachment may just be part of the natural history of neovascular AMD. The identification of a deep hypofluorescent triangular area on FA (easily confirmed on ICG) is crucial (Fig. 14.2.9 A, B, and C).

Acute RPE tears occur most frequently after PDT for a fibrovascular PED (Fig. 14.2.10); the straight line of rolled RPE on OCT adjacent to a homogenous persistent hyperfluorescent crescent on FA confirms the diagnosis. At an early stage, however, the diagnostic area may be hidden by a profuse hemorrhage and becomes connected to the event only after its resorption (24). A greenish macular lesion is reported as an adverse event of PDT.

CONCLUSIONS

Fluorescein angiography is the most important method of assessing and classifying CNV to determine whether PDT with verteporfin is indicated. In addition, FA is crucial to assess treatment outcomes and determine whether retreatment is needed. In some cases, OCT can provide not only confirmation but also useful additional information, particularly in eyes with occult CNV. For example, in MPS type II occult CNV, although neovascularization may not be ascertained on FA, fluid accumulation may be disclosed on OCT. Achieving the greatest possible benefits for patients with CNV owing to AMD requires careful assessment of FA, which can be supported in some cases by the use of ICG and OCT.

REFERENCES

1. Soubrane G, Bressler NM. Treatment of subfoveal choroidal neovascularization in age related macular degeneration: focus on clinical application of verteporfin photodynamic therapy. *Br J Ophthalmol* 2001;85:483–495.
2. Treatment of Age-Related Macular Degeneration with Photodynamic Therapy (TAP) Study Group. Photodynamic therapy of subfoveal choroidal neovascularization in age-related macular degeneration with verteporfin. One-year results of 2 randomized clinical trials. *Arch Ophthalmol* 1999;117:1329–1345.
3. Puliafito CA, Hee MR, Lin CP, et al. Imaging of macular diseases with optical coherence tomography. *Ophthalmology* 1995;102: 217–229.
4. The Macular Photocoagulation Study Group. The use of fundus photographs and fluorescein angiograms in the identification and treatment of choroidal neovascularization in the Macular Photocoagulation Study. *Ophthalmology* 1989;96:1526–1534.
5. Yannuzzi LA, Slakter JS, Sorenson JA, et al. Digital indocyanine green videoangiography and choroidal neovascularization. *Retina* 1992;12:191–223.
6. Coscas G, Glaser B, Green WR, et al. *Dégénerescences maculaires liées à l'âge et néovaisseaux rétiniens.* Paris: Masson, 1991.
7. Gass JDM. Pathogenesis of disciform detachment of the neuroepithelium. IV. Fluorescein angiographic study of senile disciform macular degeneration. *Am J Ophthalmol* 1967;63: 644–659.
8. Macular Photocoagulation Study Group. Subfoveal neovascular lesions in age-related macular degeneration. Guidelines for evaluation and treatment in the Macular Photocoagulation Study. *Arch Ophthalmol* 1991;109:1242–1257.
9. Soubrane G, Coscas G, Koenig F, et al. Natural history of occult subretinal new vessels in age-related macular degeneration. *Doc Ophthal Proc Series* 1987;50:219–222.
10. Bressler NM, Frost LA, Bressler SB, et al. Natural course of poorly defined choroidal neovascularization associated with macular degeneration. *Arch Ophthalmol* 1988;106:1537–1542.
11. Soubrane G, Coscas G, Francais C, et al. Occult subretinal new vessels in age-related macular degeneration. Natural history and early laser treatment. *Ophthalmology* 1990;97:649–657.
12. Scheider A, Kaboth A, Neuhauser L. Detection of subretinal neovascular membranes with indocyanine green and an infrared scanning laser ophthalmoscope. *Am J Ophthalmol* 1992;113: 45–51.
13. Soubrane G, Arnold J, Quaranta M. Atteintes dégénératives de l'épithélium pigmentaire. In: Soubrane G, ed. *Les affections acquises de l'épithélium pigmentaire.* Marseille: Fuery-Lamy, 1995:169–204.
14. Kuhn D, Meunier I, Soubrane G, et al. Imaging a chorioretinal anastomoses in vascularized retinal pigment epithelium detachments. *Arch Ophthalmol* 1995;113:1392–1398.
15. Spaide RF, Yannuzzi LA, Slakter JS, et al. Indocyanine green videoangiography of idiopathic polypoidal choroidal vasculopathy. *Retina* 1995;15:100–110.
16. Hee MR, Baumal CR, Puliafito CA, et al. Optical coherence tomography of age-related macular degeneration and choroidal neovascularization. *Ophthalmology* 1996;103:1260–1270.
17. Giovanni A, Amato GP, Mariotti C, et al. OCT imaging of choroidal neovascularization and its role in the determination of patients' eligibility for surgery. *Br J Ophthalmol* 1999;83:438–442.
18. Gass JD. Biomicroscopic and histopathologic considerations regarding the feasibility of surgical excision of subfoveal neovascular membranes. *Am J Ophthalmol* 1994;118:285–298.
19. Vander JF, Morgan CM, Schatz H. Growth rate of subretinal neovascularization in age-related macular degeneration. *Ophthalmology* 1989;96:1422–1426.
20. Stevens TS, Bressler NM, Maguire MG, et al. Occult choroidal neovascularization in age-related macular degeneration. A natural history study. *Arch Ophthalmol* 1997;115:345–350.
21. Macular Photocoagulation Study Group. Occult choroidal neovascularization. Influence on visual outcome in patients with age-related macular degeneration. *Arch Ophthalmol* 1996;114: 400–412.
22. Pharmacological therapy for macular degeneration study group. Interferon 2α is ineffective for patients with choroidal neovascularization secondary to age-related macular degeneration—Results of a prospective randomized placebo-controlled clinical trial. *Arch Ophthalmol* 1997;115:865–872.
23. Verteporfin in Photodynamic Therapy Study Group. Verteporfin therapy of subfoveal choroidal neovascularization in age-related macular degeneration: two year results of a randomized clinical trial including lesions with occult with no classic choroidal neovascularization. *Am J Ophthalmol* 2001;131:541–560.
24. Coscas G, Koenig F, Soubrane G. The pretear characteristics of pigment epithelial detachments. A study of 40 eyes. *Arch Ophthalmol* 1990;108:1687–1693.
25. Kramer M, Miller JW, Michaud N, et al. Liposomal benzoporphyrin derivative verteporfin photodynamic therapy. Selective treatment of choroidal neovascularization in monkeys. *Ophthalmology* 1996;103:427–438.
26. Miller JW, Schmidt-Erfurth U, Sickenberg M, et al. Photodynamic therapy with verteporfin for choroidal neovascularization caused by age-related macular degeneration: results of a single treatment in a phase 1 and 2 study. *Arch Ophthalmol* 1999;117: 1161–1173.
27. Schmidt-Erfurth U, Miller JW, Sickenberg M, et al. Photodynamic therapy with verteporfin for choroidal neovascularization caused by age-related macular degeneration: results of retreatments in a phase 1 and 2 study. *Arch Ophthalmol* 1999;117: 1177–1187.
28. Treatment of Age-Related Macular Degeneration with Photodynamic Therapy (TAP) Study Group. Photodynamic therapy of subfoveal choroidal neovascularization in age-related macular degeneration with verteporfin. Two-year results of 2 randomized clinical trials. *Arch Ophthalmol* 2001;119:198–207.
29. Rosenfeld PJ, Treatment of Age-Related Macular Degeneration with Photodynamic Therapy (TAP) Study Group. Visual outcomes in patients with minimally classic choroidal neovascularization (CNV): rationale for the Visudyne in Minimally classic CNV (VIM) Trial. *Invest Ophthalmol Vis Sci* 2001;42:S512.
30. Stur M, VER Study Group. Rationale for and design of the Visudyne in Early Retreatment (VER) Trial. *Invest Ophthalmol Vis Sci* 2001;42:S442.
31. Verteporfin Therapy for Subfoveal Choroidal Neurovascularization in Age-Related Macular Degeneration. Three-year results of an open-label extension of 2 randomized clinical trials—TAP report No. 5. *Arch Ophthalmol* 2002;120:1307–1314.
32. Kvanta A, Algvere PV, Berglin L, et al. Subfoveal fibrovascular membranes in age-related macular degeneration express vascular endothelial growth factor. *Invest Ophthalmol Vis Sci* 1996;37: 1929–1934.
33. Lutty GA, McLeod DS, Merges C, et al. Localization of vascular endothelial growth factor in human retina and choroids. *Arch Ophthalmol* 1996;114:971–977.

Part 3: Indocyanine Green Angiography in Photodynamic Therapy of Choroidal Neovascularization

ANTONIO P. CIARDELLA
JASON S. SLAKTER
LAWRENCE A. YANNUZZI

Indocyanine green (ICG) is a sterile, water-soluble tricarbocyanine dye that absorbs and fluoresces in the near-infrared range between 790 and 805 nm (1–9). Because of the special characteristics of the dye, there is less blockage by the normal eye pigments, which allows enhanced imaging of the choroid and any associated abnormalities through overlying hemorrhage, serous fluid, lipid, and pigment. This property allows enhanced imaging of occult choroidal neovascularization (CNV) and pigment epithelial detachment (PED) (10,11).

Indocyanine green angiography may be helpful in PDT of CNV both in recognizing different subtypes of CNV, which could have different responses to PDT, and in evaluating the effects of PDT on CNV and the choroid. Indocyanine green angiography may be especially useful in the evaluation of patients with occult or minimally classic CNV by fluorescein angiography (FA). Four different subtypes of CNV in AMD have been identified with the help of ICG angiography: hot spots, plaques, polypoidal choroidal vasculopathy (PCV), and retinal angiomatous proliferation (RAP).

A hot spot is a well-defined area of hyperfluorescence that usually appears in the early to mid-phase of the ICG study, and leaks in the late phase. It represents an area of active CNV (Fig. 14.3.1). We found, in a prospective consecutive series of AMD patients, that a hot spot on ICG angiography represents focal occult CNV in 8% of cases, PCV in 60% of cases, and RAP in 32% of cases (Freund KB, unpublished data). A plaque of CNV is a less well-demarcated area of late staining of ICG dye measuring greater than 1 disc area in size. It represents a less active component of the CNV complex (Figs. 14.3.2 through 14.3.4).

Polypoidal choroidal vasculopathy is a primary abnormality of the choroidal circulation characterized by an inner choroidal vascular network of vessels ending in a aneurysmal bulge or outward projection, visible clinically as a reddish orange, spheroid, polyplike structure. The disorder is associated with multiple, recurrent, serosanguineous detachments of the retinal pigment epithelium (RPE) and neurosensory retina, secondary to leakage and bleeding from the peculiar choroidal vascular abnormality (12–15). Indocyanine green angiography has been used to detect and characterize the PCV abnormality with enhanced sensitivity and specificity (Fig. 14.3.5) (15–17). A distinct network of vessels within the choroid becomes visible in the initial

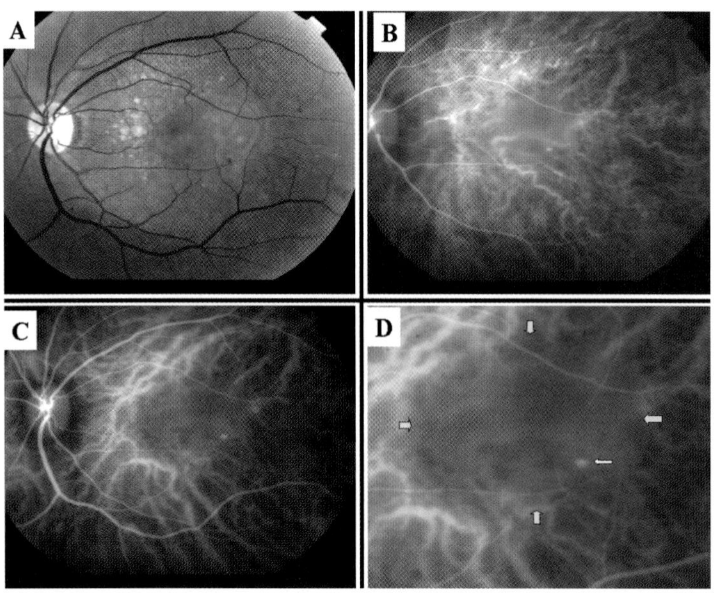

FIGURE 14.3.1. Hot spot. **A:** Red-free photograph of the left eye of a patient with CNV showing large drusen, pigment epithelial detachment (PED), and a small subretinal hemorrhage. **B:** Early-phase indocyanine green angiography study reveals the presence of a PED and a hyperfluorescent hot spot. **C:** Mid-phase indocyanine green study of the same eye better shows a well-delineated, hypofluorescent PED and a hot spot at its inferotemporal border. **D:** High magnification of the photograph in **C** that better shows the hot spot of active CNV *(white arrow)* at the edge of the PED *(yellow arrows)*.

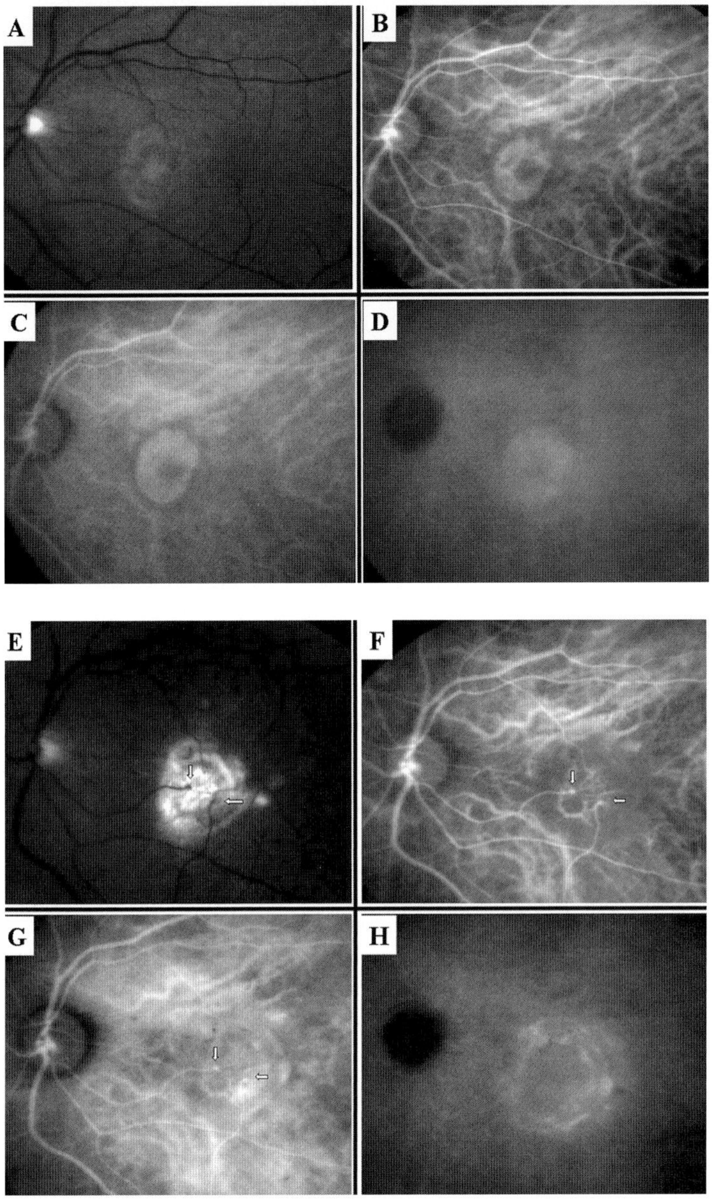

FIGURE 14.3.2. Plaque. This patient was enrolled in the Treatment of Age-Related Macular Degeneration with Photodynamic Therapy study and received placebo. **A through D:** Baseline. Red-free photograph of the left eye reveals the presence of macular neurosensory detachment. Early- and mid-phase indocyanine green (ICG) angiography of the same eye shows a well-demarcated area of CNV. A plaque of CNV is apparent in the late phase of the study. Visual acuity was 20/126. **E through H:** One-year follow-up study of the same patients. There was progression of the CNV complex with formation of a disciform scar in the macula. Note the presence of two retino-choroidal anastomoses *(arrows)* in the red-free photograph. Early- and mid-phase ICG study better shows the two areas of anastomosis of the retinal vessels with the deeper CNV complex. Late-phase ICG study shows enlargement of the plaque of CNV. Visual acuity was 20/250.

phases of an ICG study. In patients with juxtapapillary involvement, the vascular channels extend in a radial, arching pattern and are interconnected with smaller spanning branches that become more evident and numerous at the edge of the PCV lesion. Early in the course of the ICG study, the larger vessels of the PCV network start to fill before the retinal vessels, but the area within and surrounding the network is relatively hypofluorescent compared with the uninvolved choroid. The vessels of the network appear to fill more slowly than the retinal vessels. Shortly after the network can be identified on the ICG angiogram, small hyperfluorescent "polyps" become visible within the choroid. These polypoidal structures correspond to the reddish, orange choroidal excrescences seen on clinical examination. They appear to leak slowly as the surrounding hypofluorescent area becomes increasingly hyperfluorescent. In the later phase of the angiogram, there is a uniform disappearance of the dye ("washout") from the bulging polypoidal lesions. The late ICG staining characteristic of occult CNV is not seen in the PCV vascular abnormality. Although the first reports of PCV were in middle-aged black females, it is now recognized that PCV may be a variant of CNV seen in white patients with AMD, it may be localized in the macular area without any peripapillary component, and it may be formed by a network of small branching vessels ending in polypoidal dilation difficult to image without ICG angiography (18,19). It is possible that in this form of CNV, PDT is able to effectively close the

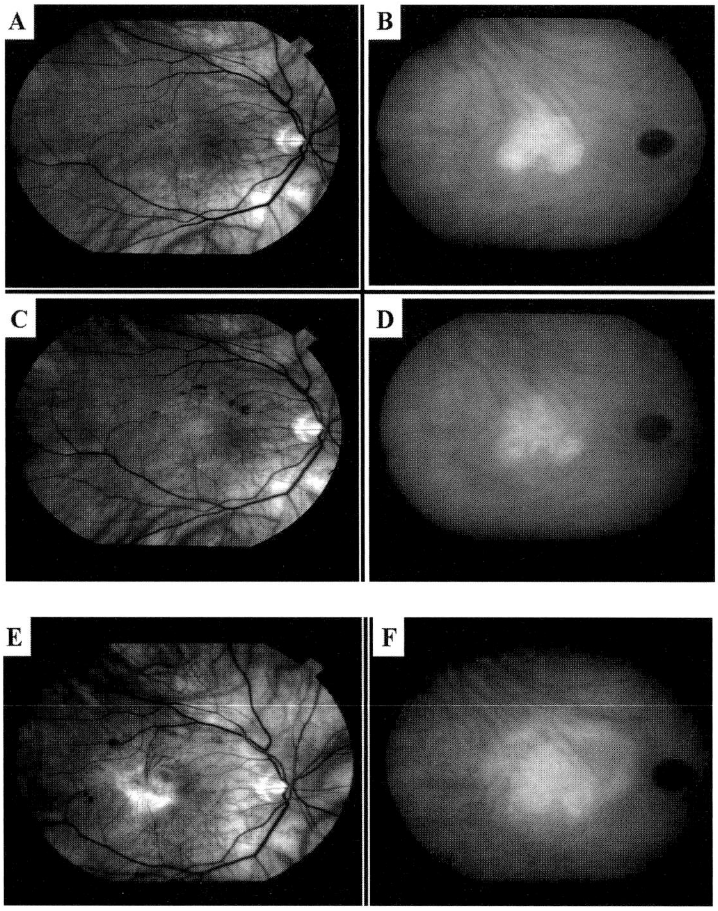

FIGURE 14.3.3. Plaque. This patient was enrolled in the Treatment of Age-Related Macular Degeneration with Photodynamic Therapy study and received placebo. **A,B:** Baseline. **C,D:** Three-month follow up. **E,F:** One-year follow up. **A:** Red-free photograph of the right eye at baseline examination demonstrating the presence of macular neurosensory detachment, and subretinal hemorrhage. Visual acuity was 20/80. **B:** Late-phase indocyanine green (ICG) angiography study of the same eye shows a well-defined plaque of choroidal neovascularization. **C:** Red-free photograph at 3-month follow up shows enlargement of the neurosensory detachment and more subretinal blood. Visual acuity was 20/80. **D:** Late-phase ICG angiography study shows enlargement of the plaque of choroidal neovascularization. **E:** Red-free photograph at 1-year follow up reveals further extension of the neurosensory detachment. There is also development of subretinal fibrosis. Visual acuity was 20/80. **F:** Late-phase ICG angiography study of demonstrates further growth of the plaque of CNV.

large, dilated choroidal vascular channels that form the CNV complex. Studies to assess the efficacy of PDT for PCV are under way.

Retinal angiomatous proliferation is a distinct subgroup of neovascular AMD. Angiomatous proliferation within the retina is the first manifestation of the neovascularized process in this form of neovascular AMD (20–24). Dilated retinal vessels and preretinal, intraretinal, and subretinal hemorrhages and exudates evolve surrounding the angiomatous proliferation as the process extends into the deep retina and subretinal space. One or more dilated compensatory retinal vessels perfuse and drain the neovascularization, sometimes forming a retinal-retinal anastomosis (RRA). Fluorescein angiography in these patients usually reveals indistinct staining, a form of occult-CNV. Indocyanine green angiography is useful to make an accurate diagnosis in most cases (Fig. 14.3.6). It reveals a focal area of intense hyperfluorescence corresponding to the neovascularization (hot spot), and some late extension of the leakage within the retina from the intraretinal neovascularization (IRN). As the IRN progresses toward the subretinal space, the CNV becomes part of the neovascular complex. At this stage, there is often clinical and angiographic evidence of a vascularized pigment epithelium detachment (V-PED). Indocyanine green angiography better images the presence of a V-PED, because the serous component of the PED remains dark during the study and the vascular component appears as a hot spot (Fig. 14.3.3) (25–35). At this stage, ICG angiography sometimes may be able to image a direct communication between the retinal and choroidal components of the neovascularization, which form a retino-choroidal anastomosis (RCA). Lafaut and coworkers recently reported on the clinicopathologic correlation of RCA in AMD (24). They found that RCA histologically represents neovascularization growing out of the neurosensory retina, into the subretinal space, which mimics CNV.

Clinical knowledge and recognition of RAP is important because this form of neovascular AMD may have a natural course, visual prognosis, and response to treatment distinct from other forms of neovascular AMD. Because RAP may present simply as IRN or progress to be complicated by subretinal neovascularization (SRN) with or without a serous-PED, and with or without CNV and an RCA, different forms of treatment may be preferable for each stage of the disorder. For example, we have found that an uncomplicated focal area of IRN may be amenable to conventional thermal laser treatment; whereas a more advanced stage involving a vascularized PED and an RCA is not likely to

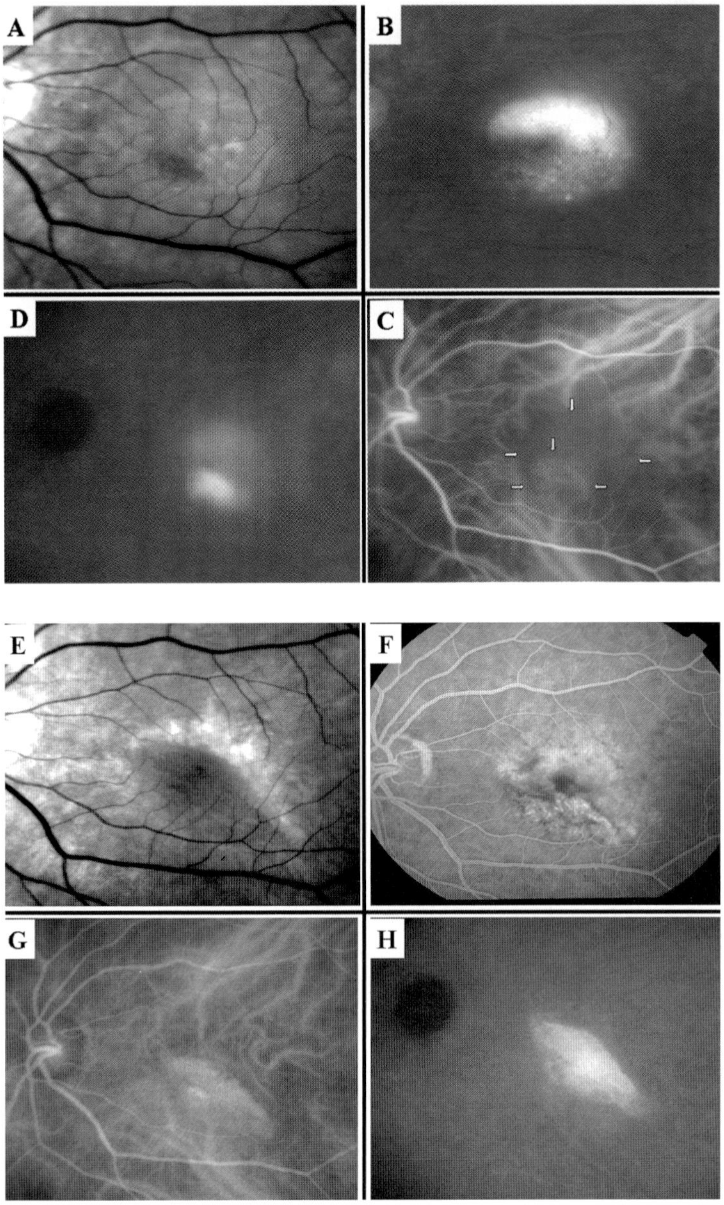

FIGURE 14.3.4. Active CNV. This patient received PDT with verteporfin (Visudyne, Novartis Pharmaceuticals, Basel, Switzerland). **A through C:** Baseline. **D through F:** One-year follow-up. **A:** Red-free photograph of the left eye shows the presence of a macular pigment epithelium detachment and a larger neurosensory detachment. Visual acuity was 20/50. **B:** Late-phase fluorescein angiography study demonstrates the presence of occult CNV and a pigment epithelial detachment (PED). **C:** Early-phase indocyanine green (ICG) angiography better demonstrates the presence of a serous PED *(white arrows).* A well-defined area of CNV is present under the PED *(yellow arrows).* **D:** Late-phase ICG study reveals an area of CNV actively leaking in the sub–retinal pigment epithelium space. **E:** Red-free photograph of the same eye at 1-year follow-up visit. There is resolution of the PED. Visual acuity was 20/26. **F:** Fluorescein angiography study shows occult CNV. **G:** Early-phase ICG study revels a larger, less well-defined area of CNV. There is no PED. **H:** Late-phase ICG study of the same eye demonstrates a quiescent plaque of CNV. There is no leakage of dye in the subretinal space.

respond to any form of currently available treatment. Also, PDT with a photosensitizing dye, such as verteporfin, may have a different effect on RAP than on patients with classic or occult CNV (36–39). Given the tendency for the ICG dye to stain the retina in eyes with RAP, there is a possibility that similar staining may occur with the verteporfin molecule, theoretically predisposing the retina to photochemical damage when exposed to the excitatory light used in PDT. This possibility obviously is still mere speculation because verteporfin has not yet been imaged successfully with good spatial and temporal definition in these cases. However, its fundamental spectral characteristics in conjunction with its affinity to bind with protein may be similar to the ICG molecule. Because eyes with RAP in AMD are generally classified as either minimally classic or pure occult CNV with FA, it is possible that patients with RAP were actually treated in the TAP and VIP trial (37,39). In this trial, ICG angiography was not routinely used to evaluate patients; therefore, the frequency of RAP in the subset of patients classified as minimally classic or occult-CNV is not known. Future studies on the expanded use of PDT with verteporfin are incorporating ICG angiography, which should be helpful in characterizing the true nature and frequency of RAP and its response to this form of treatment.

In the TAP study, a small subgroup of 56 patients underwent ICG angiography examination at baseline. At 1-year follow up, 39 of these 56 patients had ICG examinations. By ICG angiography, hot spots were present in 18% of these eyes, plaques in 86%, and RCAs in 8% (Slakter JS, unpublished data). Kusserow and colleagues (40) treated 12

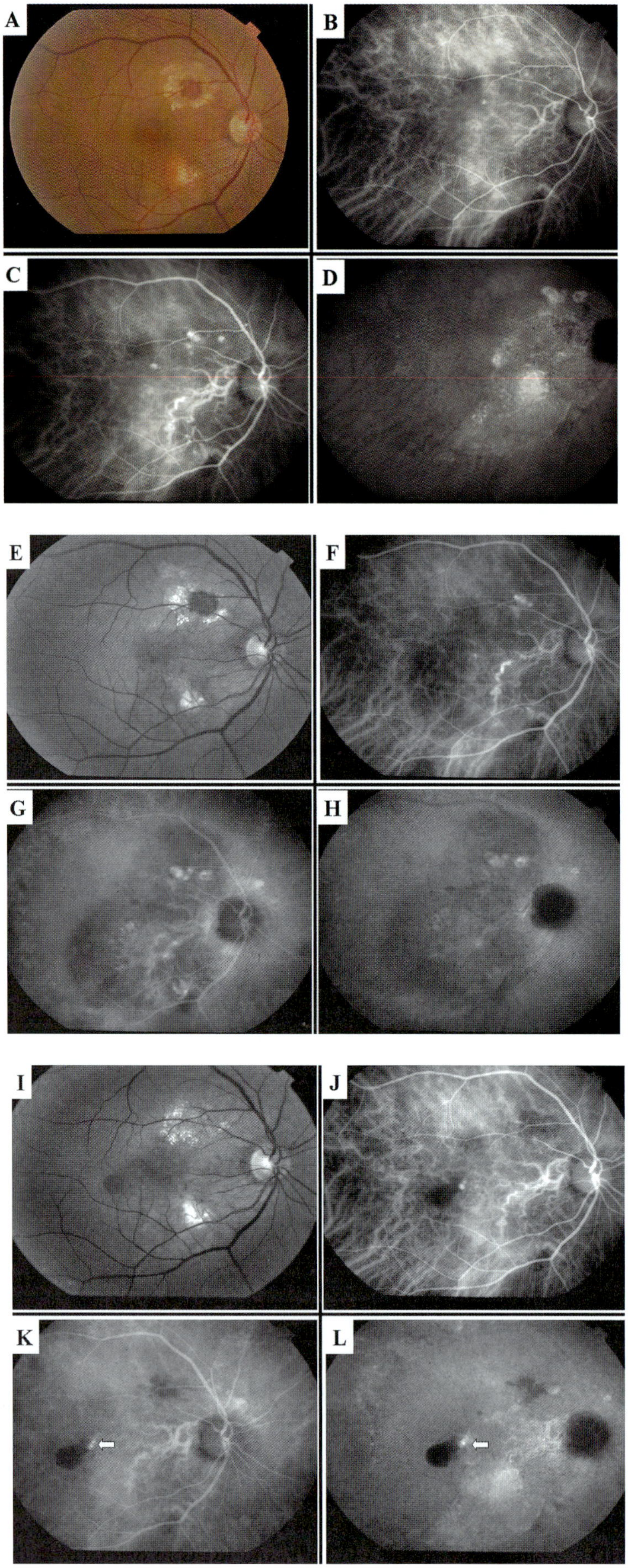

FIGURE 14.3.5. Polypoidal choroidal vasculopathy (PCV). **A through D:** Baseline. **E through H:** One week after PDT with verteporfin. **I through L:** One year after treatment. **A:** Clinical photograph of the right eye of a patient with PCV. Note the presence of a peripapillary pattern of dilated choroidal vascular channel branching toward the macula. There is reddish, large, bulging polypoidal dilation inferiorly. A smaller lesion superiorly is actively leaking and is surrounded by a circinate ring of exudates. Visual acuity was 20/60. **B:** Early-phase indocyanine green (ICG) study shows a ramified pattern of dilated choroidal vessels radiating from the peripapillary area. **C:** Mid-phase ICG study reveals the presence of numerous hot spots of actively leaking CNV. **D:** Late-phase ICG study shows a washout of the choroidal vascular abnormality. **E:** Red-free photograph of the same patient 1 week after PDT treatment. There is a neurosensory detachment in the macula and subretinal hemorrhage. Visual acuity had dropped to 20/400. **F:** Early-phase ICG study reveals the presence of a large area of hypofluorescence. This area corresponds to the area of PDT. (Three different laser spots were applied to cover the entire area.) **G:** Mid-phase ICG study shows the network of polypoidal vascular dilation. The area of hypofluorescence is better defined. **H:** Late-phase ICG study of the same patient reveals persistence of the hypofluorescent area. **I:** Red-free photograph of the same patient 1 year after treatment. There is resolution of the macular neurosensory detachment. A new subretinal hemorrhage is present in the temporal macula. Visual acuity had improved to 20/30. **J:** Early-phase ICG angiography shows the pattern of polypoidal vessels radiating from the optic nerve. **K:** Mid-phase ICG angiography photograph demonstrates closure of previously active hot spots of leaking CNV. A new hot spot is present temporally at the edge of the subretinal hemorrhage *(white arrow).* **L:** Late-phase ICG angiography reveals further leakage from the area of active CNV *(white arrow).* There is complete disappearance of the circular areas of hypofluorescence.

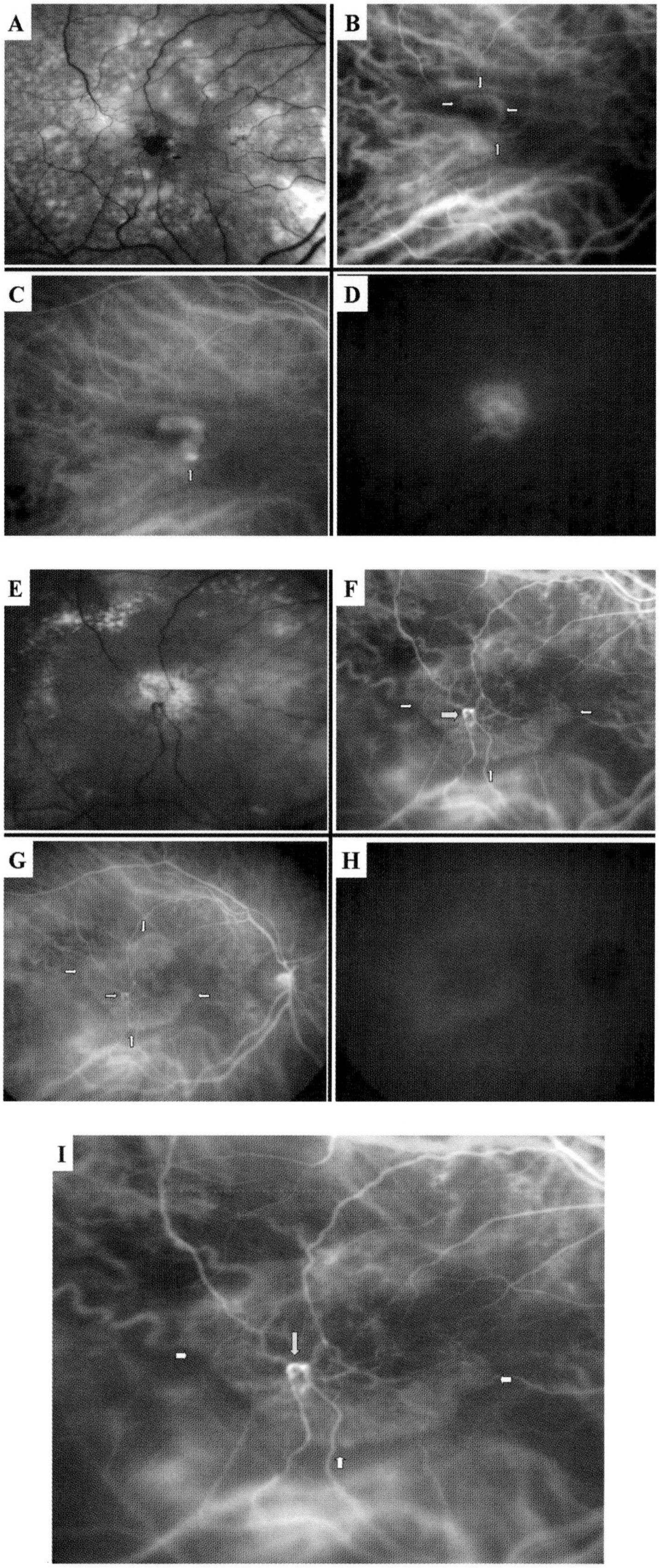

FIGURE 14.3.6. Retinal angiomatous proliferation. **A through D:** Baseline. **E through H:** One-year follow up after PDT with verteporfin. **A:** High-magnification red-free photograph of the right eye demonstrates the presence of a neurosensory macular detachment, intraretinal and subretinal hemorrhages, and large drusen. Visual acuity was 20/160. **B:** Early-phase, high-magnification indocyanine green (ICG) study of the same eye reveals the presence of a hot spot of intraretinal neovascularization (IRN) *(yellow arrow)* and a larger, less well-defined area of CNV *(white arrows).* **C:** Mid-phase ICG study better demonstrates the hot spot of IRN *(yellow arrow).* **D:** Late-phase ICG study shows intraretinal leakage of ICG. **E:** High-magnification red-free photograph of the same eye 1 year after PDT with verteporfin. There is a much larger neurosensory detachment, lipid exudation, and fibrous scarring in the fovea. Also, the presence of a retino-choroidal and retinal-retinal anastomosis is now evident. Visual acuity was 20/800. **F:** An early-phase, high-magnification ICG angiography study better demonstrates the presence of a retino-choroidal anastomosis *(yellow arrow).* Note the growth of the choroidal component of the neovascular complex *(white arrows).* **G:** Mid-phase ICG angiography study better delineates the extension of the choroidal component *(white arrows)* of neovascularization. **H:** Late-phase ICG angiography reveals a much larger plaque of CNV. **I:** Higher magnification photograph of mid-phase ICG angiography demonstrates the connection between the retinal *(yellow arrow)* and choroidal component *(white arrows)* of the neovascularization.

patients who had RCA with PDT. All patients demonstrated a drop in visual acuity of at least one line over a 6-month period. Mean baseline visual acuity was 20/126, ranging from 20/40 to 20/200. At 6 months the mean visual acuity had dropped to 20/200, ranging from 20/80 to 20/400. Early angiography demonstrated an absence of initial occlusion of the neovascular lesion, followed by continuous growth of the CNV. At 6 months, the mean size of the CNV lesion had increased from 1.3 mm^2 to 2.6 mm^2 as measured on FA.

Finally, ICG angiography is able to image hypofluorescent areas of choroidal circulation that appear to be related to verteporfin therapy (Fig. 14.3.7). Its ability to give better definition of the choroid may provide a better measure of treatment effect and safety. In the same small subgroup of TAP patients who had ICG examination at 1-year follow up, 16 of 39 (41%) showed circular areas of hypofluorescence of the choroid in the macular area. All of these eyes were part of the treatment group. No correlation was noted between the presence of choroidal hypofluorescence and visual acuity, suggesting that these choroidal changes were not indicative of a detrimental effect from PDT (Slakter JS, unpublished data).

Schmidt-Erfurth and colleagues (41,42) studied the effects of PDT on the choroidal circulation with ICG angiography performed via the Heidelberg Scanning Laser Ophthalmoscope. Indocyanine green angiography was performed before and at 5 hours, 1 day, 1 week, and 3 and 12 months post-PDT. The documented phenomena were differentiated into those effects seen at the lesion site (thera-

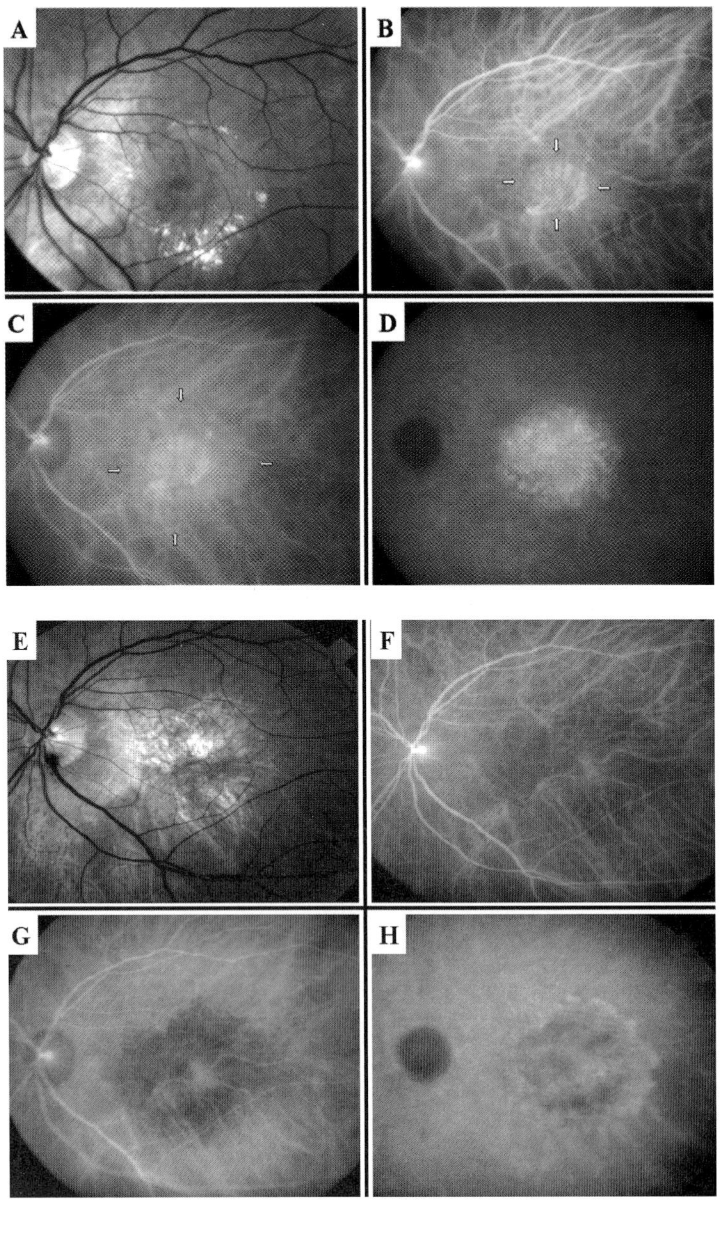

FIGURE 14.3.7. Hypofluorescence. **A through D:** Baseline. **E through H:** One-year follow up after PDT with verteporfin. **A:** Red-free photograph of the left eye reveals the presence of a neurosensory detachment and lipid exudation. Visual acuity was 20/50. **B:** Early-phase indocyanine green (ICG) angiography study shows a well-demarcated area of CNV *(white arrows).* **C:** Mid-phase ICG study demonstrates a larger component of the neovascular complex *(yellow arrows).* **D:** Late-phase ICG study reveals a large plaque of CNV. **E:** Red-free photographs at a 1-year follow-up visit after PDT shows resolution of the neurosensory detachment and the lipid exudates. Visual acuity was 20/50. **F:** Early-phase ICG angiography study reveals the presence of a round area of hypofluorescence corresponding to the spot size of the laser treatment. **G:** Mid-phase ICG study better shows the hypofluorescent area. Note the absence of well-defined CNV. **H:** Late-phase ICG angiography study shows growth of the plaque of CNV outside the border of the hypofluorescent area.

peutic effects) and the changes observed within the surrounding choroid (considered side effects). Indocyanine green angiography 5 hours after PDT showed an increase in volume of the CNV because of extravasation of dye from damaged vascular walls of the neovascular complex. One day after treatment, there was still increased exudation from the adjacent choroid and CNV. Choroidal neovascularization leakage progressively decreased during the following week. However, parts of the lesion could still be delineated as early as 1 week after PDT in half of the treated eyes. The CNV complex appeared to be progressively smaller after each PDT treatment in the follow-up period. Lesions were still detectable at 12 weeks, but mean lesion size and hyperfluorescence were markedly reduced. In addition, ICG angiography showed impressive changes, characterized by intensive postoperative hypofluorescence within the adjacent choroid. The size of the hypofluorescence correlated with the size of the spot used for light exposure. Choroidal fluorescence recovered progressively during posttreatment follow up. No pathologic changes were observed by ICG angiography after 1 to 2 years. The cause of PDT-induced hypofluorescence remains speculative in the absence of pathologic correlation. However, it is reasonable to attribute such hypofluorescence to a temporary reduction of choriocapillaris perfusion in the treated area.

In conclusion, ICG angiography is promising as a means to differentiate the various subtypes of CNV, which can have different clinical responses to PDT. In addition, ICG angiography appears useful in documenting therapeutic effects on the CNV complex and potential side effects on the normal surrounding choroidal vasculature following PDT.

REFERENCES

1. Patz A, Flower RW, Klein ML, et al. Clinical applications of indocyanine green angiography. *Doc Ophthalmol Proc Series* 1976;9:245–251.
2. Cherrick GR, Stein SW, Leevy CM, et al. Indocyanine green: observations on its physical properties, plasma decay, and hepatic extraction. *J Clin Invest* 1960;39:592.
3. Baker KJ. Binding of sulfobromophthalein (BSP) sodium and indocyanine green (ICG) by plasma a1-lipoproteins. *Proc Soc Exp Biol Med* 1966;122:957.
4. Ketterer SG, Wiengand BD. The excretion of indocyanine green and its use in the estimation of hepatic blood flow. *Clin Res* 1959; 7:71.
5. Ketterer SG, Wiengand BD. Hepatic clearance of indocyanine green. *Clin Res* 1959;7:289.
6. Probst P, Paumgartner G, Caucig H, et al. Studies on clearance and placental transfer of indocyanine green during labor. *Clin Chim Acta* 1970;29:157.
7. Goresky CA. Initial distribution and rate of uptake of sulfobromophthalein in the liver. *Am J Physiol* 1964;207:13.
8. Leevy CM, Bender J, Silverberg M, et al. Physiology of dye extraction by the liver: comparative studies of sulfobromophthalein and indocyanine green. *Ann NY Acad Sci* 1963;111:161.
9. Geeraets WJ, Berry ER. Ocular spectral characteristics as related to hazards from lasers and other light sources. *Am J Ophthalmol* 1968;66:15–20.
10. Yannuzzi LA, Slakter JS, Sorenson JS, et al. Digital indocyanine green videoangiography and choroidal neovascularization. *Retina* 1992;12:191–223.
11. Fox IJ, Wood EH. Application of dilution curves recorded from the right side of the heart or venous circulation with the aid of a new indicator dye. *Proc Mayo Clin* 1957;32:541.
12. Kleiner RC, Brucker AJ, Johnston RL. The posterior uveal bleeding syndrome. *Ophthalmology 91* 1984;(Suppl 9):110.
13. Kleiner RC, Brucker AJ, Johnston RL. The posterior uveal bleeding syndrome. *Retina* 1990;10:9–17.
14. Yannuzzi LA, Sorenson JS, Spaide RF, et al. Idiopathic polypoidal choroidal vasculopathy. *Retina* 1990;10:1–8.
15. Yannuzzi LA, Ciardella AP, Spaide RF, et al. The expanding clinical spectrum of idiopathic polypoidal choroidal vasculopathy. *Arch Ophthalmol* 1999;115:478–485.
16. Ross RD, Gitter KA, Cohen G, et al. Idiopathic polypoidal choroidal vasculopathy associated with retinal arterial macroaneurysm and hypertensive retinopathy. *Retina* 1996;16:111.
17. Spaide RF, Yannuzzi LA, Slakter JS, et al. Indocyanine green videoangiography of idiopathic polypoidal choroidal vasculopathy. *Retina* 1995;15:100–110.
18. Yannuzzi LA, Freund KB, Goldbaum M, et al. Polypoidal choroidal vasculopathy masquerading as central serous chorioretinopathy. *Ophthalmology* 2000;107:767–777.
19. Yannuzzi LA, Wong DW, Sforzolini BS, et al. Polypoidal choroidal vasculopathy and neovascularized age-related macular degeneration. *Arch Ophthalmol* 1999;117:1503–1510.
20. Yannuzzi LA, Negrao S, Iida T, et al. Retinal angiomatous proliferation in age-related macular degeneration. *Retina* 2001;21: 416–434.
21. Slakter JS, Yannuzzi LA, Scheider U, et al. Retinal choroidal anastomosis and occult choroidal neovascularization. *Ophthalmology* 2000;107:742–753.
22. Kuhn D, Meunier I, Soubrane G, et al. Imaging of chorioretinal anastomoses in vascularized retinal pigment epithelium detachments. *Arch Ophthalmol* 1995;113:1392–1396.
23. Hartnett ME, Weiter JJ, Staurenghi G, et al. Deep vascular anomalous complexes in advanced age-related macular degeneration. *Ophthalmology* 1996;103:2042–2053.
24. Lafaut BA, Aisenbrey S, Vanden Broecke C, et al. Clinicopathological correlation of deep retinal vascular complex in age related macular degeneration. *Br J Ophthalmol* 2000;84:1269–1274.
25. Schwartz S, Guyer DR, Yannuzzi LA, et al. Indocyanine green videoangiography guided laser photocoagulation of primary occult choroidal neovascularization in age-related macular degeneration. *Invest Ophthalmol Vis Sci* 1995;36:186.
26. Yannuzzi LA, Hope-Ross M, Slakter JS, et al. Analysis of vascularized pigment epithelium detachments using indocyanine green videoangiography. *Retina* 1994;14:99–113.
27. Lim JI, Stenberg P, Capone A, et al. Selective use of indocyanine green angiography for occult choroidal neovascularization. *Am J Ophthalmol* 1995;120:75–82.
28. Guyer DR, Yannuzzi LA, Slakter JS, et al. Digital indocyanine-green videoangiography of occult choroidal neovascularization. *Ophthalmology* 1994;101:1727–1737.
29. Guyer DR, Yannuzzi LA, Slakter JS, et al. Classification of choroidal neovascularization by digital indocyanine green videoangiography. *Ophthalmology* 1996;103:2054–2060.
30. Guyer DR, Yannuzzi LA, Ladas I, et al. Indocyanine green guided laser photocoagulation of focal spots at the edge of plaques of choroidal neovascularization: a pilot study. *Arch Ophthalmol* 1996;114:693–697.
31. Slakter JS, Yannuzzi LA, Sorenson JA, et al. A pilot study of indocyanine green videoangiography-guided laser photocoagulation

of occult choroidal neovascularization in age-related macular degeneration. *Arch Ophthalmol* 1994;112:465–472.
32. Mandava N, Guyer DR, Yannuzzi LA, et al. Indocyanine green videoangiography-guided laser photocoagulation of occult choroidal neovascularization. *Ophthal Surg Lasers* 1997;28:844–852.
33. Lim JI, Aaberg TM Sr, Capone A Jr, et al. Indocyanine green angiography-guided photocoagulation of choroidal neovascularization associated with retinal pigment epithelial detachment. *Am J Ophthalmol* 1997;123:524–532.
34. Freund KB, Yannuzzi LA, Sorenson JA, et al. Age-related macular degeneration and choroidal neovascularization. *Am J Ophthalmol* 1993;115:786–791.
35. Sorenson JA, Yannuzzi LA, Slakter JS, et al. A pilot study of digital indocyanine green videoangiography for recurrent occult choroidal neovascularization in age-related macular degeneration. *Arch Ophthalmol* 1994;112:473–479.
36. Schmidt-Erfurth U, Hasan T. Mechanisms of action of photodynamic therapy with vertoporphin for treatment of age-related macular degeneration. *Surv Ophthalmol* 2000;45:195–214.
37. Treatment of age-related macular degeneration with photodynamic therapy (TAP) study group. Photodynamic therapy of subfoveal choroidal neovascularization in age-related macular degeneration with verteporfin. One-year results of 2 randomized clinical trials 1. *Arch Ophthalmol* 1999;117:1329–1345.
38. Verteporfin in Photodynamic Therapy Study Group. Verteporfin therapy of subfoveal choroidal neovascularization in age-related macular degeneration: two-year results of a randomized clinical trial including lesions with occult with no classic choroidal neovascularization. *Am J Ophthalmol* 2001;131:541–560.
39. Treatment of Age-related Macular Degeneration with Photodynamic Therapy (TAP) Study Group. Photodynamic therapy of subfoveal choroidal neovascularization in age-related macular degeneration with verteporfin: two-year results of 2 randomized clinical trials. *Arch Ophthalmol* 2001;119:198–207.
40. Kusserow C, Michels S, Kollner C, et al. *Impact of chorioretinal anastomosis on prognosis in photodynamic therapy.* ARVO annual meeting, Fort Lauderdale, FL, April 29–May 4, 2001.
41. Schmidt-Erfurth UM. Indocyanine green angiography and retinal sensitivity after photodynamic treatment of subfoveal choroidal neovascularization. *Semin Ophthalmol* 1999;14:35–44.
42. Schmidt-Erfurth UM, Niemeyer M, Michels S, et al. *Three-dimensional imaging of dynamic and structural vascular changes induced by photodynamic therapy.* ARVO annual meeting, Fort Lauderdale, FL, April 29–May 4, 2001.

Part 4: Subfoveal Choroidal Blood Flow and Its Regulation After Verteporfin Photodynamic Therapy in Choroidal Neovascularization

CONSTANTIN J. POURNARAS
CHARLES E. RIVA
ERIC LOGEAN
GISÈLE SOUBRANE

Alterations of blood flow in the subfoveal choroidal circulation may be important in the development of neovascular age-related macular degeneration (AMD). Blood flow changes affect the metabolism of the adjacent external retinal layers and can lead to the development of subretinal neovascular tissue through the release of neovascular mediators (1).

Histopathologic studies reveal that abnormal new blood vessels grow from the choriocapillaris and proliferate through breaks in Bruch's membrane under the retinal pigment epithelium (RPE) and further proliferate into the subretinal space between the RPE and neurosensory retina.

Although metabolic changes of the RPE appear to be primarily caused by aging, the RPE is also affected by vascular changes in the choroid. Delayed filling of the choriocapillaris may correlate with the diffuse thickening of Bruch's membrane (2), which is often observed in eyes with neovascular AMD (3) and may lead to an increased incidence of geographic atrophy (4). In addition, evidence of increased vascular resistance in the choroidal vasculature is provided by retrobulbar hemodynamics assessment, which indicates increased pulsatility and decreased end-diastolic blood flow velocity of the short posterior ciliary arteries (5).

Photodynamic therapy (PDT) with verteporfin has been shown in randomized clinical trials to be an effective treatment for selected patients with neovascular AMD (6). It can reduce the risk of visual acuity loss by inducing the occlusion of neovascular tissue that forms during the natural progression of neovascular AMD. Fluorescein angiographic (FA) evaluation of the treated neovascular tissue reveals initial hypofluorescence followed by reperfusion of the treated area within a 4-week period. However, histopathologic data confirm the endothelial cell damage, thrombus formation, and vascular occlusion of the neovascular tissue in patients with AMD treated by PDT (7), in agreement with histopathologic data available from animal models.

Clinical observations, optical coherence tomography (OCT) findings, and FA performed 24 hours after PDT indicate that the early initial hypofluorescence could result from a masking effect produced by a protein-rich exudate lying within the treated area. However, indocyanine green angiography (ICG-A) studies indicate that large choroidal and feeder vessels persist within the treated hypofluorescent area in more than 50% of eyes (8). In these studies, hypofluorescence disappeared several weeks after PDT, either with the resolution of exudate or the restoration of vascular barrier functions. Thus, occlusion of choroidal neovascularization (CNV) might be a consequence of transient changes in the subfoveal choroidal vessel circulation. In addition, ICG-A revealed a complete recovery of the surrounding normal choriocapillaris in the majority of eyes treated with PDT with verteporfin at the 12-week follow-up examination (8).

Assessment of choroidal blood flow (ChBF) in neovascular AMD and changes in this flow following PDT may be crucial to understand hemodynamic changes within the neovascular subretinal tissue, and might be helpful with regard to further retreatment.

CHOROIDAL BLOOD FLOW

Choroidal blood flow is about 10 times higher than the flow in the gray matter of the brain and four times that of the kidney (9), even though a corresponding difference in metabolic requirements does not exist. This high rate of blood flow is probably attributable to the low resistance of the choroidal vascular system, a consequence of the unusually large caliber of the choriocapillary lumen. Eighty-five percent of the total blood flow to the eye is distributed to the choroid and only 4% to the retina. The remaining flow perfuses the ciliary body (10%) and the iris (1%) (9,10).

Consequently, the oxygen extraction from the choroidal blood is very low: The arteriovenous difference is only about 3% (11). Conversely, the oxygen content of the retinal venous blood in humans (12) and pigs (13) is about 38% lower than of arterial blood. In pigs, however, about 60% of oxygen and 75% of glucose are delivered to the retina by the choroidal circulation despite the low oxygen extraction from the choroidal blood (13).

TECHNIQUES OF CHOROIDAL BLOOD FLOW EVALUATION

Most of our knowledge about choroidal circulatory physiology comes from animal studies because until recently only invasive techniques could be used to obtain quantitative information on choroidal hemodynamics. These techniques include calorimetry (14), direct measurements from choroidal veins (15), radioactive krypton desaturation (16), labeled microspheres (10,17) and hydrogen clearance (18), of which the injection of radioactive labeled microspheres has been used most extensively to calculate tissue blood flow in animals. Most of our knowledge about human choroidal physiology is extrapolated from animal studies because this technique is not applicable to humans.

Information on choroidal blood flow and its regulation have been obtained in normal and diseased human eyes from computer-assisted analysis of fluorescein and indocyanine green (ICG) angiograms. However, the information regarding blood flow rate has remained largely qualitative.

The non-invasive laser Doppler flowmetry (LDF) (19) permits relative and continuous measurement of the subfoveal choroidal blood velocity (ChBVel), volume (ChBVol), and flow (ChBF) in healthy and diseased eyes (20–22); and the changes of these flow parameters in response to physiological stimuli, such as changes in the ocular perfusion pressure (23,24), breathing conditions (25), and state of adaptation of the eye (26). Choroidal blood flow is obtained from the relationship

$$\text{ChBF} = k \times \text{ChBVel} \times \text{ChBVol}$$

where: k is an instrumental constant.

Two types of LDF instrument have been used to measure ChBF. In the fundus camera (Topcon TRC, Tokyo, Japan)–based system, the laser beam is delivered to the eye along the illumination path of the camera. The beam originates from a diode (wavelength = 811 nm, 100 μW at the cornea) and has a diameter at the fundus of about 300 μm. The light scattered by the erythrocytes moving in the tissue volume sampled by the incident laser beam is detected at the fundus image plane of the camera by an optical fiber (approximately 150 mm diameter) at the retinal image plane. Subjects are asked to fixate this beam, which appears as a faint pointlike spot. A measurement lasts approximately 10 to 20 seconds.

Recently, a confocal LDF module (Fig. 14.4.1A) mounted on an existing topographical scanning system (TopSS, Laser Diagnostic Technologies, San Diego, CA) was described. This module allows subfoveal measurements at various choroidal depths (27). A schematic diagram of this module is shown in Figure 14.4.1B.

The probing light source is a laser diode whose beam is focused onto a 50-μm diameter pinhole. From the pinhole, the laser light passes through a beam splitter, a focusing lens, and a pair of joystick-controlled mirrors before being coupled into the normal optical path of the TopSS by a dichroic mirror. The joystick control allows placement of the probing beam in the desired location at the fundus in the x–y directions. The focusing lens allows selection of the probed volume depth within the fundus tissues. This depth is calibrated in diopters in relation to the focal plane of the TopSS imaging beam.

Light scattered from the focal plane follows the identical path back through the optics, up to the beam splitter, where

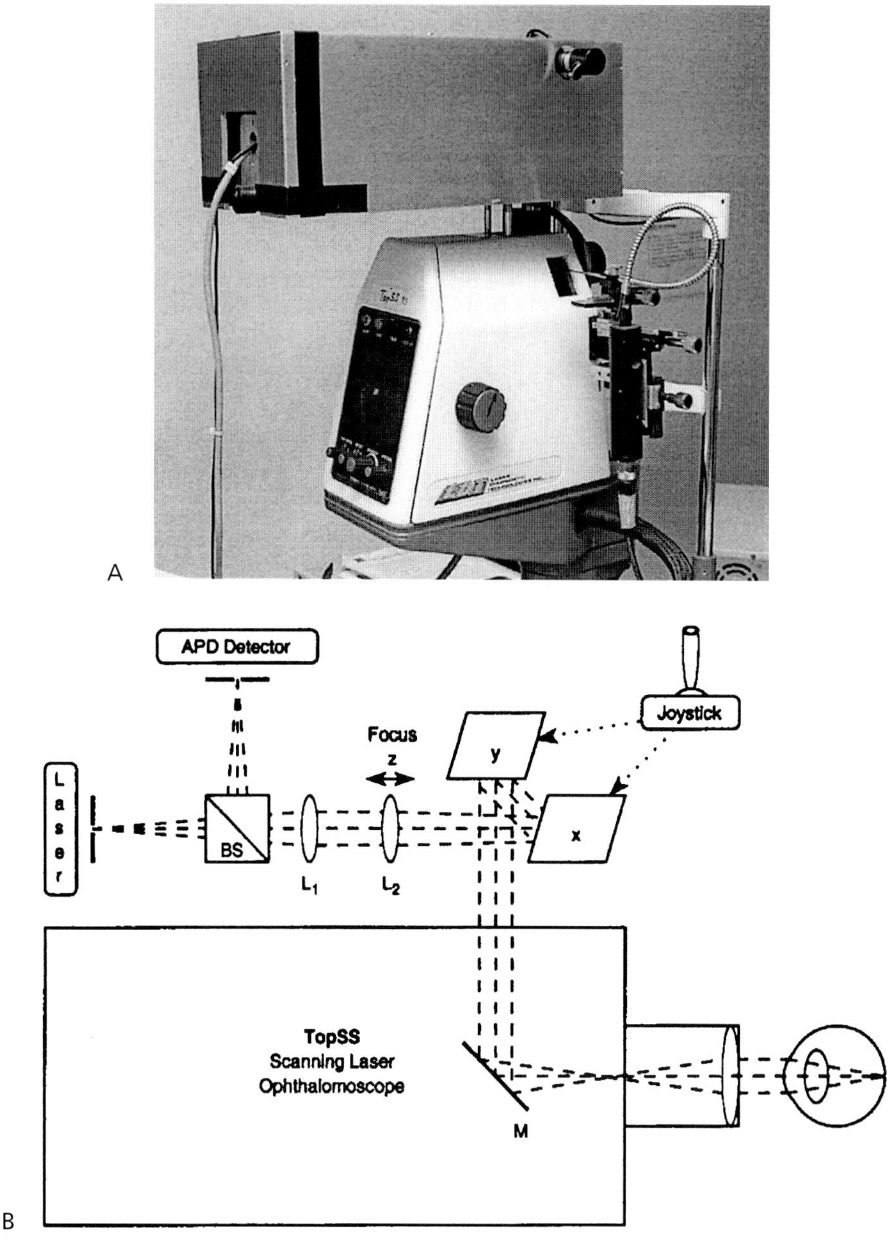

FIGURE 14.4.1. A: Laser Doppler flowmeter adapted for the TopSS scanning laser ophthalmoscope. **B:** Schematic diagram of confocal laser Doppler flowmeter inserted into the TopSS.

it is focused onto a pinhole in front of an avalanche photodiode detector. The pinhole at the detector is conjugated to the pinhole in front of the laser source (confocal design). The probing beam diameter and power at the cornea are approximately 1 mm and 30 μW, respectively.

Ten to 20 seconds are necessary to record each measurement. When the subject fixates steadily, as verified by the operator on the TopSS screen, a second operator slowly moves the CLDF focusing lens, according to the refractive error of the examined eye.

CHANGES TO CHOROIDAL BLOOD FLOW IN AGE-RELATED MACULAR DEGENERATION

Metabolic changes of the RPE owing to senescence are considered the main cause of early clinical findings in AMD. These findings include various forms of drusen, hyperpigmentation, and RPE atrophy in nonexudative AMD; and subfoveal neovascularization in exudative AMD. However, vascular changes in the choroid might have secondary deleterious effects on the RPE.

A healthy RPE is necessary for the preservation of the choriocapillaris. Indeed, it was experimentally shown in animal models that RPE loss produced by substances injected intravitreally (28) or intravenously (sodium iodate) (29), or by surgical removal (30,31) induce choriocapillaris degeneration.

In addition to environmental influences (smoking, sunlight exposure, and nutritional factors), many of the risk factors for AMD are similar to those for cardiovascular diseases, such as hypertension. This suggests a vascular role in the development of AMD.

In eyes with neovascular AMD, delayed choroidal filling (3,32,33) associated with a diffuse thickening of Bruch's membrane (2) leads to a greater incidence of geographic atrophy (4). The functional significance of delayed choroidal filling is expressed by an increased scotopic threshold on static perimetry (34), and is associated with a high risk of vision loss (4).

Recent ICG-A findings showed a statistically significant increase in the frequency of presumed macular watershed areas (assumed to be choroidal areas of hypoperfusion) in 55% of AMD patients compared with 15% of normal, control individuals. Further, the abnormal new vessels developed from the presumed macular watershed areas in 92% of eyes with CNV (35).

Indocyanine green angiography studies were performed by scanning laser ophthalmoscopy to assess choroidal perfusion and dye intensity curves in the choriocapillaris were recorded in four areas around the macular area and two areas in the temporal peripapillary retina (36,37). The results demonstrated a significant delayed and heterogeneous filling of the dye in the choriocapillaries in nonexudative AMD patients compared to control, non-AMD individuals (38). A statistically significant correlation between choroidal perfusion defects, visual acuity, and severity of non-neovascular AMD was observed as well. In addition, retrobulbar hemodynamics assessment by color Doppler imaging indicates increased pulsatility and decreased end-diastolic blood flow velocity of the short posterior ciliary arteries and the central retinal artery in AMD patients compared with controls, suggesting a more generalized perfusion defect than just the choroid (5,39).

Friedman (1,5,40) has hypothesized that there is a generalized vascular stiffening in AMD patients, leading to an increase in resistance of both choroidal and cerebral circulations. If the choroidal resistance increase subsequent to the stiffening of the vessels is bigger than the cerebral, choroidal perfusion will decrease, causing an increase in the osmotic gradient against which the RPE must pump. This increased gradient could lead to an accumulation of metabolic debris and drusen formation.

A study by Grunwald and coworkers (20), of the effect of age on choroidal blood flow demonstrated no significant correlation between ChBVel and subjects' age. However, ChBVol differed significantly between younger (up to 45 years) and older subjects (46 to 76 years). A significant decrease of ChBF with age was observed (20). These authors also demonstrated that ChBF is 37% lower in AMD patients than in age-matched control subjects. This decrease was mainly owing to a decrease of ChBVol (21). An investigation by Straubhaar and associates (22) in a larger cohort of normal subjects revealed an age-related decrease of ChBVel.

It is important to mention here that comparison between the LDF flow parameters obtained in various subjects is strictly valid only if the scattering properties of the tissue volume from which the LDF flow parameters have been obtained are identical. This is owing to the fact that the Doppler shift power spectrum depends not only on the number and velocity of red blood cells in the sampled volume, but also on the optical characteristics (i.e., the absorption and scattering coefficients) of the tissue sampled. In general, increased tissue scattering broadens the power spectrum and causes an artifactual increase in the measured mean blood velocity. It is not clear yet how the scattering of light by the tissue in the region of the fovea changes with age or the presence of AMD pathology, and therefore how it may affect the measured flow parameters (41).

Using a laser interferometric method, local fundus pulsation amplitudes (FPAs) were obtained from retinal areas associated with CNV and from healthy retinal areas adjacent to CNV in order to assess differences of pulsatile blood flow (42–44). In eyes with neovascular AMD, FPAs were consistently lower from CNV-associated retinal areas than from the surrounding healthy retina (44). This finding may reflect either a reduced pulsatile blood flow in the choroid and/or may be attributed to changes in layer structure. It also could be a consequence of a decrease of the local vascular resistance resulting from the formation of choroidal new vessels.

AGE-RELATED CHANGES OF CHOROIDAL BLOOD FLOW REGULATION

In healthy volunteers ChBF is maintained largely constant in spite of increases in the mean ocular perfusion pressure (PPm) up to 67% of the baseline value, when PPm is raised by means of isometric exercises (Fig. 14.4.2) (24). During the isometric exercise, blood pressure in the brachial artery rises in parallel with that in the ophthalmic artery, and the intraocular pressure does not change significantly (45). Consequently, as discussed by Riva and coworkers (24), the maintenance of constant ChBF in spite of the increased PPm is achieved through an increase in choroidal vascular resistance by a mechanism that probably involves the sympathetic nervous system (46–48).

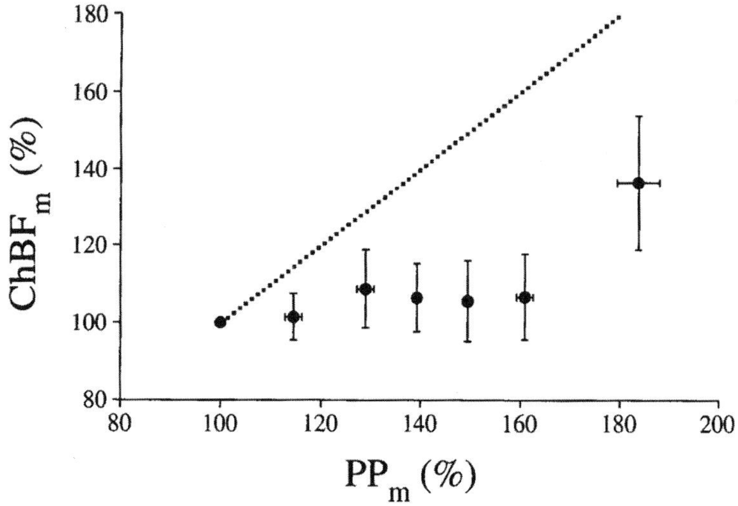

FIGURE 14.4.2. Average choroidal blood flow versus perfusion pressure during isometric exercise in 22 eyes of 11 healthy volunteers. (From: Riva CE, Titze P, Hero M, et al. Effect of acute decreases of perfusion pressure on choroidal blood flow in humans. *Invest Ophthalmol Vis Sci* 1997;38:1752–1760, with permission.)

Aging causes loss of neurons and adrenergic nerve terminations in various human systems, including the choroidal circulation (49). Further, age-related morphologic and functional changes to the vascular endothelium of the choroidal vessels probably alters the release of vasoactive substances, which in turn may affect the regulation of ChBF.

To assess the effects of early AMD on the regulation of ChBF in response to an acute increase in systemic blood pressure, a study monitored ChBF during isometric exercise designed to induce a temporary elevation of the blood pressure (50). Laser Doppler flowmetry measurements in 14 eyes of 14 patients (mean age 76.8 ± 7.7 SD years) with

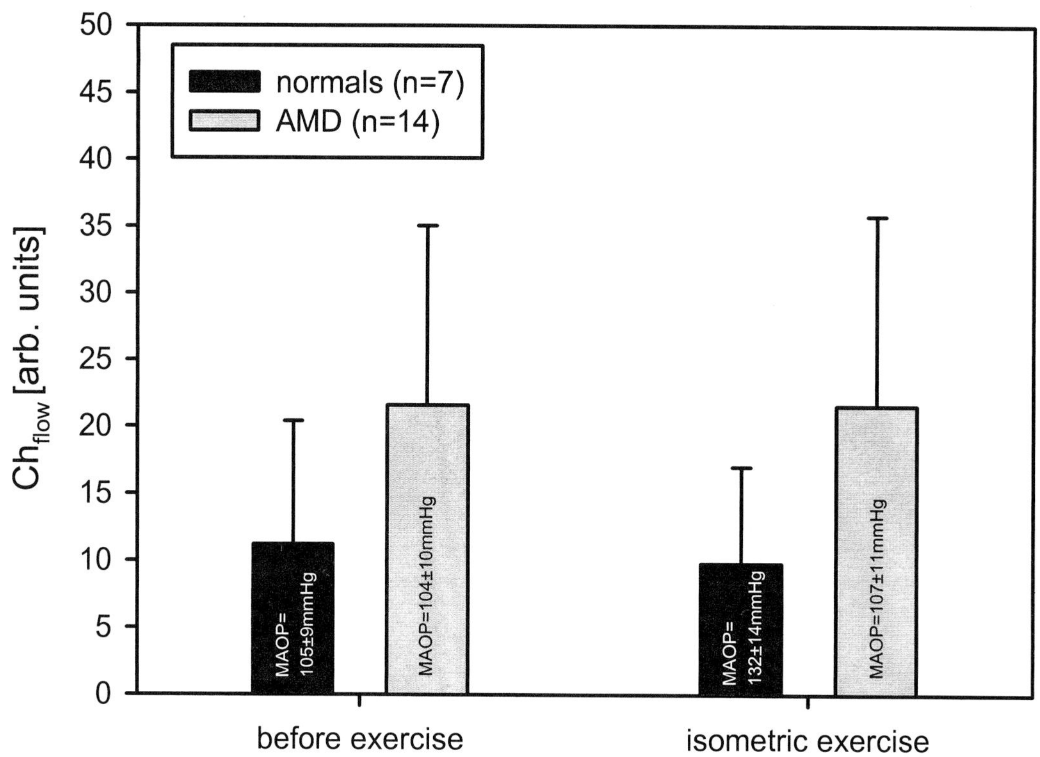

FIGURE 14.4.3. Mean choroidal blood flow ± SD at baseline, after exercise, and after recovery from exercise in age-matched healthy individuals *(black columns)* and patients with early AMD *(striate columns).* MAOP, the mean arterial ophthalmic pressure.

early degenerative macular changes, such as pigmentary changes or hard drusen, were compared with those obtained from seven eyes of seven healthy volunteers (mean age 78.1 ± 5.0 SD years). Baseline systemic blood pressure, ChBF, ChBVel, and ChBVol were measured in AMD patients and healthy volunteers at rest (sitting). Patients and volunteers were then asked to stand up and to squat for as long as possible to induce an elevation of systemic blood pressure. The same measurements were taken again when the patients and volunteers could no longer remain in the skating position. Muscular weakness was the limiting factor. A third set of measurements was taken after recovery, once blood pressure had returned to the basal level.

The mean elevation of blood pressure during isometric exercises was identical for the two groups (34% ± 13% SD). No significant differences were detected in the changes of ChBVel, ChBVol, and ChBF in subjects with or without AMD ($p > 0.05$).

As found in normal controls, acute elevation of the systemic blood pressure induced by isometric exercise does not affect choroidal blood flow in elderly subjects with early macular changes (Fig. 14.4.3). Regulation of choroidal blood flow during isometric exercise induces an acute elevation of blood pressure that seems to be preserved in the early stages of AMD and with increasing age.

Identical measurements were performed in a group of healthy individuals (>45 years old) and a group of age-matched subjects presenting with neovascular AMD. Table 14.4.1 shows the percent changes relative to resting values of PPm, vascular resistance (Rm), and LDF parameters at the end exercise in both groups. Although the mean elevation of PPm during isometric exercise was similar for the controls and the neovascular groups (19.8% ± 3.5%, and 22.6% ± 3.9% CI, two-tailed independent Student's t-test, p = 0.99% CI = 95% confidence interval, respectively), a statistically significant (14.6% + 6.2 % CI, $p = 0.006$ n = 24), increase of ChBF only in the neovascular subretinal tissue was observed. The increased blood flow in the neovascular tissue results from an insufficient increase in vascular resistance. Therefore, an overperfusion in the neovascular tissue should occur, as was reported previously in eyes with retinal neovascularization.

TABLE 14.4.1. LASER DOPPLER FLOWMETRY PARAMETERS, PPM, AND RM CHANGES DURING ISOMETRIC EXERCISE

Normals >45		New Vessels	
PPm (mm Hg)	19.8 ± 3.5	PPm (mm Hg)	22.6 ± 3.9
Vel_{Ch} (kHz)	5.1 ± 8.3	Vel_{Ch} (kHz)	12.0 ± 11.2[a]
Vol_{Ch} (AU)	−2.3 ± 6.6	Vol_{Ch} (AU)	5.2 ± 7.0
$Flow_{Ch}$ (AU)	0.5 ± 1.7	$Flow_{Ch}$ (AU)	14.6 ± 6.2[a]
Rm	19.5 ± 4.1	Rm	8.4 ± 5.3

[a]Statistically significant $p = 0.006$.

CHANGES IN CHOROIDAL BLOOD FLOW FOLLOWING PHOTODYNAMIC THERAPY

Fluorescein angiographic evaluation of subfoveal neovascular tissue treated with PDT reveals that after an initial 4-week period of hypofluorescence, a reperfusion of the treated neovascular tissue occurs. The early hypofluorescence may result from a masking effect of an exudate originating from the breakdown of the vascular/RPE barrier within the treated area. Optical coherence tomography findings have indicated an increase of subretinal fluid following PDT; however, this would be insufficient to block fluorescence and such a phenomenon should persist to the late phases of the angiogram. The subretinal neovascularization does not usually disappear after PDT, but shows an absence of leakage. ICG-A studies indicate the persistence of feeder vessels within the treated area in more than 50% of eyes. In addition, ICG-A revealed a complete recovery of the surrounding normal choriocapillaris in the majority of treated eyes at the 12-week follow-up examination after PDT (7).

Confocal laser Doppler flowmetry was used to measure the subfoveal choroidal blood flow within an area of choroidal neovascularization before and after PDT (51). The laser beam was focused to a depth of approximately 300 μm from the inner limiting membrane. The LDF parameters were measured in 17 eyes, three times for about 10 seconds each time and then averaged.

Immediately after PDT, ChBF decreased by an average of 74% ± 25% ($p < 0.001$) compared with the pretreatment level. One week after PDT, eight of the 10 patients who did not have sustained closure of the neovascular membranes following PDT had increased ChBF (group average 100%). Five of the seven patients with partially or fully closed neovascular membranes had decreased ChBF (group average 34%). There was a significant correlation between the change in ChBF (decrease or increase) and the outcome of PDT (closure or reopening) ($x^2 = 4$, $p < 0.05$). These results taken immediately after PDT indicate a significant closure of the neovascular membranes, whereas those obtained 1 week after PDT suggest that ChBF in CNV is correlated in some patients with the short-term effect of PDT (51). However, additional assessment of five eyes failed to indicate any significant changes in the LDF measurements of the subfoveal area at baseline and 1 and 4 weeks after PDT (Fig. 14.4.4).

The obvious question that arises from these results is whether regression of subretinal CNV is related to changes in blood flow regulation within the neovascular tissue. Confocal LDF measurements were taken at baseline and during an increase in PPm in 10 eyes of 10 patients with subretinal CNV (mean age 67 ± 13 years) before PDT and 2 weeks after PDT. Before PDT treatment, isometric exercise induced a significant increase in PPm (18.7% ± 5.7% CI), resulting in an increase of ChBF within the neovascular tis-

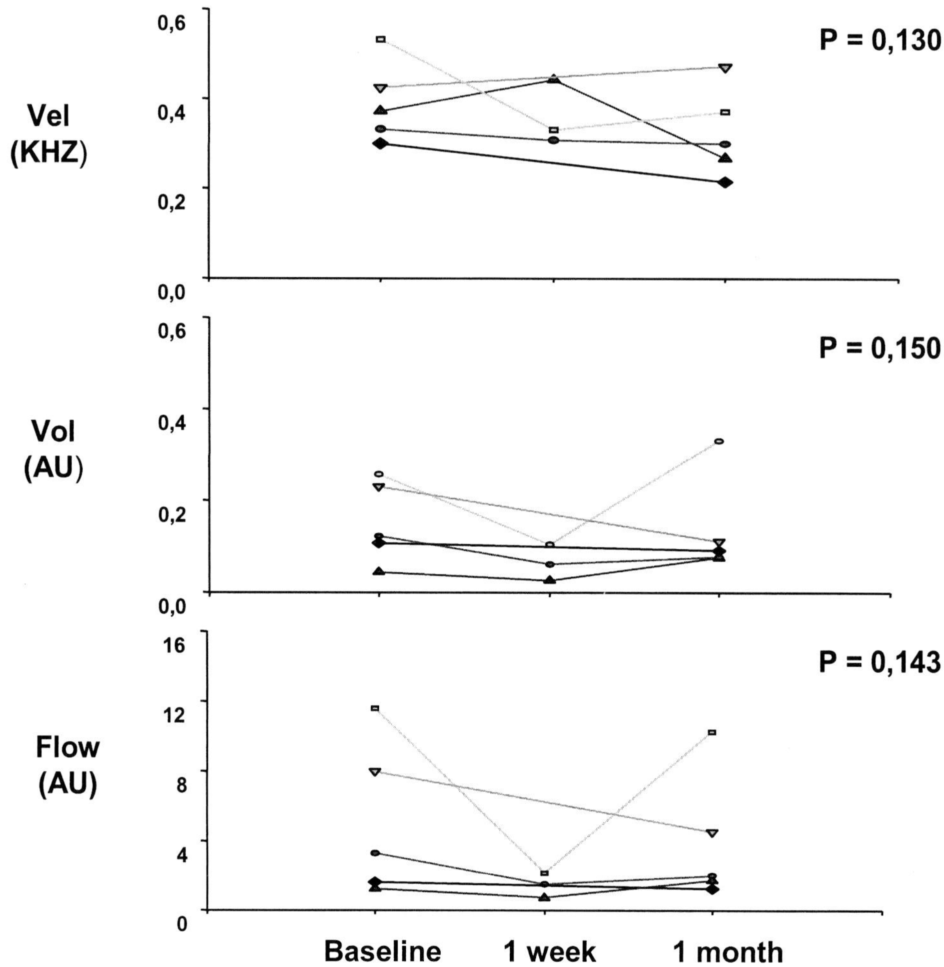

FIGURE 14.4.4. Relative change in subfoveal laser Doppler flowmeter measurements taken at baseline, and at 1 and 4 weeks after PDT (n = 5). No statistically significant changes were observed.

sue (17.4% ± 13.5% CI, two-tailed independent Student's t-test, p = 0.04). Laser Doppler flowmetry measurements were also taken in the same eyes 2 weeks after PDT (14.8 ± 7 days). During squatting, PPm increased in 28.7% ± 11.1% CI; however, the LDF measurements did not change significantly (Table 14.4.2).

Thus, the determination of the response of ChBF might allow the testing of whether or not measurements were made within an abnormal vascular bed. Laser Doppler flowmetry measurements post–PDT combined with FA findings might be useful in the evaluation of long-term efficacy of this treatment.

TABLE 14.4.2. MEAN LASER DOPPLER FLOWMETRY PARAMETERS, PPM, AND RM, AT BASELINE AND DURING ISOMETRIC EXERCISE

	Before PDT		After PDT	
	Baseline	End Exercise	Baseline	End Exercise
PPm (mm Hg)	55.0 ± 4.3	65.0 ± 6.9[a]	52.0 ± 2.1	67.0 ± 4.9[a]
Vel$_{Ch}$ (kHz)	1.37 ± 0.28	1.7 ± 0.35[a]	1.37 ± 0.28	1.25 ± 0.21
Vol$_{Ch}$ (AU)	2.74 ± 1.33	2.7 ± 1.41	77 ± 0.87	2.02 ± 1.03
Flow$_{Ch}$ (AU)	82.0 ± 46.0	90.0 ± 48.0[a]	51.0 ± 26	56 ± 32
Rm	1.19 ± 0.48	1.23 ± 0.53	1.61 ± 0.72	1.8 ± 0.75[a]

[a]Statistically significant.

CONCLUSIONS

Quantitative information on choroidal hemodynamics and regulation of ChBF in normal and diseased human eyes was obtained by computer-assisted analysis of LDF methods, which provides a relatively continuous measurement of ChBVel, ChBVol, and ChBF in the subfoveal choroid. Such information may contribute to an improved understanding of the physiologic parameters in the choroidal circulation.

Laser Doppler flowmetry findings suggest both a significant aged-related decrease of choroidal blood flow and a significant decrease of ChBF in AMD patients compared to age-matched control subjects, although these results must be interpreted with caution because ChBF is influenced by the scattering properties of the sampled volume, which may vary with age and disease. As found in normal controls, acute elevation of the systemic blood pressure induced by isometric exercises does not appear to affect ChBF in elderly subjects with early macular changes.

Acute elevation of blood pressure induces increased blood flow in neovascular tissue because vascular resistance does not increase sufficiently. This leads to an overperfusion of the neovascular tissue.

LDF measurements made 2 weeks after PDT in patients with neurovascular AMD indicated a regulation of subfoveal blood flow similar to that measured in age-matched healthy eyes, suggesting that the measurements were made in a vascular bed that recovered normal blood flow regulation.

The use of choroidal LDF to analyze ChBF regulation may determine whether measurements were made within an abnormal vascular bed. Comparison of the results of LDF with angiographic findings may be useful when evaluating the long-term efficacy of PDT for the treatment of CNV in patients with AMD.

REFERENCES

1. Friedman E. The role of the atherosclerotic process in the pathogenesis of age-related macular degeneration. *Am J Ophthalmol* 2000;130:658–663.
2. Pauleikhoff D, Chen JC, Chisholm IH, et al. Choroidal perfusion abnormality with age-related Bruch's membrane change. *Am J Ophthalmol* 1990;109:211–217.
3. Remulla JF, Gaudio AR, Miller S, et al. Foveal electroretinograms and choroidal perfusion characteristics in fellow eyes of patients with unilateral neovascular age-related macular degeneration. *Br J Ophthalmol* 1995;79:558–561.
4. Piguet B, Palmvang IB, Chisholm IH, et al. Evolution of age-related macular degeneration with choroidal perfusion abnormality. *Am J Ophthalmol* 1992;113:657–663.
5. Friedman E, Krupsky S, Lane AM, et al. Ocular blood flow velocity in age-related macular degeneration. *Ophthalmology* 1995;102:640–646.
6. Treatment of Age-related Macular Degeneration with Photodynamic Therapy (TAP) Study Group. Photodynamic therapy of subfoveal choroidal neovascularization in age-related macular degeneration with verteporfin: one-year results of 2 randomized clinical trials. *Arch Ophthalmol* 1999;117:1329–1345.
7. Ghazi NG, Jabbour NM, DeLa Cruz ZC, et al. Clinicopathologic studies of age related macular degeneration with classic subfoveal neovascularization treated with photodynamic therapy. *Retina* 2001;21(5):478–486.
8. Schmidt-Erfurth U. Indocyanine green angiography and retinal sensitivity after photodynamic therapy of subfoveal choroidal neovascularization. *Semin Ophthalmol* 1999;14:35–44.
9. Alm A, Bill A. Ocular circulation. In: Moses RA, Hart WM, eds. *Adler's physiology of the eye: clinical applications*, 8th ed. St. Louis: Mosby-Year Book, 1987:183–203.
10. Alm A, Bill A. Ocular and optic nerve blood flow at normal and increased intraocular pressure in monkeys (Macaca irus): a study with radioactively labeled microspheres including flow determinations in brain and some other tissues. *Exp Eye Res* 1973;15:15–29.
11. Alm A, Bill A. Blood flow and oxygen extraction in the cat uvea at normal and high intraocular pressures. *Acta Physiol Scand* 1970;80:19–28.
12. Hickam JB, Frayser R, Ross JC. A study of retinal venous blood oxygen saturation in human subjects by photographic means. *Circulation* 1963;27:375–385.
13. Törnquist P, Alm A. Retinal and choroidal contribution to retinal metabolism in vivo. A study in pigs. *Acta Physiol Scand* 1979;106:351–357.
14. Bill A. Calorimetric procedures for the study of the blood flow through the ciliary region and the choroid in rabbits. *Acta Ophthalmol* 1962;40:131–148.
15. Bill A. Intraocular pressure and blood flow through the uvea. *Arch Ophthalmol* 1962;67:336–348.
16. Friedman E, Kopald HH, Smith TR. Retinal and choroidal blood flow determined with krypton-85 in anesthetized animals. *Invest Ophthalmol Vis Sci* 1964;3:539–547.
17. Alm A, Bill A. The oxygen supply to the retina. II. Effects of high intraocular pressure and of increased arterial carbon dioxide on uveal and retinal blood flow in cats. A study with radioactively labeled microspheres including flow determinations in brain and some other tissues. *Acta Physiol Scand* 1972;84:306–319.
18. Yu DY, Alder VA, Cringle SJ, et al. Choroidal blood flow measured in the dog eye in vivo and in vitro by local hydrogen clearance polarography: validation of a technique and response to raised intraocular pressure. *Exp Eye Res* 1988;46:289–303.
19. Riva CE, Cranstoun SD, Grunwald JE, et al. Choroidal blood flow in the foveal region of the human ocular fundus. *Invest Ophthalmol Vis Sci* 1994;35:4273–4281.
20. Grunwald JE, Hariprasad SM, DuPont J. Effect of aging on foveolar choroidal circulation. *Arch Ophthalmol* 1998;116:150–154.
21. Grunwald JE, Hariprasad SM, DuPont J, et al. Foveolar choroidal blood flow in age-related macular degeneration. *Invest Ophthalmol Vis Sci* 1998;39:385–390.
22. Straubhaar M, Orgül S, Gugleta K, et al. Choroidal laser Doppler flowmetry in healthy subjects. *Arch Ophthalmol* 2000;118:211–215.
23. Riva CE, Titze P, Hero M, et al. Effect of acute decreases of perfusion pressure on choroidal blood flow in humans. *Invest Ophthalmol Vis Sci* 1997;38:1752–1760.
24. Riva CE, Titze P, Hero M, et al. Choroidal blood flow during isometric exercises. *Invest Ophthalmol Vis Sci* 1997;38:2338–2343.
25. Geiser M, Riva CE, Dorner GT, et al. Response of choroidal blood flow in the foveal region to hyperoxia and hyperoxia-hypercapnia. *Curr Eye Res* 2000;21:669–676.
26. Longo A, Geiser M, Riva CE. Subfoveal choroidal blood flow in response to light-dark exposure. *Invest Ophthalmol Vis Sci* 2000;41:2678–2683.
27. Petrig BL, Riva CE, Lorenz B, et al. Confocal laser Doppler sys-

tem for measurements of blood velocity in retinal vessels and flow in the optic nerve through the undilated pupil. In: *Laser and light*, vol. 8. The Hague: Kugler, 1998:137–142.
28. Takeuchi M, Itagaki T, Takahashi K, et al. Changes in the intermediate stage of retinal degeneration after intravitreal injection of ornithine. *Nippon Ganka Gakkai Zasshi* 1993;97:17–28.
29. Henkind P, Gartner S. The relationship between retinal pigment epithelium and the choriocapillaris. *Trans Ophthalmol Soc UK* 1983;103:444–447.
30. Del Priore LV, Hornbeck R, Kaplan HJ, et al. Debridement of the pig retinal pigment epithelium in vivo. *Arch Ophthalmol* 1995;113:939–944.
31. Del Priore LV, Kaplan HJ, Hornbeck R, et al. Retinal pigment epithelial debridement as a model for the pathogenesis and treatment of macular degeneration. *Am J Ophthalmol* 1996;122: 629–643.
32. Boker T, Fang T, Steinmetz R. Refractive error and choroidal perfusion characteristics in patients with choroidal neovascularization and age-related macular degeneration. *Ger J Ophthalmol* 1993;2:10–13.
33. Zhao J, Frambach DA, Lee PP, et al. Delayed macular choriocapillary circulation in age-related macular degeneration. *Int Ophthalmol* 1995;19:1–12.
34. Chen JC, Fitzke FW, Pauleikhoff D, et al. Functional loss in age-related Bruch's membrane change with choroidal perfusion defect. *Invest Ophthalmol Vis Sci* 1992;33:334–340.
35. Ross RD, Barofsky JM, Cohen G, et al. Presumed macular choroidal watershed vascular filling, choroidal neovascularization, and systemic vascular disease in patients with age-related macular degeneration. *Am J Ophthalmol* 1998;125:71–80.
36. Ciulla TA, Harris A, Danis RP. Presumed macular choroidal watershed vascular filling, choroidal neovascularization, and systemic vascular disease in patients with age-related macular degeneration. *Am J Ophthalmol* 1998;126:153–155.
37. Harris A, Chung HS, Ciulla TA, et al. Progress in measurement of ocular blood flow and relevance to our understanding of glaucoma and age-related macular degeneration. *Prog Retin Eye Res* 1999;18:669–687.
38. Ciulla TA, Harris A, Chung HS, et al. Choroidal perfusion is delayed in non-exudative age-related macular degeneration. *Br J Ophthalmol* 2002;86(2):209–213.
39. Ciulla TA, Harris A, Chung HS, et al. Color Doppler imaging discloses reduced ocular blood flow velocities in non-exudative age-related macular degeneration. *Am J Ophthalmol* 1999;128: 75–80.
40. Friedman E. A hemodynamic model of the pathogenesis of age-related macular degeneration. *Am J Ophthalmol* 1997;124: 677–682.
41. Riva CE. Basic principles of laser Doppler flowmetry and application to the ocular circulation. *Int Ophthalmol* 2001;23: 183–189.
42. Schmetterer L, Lexer F, Unfried C, et al. Topical measurement of fundus pulsations. *Opt Eng* 1995;34:711–716.
43. Schmetterer L, Wolzt M, Lexer F, et al. The effect of hyperoxia and hypercapnia on fundus pulsations in the macular and the optic disc region in healthy young men. *Exp Eye Res* 1995;61: 685–690.
44. Schmetterer L, Kruger A, Findl O, et al. Topical fundus pulsation measurements in age-related macular degeneration. *Graefes Arch Clin Exp Ophthalmol* 1998;236:160–163.
45. Robinson F, Riva CE, Gruwald JE, et al. Retinal blood flow autoregulation in response to an acute increase in blood pressure. *Invest Ophthalmol Vis Sci* 1986;27:722–726.
46. Alm A, Bill A. The effect of stimulation of the cervical sympathetic chain on retinal oxygen tension and on uveal, retinal and cerebral blood flow in cats. *Acta Physiol Scand* 1973;88:84–96.
47. Alm A. The effect of sympathetic stimulation on blood flow through the uvea, retina, and optic nerve in monkeys (Macaca irus). *Exp Eye Res* 1977;25:19–24.
48. Ernest JT. The effect of systolic hypertension on rhesus monkey eyes after ocular sympathectomy. *Am J Ophthalmol* 1977;84: 341–344.
49. Nuzzi R, Finazzo C, Grignolo FM. Modifications de l'innervation adrénergique de la choroïde pendant la sénescence. *J Fr Ophtalmol* 1996;19:89–96.
50. De Gottrau P, Pournaras CJ, Petrig BL, et al. Regulation of subfoveolar choroidal blood flow in age-related macular degeneration. *Invest Opthalmol Vis Sci* 2000;41:S159.
51. Petrig BL, Chamot S, Riva CE, et al. Subfoveal blood flow in choroidal neovascularization before and after photodynamic therapy as measured by TopSS-based confocal laser Doppler flowmeter. *Invest Opthalmol Vis Sci* 2000;41:S177.

Part 5: Results of Age-Related Macular Degeneration Trials Using Verteporfin PDT: Phases I and II

JOAN W. MILLER
EVANGELOS S. GRAGOUDAS

Preclinical studies demonstrated that verteporfin (Visudyne, Novartis Pharmaceuticals, Basel, Switzerland) photodynamic therapy (PDT) could occlude laser-injury experimental choroidal neovascularization (CNV) with cessation of angiographic leakage on fluorescein angiography (FA) and thrombotic occlusion of vessels on histologic examination (1–3). By controlling the drug dose, the light dose (fluence and irradiance), and the timing of light irradiation, the outcome could be relatively selective, with minimal effect on the choroid and surrounding retina and without injury to the retinal vessels. Typically, damage was noted at the level of the choriocapillaris and retinal pigment epithelium with minimal effects on photoreceptors. Preclinical studies also demonstrated the safety of higher irradiance treatment because standard PDT usually was performed previously at irradiances of 150 to 200 mW/cm^2 or lower, which required relatively long treatment times that were felt to be impractical for treatment of CNV. Irradiances as high as 1800 mW/cm^2 failed to produce thermal denaturation of collagen fibrils in the choroid, and 600 mW/cm^2 was selected as the treatment parameter for the clinical studies (4). In addition, preclinical studies demonstrated the recovery of normal structures (choriocapillaris and RPE) after single and repeated PDT in a dose-dependent fashion (5,6).

Based on these preclinical studies, a clinical study was designed to assess the safety of PDT and determine the maximum tolerated dose of PDT using verteporfin to treat CNV. It was later expanded by a number of treatment protocol amendments to make comparison evaluations on dosimetry. Inclusion criteria included subfoveal CNV secondary to AMD and other causes (7,8). This chapter covers the data for the 128 patients with CNV secondary to AMD. Of these, 97 patients had follow up planned through 3 months after a single treatment. Thirty-one patients were cared for with a course of multiple treatments. The remaining 13 patients had CNV secondary to other causes, which is discussed in Chapters 15 and 16.

DESIGN AND METHODOLOGY

The study was a nonrandomized, multicenter, open label trial using five different dose regimens. The inclusion and exclusion criteria are provided in Table 14.5.1, with the primary requirement of subfoveal CNV with some classic component. Standardized protocol refractions, visual acuity determinations, complete ophthalmic examinations, color fundus photography, and FA were performed at baseline (1 to 7 days prior to the day of treatment), and at follow-up weeks 1, 4, and 12. Repeat visual acuity testing without refraction also was performed on the day of treatment and 1 day after treatment. Additional testing was carried out at week 2 if any ocular adverse event was noted at week 1, or at any time between visits, if clinically indicated. In addition, each patient had vital signs measured, a physical examination, and an electrocardiogram performed at baseline and at week 12. Laboratory testing—including a complete blood count, serum cholesterol, triglycerides, blood urea nitrogen, creatinine, electrolytes, calcium, phosphorus, glucose, protein, albumin, bilirubin, liver function tests, and urinalysis—was performed at baseline and at weeks 1 and 12.

The size of the treatment spot was calculated using the baseline FA. The greatest linear dimension of the neovascular lesion was measured and this dimension was divided by 2.5 to account for the magnification of the camera systems used to yield the size of the lesion on the retina. Initially the dimension was divided by 3.0 based on MPS protocol, but this was found to be in error, and the method was modified for the PDT studies. A 600-μm border was added to the dimension on the retina to provide at least a 300-μm border at all edges. In some cases, the resulting treatment border at a given edge was greater than 300 μm, but was always less than 500 μm. This border provided adequate treatment despite small errors inherent in the size calculation because of the optics of the individual eye and any small movement by the patient or treating physician during treatment, and finally provided a border or margin beyond the CNV detected angiographically. The treatment spot was selected based on the available laser link settings (400 to 4,000 μm) and magnification of the contact lens, according to the lens manufacturer (David Dewey, personal communication).

TABLE 14.5.1. MAIN INCLUSION AND EXCLUSION CRITERIA

Inclusion criteria
Clinical signs of choroidal neovascularization (CNV) owing to any cause
CNV under the geometric center of the foveal avascular zone (subfoveal)
Some classic CNV (occult CNV could be but need not be present)
Greatest linear dimension of entire CNV ≤5,400 μm diameter
Nasal side of CNV ≥500 μm from temporal border of optic nerve
For CNV lesions recurring after standard laser therapy, foveal center must not have been included in area treated by laser
Best corrected visual acuity of 20/40 or worse
≥50 years of age
Exclusion criteria
Tears of the RPE at screening
Vitelliform-like detachment retinal pigment epithelium
Central serous retinopathy
Drusenoid pigment epithelium detachment alone
Additional retinovascular diseases compromising visual acuity of study eye
Use of investigational drugs, systemic steroids, cytokines, or photosensitive drugs in past 3 months
Significant hepatic, renal, or neurologic disease
Class III or IV cardiovascular disease (New York Heart Association functional status criteria)
Porphyria, porphyrin sensitivity, hypersensitivity to sunlight or bright artificial light
Any malignancy treatment
Any acute illness during screening or fever on day of treatment prior to verteporfin infusion
Uncontrolled hypertension
Ocular surgery within 3 months prior to study treatment

RPE, retinal pigment epithelium.

The initial study treatment regimen involved intravenous (iv) infusion of verteporfin (6 mg/m^2 or approximately 0.15 mg/kg), followed by irradiation 30 minutes after the start of dye infusion (Regimen 1) using 689-nm light delivered by a Coherent (Palo Alto, CA) Ocular Photoactivation Diode and Laser Link Slit Lamp, as described in a previous study (3). The delivered irradiance was kept constant at 600 mW/cm^2. Additional regimens were studied to determine whether more persistent closure of CNV could be obtained. These are listed in Table 14.5.2. In the first three treatment regimens, the

TABLE 14.5.2. TREATMENT REGIMENS 1 THROUGH 5 AND DURATION OF FOLLOW UP

Treatment Regimen	Verteporfin Dose (mg/m²)	No. of Minutes Over Which Infusion was Planned	Light Doses (J/cm²)	Time of Light Application After Start of Verteporfin Infusion (min)	No. of Patients	No. with 4-week Follow Up Before any Retreatment	No. with 12-week Follow Up Before any Retreatment
1	6	10 min	50, 75, 100, 150	30[a]	22	22	19[b]
2	6	10 min	50, 75, 100, 150	20	37	28[c]	17[d]
3	12	10 min	50, 75, 100, 150	30	19	19	19
4	6	10 min	50, 75, 100	15	22	22	11[e]
5	6	5 min	12.5, 25, 50	10	28	27[f]	25[g]

[a]Includes two patients in whom light administration was 39 and 55 minutes late.
[b]One patient withdrew after week 4 assessment; two patients received multiple photodynamic therapy (PDT) treatments after week 4, before week 12.
[c]Nine patients received multiple PDT treatments after week 1, before week 4.
[d]11 patients received multiple treatments after 4, before week 12.
[e]Nine patients received multiple treatments after week 4 but before week 12; two additional patients missed the week-12 follow-up visit.
[f]One patient withdrew before week 1.
[g]Two patients withdrew after week 4.
From Miller JW, Schmidt-Erfurth U, Sickenberg M, et al. Photodynamic therapy with verteporfin for choroidal neovascularization caused by age-related macular degeneration: results of a single treatment in a phase I and II study. *Arch Ophthalmol* 1999;117:1164, with permission.

light dose (fluence) was escalated from 50 to 75 to 100 to 150 J/cm², with a minimum of three patients at each light dose. In Regimen 4, the 150-J/cm² light dose was not included because of nonselective retinal vessel occlusion seen after PDT with this light dose in Regimens 2 and 3. In Regimen 5, lower light doses of 12.5, 25, and 50 J/cm² were included.

The patient was weighed on the day of treatment and the verteporfin solution was prepared as 6 or 12 mg/m². The verteporfin solution and iv tubing were wrapped in aluminum foil to protect the verteporfin from light. The verteporfin was infused using a syringe pump followed by a 5-mL flush of 5% dextrose solution (D_5W). Irradiation was performed at a specified time following the start of verteporfin infusion using the selected contact lens, and the duration of irradiation ranged from 21 to 250 seconds, depending on the light dose used (Table 14.5.2). The first 45 participants underwent cardiac monitoring during PDT using a two-lead rhythm strip, and vital signs were measured periodically. Initially, patients underwent retrobulbar injection of anesthetic of the study eye to ensure akinesia. This was discontinued after approximately 50 patients when it was judged to be unnecessary. Patients were instructed to avoid bright sunlight as much as possible over the 7 days following the procedure, and to wear special sunglasses with a low (4%) transmittance during that time.

RETREATMENT REGIMENS

Additional regimens involving retreatment at 2- and 4-week intervals were studied because preliminary results showed that the effect on angiographic leakage was only temporary. Repeated PDT treatments had been assessed in normal monkey eyes and demonstrated drug dose-dependent recovery of the RPE and choriocapillaris with minimal damage to the photoreceptors. Two sets of patients were studied, with the first group undergoing retreatment 2 to 4 weeks after the initial PDT treatment. A second set of patients had participated in the single treatment protocol. They were reenrolled in a retreatment protocol some time beyond week 12 but less than 6 months after their initial treatment if they met the criteria for retreatment at that time. Criteria for retreatment or reenrollment included the following: (a) evidence of fluorescein leakage from classic or occult CNV; (b) greatest linear dimension of leakage from CNV of less than 6,400 μm; (c) no adverse event judged to result from PDT; and (d) no additional ocular abnormality associated with visual loss identified since the first PDT. Criteria for reenrollment also required fluorescein leakage from classic CNV.

The first set of patients were given retreatment 2 to 4 weeks after the first PDT treatment. Following the first retreatment, follow-up FA was obtained and evaluated for CNV leakage 1 and 4 weeks after retreatment. If leakage had reappeared, an additional course of retreatment was applied at 2- or 4-week intervals, and a final evaluation was performed 12 weeks after the last retreatment. For the second set of patients, up to three additional courses of retreatment were to be instituted if indicated. In this group of patients, the second and third retreatments were scheduled at 4-week intervals, and final evaluation was performed 12 weeks after the last retreatment.

Treatment Regimens 2 and 4 (Table 14.5.2) were used in the retreatment protocols. The other aspects of the protocol, refraction, ophthalmic examination, PDT protocol, and follow-up were the same as for the single-treatment protocol.

OUTCOME MEASURES

Two measures were used to assess short-term efficacy and safety: (a) the extent of fluorescein leakage from the CNV (classic and occult); and (b) stabilization of the 12-week follow-up best-corrected visual acuity compared with baseline. A grading system was devised to semiquantitatively assess the effect of PDT on the extent (area) of fluorescein leakage from the CNV lesions at each follow-up visit compared with that seen at baseline (Table 14.5.3). Fluorescein leakage from classic and occult CNV was assessed without any knowledge of the PDT dosage. The extent of fluorescein leakage was graded based on the area of leakage compared to that present at baseline. The terminology in this chapter has been modified from the published study results in order to be consistent with that used subsequently to describe the findings of the Phase III trials. The different grades of fluorescein leakage from CNV were evaluated descriptively by treatment regimen and within subgroups. Comparisons between treatment regimens were performed using Fisher's exact test to assess differences in the degree of absence of leakage by visit. Two-by-two contingency tables were generated by collapsing the categories of leakage extent for each treatment regimen. Other fundus characteristics were graded from fundus photographs and angiograms, including the extent of subretinal hemorrhage, RPE atrophy, as well as retinal arteriolar, venular, and capillary nonperfusion.

Best-corrected visual acuity was obtained primarily as an indicator of safety, not efficacy, given the absence of a control group, the short period of follow up, and the known variability in the natural history of the disease. However, changes in visual acuity and angiographic leakage were used to compare the results among the regimens. A change in visual acuity of three or more lines was considered to be clinically significant. This exploratory analysis was used to select the treatment regimen for the subsequent randomized, placebo-controlled trial. Summary statistics (mean, median, and standard deviation) were generated for the change from baseline in visual acuity by treatment regimen and within subgroups. Further exploratory comparisons using ANOVA methods were performed to assess the relationship between visual acuity outcomes and baseline characteristics such as visual acuity, lesion size, lesion component, and lesion status. Adverse events, both ocular and systemic, were captured by the treating investigator and by the Reading Center review of fundus photographs and angiograms.

RESULTS

Single Treatment

One hundred twenty-eight patients with subfoveal CNV caused by AMD were treated with at least a single course of PDT, including 31 patients who later received multiple courses of PDT with Regimen 2 or 4. The baseline characteristics of the 128 patients in the Phase I and II studies indicated that most patients (80%) had a baseline visual acuity better than or equal to 20/200 in the eye to be treated, with both the mean and median baseline visual acuities measuring 20/125. The mean baseline lesion size was 5.1 macular photocoagulation study disc areas (DAs), with a range of one to 16 MPS disc areas, and was therefore larger than the lesions included in the MPS studies. Eighty-one (63%) of the CNV lesions presented with classic CNV in which the area of classic CNV was greater than or equal to 50% of the area of the lesion. Of these lesions, 41 (32%) had no occult CNV. Ten (8%) of the baseline lesions were judged to have no classic CNV on review by the Reading Center. Fibrosis was judged to be less than or equal to 50% of the lesion in 93% of the lesions.

The Phase I and II studies were designed primarily as safety trials, and in each regimen the light dose was escalated to determine a maximum tolerated dose before visual acuity changes, ocular adverse events, or systemic adverse events were noted. Dose-escalation in Regimen 1 did not result in any signs of toxicity, but also did not result in absence of fluorescein leakage from the CNV by week 12. Therefore, additional regimens were investigated with changes in the verteporfin dose, rate of verteporfin infusion, or timing of light irradiation, as well as repeated treatments to assess the effect on vision and fluorescein leakage from the CNV. At the highest light dose used (150 J/cm^2) in Regimens 2 and 3, PDT-related vision losses were observed in three patients. Two of the three patients treated using the 150 J/cm^2 light dose in Regimen 2 had significant vision loss at 12 weeks (losing five and nine lines, respectively). Two of five patients treated with 150 J/cm^2 in Regimen 3 had retinal vessel closure, one patient with occlusion of branch retinal arteries and veins in the posterior pole and 12 lines of vision loss at week 1, and one patient with extensive capillary nonperfusion (>30% of the treated area) and only minimal vision loss. Subsequently, patients were not treated at this light dose. The maximally tolerated light dose

TABLE 14.5.3. GRADING OF EXTENT OF FLUORESCEIN LEAKAGE FOLLOWING PHOTODYNAMIC THERAPY

Grade	Description
1. Absence of leakage	Absence of leakage from 100% of area of choroidal neovascularization (CNV) noted at baseline and no progression
2. Minimal leakage	Area of CNV <50% of the area of leakage noted at baseline and no progression
3. Moderate leakage	Area of CNV ≥50% of the area of leakage noted at baseline and no progression
4. Progression of leakage	Leakage from CNV beyond area of CNV noted at baseline, regardless of amount of leakage noted within area of leakage seen at baseline

TABLE 14.5.4. VISUAL ACUITY CHANGE FROM BASELINE BY VISIT AND TREATMENT REGIMEN WITH SINGLE TREATMENT

Week	Visual Acuity Change	Regimen 1 (n = 22)	Regimen 2 (n = 37)	Regimen 3 (n = 19)	Regimen 4 (n = 22)	Regimen 5 (n = 28)
1						
	≥3-Line gain	3 (14%)	6 (16%)	0 (0%)	5 (23%)	4 (15%)[a]
	No change	18 (81%)	29 (78%)	17 (89%)	15 (68%)	23 (85%)[a]
	≥3-Line loss	1 (5%)	2 (5%)	2 (11%)	2 (9%)	0 (0%)[a]
	Mean change	+0.7	+0.8	−0.9	+0.9	+1.4
	STD	1.5	2.6	2.9	2.5	2.0
	Range	−3 to +4	−7 to +8	−12 to +2	−3 to +7	−2 to +9
4						
	≥3-Line gain	3 (14%)	5 (18%)[b]	0 (0%)	3 (14%)	4 (15%)
	No change	18 (81%)	21 (75%)[b]	13 (68%)	18 (82%)	20 (74%)
	≥3-Line loss	1 (5%)	2 (7%)[b]	6 (32%)	1 (5%)	3 (11%)
	Mean change	+0.1	+0.3	−1.6	+1.1	+0.7
	STD	1.7	2.3	3.2	2.4	2.3
	Range	−3 to +4	−7 to +5	−9 to +2	−4 to +7	−4 to +7
12						
	≥3-Line gain	0 (0%)[c]	1 (6%)[d]	0 (0%)	4 (36%)[e]	3 (12%)[f]
	No change	18 (95%)[c]	12 (70%)[d]	15 (79%)	4 (36%)[e]	19 (76%)[f]
	≥3-Line loss	1 (5%)[c]	4 (24%)[d]	4 (21%)	3 (27%)[e]	3 (12%)[f]
	Mean change	−0.2	−0.9	−1.6	+0.4	+0.1
	STD	1.4	3.3	3.1	4.5	3.2
	Range	−3 to +2	−9 to +5	−9 to +2	−8 to +7	−8 to +9

STD, standard deviation.
[a]One patient withdrew before week 1.
[b]Nine patients received multiple photodynamic therapy (PDT) treatments after week 1, before week 4.
[c]One patient withdrew after week 4 assessment; two patients received multiple PDT treatments after week 4, before week 12.
[d]Eleven patients received multiple treatments after week 4, before week 12.
[e]Nine patients received multiple treatments after week 4 but before week 12: two additional patients missed the week-12 follow-up visit.
[f]Two patients withdrew after week 4.
From Miller JW, Schmidt-Erfurth U, Sickenberg M, et al. Photodynamic therapy with verteporfin for choroidal neovascularization caused by age-related macular degeneration: results of a single treatment in a phase I and II study. *Arch Ophthalmol* 1999;117:1166, with permission.

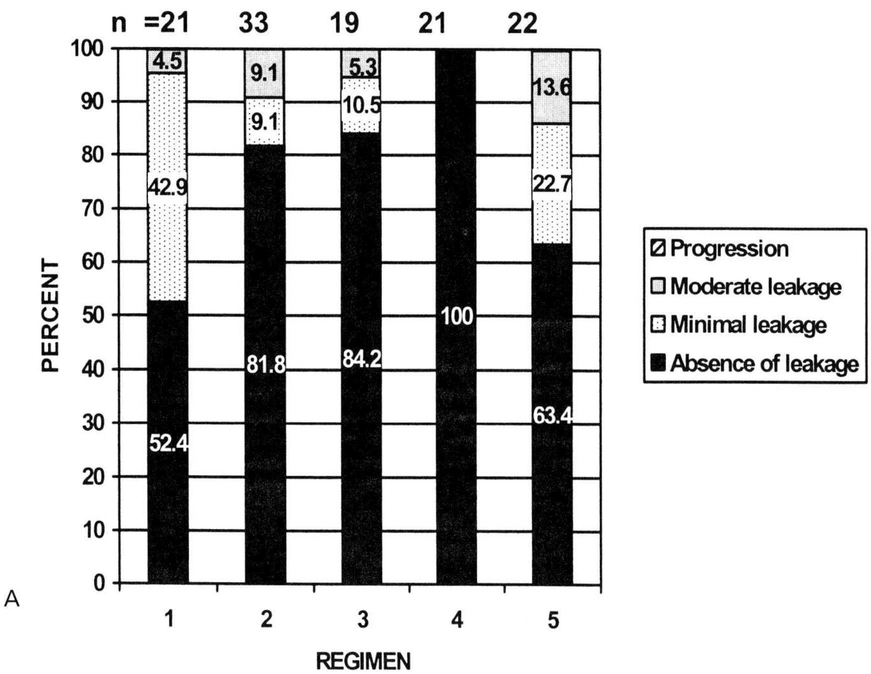

FIGURE 14.5.1. Grading of fluorescein leakage from classic choroidal neovascularization at week 1 **(A)**, week 4 **(B)**, and week 12 **(C)** in treatment Regimens 1 to 5 in patients with age-related macular degeneration after a first course of photodynamic therapy. (From: Miller J, Schmidt-Erfurth U, Sickenberg M, et al. Photodynamic therapy with verteporfin for choroidal neovascularization caused by age-related macular degeneration. Results of a single treatment in a Phase 1 and 2 study. *Arch Ophthalmol* 1999;117, with permission.)

for verteporfin treatment of CNV should be considered to be 100 J/cm^2.

The visual acuity findings are summarized in Table 14.5.4. Overall, PDT with verteporfin had no short-term effect on vision, with a mean change at week 1 of +0.7 lines. Interestingly, in a small number of patients (14%), substantial vision improvement of three or more lines was noted. There was a small but statistically significant difference in the mean visual acuity change at week 4 between Regimen 3 (−1.6 lines) and Regimen 4 (+1.1 lines), and was part of the basis for selecting Regimen 4 for subsequent trials. Exploratory analyses also demonstrated that patients with smaller lesions (≤4 MPS DA) and worse baseline vision (≤20/200) had better visual acuity outcomes. Additionally, patients with lesions composed of classic CNV only, showed a better visual acuity outcome at 12 weeks than those with lesions containing some occult component, gaining 0.6 lines compared to losing 0.8 lines. Some of these early findings were later corroborated in the Phase III clinical trials with 2-year follow up and placebo-controlled, randomized design.

Photodynamic therapy with verteporfin did have a demonstrable effect on fluorescein leakage from CNV. Figure 14.5.1

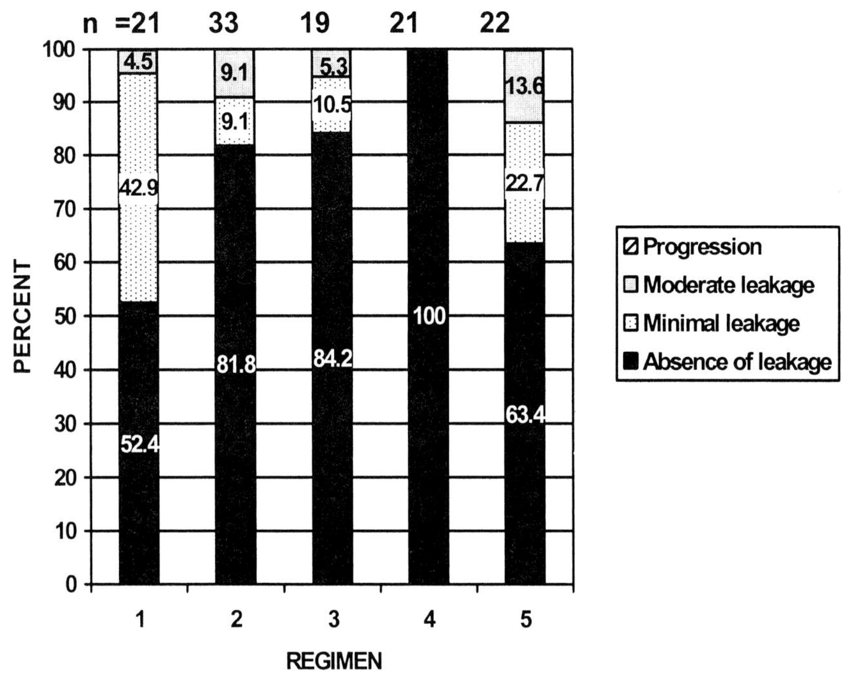

B

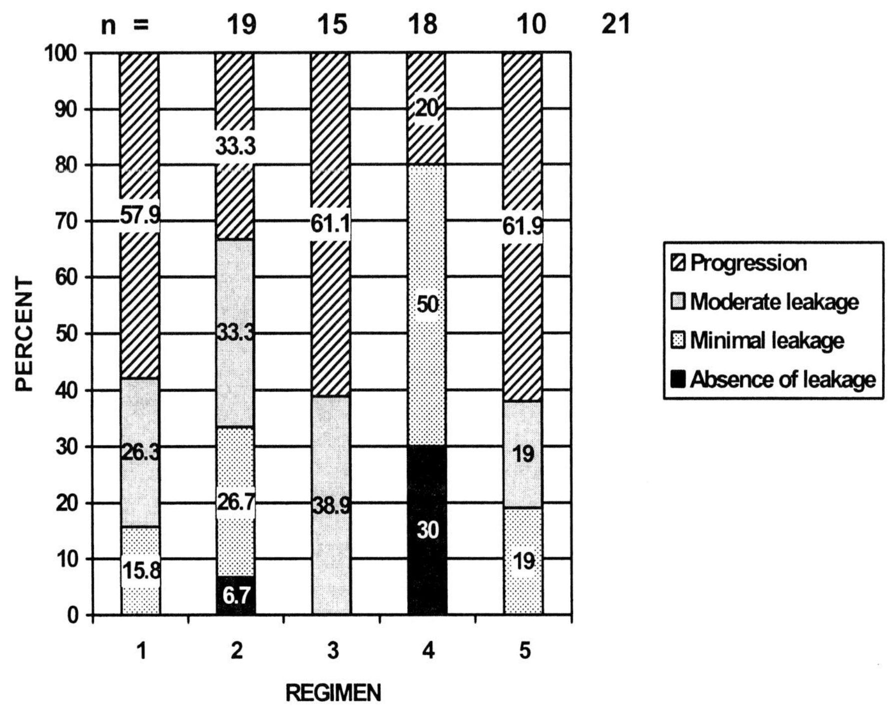

C

FIGURE 14.5.1 *(continued).*

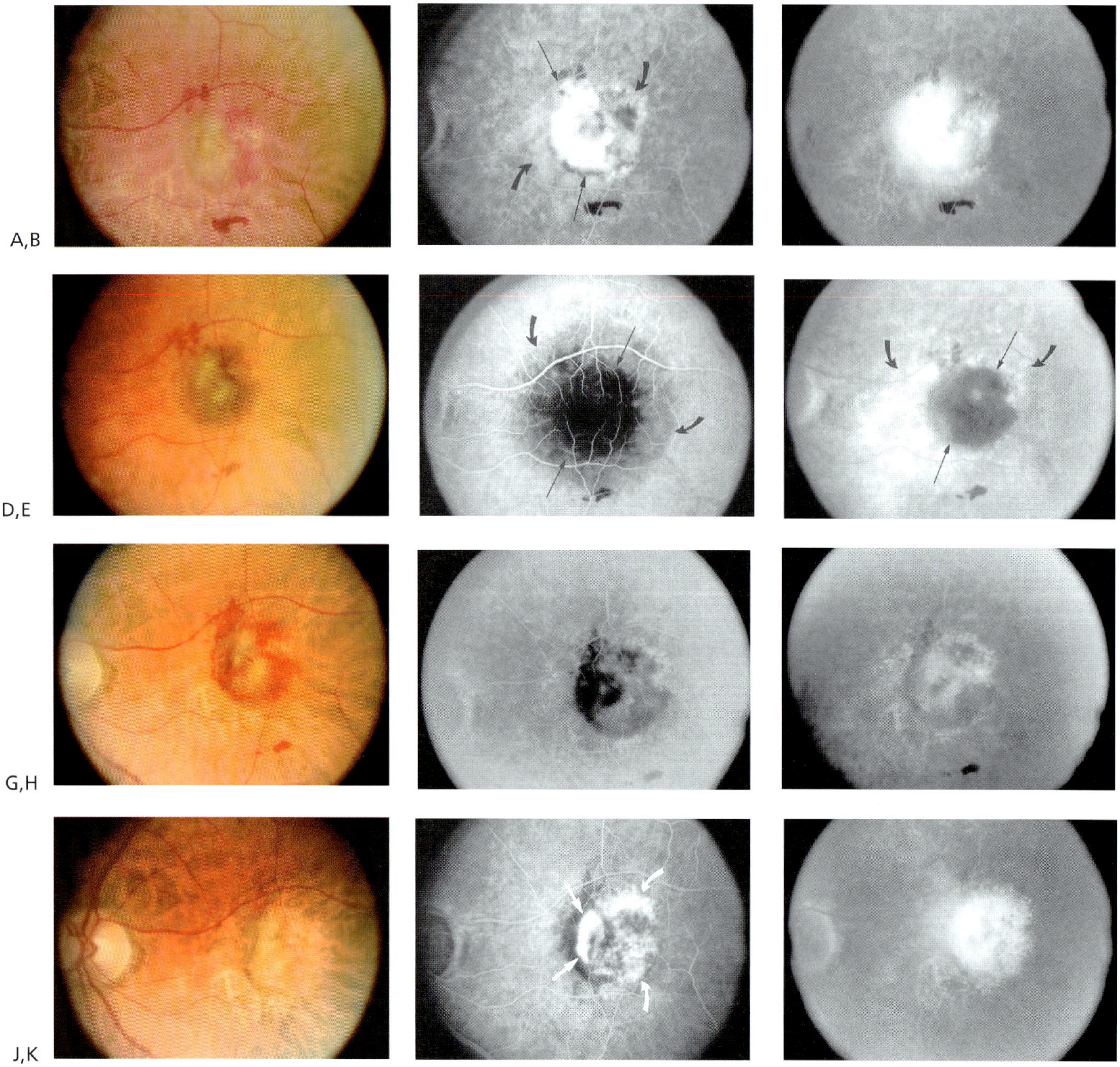

FIGURE 14.5.2. Baseline and follow-up images of a patient receiving a single treatment of photodynamic therapy (PDT) with verteporfin using Regimen 3 (light dose of 100 J/cm^2). Color fundus photograph from initial visit (visual acuity 20/50) **(A)** shows fibrovascular tissue with subretinal fluid and hemorrhage. Early phase fluorescein angiogram **(B)** shows a bright area of hyperfluorescence corresponding to classic choroidal neovascularization (CNV) *(straight arrows)*, with additional hyperfluorescence *(curved arrows)* corresponding to occult CNV. Both areas demonstrate leakage on late phase frame **(C)**. One week after PDT (visual acuity 20/64), color fundus photograph shows darker appearance of fibrovascular tissue **(D)**. Corresponding fluorescein angiogram, early-phase frame **(E)** shows a hypofluorescent area in the area of treatment with a darker center *(straight arrows)* and an additional area *(curved arrows)* of relatively less hypofluorescence. Late-phase frame **(F)** shows persistence of the central hypofluorescent area *(straight arrows)*. A hyperfluorescent area of staining *(curved arrows)* surrounds the hypofluorescence. Four weeks after PDT (visual acuity 20/50), color fundus photograph **(G)** shows a central fibrous component surrounded by hemorrhage. Corresponding fluorescein angiogram shows some hypofluorescence within the area of previous leakage **(H)**, with no leakage from classic CNV and minimal leakage from occult CNV seen in the late-phase frame **(I)** within the area previously occupied by classic and occult CNV. Twelve weeks after PDT (visual acuity 20/50), color fundus photograph **(J)** shows subretinal fibrosis and atrophy with complete clearing of subretinal hemorrhage. Corresponding fluorescein angiogram shows minimal leakage from classic CNV *(straight arrows)* and moderate leakage from occult CNV *(curved arrows)* in early- **(K)** and late-phase **(L)** frames, within the area occupied by classic and occult CNV at baseline **(B and C)**.

summarizes the change in fluorescein leakage from classic CNV for Regimens 1 through 5 at weeks 1, 4, and 12 (excluding patients with no classic CNV at baseline). At week 1, some cessation of fluorescein leakage was observed angiographically in all patients (Fig. 14.5.2). Absence of fluorescein leakage from classic CNV at week 1 occurred in 52% to 100% of patients, depending on the regimen used. Leakage typically reappeared in a portion of the CNV by week 4 in most patients in all regimens (Fig. 14.5.2). Regimen 4 resulted in the largest proportion of cases, with absence of leakage at week 1 (Fig. 14.5.1). Within Regimen 4, the 50 J/cm^2 light dose was associated with the highest percentage of patients with complete absence of leakage at week 4 and the lowest percentage of patients with progression of classic CNV at 12 weeks. These slight advantages, combined with the visual acuity differences observed, formed the basis for the selection of Regimen 4 using 50 J/cm^2 for the Phase III clinical trials. Otherwise, there was no obvious light-dose–response relationship in the ability to stop fluorescein leakage from classic CNV. Angiographic analysis identified a minimally effective dose because the lowest light doses of 12.5 and 25 J/cm^2 were ineffective in eliminating angiographic leakage. In addition, cases with leakage at week 4 were more likely to show progression at week 12, and once again Regimen 4 showed the lowest rate of leakage at week 4 and progression at week 12.

Leakage from occult CNV was qualitatively more difficult to grade. All eyes showed some fluorescence of the treated fibrovascular tissue or retina immediately surrounding the CNV in the late phase of the angiogram (Fig. 14.5.2). This staining was difficult to distinguish from the staining and leaking characteristics of occult CNV in many cases.

The extent of posttreatment fluorescein leakage from CNV relative to baseline also appeared to be correlated with visual acuity outcome. The 33 patients with lesions that showed a reduced area of leakage from both classic and occult CNV at 12 weeks, compared with baseline, had a mean change in visual acuity of +0.8 lines. In comparison, the 49 patients with lesions that developed progression of either classic, or occult, CNV by 12 weeks, lost 0.8 lines of vision. This difference was statistically significant (p = 0.012). This finding suggests that patients who demonstrate stabilization of fluorescein leakage from CNV after PDT may have a beneficial visual outcome if this stabilization can be maintained.

SAFETY

Thirty-eight (24%) of the 128 patients receiving a single course of PDT had an adverse event in the treatment eye, as reported by the treating ophthalmologists. Thirty-one of these patients had events that were judged to be possibly or probably treatment-related. Independent of the relationship to therapy, the highest incidence of adverse events in the treated eyes were as follows: increased subretinal hemorrhage (8.6%), increased fibrosis associated with CNV (8.6%), increased RPE atrophy (3.9%), subretinal hemorrhage (3.1%), eye pain (3.1%), fibrosis (3.1%), branch retinal arteriolar/venular nonperfusion (2.3%), choroidal vessel staining (1.6%), increased hemorrhage (1.6%), and vitreous hemorrhage (1.6%).

RETREATMENTS

Thirty-six patients with subfoveal CNV secondary to AMD were treated with multiple courses of PDT using verteporfin. Up to four treatments in total were performed, with two PDT regimens and two different retreatment intervals (2 and 4 weeks). The changes in visual acuity for patients undergoing retreatment with Regimens 2 and 4 are shown in Tables 14.5.5 and 14.5.6. The mean visual acuity remained stable after PDT treatment, and visual acuity was not reduced even after a second or third PDT application, and in fact showed a small improvement. Twelve weeks after the last retreatment for the 16 participants in Regimen 2, the average visual acuity was not changed (+0.1 lines) from baseline. Regimen 4 gave similar results, with a small initial increase and an average visual acuity decrease by one line from baseline, 12 weeks after the last retreatment.

Overall, retreatments at 2- and 4-week intervals did not lead to any more prolonged cessation of angiographic leakage. Fluorescein leakage was absent 1 week after the first treatment in almost all participants in Regimen 2 and in all participants in Regimen 4. Independent of the regimen, leakage from classic CNV was absent at 1 week after each retreatment. Typical recurrence of leakage was noted in a portion of the classic CNV 4 weeks after each PDT course. Recurrence with progression (beyond the original borders) ranged from 17% to 25% in Regimen 2, and was as high as 30% in Regimen 4. This was somewhat higher than the progression rate noted in the single-treatment study, but numbers were small and as noted before, patients were not randomly assigned to the different regimens, which made comparisons difficult. Twelve weeks after the last treatment, progression rates from classic CNV were 44% in Regimen 2, and 89% in Regimen 4. There was a notable on/off effect of PDT on fluorescein leakage with recurrence occurring after each treatment, but the area of leakage typically decreased over the retreatment schedule and was typically less at the last follow-up compared to baseline. A correlation of angiographic effects with visual acuity outcome was apparent in the retreatment study; an increase in mean visual acuity seemed to be associated with repeated achievement of eradication of leakage from classic CNV. As with the single-treatment study, lesions with only classic CNV seemed to respond best to retreatments, as demonstrated both angiographically and via visual acuity.

Safety evaluation in the retreatment study showed no arteriolar or venular nonperfusion, or any vitreous hemorrhage, and the highest light dose (150 J/cm^2) was not used in the

TABLE 14.5.5. CHANGE FROM BASELINE IN VISUAL ACUITY FOR PATIENTS RECEIVING MULTIPLE PHOTODYNAMIC THERAPY (PDT) TREATMENTS WITH REGIMEN 2

		Time After Most Recent PDT			
		Week 1		Week 4	
PDT Treatment	Number of Patients	Mean	Range	Mean	Range
First	16	−0.25	−5 to +4	−0.3[a]	−2 to +3
Second	16	+1.3	−2 to +5	+0.7[b]	−3 to +5
Third	12[c]	+1.2	−2 to +5	+0.3	−3 to +5
Last follow-up[d]	16	+0.1	−4 to +4		

[a]Four participants were retreated before week 4 and are not included in the week 4 mean or range for the "first treatment" row. Also, the five "reenrolled" patients are not included.
[b]No visual acuity data are available at this visit for one participant.
[c]Four participants did not receive a third treatment.
[d]Last follow up was week 16 after baseline for participants who had two treatments and week 20 for participants who had three treatments.
From Miller JW, Schmidt-Erfurth U, Sickenberg M, et al. Photodynamic therapy with verteporfin for choroidal neovascularization caused by age-related macular degeneration: results of a single treatment in a phase I and II study. *Arch Ophthalmol* 1999;117:1180, with permission.

retreatment study. Retinal capillary nonperfusion (<30% of the treated area) was seen in four patients and retinal vascular leakage in three patients. There was an increase in RPE atrophy noted in 11 patients (39%). A correlation with the number of retreatments and progression of RPE atrophy was not seen, but the number of patients receiving more than one retreatment (n = 14) was probably too small.

The findings of the Phase I and II Studies of Verteporfin PDT can be summarized as follows.

1. Verteporfin PDT can lead to cessation of fluorescein leakage from CNV for 1 to 4 weeks, with stabilization or improvement of vision for 12 weeks.
2. The maximum tolerated light dose appears to be less than 150 J/cm^2, and the minimally effective dose is greater than 25 J/cm^2.
3. Fluorescein leakage, in at least a portion of the CNV, returns in most cases by 4 weeks, with progression in some cases by 12 weeks.

TABLE 14.5.6. CHANGE FROM BASELINE IN VISUAL ACUITY FOR PATIENTS RECEIVING MULTIPLE PHOTODYNAMIC THERAPY (PDT) TREATMENTS WITH REGIMEN 4

		Time After Most Recent PDT			
		Week 1		Week 4	
PDT Treatment	Number of Patients	Mean	Range	Mean	Range
First	10	+1.2	−3 to +5	+1.1	−2 to +3
Second	10	+0.8	−3 to +3	0	−5 to +5
Last follow-up[b]	9[c]	−1.0	−5 to +3		

[a]Two patients had a third PDT treatment with no change from baseline in visual acuity for both patients 1 week after third treatment; 4 weeks after the third treatment, visual acuity change from baseline was +1.0 and 0 for the two patients.
[b]Last follow-up was week 16 after baseline for participants who had two treatments and week 20 for participants who had three treatments.
[c]One patient had no final follow-up assessment because of hip replacement surgery, which was unrelated to treatment.
From Miller JW, Schmidt-Erfurth U, Sickenberg M, et al. Photodynamic therapy with verteporfin for choroidal neovascularization caused by age-related macular degeneration: results of a single treatment in a phase I and II study. *Arch Ophthalmol* 1999;117:1180, with permission.

4. Retreatments appear to be safe and although recurrence of leakage was noted with retreatments, the area of leakage decreased with subsequent PDT applications.
5. Exploratory analyses demonstrated an association between preserved vision and a smaller extent of CNV leakage at 12 weeks, suggesting that confining the CNV growth using PDT might preserve vision.
6. Exploratory analyses suggested that smaller lesions and lesions composed of classic CNV only had better vision outcomes.

Randomized, placebo-controlled, larger investigations with longer follow up (described in Chapter 14 part 6) were designed to answer the question of whether PDT using verteporfin could be effective at confining CNV growth and leakage and preserve vision in patients with neovascular AMD (9–11).

REFERENCES

1. Miller JW, Walsh AW, Kramer M, et al. Photodynamic therapy of experimental choroidal neovascularization using lipoprotein-delivered benzoporphyrin. *Arch Ophthalmol* 1995;113:810–818.
2. Kramer M, Miller JW, Michaud N, et al. Liposomal BPD verteporfin photodynamic therapy: selective treatment of choroidal neovascularization in monkeys. *Ophthalmology* 1996;103: 427–438.
3. Husain D, Miller JW, Michaud N, et al. Intravenous infusion using liposomal benzoporphyrin derivative verteporfin for photodynamic therapy of experimental choroidal neovascularization. *Arch Ophthalmol* 1996;114(8):978–985.
4. Moulton RS, et al. Response of retinal and choroidal vessels to photodynamic therapy using benzoporphyrin derivative monoacid. *Invest Ophthalmol Vis Sci* 1993;34:1169A.
5. Husain D, Kramer M, Kenny AG, et al. Effects of photodynamic therapy using verteporfin on experimental choroidal neovascularization and normal retina and choroid up to seven weeks after treatment. *Invest Ophthalmol Vis Sci* 1999;40:2322–2331.
6. Reinke M, et al. Photodynamic therapy (PDT) retreatment of normal retina and choroid in the primate. *Invest Ophthalmol Vis Sci* 1997;38:S17.
7. Miller J, Schmidt-Erfurth U, Sickenberg M, et al. Photodynamic therapy with verteporfin for choroidal neovascularization caused by age-related macular degeneration. Results of a single treatment in a Phase 1 and 2 study. *Arch Ophthalmol* 1999;117: 1161–1173.
8. Schmidt-Erfurth U, Miller JW, Sickenberg M, et al. Photodynamic therapy with verteporfin for choroidal neovascularization caused by age-related macular degeneration. Results of retreatments in a Phase 1 and 2 study. *Arch Ophthalmol* 1999;117: 1177–1187.
9. Treatment of Age-related Macular Degeneration with Photodynamic Therapy (TAP) Study Group. Verteporfin (Visudyne) therapy of subfoveal choroidal neovascularization in age-related macular degeneration. One year results of two randomized clinical trials. *Arch Ophthalmol* 1999;117:1329–1345.
10. Verteporfin in Photodynamic Therapy (VIP) Study Group. Verteporfin therapy of subfoveal choroidal neovascularization in age-related macular degeneration: two-year results of a randomized clinical trial including lesions with occult with no classic choroidal neovascularization. *Am J Ophthalmol* 2001;131:541–560.
11. Treatment of Age-related Macular Degeneration with Photodynamic Therapy (TAP) Study Group. Photodynamic therapy of subfoveal choroidal neovascularization in age-related macular degeneration with verteporfin. Two-year vision results of two randomized clinical trials. *Arch Ophthalmol* 2001;119:198–207.

Part 6: Results of Age-Related Macular Degeneration Trials Using Verteporfin PDT (Visudyne): the Treatment of Age-Related Macular Degeneration with Photodynamic Therapy and Verteporfin in Photodynamic Therapy Trials

JENNIFER JOAN ARNOLD

The clinical application of photodynamic therapy (PDT) with verteporfin (Visudyne, Novartis Pharmaceuticals, Basel, Switzerland) to subfoveal choroidal neovascularization (CNV) in age-related macular degeneration (AMD) has been studied in a series of large multicenter double-masked placebo controlled randomized clinical trials. The Treatment of Age-Related Macular Degeneration with Photodynamic Therapy (TAP) investigation consisted of two identically designed clinical trials that studied PDT in new and recurrent subfoveal CNV containing some classic CNV. Combined data from these two studies are available for 12- and 24-month follow up (1–3). The Verteporfin in Photodynamic Therapy (VIP) trial studied PDT in a wider range of exudative AMD as well as in pathologic myopia. Age-related macular degeneration patients had either occult with no classic CNV or with presumed early onset CNV and good visual acuity. Twenty-four month follow-up data are available for the VIP-AMD trial (4,5). The quality of clinical evidence presented in these reports has been reviewed independently and commented on by the Cochrane Libraries (6) and the American Academy of Ophthalmology (7).

STUDY DESIGN AND PROTOCOL

The study design and treatment protocols, apart from eligibility criteria, were identical in the TAP and VIP trials; therefore, they are described together.

Each study was an international multicenter study carried out in 22 (TAP) and 28 (VIP) ophthalmology practices in Europe and North America with strict adherence to the protocol being assured through standardized procedures and accreditation of all study personnel. The studies were supervised through an independent Data and Safety Monitoring Committee.

Patient Selection and Eligibility Criteria

Eligibility criteria for TAP and VIP are given in Tables 14.6.1 and 14.6.2, respectively. Both TAP and VIP studies enrolled new and recurrent subfoveal CNV in AMD. The area of the CNV must occupy at least 50% of the area of the entire neovascular lesion: for this reason patients with massive subretinal and subretinal pigment epithelial hemorrhage as well as those with serous pigment epithelial detachment were generally ineligible. The greatest linear dimension (GLD) of the CNV lesion must be less than or equal to 5,400 μm in size, this limitation resulting from the upper limit of laser spot size deliverable by the prototype lasers available for the study.

Further angiographic and visual acuity criteria for each study were defined. For the TAP study (Table 14.6.1), visual acuity must be between 73 and 34 letters on the ETDRS chart (approximate Snellen equivalent 20/40 through 20/200) and there must be some evidence of classic CNV on stereoscopic fluorescein angiography (FA). The VIP study (Table 14.6.2) had two groups of eligible patients. If classic CNV is present, the visual acuity must be better than 70 letters (approximate Snellen equivalent 20/40). If there is no evidence of classic CNV, then the visual acuity must be better than 50 letters (approximate Snellen equivalent 20/100) and there must be either the presence of CNV-associated hemorrhage, or angiographic or visual progression within the preceding 3 months. These

TABLE 14.6.1. ELIGIBILITY CRITERIA IN THE TREATMENT OF AGE-RELATED MACULAR DEGENERATION WITH PHOTODYNAMIC THERAPY (TAP) STUDY

Inclusion criteria
- Choroidal neovascularization (CNV) secondary to age-related macular degeneration
- CNV under the geometric center of the foveal avascular zone
- Evidence of classic CNV on fluorescein angiography
- Area of CNV at least 50% of the area of the total neovascular lesion
- Greatest linear dimension of lesion ≤5,400 μm (not including any area of prior laser photocoagulation)
- Best-corrected TAP protocol visual acuity of 73 through 34 letters (Snellen equivalent approximately 20/40 through 20/200)
- Age ≥50 years
- Willing and able to provide written informed consent

Exclusion criteria
- Tear (rip) of retinal pigment epithelium
- Any significant ocular disease (other than CNV) that has compromised or could compromise vision in the study eye and confound analysis of the primary outcome
- Inability to obtain photographs to document CNV, including difficulty with venous access
- History of treatment for CNV in study eye other than nonfoveal confluent laser photocoagulation
- Participation in another ophthalmic clinical trial or use of any other investigational new drugs within 12 weeks prior to the start of study treatment
- Active hepatitis or clinically significant liver disease
- Porphyria or other porphyrin sensitivity
- Prior photodynamic therapy for CNV
- Intraocular surgery within last 2 months or capulotomy within last month in study eye

TABLE 14.6.2. ELIGIBILITY CRITERIA IN THE VERTEPORFIN IN PHOTODYNAMIC THERAPY STUDY

Inclusion criteria
- Choroidal neovascularization (CNV) under the geometric center of the foveal avascular zone
- Area of CNV at least 50% of the area of the total neovascular lesion
- Greatest linear dimension >5,400 μm (not including any area of prior laser photocoagulation)
- If evidence of classic CNV, then visual acuity letter score >70
- If no evidence of classic CNV, then presumed to have recent disease progression because of deterioration (visually or anatomically) within last 3 months or evidence of hemorrhage from CNV
- Best-corrected protocol visual acuity letter score of at least 50 (Snellen equivalent approximately 20/100 or better)
- Willing and able to provide written informed consent

Exclusion criteria
- Features of any condition other than age-related macular degeneration (e.g., pathologic myopia) associated with CNV in study eye
- Tear (rip) of the retinal pigment epithelium
- Any significant ocular disease (other than CNV) that has compromised or could compromise vision in the study eye and confound analysis of the primary outcome
- Inability to obtain photographs to document CNV, including difficulty with venous access
- History of treatment for CNV in study eye other than nonfoveal confluent laser photocoagulation
- Participation in another ophthalmic clinical trial or use of any other investigational new drugs within 12 weeks before the start of study treatment
- Active hepatitis or clinically significant liver disease
- Porphyria or other porphyrin sensitivity
- Prior photodynamic therapy for CNV
- Intraocular surgery within last 2 months or capulotomy within last month in study eye

criteria were aimed to include cases of occult-only lesions with presumed recent disease progression.

Best-corrected visual acuity was measured using Early Treatment Diabetic Retinopathy Study (ETDRS) charts after a protocol refraction. Contrast sensitivity was measured using Pelli-Robson charts. Stereoscopic fundus photography and FA were performed.

Eligible patients were randomized in a ratio of 2:1 to verteporfin treatment or placebo. Both the patient and all study personnel responsible for the assessment and treatment of the patient were masked to the randomization state of the patient.

Treatment Protocol

Verteporfin treatment was performed according to a standard protocol based on the results of the Phase I/II dosimetry studies (8,9). Verteporfin at a dose of 6 mg/mm_2 body surface area was infused intravenously over 10 minutes. Placebo patients received a sham infusion of 5% dextrose water over 10 minutes. Laser light of 689 nm was applied to the macula 15 minutes after the start of the infusion in both treated and placebo patients at an intensity of 600 mW/cm^2 over 83 seconds to deliver a total light dose of 50 J/cm^2. The laser spot size was calculated by adding a 500-µm margin to the greatest linear dimension of the CNV lesion on stereo fundus angiography.

Patient Follow Up and Retreatments

All patients were reviewed every 3 months for 2 years. At each visit medical and medication history was taken and protocol refraction, visual acuity and contrast sensitivity measurement, ophthalmic examination, and stereoscopic fundus photography and FA were performed. The patient was retreated if there was any leak caused by CNV visible on FA. Patients were telephoned within 2 to 4 days after each treatment and were reviewed if any adverse visual or systemic event was reported.

RESULTS

Outcome Measures

Both visual and angiographic outcomes were assessed in the TAP and VIP studies. Moderate and severe visual loss were defined as a loss of 15 letters (three lines) and 30 letters (six lines), respectively, on the ETDRS chart, representing a doubling and quadrupling of the visual angle. Photographic eligibility and assessment of angiographic outcomes were performed by the Photographic Reading Center at the Johns Hopkins Medical Institutions and graded with reference to the baseline angiograms. Progression of leakage was defined as CNV beyond the borders of the entire CNV lesion noted at baseline. The amount of CNV leakage within the area of CNV lesion seen at baseline was graded if there was no CNV progression. Moderate leakage was defined as an area of CNV occupying greater than or equal to 50% of CNV area at baseline, minimal leakage was defined as an area of CNV occupying less than 50% of CNV area at baseline, and absence of leakage was defined when there was no CNV leakage within the CNV area at baseline. Choroidal neovascularization leakage was graded separately for both classic and occult CNV.

The principal efficacy outcome measure was the proportion of eyes that had 15 or more letters lost compared to baseline (moderate visual loss). Secondary visual acuity outcome measures included: Thirty or more letters lost (severe visual loss), mean change in visual acuity, mean change in contrast threshold, and proportion of eyes with fewer than 34 letters vision score (Snellen equivalent ≤20/200, legal blindness). Secondary angiographic outcome measures included size of CNV lesion, progression of CNV, and (in the VIP study) the proportion developing classic CNV.

All statistical analyses were based on a strict intent-to-treat scrutiny with lost observations carried forward.

Follow Up

A high rate of follow up for each 3-month visit was achieved for both treatment and placebo groups in all studies. In the TAP study, 86% of treated patients and 87% of placebo patients completed a 24-month follow up. In the VIP study, 87% of treated patients and 86% of placebo patients completed a 24-month follow up.

RESULTS OF THE TAP STUDY

Six hundred nine people were enrolled in the TAP study between December, 1996 and October, 1997 with 402 eyes assigned to verteporfin treatment and 207 eyes to placebo.

Baseline lesion characteristics were statistically balanced between treatment and placebo groups except that more women and more patients with lesions with blood were assigned to placebo, and more past or current smokers were assigned to verteporfin treatment.

The TAP and VIP study protocols specified that PDT with verteporfin was to be applied if any leakage from CNV was detected on FA, without consideration of the clinical relevance of that leakage. At each follow-up visit through 24 months, fewer verteporfin-treated eyes than placebo eyes were assessed by the treating ophthalmologist as requiring treatment: 45% of treated compared to 65% of placebo eyes received treatment at the last treatment visit (21-month follow up). An average of 5.6 treatments (3.4 in the first year and 2.1 in the second year) out of a total possible of eight were given to the verteporfin group. Given that the treating ophthalmologists remained masked to the randomization state of the patient, this

TABLE 14.6.3. VISUAL AND ANGIOGRAPHIC OUTCOMES AT MONTH 24 IN TREATMENT OF AGE-RELATED MACULAR DEGENERATION WITH PHOTODYNAMIC THERAPY (TAP) STUDY FOR THE TOTAL STUDY POPULATION AND FOR SUBGROUPS WITH PREDOMINANTLY CLASSIC AND MINIMALLY CLASSIC CHOROIDAL NEOVASCULARIZATION

	Total Study Population			Predominantly Classic Subgroup			Minimally Classic Subgroup		
	Treated (n = 402)	Placebo (n = 207)	p-value	Treated (n = 159)	Placebo (n = 83)	p-value	Treated (n = 202)	Placebo (n = 104)	p-value
Visual acuity outcomes									
Moderate vision loss: Loss of 15 letters or more	189/ 47.0%	129/ 62.3%	$p < .001$	65/40.9%	57/ 68.7%	$p < .001$	106/ 52.5%	58/ 55.7%	$p = 0.58$
Severe vision loss: Loss of 30 letters or more	73/ 18.2%	62/ 30.0%	$p < .001$	24/ 15.1%	30/ 36.1%	$p < .001$	40/ 19.8%	28/ 26.9%	
Moderate vision improvement: Gain of 15 letters or more	36/ 9.0%	8/ 3.9%		14/ 8.8%	3/ 3.6%		17/ 8.4%	5/ 4.8%	
Mean letters of vision (Snellen equivalent)	39 (20/ 160 + 1)	33 (20/ 200 − 2)		38 (20/ 160 − 2)	28 (20/ 250 − 2)	$p < .001$	40 (20/ 160 + 2)	37 (20/ 200 + 2)	$p = 0.26$
Mean lines (letters) of vision lost	2.7 (13.4)	3.9 (19.6)		2.4 (11.7)	4.6 (22.6)	$p < .001$	3.0 (14.9)	3.4 (17.0)	
Visual acuity <34 letters (20/200 or less)	165/ 41.0%	114/ 55.1%	$p = .001$	70/ 44.0%	56/ 67.5%	$p = .001$	81/ 40.1%	48/ 46.2%	$p = .18$
Contrast sensitivity: Mean letters lost	1.3	5.2	$p < .001$	0.2	6.4	$p < .001$	2.0	4.4	$p = 0.02$
Angiographic outcomes									
Progression of classic Choroidal neovascularization (CNV) leakage	23.1%	53.6%	$p < .001$	46/ 28.9%	54/ 65.1%	$p < .001$	20%	47%	
Absence of classic CNV leakage	51.2%	28.5%	$p < .001$	71/ 44.7%	17/ 20.5%	$p < .001$	54%	30%	
Lesion size >6 disc areas	43%	73%		61/ 38.4%	59/ 71.1%	$p < .001$	49%	73%	

indicates that some clinically evident benefit of treatment was apparent.

At each follow-up visit up to 24 months, all outcome measures were clinically and statistically significantly better in the treatment than in the control group, demonstrating a consistent and sustained benefit of PDT with verteporfin compared to placebo. At no follow-up point did treated eyes fare worse than placebo eyes. Table 14.6.3 presents data on primary and secondary outcomes at 24 months for the entire study population.

Vision Outcomes

The percentage with moderate vision loss in verteporfin treatment and placebo groups at each 3-month follow up through 24 months in the TAP study is shown in Figure 14.6.1. Much of the vision loss in both treatment and control groups occurred in the first 6 months, with slower rate of loss continuing throughout the follow up. At the 12 month follow-up visit, significantly fewer verteporfin-treated eyes had lost 15 letters or more of vision: 156 of 402 (39%) verteporfin-treated eyes versus 111 of 207 (54%) of placebo eyes. Only 8% more eyes in each group had moderate vision loss in the second year, giving the 24-month follow-up outcomes as 189 of 402 (47%) treated eyes versus 129 of 207 (62%) control eyes ($p < 0.001$). The number needed to treat (NNT) to prevent one person losing at least 15 letters of vision at 24-month follow up was 6.5.

Severe vision loss of 30 letters (six lines) or more was also significantly lower in the treatment group and was seen in 73 of 402 (18%) verteporfin-treated versus 62 of 207 (30%) control eyes at 24 months, an increase of 3% and 6%, respectively, over the 12-month data. The number needed to treat to prevent one person losing at least 30 letters of vision at 24-month follow up was 8.5. Significant benefits of verteporfin treatment were demonstrated at both the 12- and 24-month follow-up analyses for mean vision acuity, mean number of letters lost, percentage with vision less than or equal to 20/200, and mean numbers of contrast sensitivity letters lost (Table 14.6.3).

Most of the treatment benefit demonstrated was in the prevention of vision loss; only a small percentage of eyes in either group improved: 36 of 402 (9%) treated and eight of 207 (3.9%) control eyes had 15 letters (three lines) or more improvement at 24-month follow up. Figure 14.6.2 shows the lines of change of visual acuity between baseline and 24-

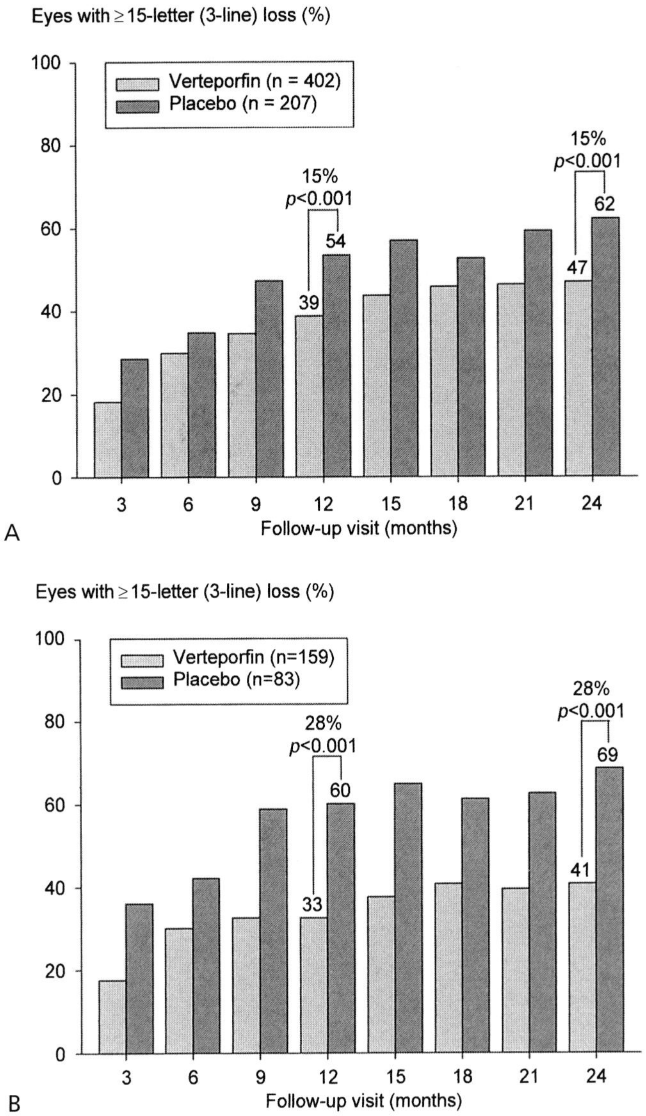

FIGURE 14.6.1. Primary efficacy outcome for the TAP study. Percentage of eyes with moderate vision loss (loss of ≥15 letters) at each 3-month study visit over time assigned to verteporfin treatment and placebo, with last observation carried forward for missing values. **A:** Total study population. **B:** Subgroup of eyes with predominantly classic CNV at baseline.

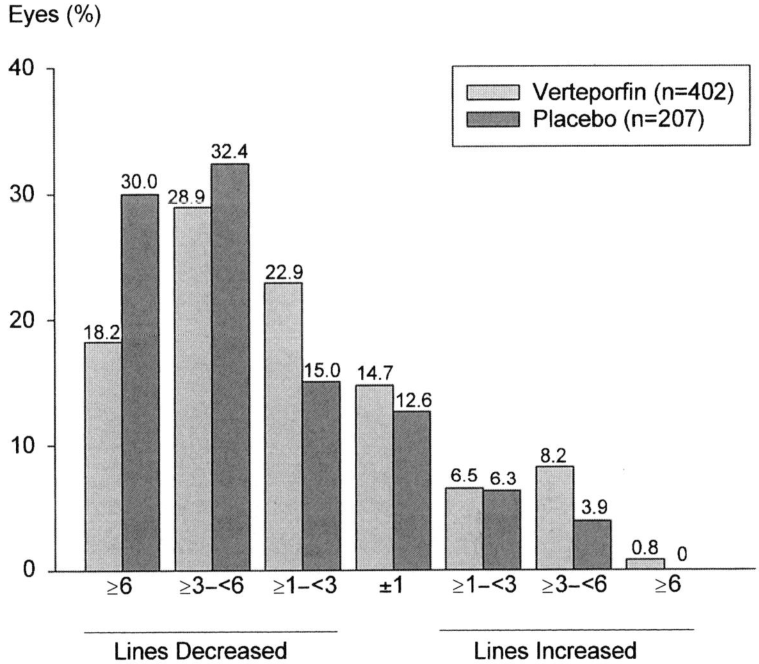

FIGURE 14.6.2. Vision outcome in the TAP study. Frequency distribution of changes in lines of visual acuity from baseline in eyes assigned to verteporfin treatment and placebo at 24-month follow up.

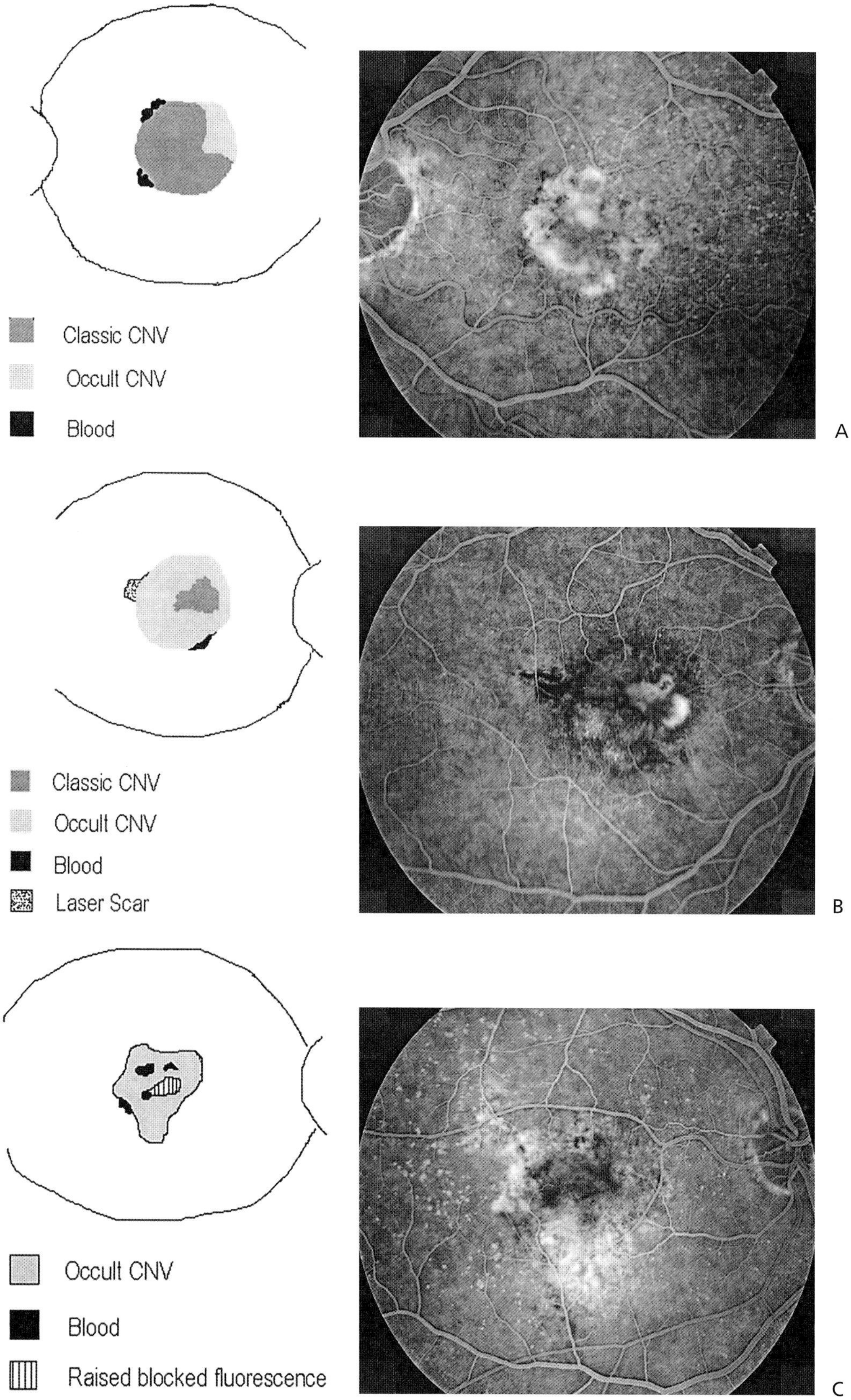

FIGURE 14.6.3. Classification of lesion components on baseline angiography in TAP and VIP studies. Early-phase fluorescein angiograms and line drawings illustrate **(A)** predominantly classic CNV (classic CNV occupies ≥50% of total CNV lesion area), **(B)** minimally classic CNV (classic CNV occupies <50% of total CNV lesion area), and **(C)** occult with no classic CNV.

month follow up for verteporfin-treated and placebo groups. The graph of the verteporfin group is shifted toward the right (less loss, more improvement) compared to the graph of the control group, demonstrating overall treatment benefit.

Angiographic Outcomes

Angiographic outcomes demonstrated a clinically and statistically significantly benefit for verteporfin-treated compared to placebo-treated eyes at both 12- and 24-month follow up (Table 14.6.3). Visual acuity benefits of treatment were achieved despite continued growth and leakage of classic CNV. Progression of classic CNV beyond the area of CNV lesion at baseline was common in both groups, but the percentage was significantly lower in the verteporfin-treated compared to placebo eyes. By 12 months, 46% of treated and 71% of placebo eyes had classic CNV progression. By 24 months, these numbers were reduced to 23% treated versus 54% control, indicating some regression of classic CNV in the second year in both groups. Absent leakage from classic CNV was uncommon at 12 months (19% treated versus 9% control), but increased to 51% of verteporfin-treated eyes and 29% of placebo-treated eyes by 24 months. Lesion size was significantly smaller in the verteporfin-treated group. Placebo-treated eyes were almost twice as likely to be more than six disc areas in size, and 2.5 times as likely to be greater than nine disc areas in size.

Subgroup Analysis

A most important finding of the TAP study was a differential benefit of verteporfin treatment depending on the amount of classic and occult CNV present in the lesion at baseline. This was the only baseline characteristic found to have a significant impact on the primary efficacy outcome (moderate visual loss) in predefined statistical subgroup analyses. Other baseline characteristics, including patient age, micronutrient use, phakic status, and previous laser photocoagulation, had no impact on the magnitude of treatment benefit (3). Most important, no evidence of harm was found, and no subgroups were identified in which the placebo eyes had a better outcome than treated eyes.

In the subgroup analysis, eyes were classified on baseline angiography into three groups based on the area (rather than the linear dimension) of the total CNV lesion occupied by classic CNV components (Fig. 14.6.3): predominantly classic, when the classic CNV occupied greater than or equal to 50% of the entire CNV lesion area; minimally classic, when classic CNV occupied less than 50% of the entire CNV lesion area; and occult, with no classic CNV. Forty percent of eyes had predominantly classic, 50% of the eyes had minimally classic, 9% of eyes had no classic CNV, and 1% of eyes could not be graded and the distribution of

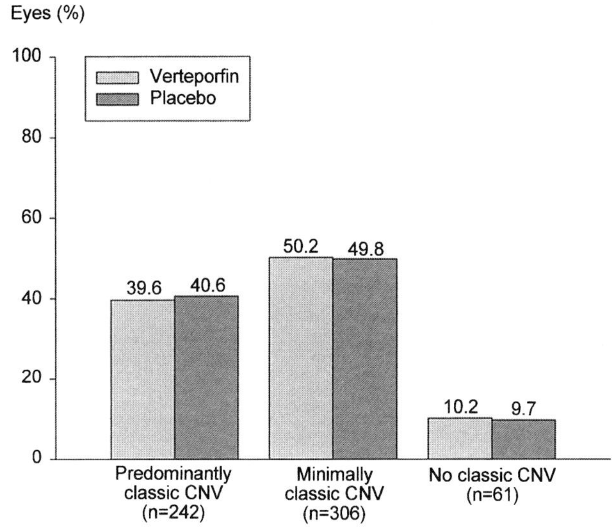

FIGURE 14.6.4. TAP study. Baseline angiographic classification of eyes in verteporfin- and placebo-treated groups.

lesions was similar between the verteporfin and placebo groups (Fig. 14.6.4). It is unlikely that lesions with no classic CNV included in the TAP study are representative of the general population of eyes with occult-only lesions in AMD, because they were considered to contain classic CNV by the treating ophthalmologist but not by the reading center and were judged to be ineligible. Therefore, results for this small subgroup are not discussed further.

Although not stratified at baseline, baseline characteristics were similar between treatment and placebo groups for predominantly and minimally classic CNV. Compared to minimally classic CNV lesions, predominantly classic CNV lesions had a smaller lesion size, worse initial visual acuity, and were more likely to have lesions containing blood (3).

Treatment benefit was found to be greater for people with predominantly classic CNV than for the total study population for all primary and secondary outcomes at both 12- and 24-month follow up (Table 14.6.3; Figs. 14.6.1 and 14.6.5 through 14.6.9). Moderate vision loss of 15 letters or more occurred in 65 of 159 (41%) treated and 57 of 83 (69%) control eyes with predominantly classic CNV at 24-month follow up (Fig. 14.6.1B). The number needed to treat to prevent one person losing 15 letters or more at 24-month follow up was 3.6. One hundred forty-three eyes (94 treated and 49 control) had lesions containing classic with no occult CNV, representing 24% of enrolled patients. Treatment benefit was of the greatest magnitude in this subgroup with moderate vision loss occurring in only 28 (30%) of treated compared to 35 (71%) of placebo eyes at 24-month follow up (NNT 2.4).

The impact of verteporfin treatment on eyes with minimally classic CNV was less marked. No significant visual

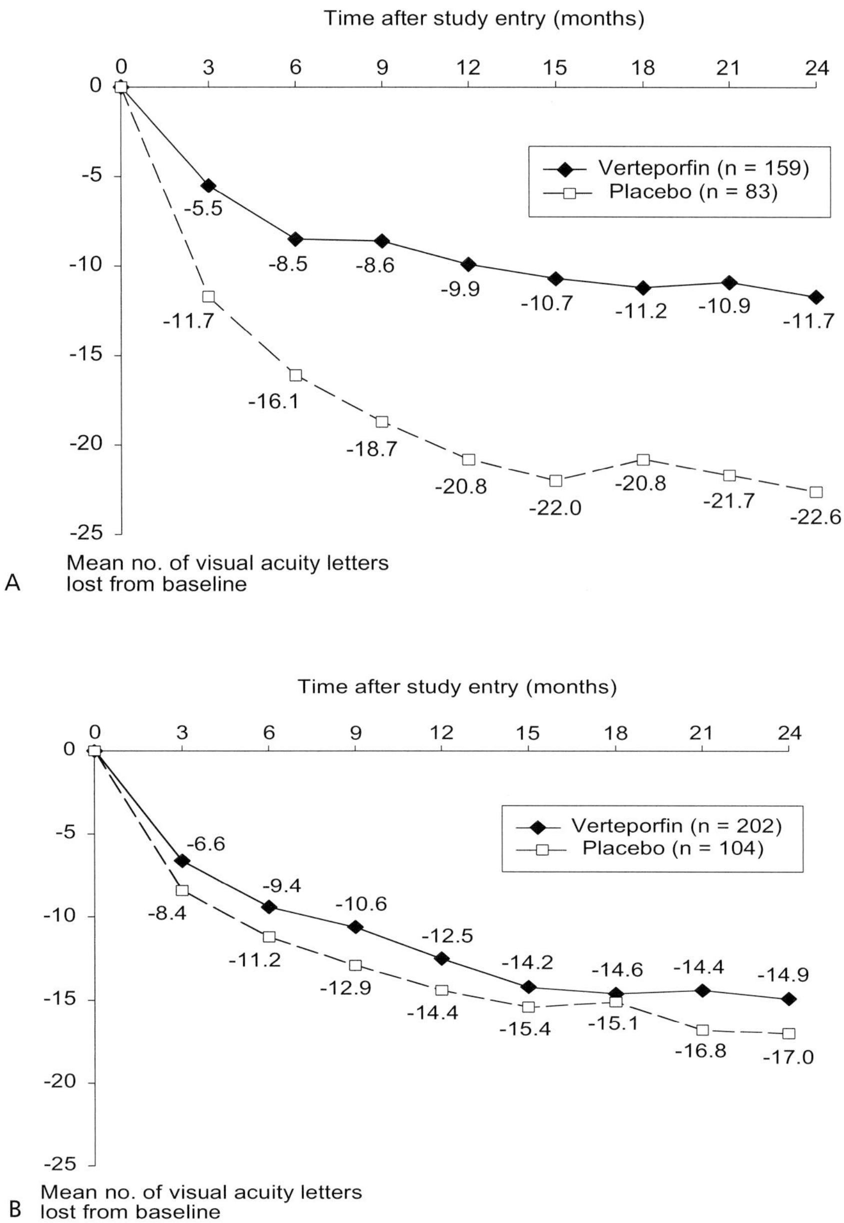

FIGURE 14.6.5. Vision outcomes in subgroup analysis in the TAP study. Mean number of letters of visual acuity lost from baseline at each 3-month study visit over time for eyes assigned to verteporfin treatment or placebo, with last observation carried forward for missing values. **A:** Lesions with predominantly classic CNV at baseline. **B:** Lesions with minimally classic CNV at baseline.

acuity benefit was demonstrated for these eyes at either 12- or 24-month follow up (Table 14.6.3). Moderate vision loss of 15 letters or more was seen in 44% of treated and 45% of control eyes at 12 months, and 106 of 202 (52.5%) versus 58 of 104 (55.8%) at 24 months (p = 0.58). The treated group lost a mean of 2.1 fewer letters than the control group at 24-month follow up (p = 0.26) (Fig. 14.6.5B). Despite the lack of visual benefit, significant benefit at both 12- and 24-month follow up was seen for the minimally classic subgroup for contrast sensitivity (Fig. 14.6.6) and angiographic outcomes, including lesion size (Fig. 14.6.7) progression of classic CNV (Fig. 14.6.8), and absence of classic CNV leakage (Fig. 14.6.9).

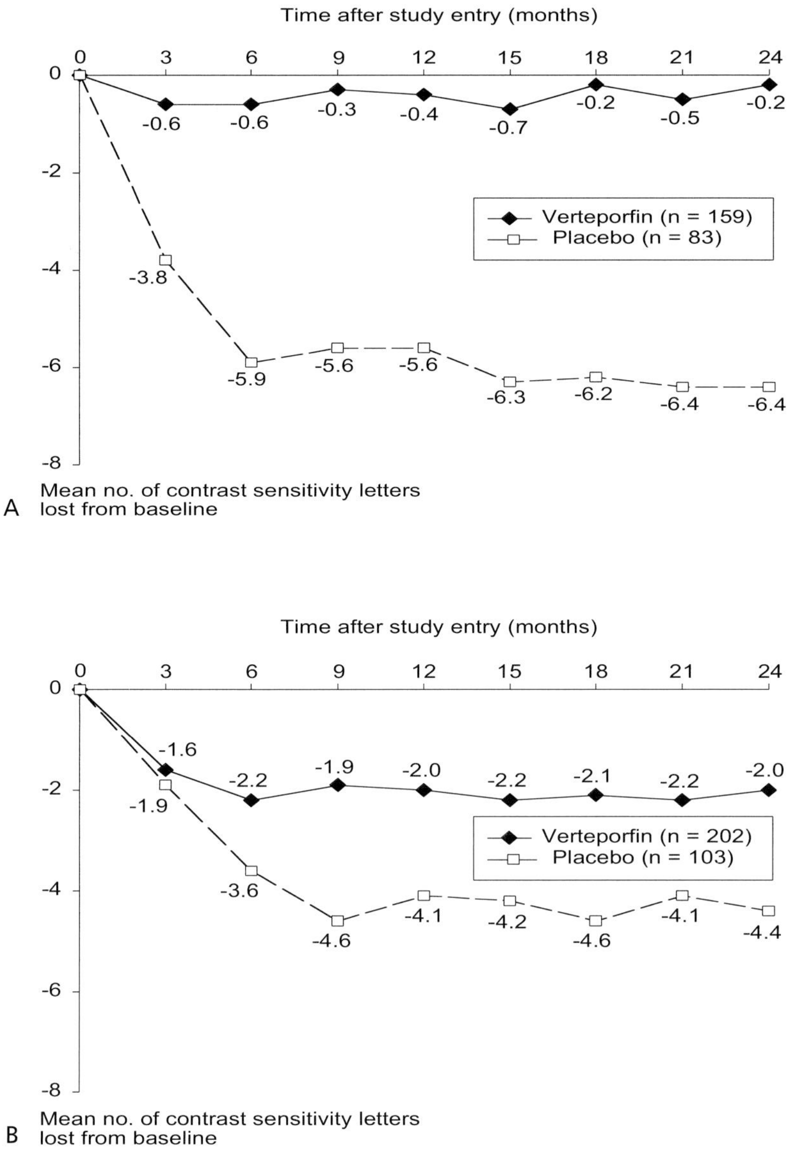

FIGURE 14.6.6. Vision outcomes in subgroup analysis in the TAP study. Mean number of letters of contrast sensitivity lost from baseline at each 3-month study visit over time for eyes assigned to verteporfin treatment or placebo, with last observation carried forward for missing values. **A:** Lesions with predominantly classic CNV at baseline. **B:** Lesions with minimally classic CNV at baseline.

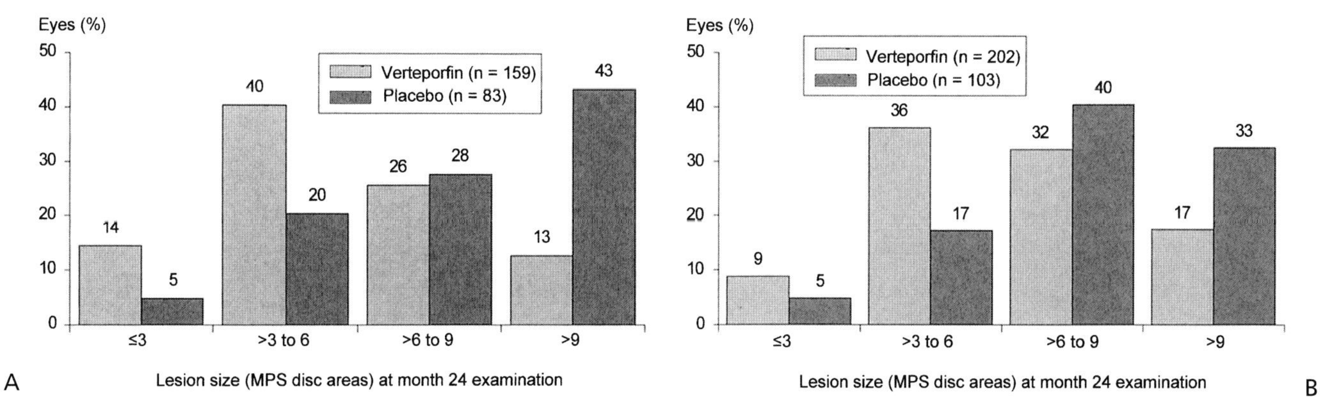

FIGURE 14.6.7. Angiographic outcomes in subgroup analysis in the TAP study. Frequency distribution of lesion sizes at 24-month examination for eyes assigned to verteporfin treatment or placebo, with last observation carried forward for missing values. **A:** Lesions with predominantly classic CNV at baseline. **B:** Lesions with minimally classic CNV at baseline.

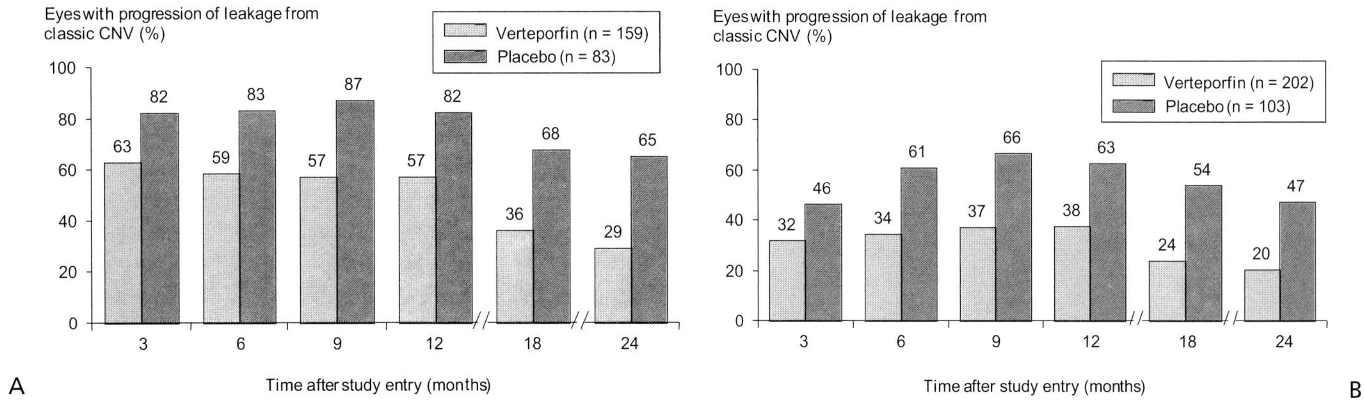

FIGURE 14.6.8. Angiographic outcomes in subgroup analysis in the TAP study. Percentage of eyes with progression of classic CNV beyond area of the lesion at baseline over time for eyes assigned to verteporfin treatment or placebo, with last observation carried forward for missing values. **A:** Lesions with predominantly classic CNV at baseline. **B:** Lesions with minimally classic CNV at baseline.

RESULTS OF THE VIP-AMD STUDY

Three hundred thirty-nine people were enrolled in the VIP-AMD study between March, 1998 and September, 1998 with 225 eyes assigned to verteporfin treatment and 114 eyes to placebo. Nearly 80% of eyes enrolled had occult with no classic CNV: 166 (74%) of verteporfin-treated and 92 (81%) of placebo-treated eyes. Detailed analyses were carried out on this large subgroup given the findings of the TAP study that baseline lesion composition influenced verteporfin treatment effect. Subgroups containing some classic CNV were too small for analysis: 16 (7%) of verteporfin-treated eyes and three (3%) of placebo-treated eyes had predominantly classic CNV lesions at baseline, and 38 (17%) of verteporfin-treated and 18 (16%) of placebo-treated eyes had minimally classic CNV.

Baseline lesion characteristics were statistically balanced between treatment and placebo groups for both the entire study population and the subgroup with occult with no classic CNV.

At each follow-up visit through 24 months, fewer verteporfin-treated eyes than placebo eyes were assessed by the treating ophthalmologist as requiring treatment, 33% of treated compared to 45% of placebo eyes received treatment at the last treatment visit (21-month follow up). These proportions were identical for the subgroup with occult with no classic CNV, with an average of 4.9 treatments (3.1 in the first year and 1.8 in the second year) out of a total possible of eight given to the verteporfin group.

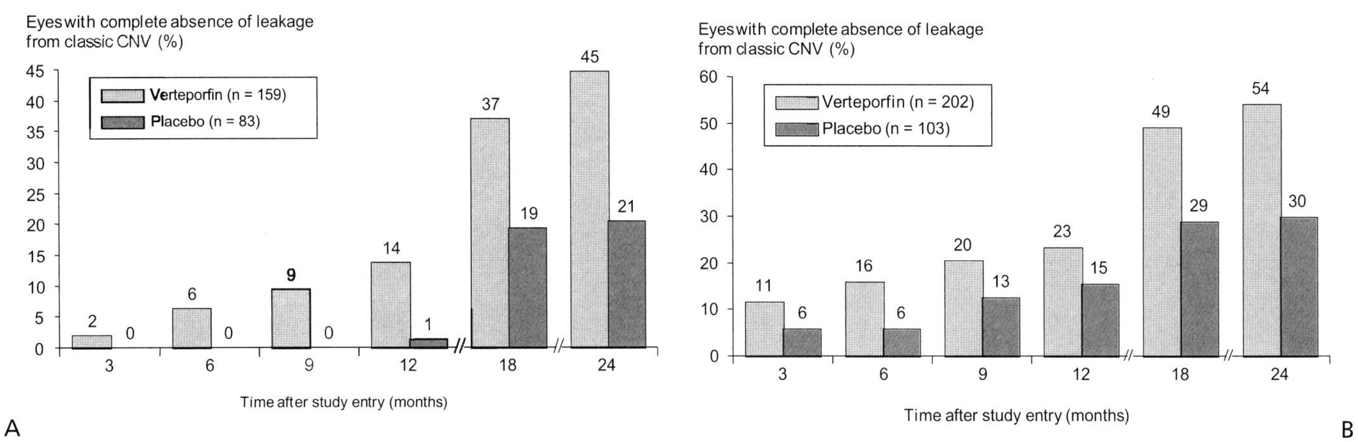

FIGURE 14.6.9. Angiographic outcomes in subgroup analysis in the TAP study. Percentage of eyes with complete absence of leakage from classic CNV over time for eyes assigned to verteporfin treatment or placebo, with last observation carried forward for missing values. **A:** Lesions with predominantly classic CNV at baseline. **B:** Lesions with minimally classic CNV at baseline.

TABLE 14.6.4. VISUAL AND ANGIOGRAPHIC OUTCOMES AT MONTH 24 IN VERTEPORFIN IN PHOTODYNAMIC THERAPY STUDY FOR THE TOTAL STUDY POPULATION AND FOR THE SUBGROUP WITH OCCULT BUT NO CLASSIC CHOROIDAL NEOVASCULARIZATION

	Total Study Population			Occult with No Classic CNV Subgroup		
	Treated n = 225	Placebo n = 114		Treated n = 166	Placebo n = 92	
Visual acuity outcomes						
Moderate vision loss: Loss of 15 letters or more	121/54%	76/67%	$p = .023$[a]	91/55%	63/68%	$p = .032$[a]
Severe vision loss: Loss of 30 letters or more	67/30%	54/47%	$p = .001$	48/29%	43/47%	$p = .004$
Moderate vision improvement: Gain of 15 letters or more				8/5%	1/1%	
Mean letters of vision (Snellen equivalent)				47 (20/126 + 2)	40 (20/160)	
Mean lines (letters) of vision lost				3.8 (19.0)	5.1 (25.5)	
Visual acuity <34 letters (20/200 or less)				46/28%	41/45%	$p = .006$
Contrast sensitivity:[b] Loss of 9 or more letters				32 of 161 (20%)	31 of 90 (34%)	$p = .01$
Angiographic outcomes						
Development of classic CNV				45/27%	45/49%	$p = .001$
Development of classic CNV that progressed beyond baseline lesion				29/17%	35/38%	
Progression of occult CNV leakage				77/46%	52/57%	$p = .12$
Absence of occult CNV leakage				70/42%	27/29%	$p = .04$
Absence of any CNV leakage (classic or occult)				58/35%	13/14%	$p < .001$
Lesion size >6 disc areas				44%	63%	

[a]Difference between treated and placebo groups not significant at 12 month follow up.
[b]Contrast sensitivity was not measured at baseline in five treated and two control eyes.

Vision Outcomes

At 24-month follow up, a statistically significant benefit of verteporfin treatment was demonstrated for vision and angiographic outcomes for both the entire study population and the subgroup with occult with no classic CNV, although the benefit was more modest than that demonstrated in the TAP study (Table 14.6.4). The benefit for the primary vision outcome of moderate vision loss was not manifest until the second year of treatment, when verteporfin eyes tended to stabilize, whereas placebo eyes continued to deteriorate (Fig. 14.6.10). At 12-month follow up, 114 of 225 (51%) verteporfin-treated compared to 62 of 114 (54%) placebo eyes lost 15 letters or more (p = .52). By 24 months, the treatment benefit had increased to reach statistical significance: 121 of 225 (54%) treated eyes versus 76 of 114 (67%) control (p = .023, NNT 7.8). A comparable treatment benefit was demonstrated for the subgroup with occult with no classic CNV: at 24-month follow up, 91 of 166 (55%) treated versus 63 of 92 (68%) control eyes had lost 15 or more letters of vision (p = .032) (Fig. 14.6.11A). The number needed to treat to prevent moderate vision loss at 24 months in one patient with occult with no classic CNV was 7.3. Figure 14.6.12 shows

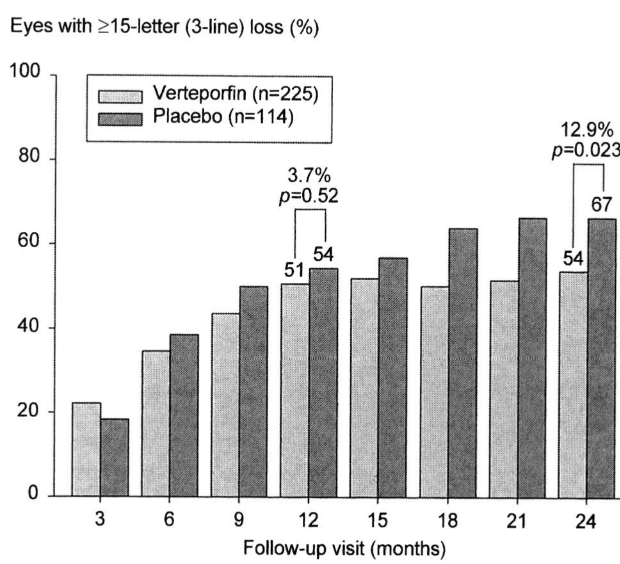

FIGURE 14.6.10. Primary efficacy outcome for the VIP study. Percentage of eyes with moderate vision loss (loss of ≥15 letters) at each 3-month study visit over time assigned to verteporfin treatment or placebo, with last observation carried forward for missing values.

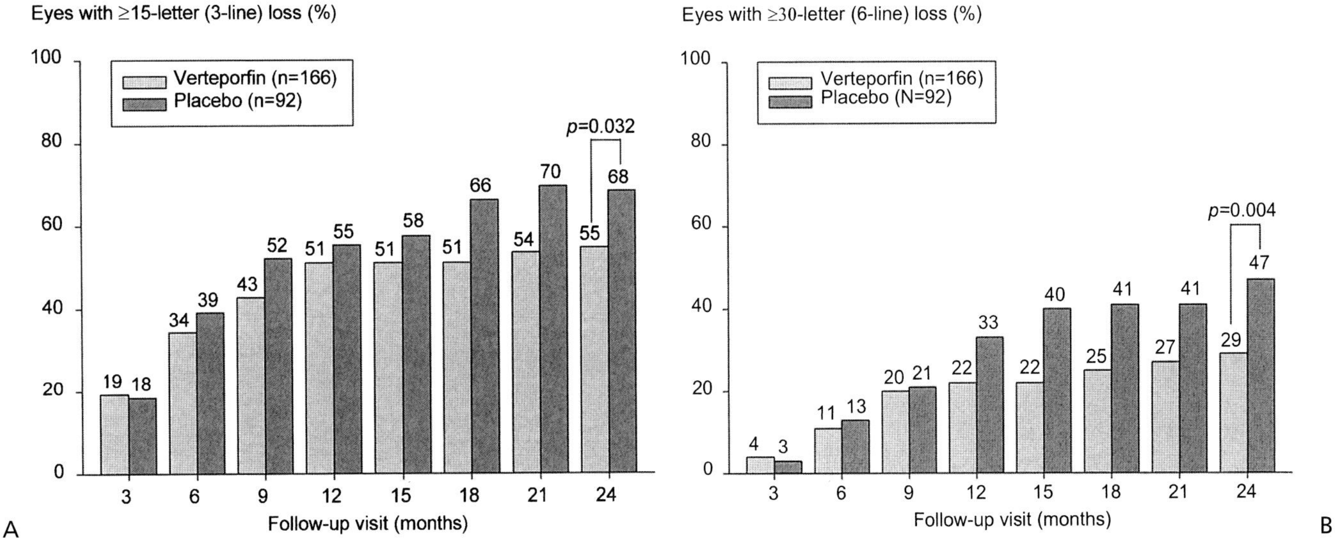

FIGURE 14.6.11. VIP study. Vision outcome in eyes with occult and no classic CNV. Percentage of eyes with **(A)** moderate vision loss (loss of ≥15 letters), and **(B)** severe vision loss (loss of ≥30) at each 3-month study visit over time for eyes assigned to verteporfin treatment or placebo, with last observation carried forward for missing values.

the lines of change of visual acuity between baseline and 24-month follow up for verteporfin treatment and placebo groups for the eyes with occult and no classic CNV.

The percentage of eyes with severe vision loss of 30 letters or more at 24 months was also significantly lower in verteporfin-treated compared to placebo eyes for both the entire study population and the subgroup with occult with no classic CNV (Table 14.6.4; Fig. 14.6.11B): 30% treated versus 47% placebo ($p = .001$) and 29% treated versus 47% control ($p = .004$), respectively. The number needed to treat to prevent severe vision loss at 24 months in one patient with occult with no classic CNV was 5.6.

The treatment benefit in other secondary visual outcomes was significant at both 12- and 24-month follow up for the entire population (data not given) and for the subgroup with occult with no classic CNV (Table 14.6.4). These include mean change in visual acuity, visual acuity distribution, percentage of eyes with vision less than 34 letters (≤20/200), and contrast sensitivity.

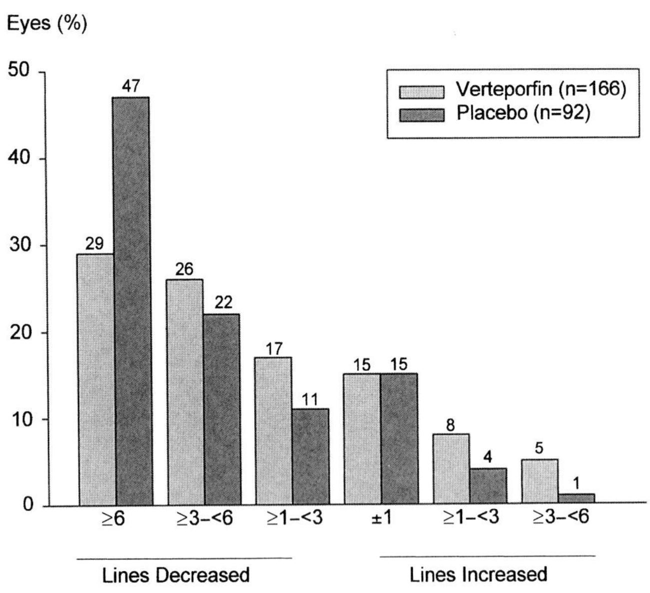

FIGURE 14.6.12. VIP study. Vision outcome in eyes with occult and no classic CNV. Frequency distribution of changes in lines of visual acuity from baseline in eyes assigned to verteporfin treatment and placebo at 24-month follow up.

Angiographic Outcomes

Angiographic outcomes also demonstrated a clinically and statistically significantly benefit for verteporfin-treated compared to placebo-treated eyes at both 12- and 24-month follow up for the entire study population (data not given) as well as for the subgroup with occult with no classic CNV (Table 14.6.4). As the TAP study demonstrated, visual benefits were achieved despite continued growth and leakage of CNV. In the subgroup with occult with no classic CNV, progression of occult was seen in 55% of treated and 73% of control eyes at 12-month follow up ($p = .004$) reducing to 46% of treated and 57% of control eyes by 24-month follow up ($p = .12$). At both time points, verteporfin-treated eyes were nearly half as likely to develop classic CNV either within or beyond the original lesion

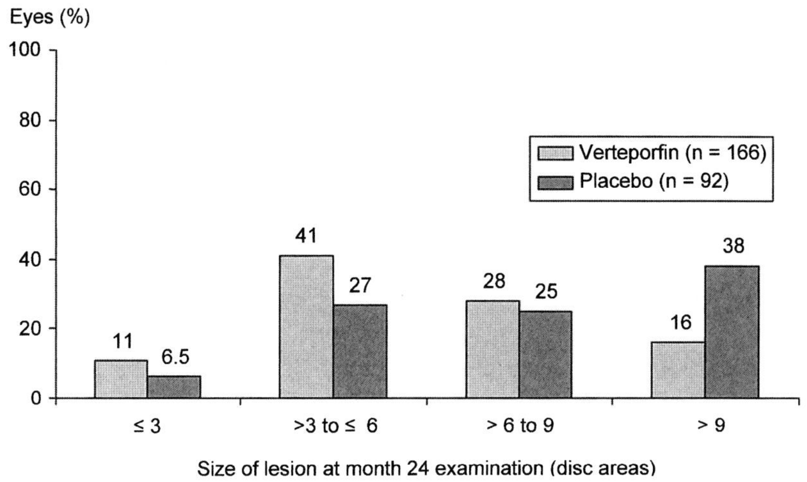

FIGURE 14.6.13. VIP study. Angiographic outcome in eyes with occult and no classic CNV. Frequency distribution of lesion sizes at the 24-month examination for eyes assigned to verteporfin treatment or placebo, with last observation carried forward for missing values.

boundary. Absent leakage from either classic or occult CNV was uncommon at 12-month follow up (14% treated versus 4% control $p = .02$) but increased by the 24-month follow up (35% treated versus 14% control, $p < .001$). Verteporfin-treated eyes had significantly smaller lesions at 24 months than placebo eyes (Fig. 14.6.13).

Subgroup Analysis

Within the population of occult with no classic in the VIP study, further exploratory analyses revealed that both initial visual acuity and baseline lesion size influenced the magnitude of treatment outcome. The results should be interpreted with caution because they are based on small subgroups of between 52 and 70 eyes; however, they suggest that the benefit of verteporfin treatment was greater in eyes with smaller lesions (defined as four Macular Photocoagulation Study [MPS] disc areas or less) or with lower levels of visual acuity (letter score < 65, approximate Snellen equivalent 20/50 – 1 or less). This range is within the population of eyes with occult but no classic enrolled in the VIP study that at baseline, following VIP study eligibility criteria, had lesions smaller than 5,400 μm GLD (around six MPS disc areas) and vision acuity better than 50 letters (approximate Snellen equivalent 20/100). Differences in risk of moderate visual loss for occult but not classic CNV according to baseline size and visual acuity are given in Table 14.6.5, and of severe vision loss in Table 14.6.6. These tables demonstrate a benefit for verteporfin therapy in eyes with smaller lesions, regardless of baseline vision, and with poorer initial vision, regardless of lesion size. There were 123 verteporfin-treated and 64 placebo-treated eyes with either lesions less than or equal to four disc areas or visual acuity less than 65 letters at baseline, representing 72% of the total subgroup with occult with no classic CNV. In this group of eyes, moderate vision loss at 24 months occurred in 60 (49%) of treated versus 48 (75%) of control eye ($p < .001$) and severe vision loss in 26 (21%) of treated versus 31 (48%) of control eyes (Fig. 14.6.14). The analysis also suggests that verteporfin may not be effective in eyes with occult but no classic lesions that are larger than four disc areas and have vision better than 20/50.

TABLE 14.6.5. VISUAL OUTCOME IN OCCULT BUT NO CLASSIC CHOROIDAL NEOVASCULARIZATION IN THE VERTEPORFIN IN PHOTODYNAMIC THERAPY STUDY

	"Poor" Visual Acuity ≤20/50 – 1 (<65 letters)			"Good" Visual Acuity ≥20/50 (≥65 Letters)		
Lesion Size	Verteporfin	Placebo	Difference	Verteporfin	Placebo	Difference
"Smaller" lesions ≤4 disc areas[a]	9/36 (25%)	11/16 (69%)	44%	27/44 (61%)	17/23 (74%)	13%
"Larger" lesions >4 disc areas[a]	24/41 (59%)	20/25 (80%)	21%	31/43 (72%)	14/27 (52%)	–20%

Loss of 15 letters or more by baseline lesion size and initial visual acuity in verteporfin-treated compared to placebo-treated patients at 24-month follow up.
[a]Macular photocoagulation study disc areas.

TABLE 14.6.6. VISUAL OUTCOME IN OCCULT BUT NO CLASSIC CHOROIDAL NEOVASCULARIZATION IN THE VERTEPORFIN IN PHOTODYNAMIC THERAPY STUDY

	"Poor" Visual Acuity ≤20/50 – 1 (<65 letters)			"Good" Visual Acuity ≥20/50 (≥65 Letters)		
Lesion Size	**Verteporfin**	**Placebo**	**Difference**	**Verteporfin**	**Placebo**	**Difference**
"Smaller" lesions ≤4 disc areas[a]	2/36 (6%)	4/16 (25%)	19%	15/44 (34%)	14/23 (61%)	27%
"Larger" lesions >4 disc areas[a]	9/41 (22%)	13/25 (52%)	30%	22/43 (51%)	11/27 (41%)	–10%

Loss of 30 letters or more by baseline lesion size and initial visual acuity in verteporfin-treated compared to placebo-treated patients at 24-month follow up.
[a]Macular photocoagulation study disc areas.

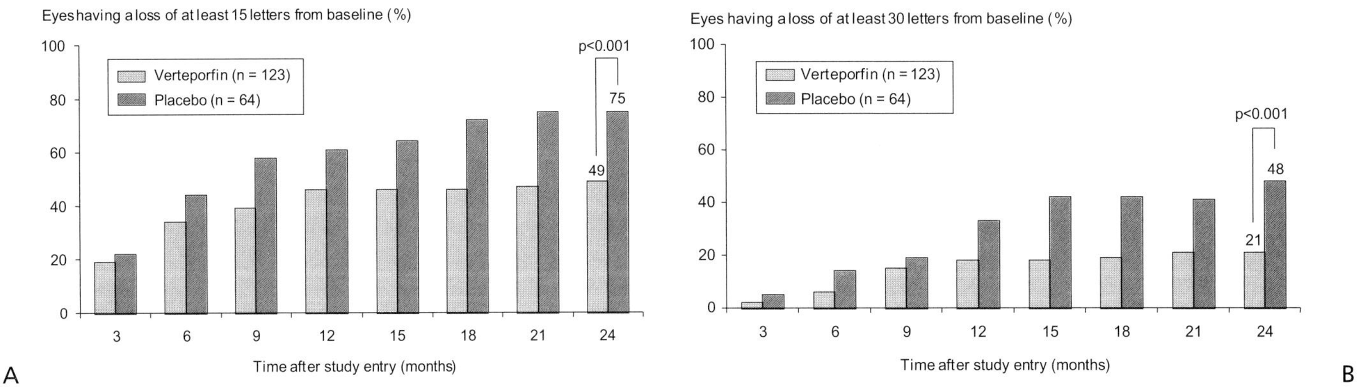

FIGURE 14.6.14. VIP study. Vision outcomes in subgroup of eyes with occult and no classic CNV with either smaller lesions or lower levels of visual acuity at baseline. Percentage of eyes with **(A)** moderate vision loss (loss of ≥15 letters), and **(B)** severe vision loss (loss of ≥30) at each 3-month study visit over time for eyes assigned to verteporfin treatment or placebo, with last observation carried forward for missing values.

TABLE 14.6.7. CLINICALLY RELEVANT ADVERSE EVENTS IN THE TREATMENT OF AGE-RELATED MACULAR DEGENERATION WITH PHOTODYNAMIC THERAPY (TAP) AND VERTEPORFIN IN PHOTODYNAMIC THERAPY (VIP) TRIALS, IRRESPECTIVE OF RELATIONSHIP TO TREATMENT

	TAP Study		VIP Study	
	Treatment n = 402	**Placebo n = 207**	**Treatment n = 225**	**Placebo n = 114**
Injection site adverse events	64 (15.9%)	12 (5.8%)	18 (8%)	6 (5%)
Infusion related back pain	10 (2.5%)	0 (0%)	5 (2.2%)	0 (0%)
Photosensitivity reactions	14 (3.5%)	0 (0%)	1 (<1%)	1 (1%)
Allergic reactions	8 (2.0%)	3 (3.9%)	3 (1%)	3 (3%)
Any visual disturbance	89 (22.1%)	32 (15.5%)	94 (42%)	26 (23%)
Severe vision decrease: within 7 days of treatment	3 (0.75%)	0 (0%)	10 (4.4%)	0 (0%)

SAFETY

The safety of photodynamic therapy with verteporfin through 24 months of follow up and treatment in both the TAP and VIP studies was good. The treatment was well tolerated and there were minimal adverse events attributable to treatment (Table 14.6.7), although the possibility of important rare or longer-term adverse events remains. There were no deaths relating to study treatment and allergic reactions were rare, being more common in the placebo group. Verteporfin is a photosensitive dye and care must be taken to avoid tissue extravasation during infusion and exposure to bright light for 48 hours after treatment. In both studies, photosensitivity reactions and injection site reactions were more common in treatment than placebo groups. The only other nonocular adverse event caused by treatment was lower back pain during verteporfin infusion, which occurred in 15 people.

Some visual disturbance following treatment was common in both verteporfin- and placebo-treated eyes (Table 14.6.7). Rarely, verteporfin treatment caused a severe decrease in vision, defined as a loss of 20 letters (four lines) or more within 7 days of treatment. The risk appears to be higher in eyes with occult and no classic CNV, occurring in three (0.75%) people in the TAP study and 10 (4.4%) people in the VIP study. The number of people needed to be treated before causing severe vision loss in one person (number needed to harm) was 134 for TAP study and 22 for the VIP study. Of the 10 events in the VIP trial, nine occurred after the first exposure and one after the second exposure to verteporfin; the visual loss was associated with the development of extensive subretinal fluid with choroidal hypofluorescence in one event, with subretinal pigment epithelial hemorrhage in three events, and with no obvious cause in six events. Vision recovered to less than 20 letters lost in five of the 10 events. Verteporfin may be taken up by the retinal pigment epithelium (RPE) (10), but no evidence of worsening atrophy of the RPE was detected. In the TAP study, the distribution of lesion sizes when atrophy of the RPE was included did not differ from the distribution of lesion sizes without atrophy.

CONCLUSION

Evidence provided from these high-quality multicenter placebo-controlled randomized clinical trials shows that standard protocol verteporfin treatment can significantly reduce the risk of vision loss in selected patients with subfoveal CNV and AMD. The treatment benefit was clear and consistent across a range of visual and angiographic outcome measures for defined subgroups within the populations of patients who were enrolled in the studies. Relative and absolute risk reductions for the TAP and VIP studies, including important subgroups, are summarized in Table 14.6.8. The numbers needed to treat are low in each case, making photodynamic therapy with verteporfin an effective treatment.

Certain key understandings emerge from these studies. First, the treatment benefit in terms of vision outcomes is achieved despite the presence of continued CNV leakage, and frequently despite progression of that leakage, particularly in the first year of treatment. It is clear that these angiographic features, particularly in the first year, should not be interpreted as indicating a failure or lack of response to treatment, nor that continuing treatment should be abandoned.

TABLE 14.6.8. REDUCTION IN RELATIVE AND ABSOLUTE RISK AND NUMBERS NEEDED TO TREAT FOR MODERATE AND SEVERE VISION LOSS IN THE TREATMENT OF AGE-RELATED MACULAR DEGENERATION WITH PHOTODYNAMIC THERAPY (TAP) AND VERTEPORFIN IN PHOTODYNAMIC THERAPY (VIP) STUDIES

	Moderate Vision Loss: 15 Letters or More			Severe Vision Loss: 30 Letters or More		
	Relative Risk Reduction[a]	Absolute Risk Reduction[b]	Number Needed to Treat[c]	Relative Risk Reduction	Absolute Risk Reduction	Number Needed to Treat
TAP study						
Total study group	0.75	0.15	6.5	0.61	0.13	8.5
Predominantly classic	0.60	0.28	3.6	0.42	0.21	4.8
Classic with no occult	0.42	0.42	2.4	—	—	—
VIP study						
Total study group	0.81	0.13	7.8	0.63	0.17	5.9
Occult but no classic	0.80	0.13	7.3	0.62	0.18	5.6

[a]Relative risk reduction: Number of times less likely moderate or severe vision loss is to happen in verteporfin-treated eyes than placebo-treated eyes.
[b]Absolute risk reduction: Difference between risk of moderate or severe vision loss in verteporfin-treated compared to placebo-treated eyes.
[c]Number needed to treat. Number of people needed to treat to prevent moderate or severe vision loss in one person.

Second, the treatment benefit of PDT with verteporfin is influenced by the angiographic classification of classic and occult CNV lesion components at baseline, with evidence that the higher the proportion of classic CNV, the stronger the treatment benefit. For lesions containing classic CNV, treatment benefit was seen when the classic CNV occupied at least 50% of the total area CNV lesion (predominantly classic), with benefit already evident by 12 months: predominantly classic eyes treated with verteporfin were 1.9 times more likely to avoid moderate vision loss and 1.3 times more likely to avoid a severe vision loss at 24 months than control eyes. Treatment benefit was even stronger when there was no occult CNV present, a result based on analysis of 143 eyes in the TAP study: Eyes with classic and no occult CNV treated with verteporfin were 2.4 times more likely to avoid a moderate vision loss at 24 months than control eyes. No significant decreased risk of vision loss at 24 months was seen in eyes with lesser amounts of classic CNV (minimally classic CNV lesions), although it is possible that a benefit might be demonstrated with longer follow up because other outcomes, including contrast sensitivity and angiographic outcomes of progression and size of lesion, significantly favored the verteporfin group at 24-month follow up. Photodynamic therapy with verteporfin is recommended currently for eyes with predominantly classic subfoveal CNV, especially when no occult CNV is present (2,11).

In eyes without any classic CNV, a clear treatment benefit in both visual and angiographic outcomes was demonstrated in the second year of verteporfin treatment: Eyes with occult and no classic CNV treated with verteporfin were 1.4 times more likely to avoid moderate vision loss at 24 months than control eyes. Again, it appears likely that a differential effect is apparent, with baseline vision and lesion size influencing treatment effect. Eyes with smaller lesions (four MPS disc areas or less) or with lower levels of visual acuity (letter score < 65, approximate Snellen equivalent 20/50 − 1 or less) treated with verteporfin were 2.1 times as likely to avoid a moderate vision loss at 24 months than control eyes. Eligibility criteria should be remembered when interpreting the results of the VIP study because applying the study results to the general population of AMD patients with occult with no classic CNV is complex. Many patients with occult disease were not eligible for inclusion in the VIP study owing to the lack of recent progression or the predominant presence of other lesion components such as blood or serous pigment epithelial detachment. The treatment effect of PDT with verteporfin remains unknown in these cases. The current recommendation is to consider treatment for eyes with occult and no classic CNV, especially in eyes with poorer vision or with smaller lesions (4).

The data from the TAP and VIP studies also provide the starting point for future work. It may be possible that additional diagnostic and investigational tools, such as indocyanine green angiography or ocular coherence tomography, and classification of CNV on the cellular and microbiologic level may deepen our understanding of the differential effects of treatment, and serve to refine treatment decisions. It may be possible to alter the verteporfin treatment protocol or combine verteporfin therapy with adjuvant treatments to widen the range of patients with treatment benefit or to maximize the effect of treatment in the first 6 months, when much of the visual loss occurs. In the meantime, the TAP and VIP-AMD studies provide quality clinical evidence for the use and effect of PDT with verteporfin in the management of patients with subfoveal CNV and AMD.

REFERENCES

1. Treatment of Age-related Macular Degeneration with Photodynamic Therapy (TAP) Study Group. Photodynamic therapy of subfoveal choroidal neovascularisation in age-related macular degeneration with verteporfin: one-year results of 2 randomized clinical trials. *Arch Ophthalmol* 1999;117:1329–1345.
2. Treatment of Age-related Macular Degeneration with Photodynamic Therapy (TAP) Study Group. Photodynamic therapy of subfoveal choroidal neovascularisation in age-related macular degeneration with verteporfin: two-year results of 2 randomized clinical trials. *Arch Ophthalmol* 2001;119:198–207.
3. Treatment of Age-related Macular Degeneration with Photodynamic Therapy (TAP) Study Group. Verteporfin (Visudyne) therapy of subfoveal choroidal neovascularization in patients with age-related macular degeneration: Additional information regarding baseline lesion composition's impact on vision outcomes—TAP Report No. 3. *Arch Ophthalmol* 2002;120:1443–1454.
4. Verteporfin in Photodynamic Therapy Study Group. Verteporfin therapy of subfoveal choroidal neovascularization in age-related macular degeneration: two-year results of a randomized clinical trial including lesions with occult with no classic choroidal neovascularization. *Am J Ophthalmol* 2001;131:541–560.
5. Bressler NB, for The Verteporfin in Photodynamic Therapy Study Group Report No 2 Writing Committee. Letter to editor. *Am J Ophthalmol* 2001, submitted.
6. Wormald R, Evans J, Smeeth L. Photodynamic therapy for neovascular age-related macular degeneration (Cochrane Review). In *The Cochrane Library*, issue 2, 2003. Oxford: Update Software.
7. American Academy of Ophthalmology. Photodynamic therapy with verteporfin for age-related macular degeneration. *Ophthalmology* 2000;107:2314–2317.
8. Miller JW, Schmidt-Erfurth U, Sickenberg M, et al. Photodynamic therapy with verteporfin for choroidal neovascularisation caused by age-related macular degeneration. Results of a single treatment in a Phase 1 and 2 study. *Arch Ophthalmol* 1999;117:1161–1173.
9. Schmidt-Erfurth U, Miller J, Sickenberg M, et al. Photodynamic therapy with verteporfin for choroidal neovascularisation caused by age-related macular degeneration. Results of retreatments in a Phase 1 and 2 study. *Arch Ophthalmol* 1999;117:1177–1187.
10. Haimovici R, Kramer M, Miller JW, et al. Localisation of lipoprotein-delivered benzoporphyrin derivative in the rabbit eye. *Curr Eye Res* 1997;16:83–90.

15

VERTEPORFIN PHOTODYNAMIC THERAPY IN PATHOLOGIC MYOPIA

JORDI M. MONÉS

The prevalence of myopia varies considerably depending on the geographic location (1). It was estimated to be 25% in United States (2), 21% in Iceland, and 9% in Sweden (3). The prevalence of myopia is significantly higher in Asia, especially Japan and China, where it may reach 75% by age 15 years (1,4). Distribution of myopia is also affected by country-specific differences, sex, and race; it is higher in women and Asians, and lower in Africans and African-Americans (1,2,5,6). The prevalence of myopia can be as low as 2% to 5% in Australian aborigines and Solomon Islanders (7,8).

Both environmental and genetic factors have been associated with the onset and progression of myopia. However, their mechanisms and relative contributions are not well known (1,9).

Pathologic myopia greater than 6 diopters (D) affects 6% to 18% of the entire myopic population; thus, it is estimated to be present in 0.5% to 2% of the general population of the United States and Europe, and is the seventh leading cause of blindness (2,10). Pathologic myopia is characterized by excessive progressive elongation of the globe and a number of degenerative changes in the sclera, choroid, Bruch's membrane, retinal pigment epithelium (RPE), and retina. Patients with myopia of 6 D or greater or axial length of 25 mm or greater are more likely to suffer retinal abnormalities. This enlargement results in an ocular volume 50% greater than that of the normal eye (11). Funduscopic changes of pathologic myopia include a temporal peripapillary atrophic crescent, tilting of the optic disc, posterior staphyloma, stretched retinal vessels, lacquer cracks or ruptures in Bruch's membrane, subretinal hemorrhage, areas of atrophy of the RPE and choroid, and choroidal neovascularization (CNV) (12,13).

Choroidal neovascularization is a major vision-threatening complication in pathologic myopia, together with retinal detachment and chorioretinal atrophy (12). The incidence of CNV in pathologic myopia may range from 4% to 11% (14–19). In addition to the emotional and personal consequences in quality of life of central visual loss, the impact of this disease is of special importance because it affects relatively young patients with active work duties and family responsibilities.

The features of CNV in pathologic myopia differ from those of other etiologies. The neovascular membranes are usually small, and the serous retinal detachment is very limited and hard to detect on biomicroscopic examination and even in stereoscopic photographs. Leakage is minimal on fluorescein angiography (FA), although the characteristics are characteristic of classic CNV (20,21).

In spite of their small size (82% have less than one half disc diameters), CNV in pathologic myopia often results in an initial severe visual loss owing to frequent subfoveal location (89% are less than 200 μ from the foveola) (20).

Several natural history studies have reported a range of visual acuity outcomes in CNV associated with pathologic myopia. Avila and coworkers (21) described that the vascular complex regressed into an atrophic nonexudative scar in 96% of cases, especially in a subgroup of eyes in which fluorescein did not leak beyond the CNV, suggesting a self-limited course for CNV in these myopic eyes. These authors hypothesized that the attenuated nature of the choroidal blood flow supply in these eyes was the cause. However, Hotchkiss and Fine (16) reported deterioration of visual acuity in 51% of eyes, and Hampton and associates in 43% (23). In other studies of the natural history of CNV in pathologic myopia, visual acuity outcomes of 20/200 or less occurred in 41% to 60% of eyes (12,16,21–23). Secretan and associates (20) in a series of 50 eyes with myopic CNV reported that an initial visual loss was followed by transient relative stabilization of vision for 2 years. However, afterward there was a further progressive deterioration in vision. Tabandeh and colleagues (12) found that CNV in pathologic myopia had an even poorer outcome in patients 50 years of age or older. In their series, 73% of eyes had a final visual acuity of 20/200 or less, and some of the study eyes showed "significant" subretinal fibrosis. These authors suggested that highly myopic older patients might manifest features of both age-related macular degeneration (AMD) and high myopia.

Laser photocoagulation has no benefit for subfoveal CNV because of the vision loss induced by the treatment. Laser results in extrafoveal or juxtafoveal lesions can be encouraging in the short term; however, the initial benefit may be lost within 1 or 2 years after the development of subfoveal recurrent CNV or enlargement of the laser scar (21,20,24–28). Even in cases of extrafoveal lesions that were successfully treated with initially good visual results, the progressive enlargement of the laser scar may extend under the fovea and cause severe visual loss (29). Jalkh and coworkers (29) reported worsening of visual acuity in 68% of laser-treated extrafoveal lesions, and 89% of the eyes showed a wide ring of deep choroidal atrophy owing to progressive enlargement of the initial scar after an average period of 13.4 months. It has been suggested that laser scar enlargement is a consequence of a further thermal laser-induced weakness of the choroid, associated with the permanent stretch caused by progressive degenerative myopia (21,29). Also, laser photocoagulation might result in the development of new lacquer cracks or elongation of preexisting cracks (30). Recurrent CNV also has been reported to occur as frequently as 72% of the eyes treated with laser photocoagulation (20).

Photodynamic therapy with verteporfin (verteporfin PDT) was proposed as a potential therapeutic alternative that might overcome the limitations of laser photocoagulation. Based on the preliminary verteporfin PDT results of a Phase I and II investigation, and given the safety data then available from the TAP Study of patients with subfoveal CNV secondary to AMD a randomized clinical trial of verteporfin PDT was started for selected patients with CNV secondary to pathologic myopia. The objective of this clinical trial, called the Verteporfin in Photodynamic Therapy (VIP) Study, was to determine if verteporfin PDT could stabilize or improve vision in patients with subfoveal CNV secondary to pathologic myopia compared to placebo. The VIP study was a multicenter, double-masked, placebo-controlled, randomized trial in 28 ophthalmology practices in Europe and North America.

One hundred twenty eyes in as many patients were enrolled in the VIP Study and randomized in a 2 to 1 ratio to verteporfin therapy or placebo. Basically, the inclusion criteria were lesions with CNV secondary to proven pathologic myopia extending under the geometric center of the avascular zone at the FA, not larger than 5,400 μm, and with best corrected visual acuity of at least 50 Early Treatment Diabetic Retinopathy Study (ETDRS) letters, approximately 20/100 or better. Patients with ocular conditions other than pathologic myopia, rips of the retinal pigment epithelium (RPE), significant ocular disease, or any previous treatment different than confluent photocoagulation for CNV were excluded. Other exclusion criteria were significant liver disease, porphyria or porphyrin sensitivity, and pregnancy. Because eyes with subfoveal CNV secondary to pathologic myopia are likely to lose less vision than eyes with subfoveal exudative CNV secondary to AMD (31), the primary efficacy outcome was defined as the proportion of eyes that lost fewer than eight ETDRS letters, approximately 1.5 ETDRS lines, differing from the primary efficacy outcome, which was defined as moderate visual loss in the TAP investigation, 15 ETDRS letters of visual loss, or approximately three ETDRS lines.

Baseline characteristics were balanced and the completion of follow-up at 12 and 24 months was very high in both treatment and placebo groups. The VIP study demonstrated that verteporfin PDT increased the chance of stabilizing or improving vision when compared with placebo. During the 24 months of follow up, the verteporfin-treated group was more likely to remain stable (losing less than eight letters) compared with the placebo-treated group. However, this beneficial difference favoring treatment was statistically significant only during the first 12 months. At the 3-month follow-up visit, 62 eyes (77%) of the verteporfin-treated group compared with 22 eyes (56%) of the placebo-treated group (p = 0.02) lost fewer than eight letters, a 21% absolute difference favoring treatment. By the 12-month follow-up visit, the difference was 28% favoring treatment, with 58 eyes (72%) treated and 17 eyes (44%) in the placebo group losing fewer than eight letters (less than 0.01). The percentage difference in losing fewer than 15 letters dropped over the second year, from 19% to 7% in favor of verteporfin PDT (p = 0.38). However, eyes receiving treatment were more likely to have improved vision compared with placebo-treated eyes; especially after 2 years, when the absolute differences became larger (Table 15.1). At the 24-month follow-up visit, 32 eyes (40%) in the treated group gained at least one ETDRS line compared with five eyes (13%) in the placebo group (p = 0,003). Ten eyes (12%) in the treated group had an improvement of three or more ETDRS lines, compared with no eyes in the placebo group (p = 0.03). The positive visual acuity results

TABLE 15.1. IMPROVING OF VISUAL ACUITY IN THE VERTEPORFIN IN PHOTODYNAMIC THERAPY STUDY FOR CHOROIDAL NEOVASCULARIZATION IN PATHOLOGIC MYOPIA

	Verteporfin (n = 81)	Placebo (n = 39)	P value
Gain >1 lines			
Month 12	26 (32%)	6 (16%)	<0.01
Month 24	32 (40%)	5 (13%)	0.003
Gain >3 lines			
Month 12	5 (6%)	1 (3%)	<0.01
Month 24	10 (12%)	0 (0%)	0.03

were further supported by the contrast sensitivity outcomes; the verteporfin-treated group was more likely to improve at least three letters (29%) compared with the placebo-treated group (9%) at the 12-month examination. Fluorescein angiographic outcomes showed that the verteporfin-treated group was less likely to have progression of or leakage from classic CNV, and more likely to have small lesions at the 12-month examination (32).

Few ocular or other systemic adverse events were associated with verteporfin therapy compared with placebo treatment (32). Unlike in the TAP investigation (33), there were no cases of severe vision decrease within a few days of the treatment and no cases of infusion-related back pain. Visual disturbances were similar in both groups (21%, including abnormal vision, decreased vision, and visual field defects): Injection-site events were lower than in the TAP Study (7% in the verteporfin-treated group and 5% in the placebo-treated group); allergic reactions were 4% and 3%, respectively, as were photosensitivity reactions.

In the VIP Study, investigators were asked to treat based only on the presence of leakage on the FA. In equivocal cases, investigators were supposed to treat lesion. The rate of treatment in the VIP Study is shown in Figure 15.1. Since the positive study results became available, many patients with CNV secondary to pathologic myopia have been treated around the world. The issue of retreatment is one of the recurring questions in the clinical application of verteporfin PDT in this group. If leakage assessment of CNV in pathologic myopia is difficult at baseline, it becomes further complicated after Verteporfin PDT. Few patients clearly show leakage or absence of leakage at follow-up visits (Figs. 15.2 and 15.3). Indeed, most show questionable leakage. In addition, biomicroscopy cannot be used as a tool in cases of doubtful or questionable leakage because neurosensory detachment is undetectable, even in fresh untreated lesions. Thus, retreatment decision making has become more challenging and difficult than verteporfin PDT in neovascular AMD. It is our impression in several cases that lesions that were apparently not leaky and thus were not treated showed a marked progression of CNV at the next follow-up visit. Optic coherent tomography (OCT) might be considered helpful in some cases; however, it is inconclusive in lesions where only a shallow neurosensory detachment exists. Thus, another approach to avoid unnecessary retreatments (which could occur if one treats all cases of questionable leakage) is to use a much closer follow-up schedule to pick up any angiographically leaky lesion. Also, subjective changes in vision such as metamorphopsia can be helpful. In our institution, we consider subjective metamorphopsia together with visual acuity evolution as useful criteria to determine the necessity of retreatment when FA is unclear. For example, if a patient has improved vision and doubtful leakage and reports less metamorphopsia, then retreatment is not recommended. The next follow-up visit is scheduled within 4 weeks or when the patient notices a worsening in the metamorphopsia (Figs. 15.4 and 15.5). In contrast, if the patient in the same situation reports recent worsening in the metamorphopsia, then retreatment is recommended in spite of an apparently not leaky lesion or visual improvement (Fig. 15.6). Our preliminary results on the first 66 patients (unpublished data) showed a marked decrease in the retreatment rate in comparison with the VIP Study (Fig. 15.1), although the results should be considered with cau-

(text continues on page 205)

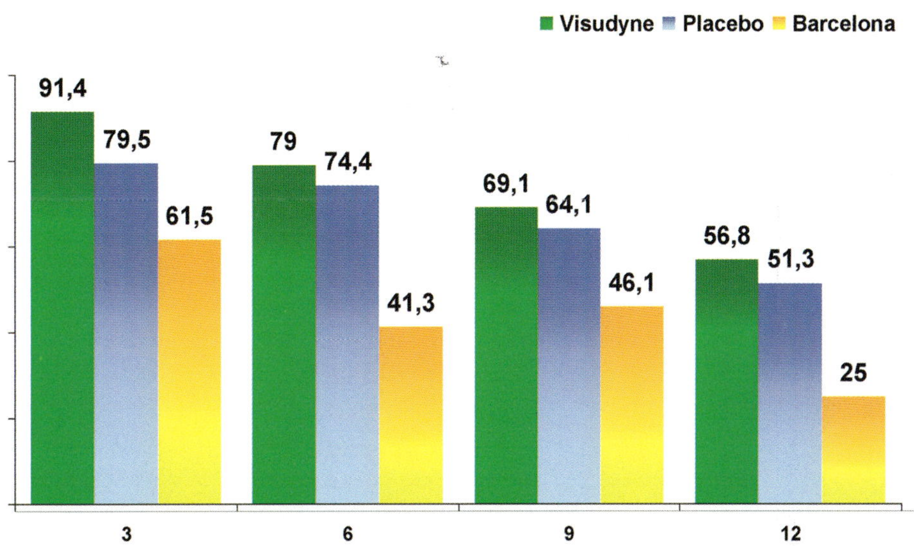

FIGURE 15.1. Treatment rate on the VIP Study (in green the treated-group, and in blue the placebo group) and rate of treatments of patients outside the Trials in Barcelona.

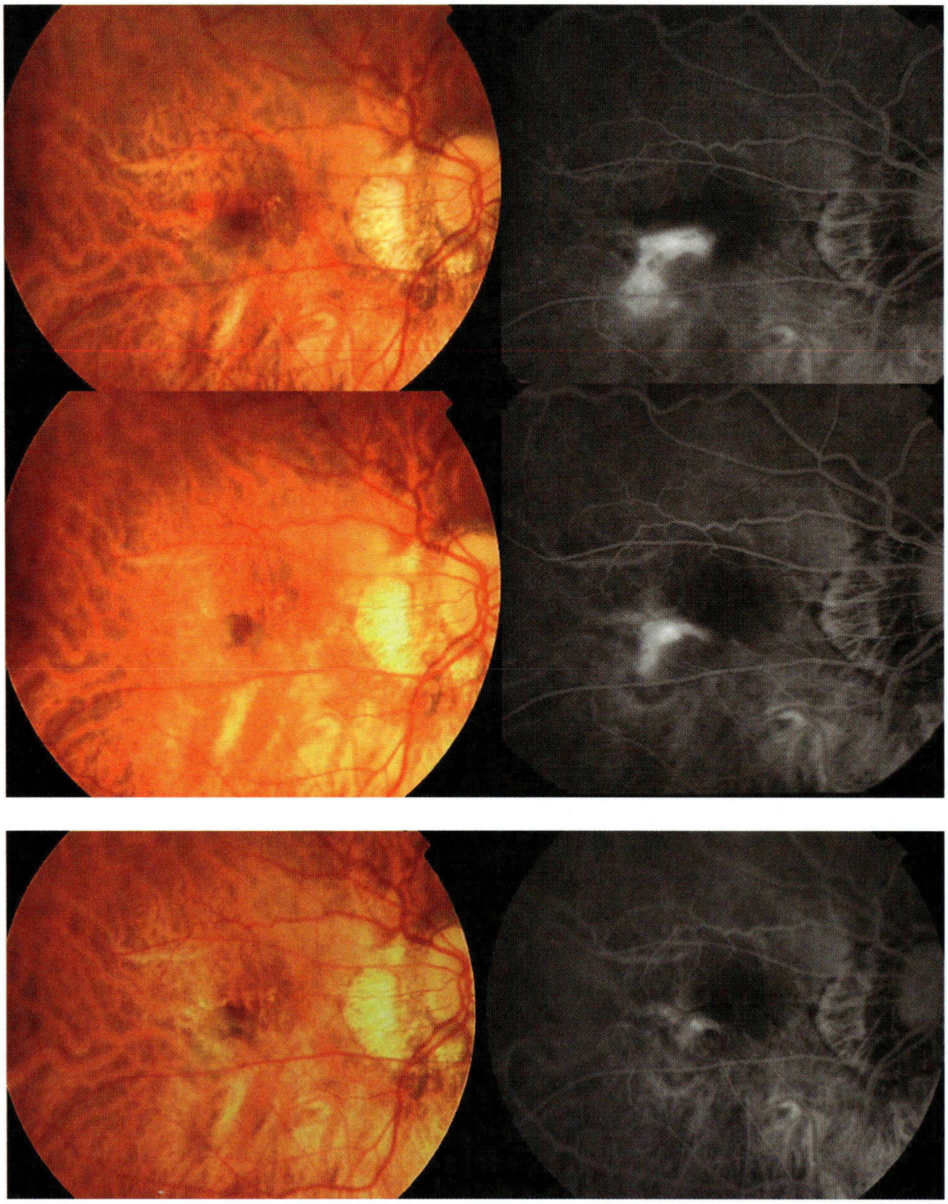

FIGURE 15.2. *Upper row:* Fundus photography and fluorescein angiography (FA) of a 52-year-old 6-diopter myopic female patient with subfoveal choroidal neovascularization (CNV). Visual acuity at baseline was 20/160. Exudation is very evident in the FA. Photodynamic therapy was performed. *Middle row:* Visual acuity was 20/64 at the 3-month follow-up visit. Exudation is easily identified at FA. The patient was retreated. *Lower row:* At the 6-month follow-up visit visual acuity was 20/32. Fluorescein angiography clearly showed staining of the lesion. The patient was not treated. The lesion features were maintained unchanged after two treatments showing only staining and achieving a visual acuity of 20/32 at the 12-month follow-up visit.

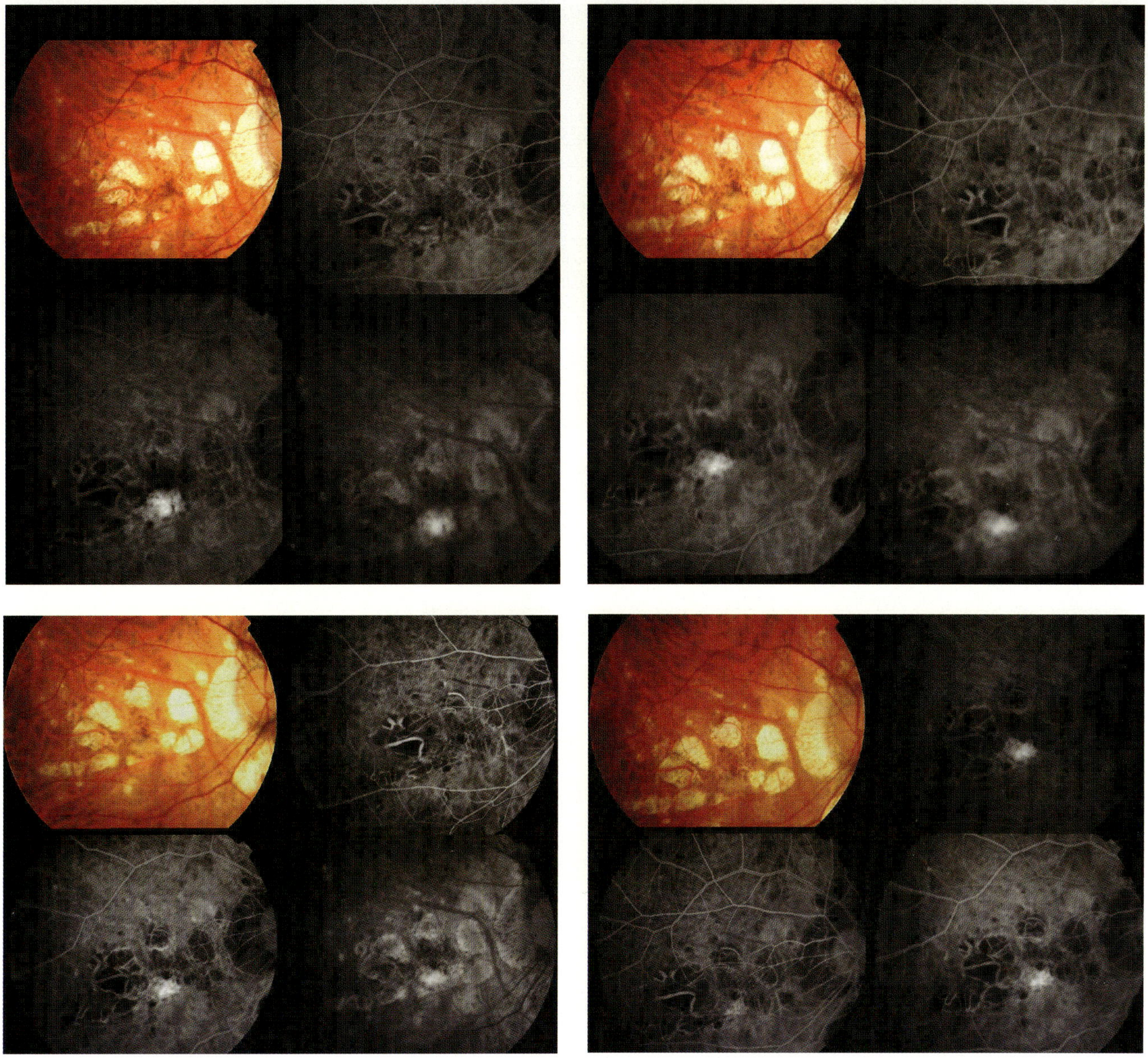

A B C D

FIGURE 15.3. A: Fundus photography and fluorescein angiography (FA) transit of a 65-year-old myopic female patient with subfoveal choroidal neovascularization (CNV). Visual acuity at baseline was 20/125. Exudation is well identified in the late frames. Photodynamic therapy was performed. **B:** Fundus photography and FA transit at the 3-month follow-up visit. Visual acuity had improved to 20/64. Leakage is still easy to observe in the late frames. Retreatment was performed. **C:** Fundus photography and FA transit at the 6-month follow-up visit. Visual acuity had improved to 20/50. At the late frames, the lesion showed distinct geographic margins. No leakage was identified. **D:** At the 12-month follow-up visit, visual acuity improved to 20/40. The lesion was unchanged, showing only staining at the FA. The patient had received two treatments in total.

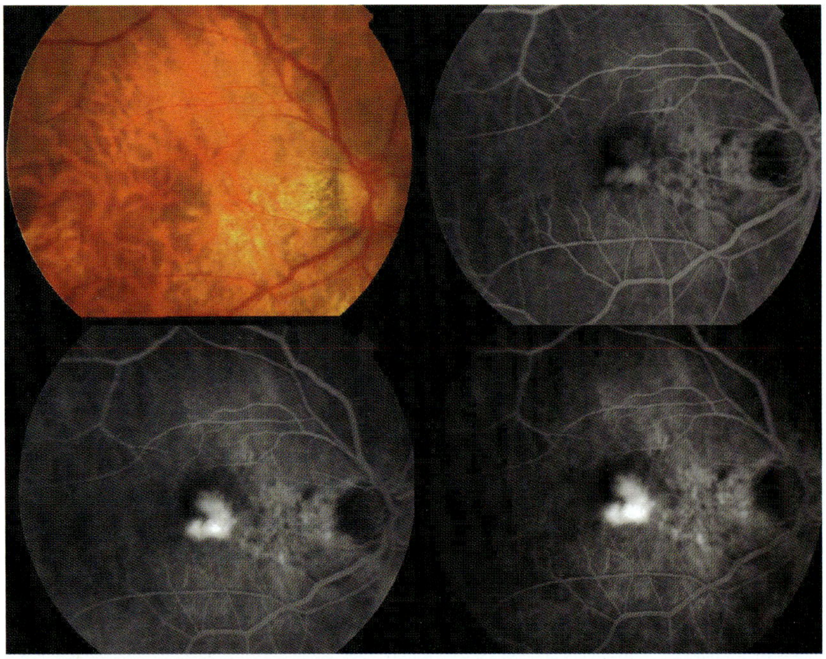

A

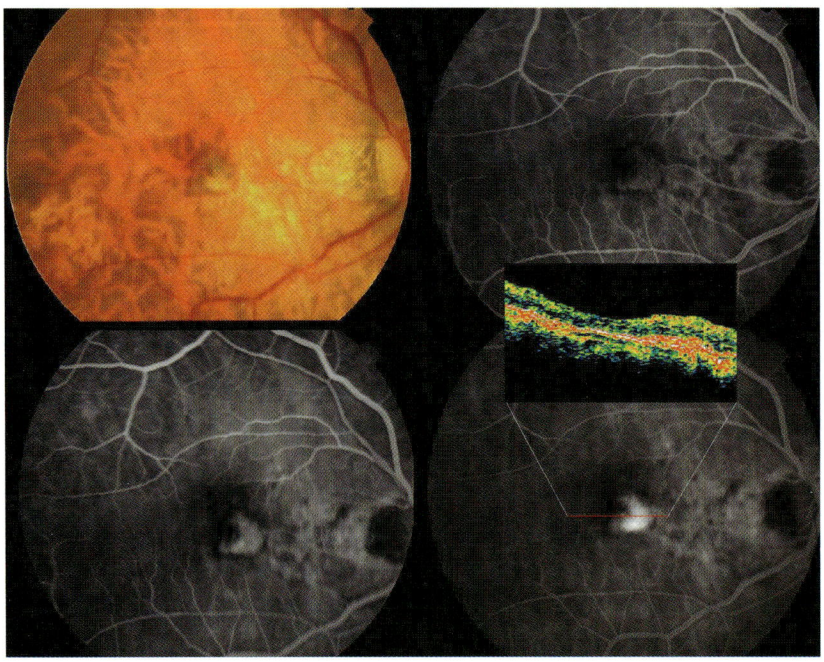

B

FIGURE 15.4. A: Fundus photography and fluorescein angiography (FA) transit of a 54-year-old myopic female patient with subfoveal choroidal neovascularization (CNV). Visual acuity at baseline was 20/80. Exudation is well identified in the late frames. Photodynamic therapy was performed. **B:** At the 3-month follow-up visit, visual acuity had improved to 20/50. Biomicroscopy examination showed no neurosensory detachment and no subretinal blood. Leakage was questionable at late frames of FA. No neurosensory detachment could be identified on optic coherent tomography examination. The patient was not treated and rescheduled in 4 to 6 weeks or earlier if she felt any worsening in the metamorphopsia or visual acuity.

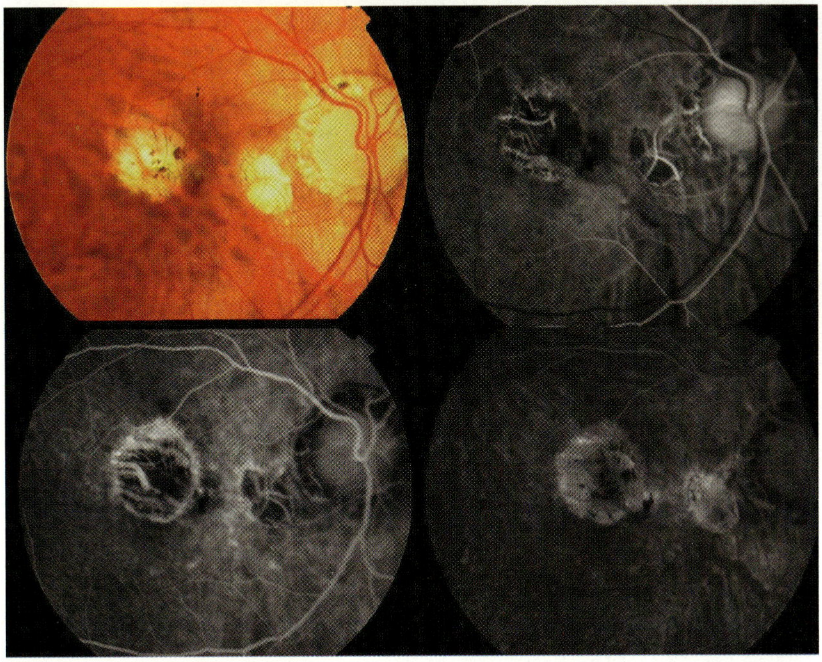

A

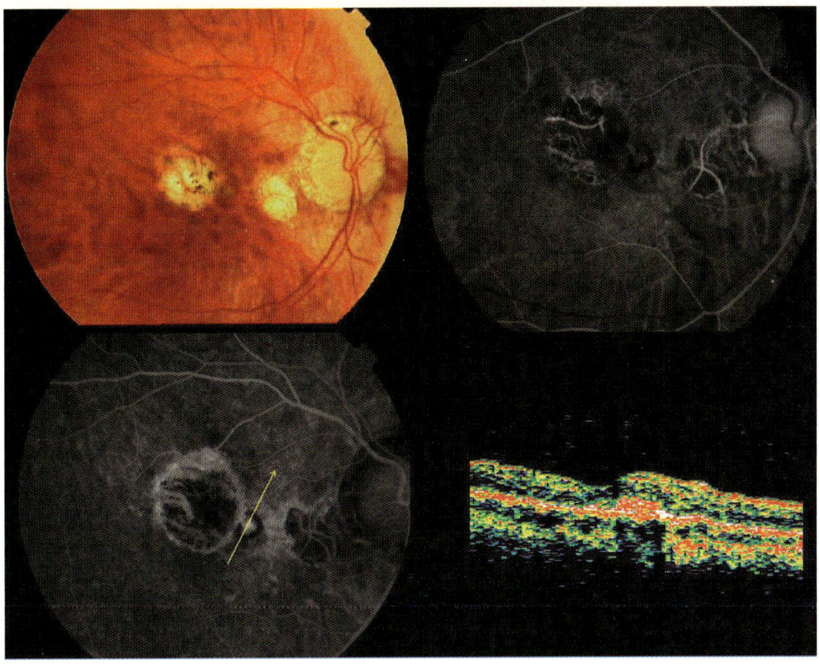

B

FIGURE 15.5. A: Color and fluorescein angiography (FA) transit of a 36-year-old myopic female patient complaining of metamorphopsia. Visual acuity was 20/32. Patient was successfully treated 1 year ago for a subfoveal CNV secondary to pathologic myopia with macular translocation and laser photocoagulation afterward. Biomicroscopy and FA showed subfoveal blood and leakage at the foveal edge of the laser scar. Photodynamic therapy was performed with a spot area of 1,600 μm. **B:** At the 3-month follow-up visit, the CNV lesion had more distinct borders and leakage was questionable in the late frames. Biomicroscopic examination did not reveal any subfoveal blood or neurosensory detachment. Patient had no metamorphopsia and visual acuity had improved one line, to 20/26. On optical coherence tomographic examination a barely subfoveal lesion was evidenced without any associated visible neurosensory detachment. Patient was not treated and rescheduled in 4 to 6 weeks or earlier if she felt any worsening in the metamorphopsia or in the visual acuity.

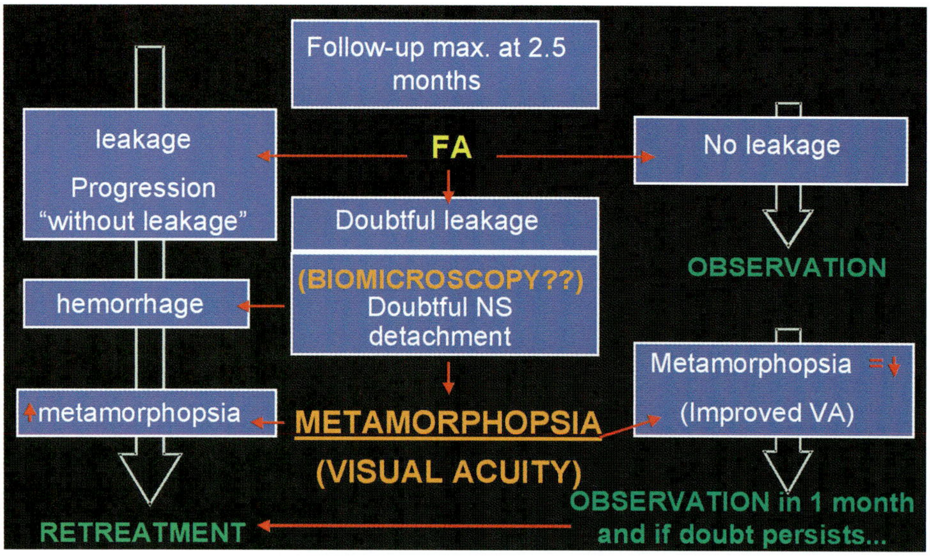

FIGURE 15.6. Algorithm of verteporfin photodynamic therapy retreatment criteria in choroidal neovascularization secondary to pathologic myopia.

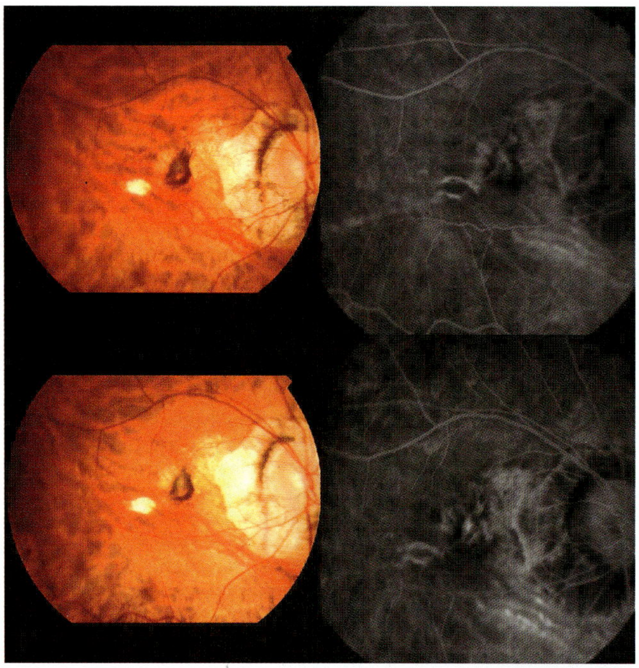

A

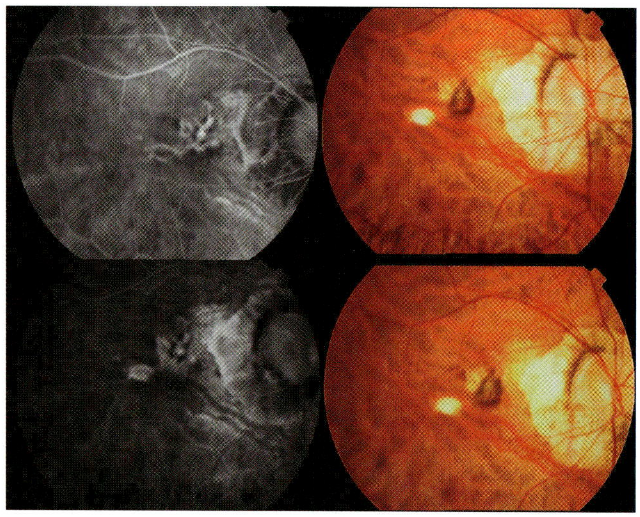

B

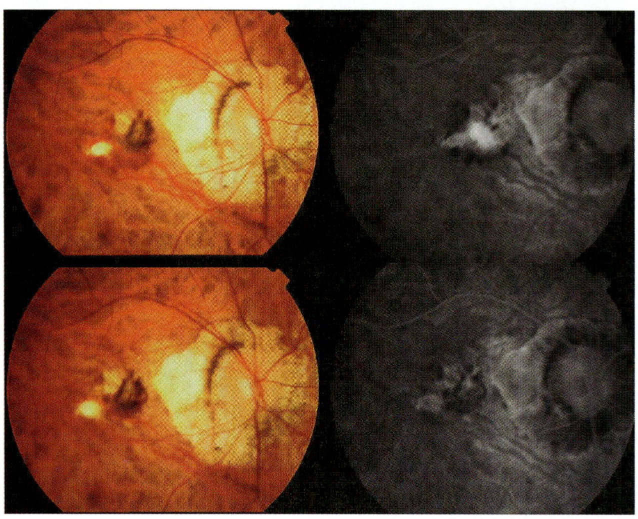

C

FIGURE 15.7. A: *Upper row:* Fundus photography and fluorescein angiography (FA) of a 57-year-old myopic female patient complaining of recent visual loss and metamorphopsia with subfoveal choroidal neovascularization (CNV). Visual acuity at baseline was 20/80. Leakage was even questionable at baseline. Photodynamic therapy was performed. *Middle row:* At the 3-month follow-up visit visual acuity did not changed. At FA leakage was identified at the nasal side of the lesion. Patient was retreated. **B:** *Upper row:* At the 6-month follow-up visit FA was interpreted not to show leakage. Biomicroscopy evidenced a flat lesion with no neurosensory detachment. Visual acuity was 20/125. The patient was not treated. *Lower row:* At the 9-month follow-up visit biomicroscopic and FA findings were similar. Visual acuity was 20/160. The patient was not treated. **C:** *Upper row:* At the 12-month follow-up visit a marked progression of the CNV was observed with significant amount of subretinal blood and prominent leakage. Visual acuity was 20/125. It is noteworthy that the lesion had never clearly showed leakage or subretinal blood. Patient was treated with verteporfin PDT. *Lower row:* At the 15-month follow-up visit the subretinal blood disappeared as well as the leakage at the FA. Lesion only showed staining and visual acuity was 20/100.

tion because other criteria (as mentioned) must be considered and the follow up is still incomplete for all the patients. Also, the timing of recurrence is unpredictable and may occur at different intervals after leakage cessation.

If it is true that unnecessary treatments should be avoided because visual loss is a potential although infrequent complication, then it is also true that misinterpreting fluorescein leakage or underestimating CNV activity may lead to a progression of the CNV. In some cases, an "AMD-like" progression of the CNV (progression of classic CNV with marked exudation and leakage outside its boundaries) has been observed (Fig. 15.7). Thus, CNV should be watched carefully and frequently after starting verteporfin PDT.

The shape of some of the neovascular membranes is another issue specific for CNV secondary to pathologic myopia. Myopic neovascular lesions sometimes are long and narrow. Thus, when the diameter of the treatment spot is applied according to the calculated greatest linear dimension of the lesion, a very large area of normal retina and retinal pigment epithelium is treated at both sides on the shortest linear dimension. To minimize these extra areas of treatment on normal fundus, in some cases we have performed multiple contiguous spots of treatment, with careful attention to avoid overlap of treatment areas. We have not found any adverse event related to this manner of treating long lesions (Fig. 15.8). The same rationale has been used successfully in cases of multiple lesions (Fig. 15.9).

Surgical alternatives have been suggested for CNV since 1985, such as surgical excision of the CNV membranes (34–36) or macular translocation (37,38). Results of surgical excision in CNV associated to pathologic myopia have not been particularly encouraging because of damage to the RPE (36). Macular translocation moves the fovea away from the CNV to a new location over an area of normal RPE and choroid. The first experimental reports in 1983 and 1985 described successful shifting of the retina using large retinotomies, but complicated by proliferative vitreoretinopathy and retinal detachment (39,40). Machemer and Steinhorst described an animal model in which the retina was completely detached, and a 360-degree peripheral retinotomy was used to rotate the retina up to 60 degrees (37,38). They also reported a similar procedure in three patients; however, proliferative vitreoretinopathy eventually developed in all of them. Macular translocation with a 180-degree retinotomy was described in 1996,

A

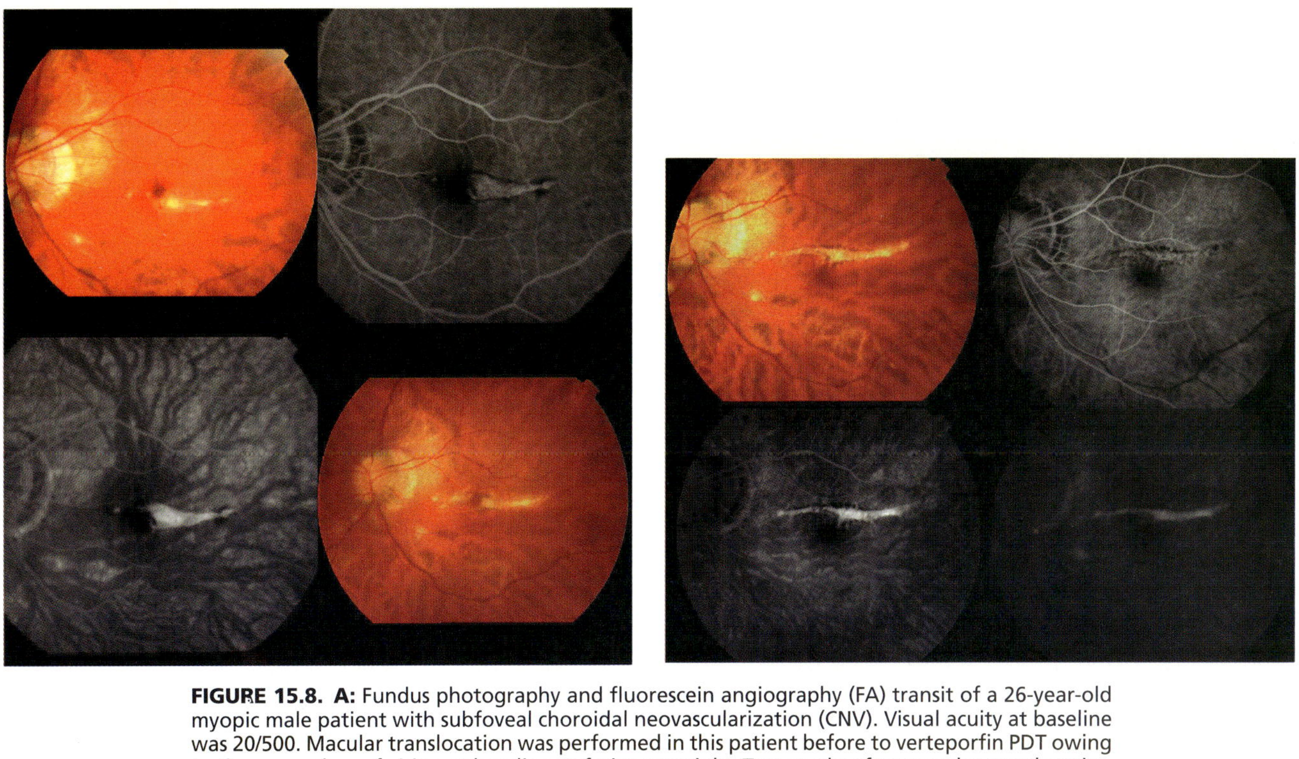

B

FIGURE 15.8. A: Fundus photography and fluorescein angiography (FA) transit of a 26-year-old myopic male patient with subfoveal choroidal neovascularization (CNV). Visual acuity at baseline was 20/500. Macular translocation was performed in this patient before to verteporfin PDT owing to the severe loss of vision at baseline. *Inferior row right:* Two weeks after macular translocation the fovea was located well below the lesion and PDT was done. Owing to the elongated shape of the CNV verteporfin PDT was performed with two immediate consecutive areas of laser exposure of 1,500 and 1,800 mm to avoid treating unnecessary large areas of retinal pigment epithelium above and below the lesion. At the 3-, 6-, and 9-month follow-up visits **(B)** the lesion showed staining at FA and was located above the fovea. The visual acuity was 20/50. The patient had received only one treatment with two consecutive spots.

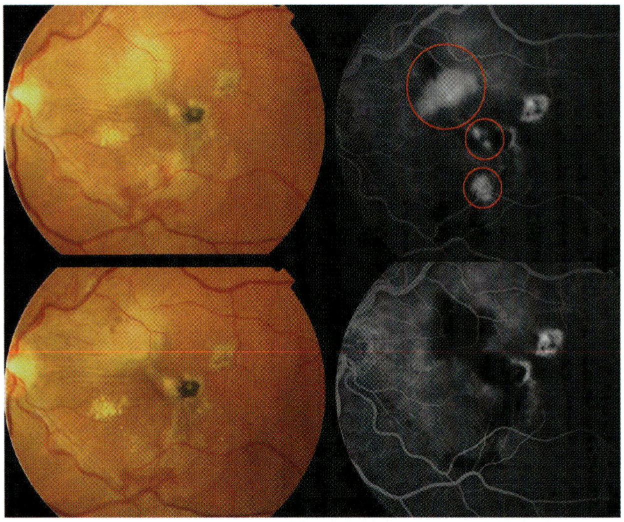

A

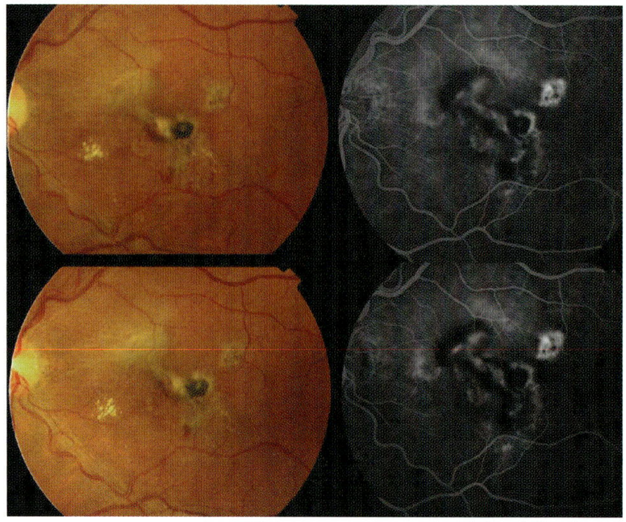

B

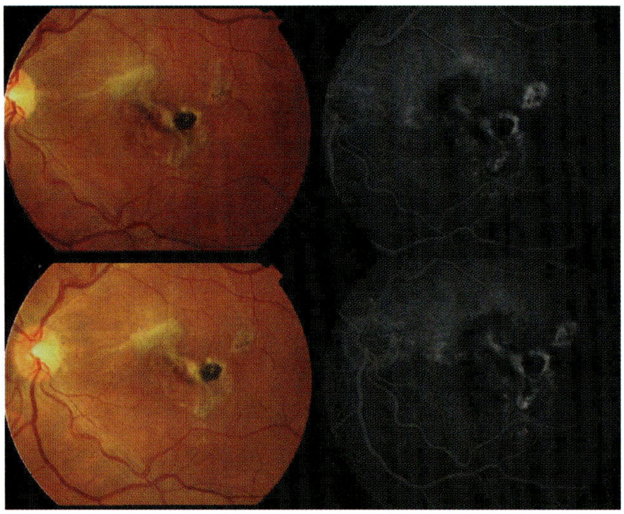

C

FIGURE 15.9. A: *Upper row:* A 28-year-old myopic female patient complaining of recent metamorphopsia and loss of vision. Visual acuity was 20/80. A subfoveal choroidal neovascularization (CNV) had been successfully excised surgically some months ago. Biomicroscopy and fluorescein angiography (FA) showed subfoveal blood and prominent leakage from three different sources. Photodynamic therapy was performed with three consecutive different spots of 2,400, 1,100, and 1,100 μm. *Lower row:* At a 1-week follow-up visit, no unexpected or adverse event was identified. Leakage ceased at the three sources. **B:** *Upper and lower rows:* Biomicroscopy at 1- and 3-month follow-up visits showed less subretinal blood, and less neurosensory detachment. Visual acuity had improved to 20/50. At FA some leakage was present again at the upper lesion. Photodynamic therapy then was performed with one-spot treatment area over leaky area. **C:** *Upper and lower row:* Biomicroscopy at 6- and 9-month follow-up visits showed absence of blood and no neurosensory detachment. Minimal residual lipid exudation was observed. Visual acuity improved and was maintained at 20/20. This patient only received two treatments, the first one being triple-spot.

although the risk of developing proliferative vitreoretinopathy was not solved (41). In 1996 Imai and de Juan developed a new approach to translocate the fovea by means of scleral resection without a retinotomy, the limited macular translocation (42). Subsequently, these authors and others have performed this technique for subfoveal CNV secondary to AMD or other causes, such as pathologic myopia (43–46).

Photodynamic therapy with verteporfin also can be considered combined with macular translocation. Theoretically, patients with poor vision might benefit initially by macular translocation, achieving an improvement in vision that might then be stabilized or further improved by verteporfin PDT. Macular translocation may achieve varying degrees of foveal displacement, with a mean of 854 μm (46). However, if the CNV is treated with laser photocoagulation the potential complication of laser scar enlargement with increase in scotoma size as well as an eventual foveal involvement with severe visual loss arises again. Photodynamic therapy with verteporfin might be beneficial by inactivating the displaced CNV and avoiding the laser complications (Figs. 15.8 and 15.10). Long-term randomized clinical trials may be warranted to assess the role of macular translocation in comparison to verteporfin PDT for efficacy as well as safety.

Photodynamic therapy may be beneficial in cases of subfoveal or juxtafoveal recurrent CNV after laser photocoagulation, with or without previous macular translocation, or in recurrent CNV after surgical excision (Fig. 15.5).

In summary, verteporfin PDT has been proved to improve or stabilize vision in patients with CNV secondary to pathologic myopia, without safety concerns. Retreatment decision making is challenging and criteria other than FA may be taken into account. Close follow up is warranted in order to detect recurrent CNV at early stages that may occur at different intervals after verteporfin PDT. In addition, verteporfin PDT may be useful when combined with other strategies.

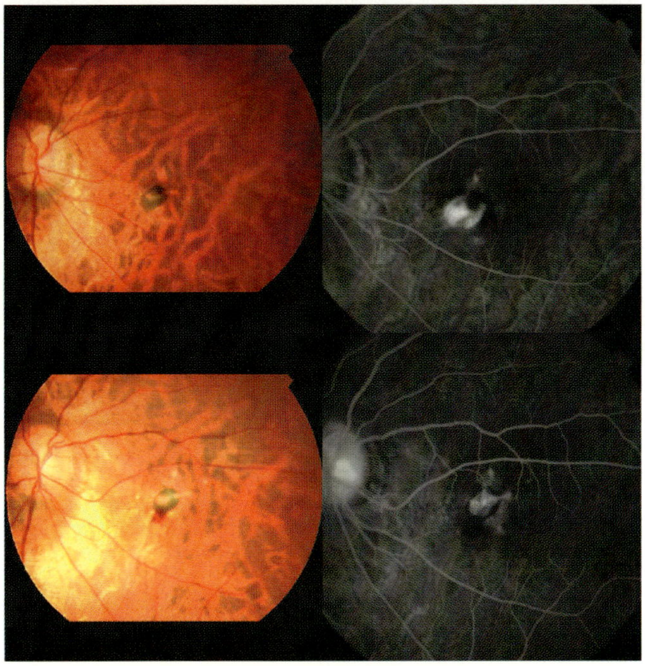

A

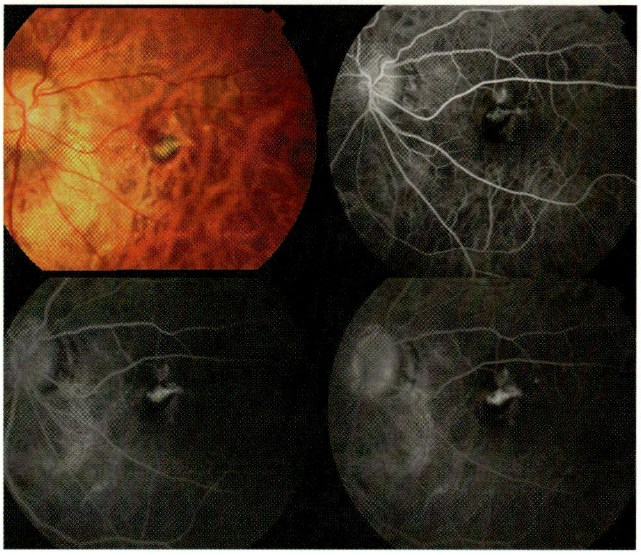

B

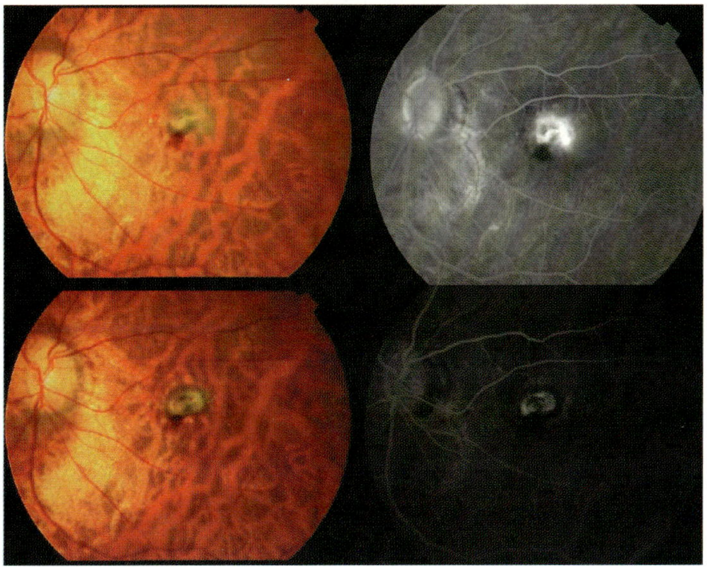

C

FIGURE 15.10. **A:** *Upper row:* Fundus photography and fluorescein angiography (FA) of a 24-year-old myopic female patient with subfoveal choroidal neovascularization (CNV). Visual acuity at baseline was 20/400. Macular translocation was performed in this patient before to verteporfin photodynamic therapy (PDT) owing to the severe loss of vision at baseline. *Lower row:* Two weeks after macular translocation the fovea was located well below the lesion and PDT was done. Visual acuity was 20/125. The lesion already showed less leakage and subretinal blood. **B:** At the 3-month follow-up visit, the visual acuity was 20/100. No blood was observed at the biomicroscopic examination (the red dot at the center is a photographic artefact) and at the FA the lesion was interpreted as not leaking and just staining. Treatment was not performed. **C:** *Upper row:* At the 6-month follow-up visit the visual acuity had unexpectedly improved to 20/80 in spite of a marked CNV progression, with intense leakage and a very evident neurosensory detachment. It is noteworthy that this patient was young and this progression of CNV cannot be influenced by the age factor as it could be hypothesized in the old-group of myopic patients. Treatment was performed. *Lower row:* At the 9-month follow-up the leakage ceased and vision was 20/100. At the 12-month follow-up visit the cessation of leakage was maintained and vision returned to 20/80.

APPENDIX: PATHOLOGIC MYOPIA CASE REPORT

Joan W. Miller

Case Report

Eight years of follow up using verteporfin PDT for subfoveal CNV secondary to pathologic myopia.[1]

A 33-year-old man with pathologic myopia (−18-D spherical equivalent) presented with loss of vision and metamorphopsia in the right eye. He had previously lost vision in the left eye to the level of counting fingers from CNV secondary to pathologic myopia. His visual acuity with refraction was 20/64 at baseline. Ophthalmoscopy revealed a pigmented subretinal membrane, and angiography demonstrated classic subfoveal CNV measuring 1,110 μm in its greatest linear diameter (Fig. 15.11). After discussing treatment options, including submacular surgery, the patient was enrolled in the Phase I clinical trial of verteporfin PDT and underwent PDT using 6 mg/m^2 of verteporfin and fluence of 50 J/cm^2. One week after the

[1] This case was presented in part by Sickenberg, et al. *Arch Ophthalmol* 2000;117:327–336. See p. 211 for a complete reference (47).

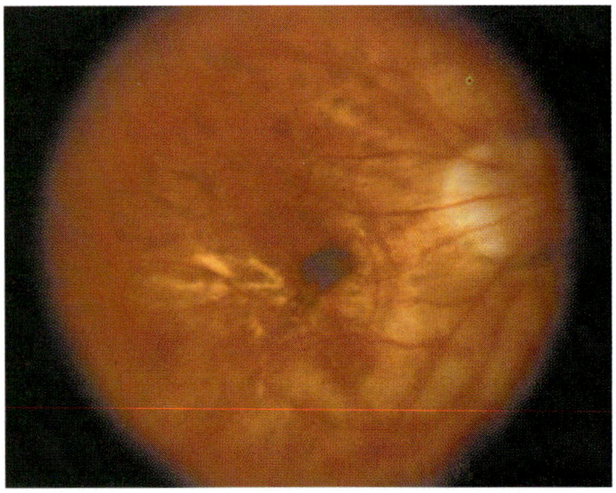

FIGURE 15.11. Initial verteporfin photodynamic therapy. Before treatment, a color fundus photograph shows a pigmented lesion under the center of the foveal avascular zone. Fluorescein angiography at that time demonstrated classic choroidal neovascularization with a bright area of hyperfluorescence in the early phase surrounded by some hypofluorescence corresponding to pigment and blood, with leakage in the late phase.

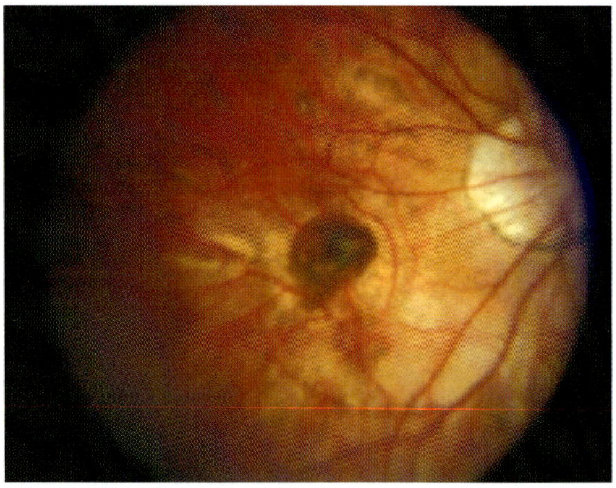

FIGURE 15.13. The patient was re-enrolled in verteporfin photodynamic therapy trials to investigate the effect of repeated treatments. A color fundus photograph shows an increase in size of the pigmented subretinal tissue and fluorescein angiography demonstrated leakage from choroidal neovascularization.

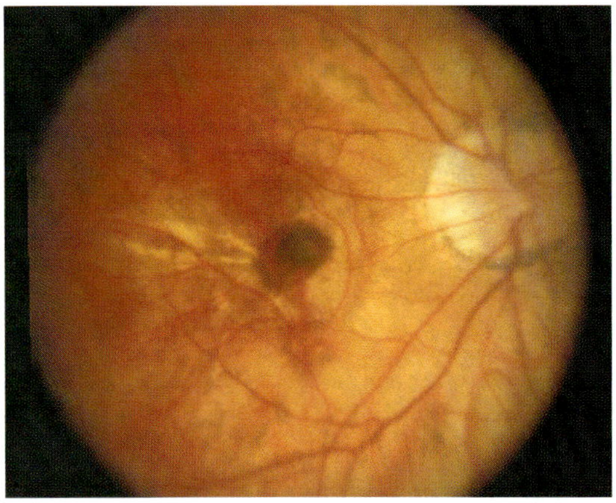

FIGURE 15.12. Twelve weeks after treatment, the pigmented subretinal tissue is visible in the color fundus photograph. The blood has resolved. Fluorescein angiography demonstrated leakage from choroidal neovascularization in the late phase.

first treatment, his vision improved to 20/50 and CNV leakage was graded as minimal. Vision continued to improve to 20/40 4 weeks after the treatment. However, by 12 weeks (the end point of the clinical study), vision had dropped again to 20/160 and CNV leakage was graded as moderate (Fig. 15.12).

The patient was re-enrolled in the Phase I study of repeat verteporfin PDT at 20 weeks after his initial treatment (Fig. 15.13), and 1 week after a second PDT his vision again improved to 20/100. Fluorescein angiography demonstrated leakage after 4 weeks, and repeat treatment was applied at 6 weeks. Four weeks after this treatment, his vision improved to 20/64. A fourth treatment was applied, and visual acuity improved to 20/40 by 4 weeks. At the end of follow up for this phase of the study (12 weeks after re-enrollment), visual acuity was 20/50 and angiography still demonstrated CNV leakage.

Fourteen months after completing the multiple treatment study, compassionate-use verteporfin therapy was permitted for patients previously enrolled in the PDT studies who demonstrated both recurrent CNV leakage angiographically and the potential to benefit from therapy.

FIGURE 15.15. Seven years after initial presentation the patient's vision was 20/50 and a color fundus photograph **(A)** shows some residual pigmented subretinal tissue that has diminished in size. Some loss of pigmentation consistent with atrophic change is noted in the surrounding retina. Fluorescein angiograms show some loss of choroidal perfusion (**B,** at 21 seconds) with perfusion of choroidal neovascularization (CNV) noted in later frames (**C,** at 1 min) and staining of tissue without leakage (**D,** at 10 min). The patient did not receive verteporfin photodynamic therapy at this time.

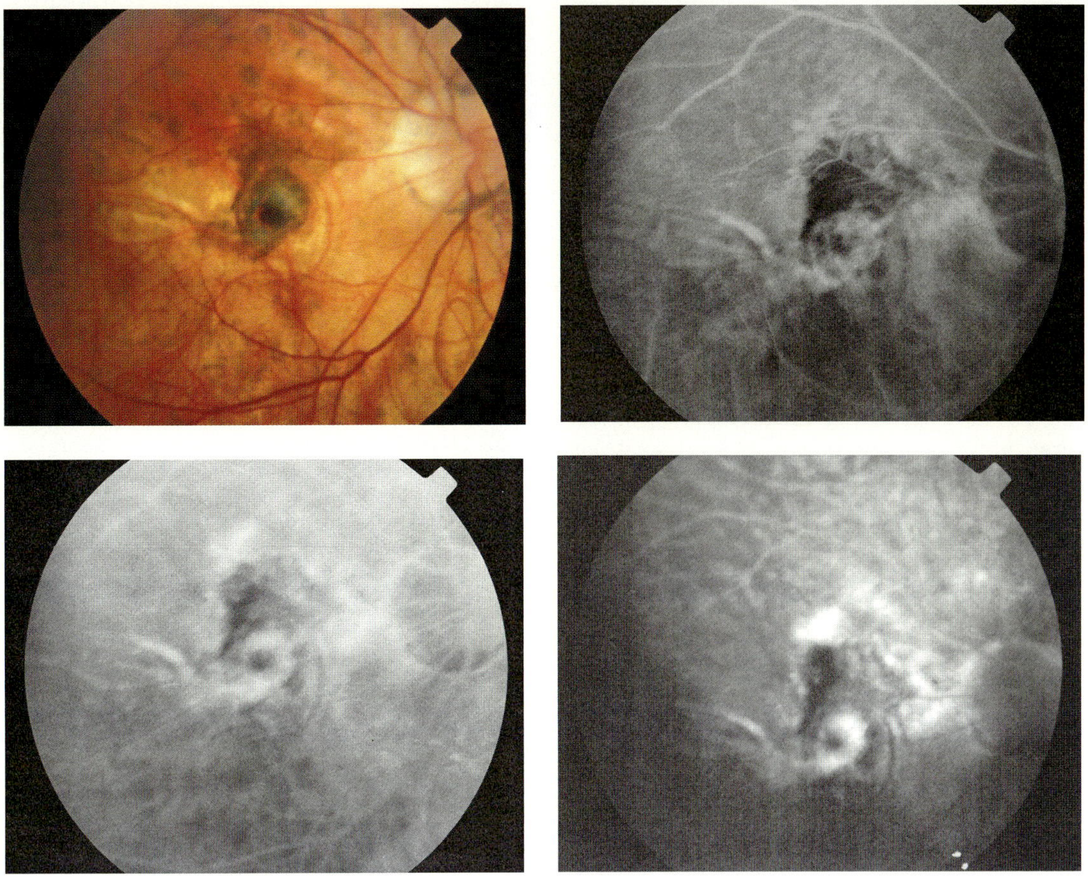

FIGURE 15.14. Two years after initial presentation the patient noted decreased vision. Visual acuity measured 20/40 and a color fundus photograph **(A)** shows subretinal blood and a slight increase in subretinal fibrosis. Fluorescein angiography demonstrates perfusion of choroidal neovascularization (CNV) (**B** at 33 s) with leakage from CNV (**C,** at 1 min 33 s and **D,** at 4 min 52 s).

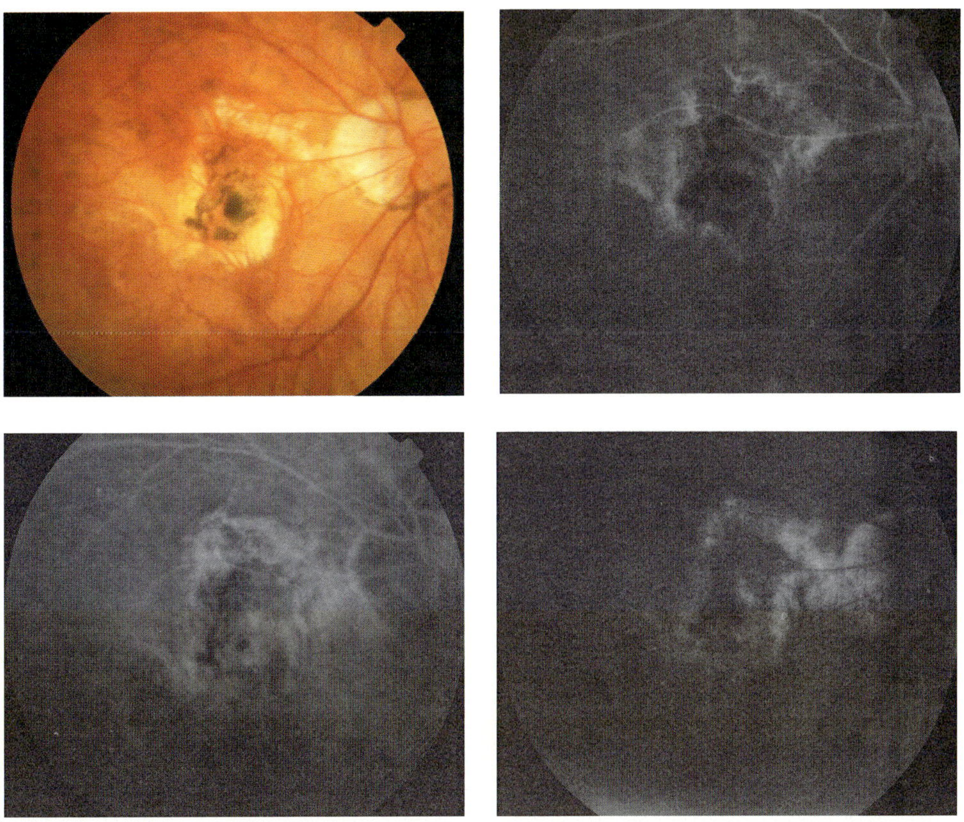

Vision at the time measured 20/40 (no longer measured using protocol refraction), angiography demonstrated mild leakage, and verteporfin PDT was repeated. Over the next 5 1/2 years, the patient underwent 12 additional treatments with verteporfin PDT, never more frequently than every 3 months, and typically when the patient noted new distortion and angiography demonstrated some leakage from CNV (Fig. 15.4). Three treatments were applied in each of years 3 (counting from presentation), 4, 5, and 6; one treatment in year 7 and none since (Fig. 15.15). Visual acuity at 2 years after the initial presentation was 20/40, 20/50 at year 3, and 20/40 to 20/50 for the remainder of his course. At the most recent follow up, the patient's visual acuity was 20/50 8 years after presentation and after 17 applications of verteporfin PDT. Ophthalmoscopy revealed pigmented subretinal tissue without evident fluid or hemorrhage, and angiography was not performed. Mild pigmentary abnormalities and atrophic changes were noted in the central macula, owing to either progression of the pathologic myopia and/or repeated verteporfin PDT. No systemic adverse events were noted with repeated treatments, although the patient had recurrent kidney stones in years 1 and 6.

REFERENCES

1. Saw SM, Katz J, Schein D, et al. Epidemiology of myopia. *Epidemiol Rev* 1996;18:175–182.
2. Sperduto RD, Deigel D, Roberts J, et al. Prevalence of myopia in the United States. *Arch Ophthalmol* 1983;101:405–407.
3. Fledelius H. Myopia prevalence in Scandinavia: a survey with emphasis on factors of relevance for epidemiological studies in general. *Acta Opthalmol Suppl* 1988;185:44–50.
4. Linn LL, Chen CJ, Hung PT, et al. Nation-wide survey of myopia among schoolchildren in Taiwan, 1986. *Acta Ophthalmol Suppl* 1988;198:29–33.
5. Wang Q, Klein BE, Klein R, et al. Refractive status in the Beaver Dam Eye Study. *Invest Ophthalmol Vis Sci* 1994;35:4344–4347.
6. Rajan U, Tan FT, Chan TK, et al. Increasing prevalence of myopia in Singapore school children. In: Chew SJ, Weintraub J, eds. *Proceedings of the Fifth International Conference on Myopia.* Toronto, Ontario, Canada, June 22–24, 1994.
7. Taylor HR. Racial variations in vision. *Am J Epidemiol* 1981;113: 62–80.
8. Verlee DL. Ophthalmic Survey in the Solomon Islands. *Am J Ophthalmol* 1968;66:304–319.
9. Wallman J. Nature and nurture of myopia. *Nature* 1994;371: 201–202.
10. Curtin BJ. *The myopias. Basic sciences and clinical management.* Philadelphia: Harper & Row, 1985:237–245.
11. Blach RK. Degenerative myopia. In: Krill AE, Archer DB, eds. *Krill's hereditary retinal and choroidal diseases,* vol II. *Clinical characteristics.* Hagerstown, MD: Harper & Row, 1977:911–937.
12. Tabandeh H, Flynn HW, Scott IU, et al. Visual acuity outcomes of patients 50 years of age and older with high myopia and untreated choroidal neovascularization. *Ophthalmology* 1999; 106:2063–2067.
13. Gass JDM. Disciform detachment associated with myopic choroidal degeneration. In: *Stereoscopic atlas of macular diseases. Diagnosis and treatment,* vol 1, 2nd ed. St. Louis: Mosby, 1977:86.
14. Levy JH, Pollock HM, Curtin BJ. The Fuchs' spot: an ophthalmoscopic and fluorescein angiographic study. *Ann Ophthalmol* 1977;9:1433–1443.
15. Curtin BJ, Carlin DB. Axial length measurements and fundus changes of the myopic eye. *Am J Ophthalmol* 1971;1:42–53.
16. Hotchkiss ML, Fine SL. Pathologic myopia and choroidal neovascularization. *Am J Ophthalmol* 1981;91:177–183.
17. Grossniklaus HE, Green WR. Pathologic findings in pathologic myopia. *Retina* 1992;12:127–133.
18. Curtin BJ. The posterior staphyloma of pathologic myopia. *Trans Am Ophthalmol Soc* 1977;75:67–86.
19. Blatt N. Augenhintergrundveränderungen bei hochgradinger Myopie. *Klin Monatsbl Augenheilkd* 1965;146:391–411.
20. Secretan M, Kuhn D, Sobrane G, et al. Long-term visual outcome of choroidal neovascularization in pathologic myopia: natural history and laser treatment. *Eur J Ophthalmol* 1997;7: 307–316.
21. Avila MP, Weiter JJ, Jalkh AE, et al. Natural history of choroidal neovascularization in degenerative myopia. *Ophthalmology* 1984; 91:1573–1581.
22. Fried M, Siebert A, Meyer-Schwickerath G, et al. Natural history of Fuchs' spot: a long-term follow-up study. In: Fledelius HC, Alsbirk PH, Goldschmidt E, eds. *Third International Conference on Myopia, 1980.* The Hague: Dr. W Junk, 1981:215–221.
23. Hampton GR, Kohen D, Bird AC. Visual prognosis of disciform degeneration in myopia. *Ophthalmology* 1983;90:923–926.
24. Pece A, Serini P, Avanza P, Brancato R. Myopie dégénérative: récidives de néovaisseaux sous-rétiniens après photocoagulation au laser. *J Fr Ophthalmol* 1990;13:24–28.
25. Brancato R, Pece A, Avanza A, et al. Photocoagulation scar expansion after laser therapy for choroidal neovascularization in degenerative myopia. *Retina* 1990;10:239–243.
26. Bressler SB, Pieramici D, Marsh MJ, et al. Laser scar expansion on pathologic myopia and ocular histoplasmosis following treatment of choroidal neovascularization. *Invest Ophthalmol Vis Sci* 1992;33:1207.
27. Tanev V, Ilieva E. La tache de Fuchs chez le myope grave. Aspects angiofluorographiques et traitmement au laser. *Bull Soc Ophthalmol Fr* 1985;85:369–370.
28. Deutman AF, Hendrikse F. Traitement des néovaisseauz sous rétiniens dans la myopie dégénérative. *Ophthalmologie* 1989;3: 299–301.
29. Jalkh AE, Weiter JJ, Trempe CL, et al. Choroidal neovascularization in degenerative myopia: role of laser photocoagulation. *Ophthalmic Surg* 1987;18:721–725.
30. Johnson DA, Yannuzzi LA, Shakin JL, et al. Lacquer cracks following laser treatment of choroid neovascularization in pathologic myopia. *Retina* 1998;18:118–124.
31. Gass JDM. *Stereoscopic atlas of macular diseases: diagnosis and treatment.* St. Louis: Mosby, 1987.
32. Verteporfin in Photodynamic Therapy (VIP) Study Group. Photodynamic therapy of subfoveal choroidal neovascularization in pathologic myopia with verteporfin: one-year results of a randomized clinical trial. *Ophthalmology* 2001;108:841–852.
33. Treatment of Age-Related Macular Degeneration with Photodynamic Therapy (TAP) Study Group. Photodynamic therapy of subfoveal choroidal neovascularization in age-related macular degeneration with verteporfin. One-year results of 2 randomized clinical trials. *Arch Ophthalmol* 1999;117:1329–1345.
34. Thomas MA, Kaplan HJ. Surgical removal of subfoveal neovascularization in the presumed ocular histoplasmosis syndrome. *Am J Ophthalmol* 1991;111:1–7.
35. Thomas MA, Grand G, Williams DF. Surgical management of subfoveal choroidal neovascularization. *Ophthalmology* 1992;99: 952–968.
36. Thomas MA, Dickinson JD, Melberg NS, et al. Visual results

after surgical removal of subfoveal choroidal neovascular membranes. *Ophthalmology* 1994;101:1384–1396.
37. Machemer R, Steinhorst UH. Retinal separation, retinotomy, and macular relocation, I: experimental studies in the rabbit eye. *Graefes Arch Clin Exp Ophthalmol* 1993;231:629–634.
38. Machemer R, Steinhorst UH. Retinal separation, retinotomy, and macular relocation, II: surgical approach for age-related macular degeneration? *Graefes Arch Clin Exp Ophthalmol* 1993;231:635–641.
39. Lindsey P, Finkelstein D, D'Anna S. Experimental retinal relocation. ARVO abstracts. *Invest Ophthalmol Vis Sci* 1983;24:242.
40. Tiedeman J, de Juan E Jr, Machemer R, et al. Surgical relocation of the macula. ARVO abstracts. *Invest Ophthalmol Vis Sci* 1985;26:59.
41. Ninomiya Y, Lewis JM, Hasegawa T, et al. Retinotomy and foveal translocation for surgical management of subfoveal choroidal neovascular membranes. *Am J Ophthalmol* 1996;122:613–621.
42. Imai K, de Juan E Jr. Experimental surgical macular relocation by scleral shortening. ARVO abstracts. *Invest Ophthalmol Vis Sci* 1996;37:S116.
43. de Juan E Jr, Lowenstein A, Bressler NM, et al. Translocation of the retina for management of subfoveal choroidal neovascularization, II: a preliminary report in humans. *Am J Ophthalmol* 1998;125:635–646.
44. Imai K, Loewenstein A, de Juan E Jr. Translocation of the retina for management of subfoveal choroidal neovascularization. I: Experimental studies in the rabbit eye. *Am J Ophthalmol* 1998;125:627–634.
45. Fujikado T, Ohji M, Saito Y, et al. Visual function after foveal translocation with scleral shortening in patients with myopic neovascular maculopathy. *Am J Ophthalmol* 1998;125:647–656.
46. Fujii GY, Humayun MS, Pieramici DJ, et al. Initial experience of inferior limited macular translocation for subfoveal choroidal neovascularization due to causes other than age-related macular degeneration. *Am J Ophthalmol* 2001;131:90–100.
47. Sickenberg M, Schmidt-Erfurth U, Miller JW, et al. A preliminary study of photodynamic therapy using verteporfin for choroidal neovascularization in pathologic myopia, ocular histoplasmosis syndrome, angioid streaks and idiopathic causes. *Arch Ophthalmol* 2000;117:327–336.

16

VERTEPORFIN PHOTODYNAMIC THERAPY OF CHOROIDAL NEOVASCULARIZATION FROM CAUSES OTHER THAN AGE-RELATED MACULAR DEGENERATION AND PATHOLOGIC MYOPIA

PHILIP J. ROSENFELD

On August 23, 2001, the United States Food and Drug Administration (FDA) expanded the approved labeling indications for ocular photodynamic therapy (OPT) with verteporfin to include patients with choroidal neovascularization (CNV) secondary to ocular histoplasmosis syndrome (OHS). This decision was based on the 1-year results from the Verteporfin in Ocular Histoplasmosis (VOH) study. Currently, there are no additional clinical studies planned to investigate verteporfin therapy for the treatment of CNV from causes other than age-related macular degeneration (AMD) and pathologic myopia. Our experience using verteporfin therapy for the treatment of CNV secondary to these other causes has evolved since the approval of verteporfin. Although no prospective controlled data are available, retrospective reports have appeared at meetings and in journals describing the expanding role of PDT for CNV.

FOOD AND DRUG ADMINISTRATION–APPROVED CLINICAL TRIALS

Phase I/II Studies Using Photodynamic Therapy with Verteporfin

The Phase I/II studies using verteporfin therapy evaluated some patients with CNV in non-AMD conditions, including pathologic myopia, angioid streaks, OHS, and idiopathy. Thirteen patients with subfoveal CNV secondary to non-AMD causes were investigated in the report by Sickenberg and associates (1). The majority of these cases were diagnosed with pathologic myopia. Different drug doses, times of light application, and number of retreatments were investigated in this population. Only one case each of CNV secondary to angioid streaks, OHS, and an idiopathic cause was investigated, and none of these cases received what is considered the standard verteporfin therapy regimen of drug dose (6 mg/m^2), time of light application following the start of drug infusion (15 minutes), and light dose (50 J/cm^2) (Table 16.1). The OHS and idiopathic cases received a higher than standard verteporfin dose of 12 mg/m^2 and the interval from infusion to light application was delayed to 30 minutes. The case of angioid streaks received the light dose 10 minutes after the start of the infusion. The idiopathic case received a higher than standard light dose (100 J/cm^2) and a total of four treatments, whereas the other two cases received only one treatment. Follow-up ranged from 12 to 35 weeks. The only patient to improve vision was the case of OHS, whereas the other two cases maintained stable visual acuity. No additional safety concerns were identified during the study. The angiographic results from these non-AMD patients demonstrated reduced leakage at the end of the follow-up period. However, in contrast to the AMD patients treated with PDT, most non-AMD patients had stable or improved visual acuity. The younger age of the non-AMD population, smaller lesion size, and higher proportion of patients with classic-only containing CNV are believed to contribute to their better visual acuity results. No definitive conclusion is possible regarding the efficacy of verteporfin therapy because of the small number of patients in this study, and variable treatment regimens and follow-up periods. However, as observed with the AMD patients, the treatment appeared to be well tolerated, and retreatment as early as every 4 weeks was shown to be safe in these non-AMD patients.

TABLE 16.1. PHOTODYNAMIC TREATMENT PARAMETERS AND OUTCOMES OF PHASE I/II STUDY PATIENTS WITH CHOROIDAL NEOVASCULARIZATION NOT CAUSED BY AGE-RELATED MACULAR DEGENERATION AND PATHOLOGIC MYOPIA

Diagnosis	Verteporfin dose (mg/m^2)	Time (min)	Light dose (J/cm^2)	No. of treatments	Follow up, (wk)	Baseline VA	Final VA
Ocular histoplasmosis syndrome	12	30	50	1	22	20/200	20/64
Idiopathic	12	30	100	4	35	20/100	20/100
Angioid streaks	6	10	50	1	12	20/64	20/64

VA, visual acuity.

Verteporfin in Ocular Histoplasmosis Study

A larger open-label, multicenter Phase II study was designed to investigate the safety and effect on visual acuity of verteporfin therapy on subfoveal CNV secondary to OHS over a 2-year period (2). This study was initiated in July, 1998 and enrollment was completed in July, 1999 when the target sample size of 26 patients was attained. All eligible patients had the diagnosis of OHS with evidence of subfoveal CNV and an approximate Snellen visual acuity of 20/40 to 20/200 (Early Treatment Diabetic Retinopathy Study letter score of between 73 and 34 letters). Any type of CNV was acceptable as long as the lesion was under the geometric center of the fovea. The standard regimen used in the TAP investigation (regimen No. 4 from the Phase I/II studies) was used for all treatments (3–5). Patients returned every 3 months for a follow-up evaluation that included fluorescein angiography. The patient received retreatment with verteporfin therapy if there was any evidence of fluorescein leakage on angiography. The study was originally planned to last 2 years, but an extension of the study allows patient follow up through 4 years.

Overall, 26 patients were enrolled in the study, but one patient was determined to be ineligible based on a failure to meet the inclusion/exclusion criteria. The remaining 25 patients continued in the study and no significant safety concerns were identified after 12 months. The median visual acuity score at month 12 increased from baseline by seven letters, with 56% gaining at least one line of vision, and 28% improving three lines or more (Table 16.2). Only one patient had a visual acuity score of 20/200 or worse. An improvement in the contrast sensitivity score was observed with a median increase from baseline of 2.0 letters. The fluorescein angiographic outcomes correlated well with the visual acuity improvements with complete absence of leakage from the classic component of the CNV in 43% of patients and progression of classic CNV beyond the area identified at baseline in only 26% of patients at 1 year. The 2-year results (unpublished data) showed continued improvement in visual acuity and angiographic outcomes.

Overall, the visual acuity and angiographic results suggest a beneficial effect of verteporfin therapy on the natural history of OHS patients with subfoveal CNV, especially when compared to historical controls. These patients probably responded much more favorably to verteporfin therapy than the AMD patients because they were younger, the lesions were smaller, and the majority of the lesions were type II classic-only CNV (Table 16.3). A

TABLE 16.2. POSSIBLE INDICATIONS FOR VERTEPORFIN THERAPY OF CHOROIDAL NEOVASCULARIZATION AND VASCULAR ABNORMALITIES CAUSED BY CONDITIONS OTHER THAN AGE-RELATED MACULAR DEGENERATION AND PATHOLOGIC MYOPIA

Ocular histoplasmosis syndrome
Idiopathic
Angioid streaks
Idiopathic polypoidal choroidal vasculopathy
Juxtafoveolar retinal telangiectasis
Inflammatory conditions (e.g., multifocal choroiditis, punctate inner choroidopathy, toxoplasmosis)
Inherited macular degenerations (e.g., Stargardt disease, Best disease, pattern dystrophy)
Central serous chorioretinopathy
Trauma (choroidal rupture)
Optic nerve abnormalities (drusen, coloboma)
Laser-induced breaks in Bruch's membrane (following macular laser for retinal edema)
Choroidal vascular and structural abnormalities (e.g., hemangioma, osteoma, nevus, melanoma)
Retinal vascular abnormalities (e.g., angioma, macroaneurysm, cavernous hemangioma)

TABLE 16.3. THE VERTEPORFIN IN OCULAR HISTOPLASMOSIS STUDY: BASELINE CHARACTERISTICS AND 1-YEAR RESULTS

Number of patients	25
Median age	50 years old
Median baseline vision	20/80 + 1 (56-letter score)
Predominantly classic CNV at baseline	73%
Classic-only CNV at baseline	65%
Median greatest linear dimension	3,040 μm
≥1-Line improvement at 1 year	56%
≥3-Line improvement at 1 year	28%
≥1-Line decrease at 1 year	16%
≥3-Line decrease at 1 year	8%
Median vision change at 1 year	+7 letters
Median contrast sensitivity change at 1 year	+2 letters

definitive treatment benefit cannot be demonstrated because of the limitations of this study, which include open-label design without a control group, short follow up, and small sample size. However, it seems unlikely that these promising results are a chance finding. An example of verteporfin therapy of CNV in an OHS patient is shown in Figure 16.1.

VERTEPORFIN THERAPY: OFF-LABEL INDICATIONS

Guidelines for the use of verteporfin therapy to treat CNV have been published based on the clinical trial experience treating CNV in patients with AMD, pathologic myopia, and OHS (6). Clinicians are now extrapolating these recommendations to include idiopathic CNV (Fig. 16.2) and other causes such as angioid streaks (Fig. 16.3), juxtafoveal retinal telangiectasis, idiopathic polypoidal choroidal vasculopathy (IPCV), trauma (choroidal rupture), inherited macular degenerations (e.g., Stargardt disease, Sorsby fundus dystrophy, Best disease, and mallatia leventinese), and inflammatory conditions such as multifocal choroiditis, punctate inner choroidopathy, and toxoplasmosis (Table 16.1). Any condition that can result in CNV may be a candidate for verteporfin therapy. However, it will never be feasible to perform clinical trials to investigate whether verteporfin therapy is beneficial for these other causes of CNV. Most of these other indications occur too infrequently to enroll sufficient patients in a short period of time for a clinical trial. Moreover, withholding verteporfin therapy may not be ethically feasible considering what we now know about the benefits of PDT in non-AMD cases, particularly with regard to the results observed in the VOH study. It seems reasonable to assume that the similar pathophysiology of these CNV lesions should result in a comparable benefit, especially if the patient is young, the lesion is small, and the CNV is of the type II variety and predominantly classic or classic-only in composition. Most of the causes listed in Table 16.1 occur in younger patients, and the CNV lesions tend to be of the type that respond well to PDT. The only exception is the CNV that arises in association with inflammation. In this situation, it may be necessary to consider antiinflammatory therapy in conjunction with PDT. Although PDT may be successful as a monotherapy, adjuvant therapy with subtenon steroid, intravitreal steroid, or topical steroid and/or nonsteroidal antiinflammatory drugs could be considered.

The evidence that verteporfin therapy of CNV owing to these other causes is beneficial is slowly accumulating in the form of published case reports, small case series, and abstracts at scientific meetings. Published reports include verteporfin therapy in individual cases of CNV secondary to inherited macular degenerations (mallatia leventinese and fundus flavimaculatus) (7,8), juxtafoveal retinal telangiectasis (9), and choroidal osteoma (10). At the most recent meeting of the Association for Research in Vision and Ophthalmology (ARVO) in May 2002 (*www.arvo.org*), additional case reports and small case series suggest that verteporfin therapy is useful in the treatment of CNV secondary to a variety of other causes. When all these reports are combined, there were positive outcomes reported in cases of CNV secondary to angioid streaks (40 eyes), polypoidal vasculopathy (21 eyes), juxtafoveal retinal telangiectasis (three eyes), and idiopathy (two eyes). Of all these indications, it seems as though the CNV secondary to angioid streaks may be the most difficult to treat with verteporfin therapy requiring frequent early retreatments secondary to recurrences and rapid growth of the CNV. Early retreatment may be necessary in this condition to achieve stabilization or minimize the extent of vision loss. We also have found that CNV secondary to angioid streaks requires aggressive management, and this should not be surprising in light of the frequent recurrences of CNV observed following thermal laser therapy. To date, these reports suggest that verteporfin therapy is useful for CNV resulting from these other causes; however, it must be realized that there is a bias in the reporting of positive results.

Verteporfin therapy may also prove useful in the treatment of retinal and choroidal vascular abnormalities. Photodynamic therapy has been used successfully for the treatment of choroidal hemangiomas in five reported cases. Barbazetto and Schmidt-Erfurth (11) modified the standard regimen used for the treatment of CNV by increasing the light dose to 100 J/cm^2. This increased light dose was achieved by increasing the exposure time during the light treatment to 168 seconds. In the two cases reported using this modified light protocol, the investigators observed resolution of the hemangiomas and improvement in vision. Madreperla (12) reported on three cases of choroidal hemangiomas treated with the standard verteporfin therapy regimen. In this report, all eyes had reduced tumor thickness and fluorescein angiographic leakage was eliminated with resolution of subretinal fluid resulting in visual acuity improvement. There also have been anecdotal reports of successful verteporfin therapy for the treatment of retinal angiomas, macroaneurysms, and other retinal vascular malformations. Thus, it appears that off-label verteporfin therapy is being expanded to include not just other causes of CNV, but also any lesion causing symptoms secondary to a vascular growth and leakage. The standard treatment regimen may suffice in most cases, but it may also be necessary to modify the regimen depending on the size and blood flow characteristics of the lesion being treated.

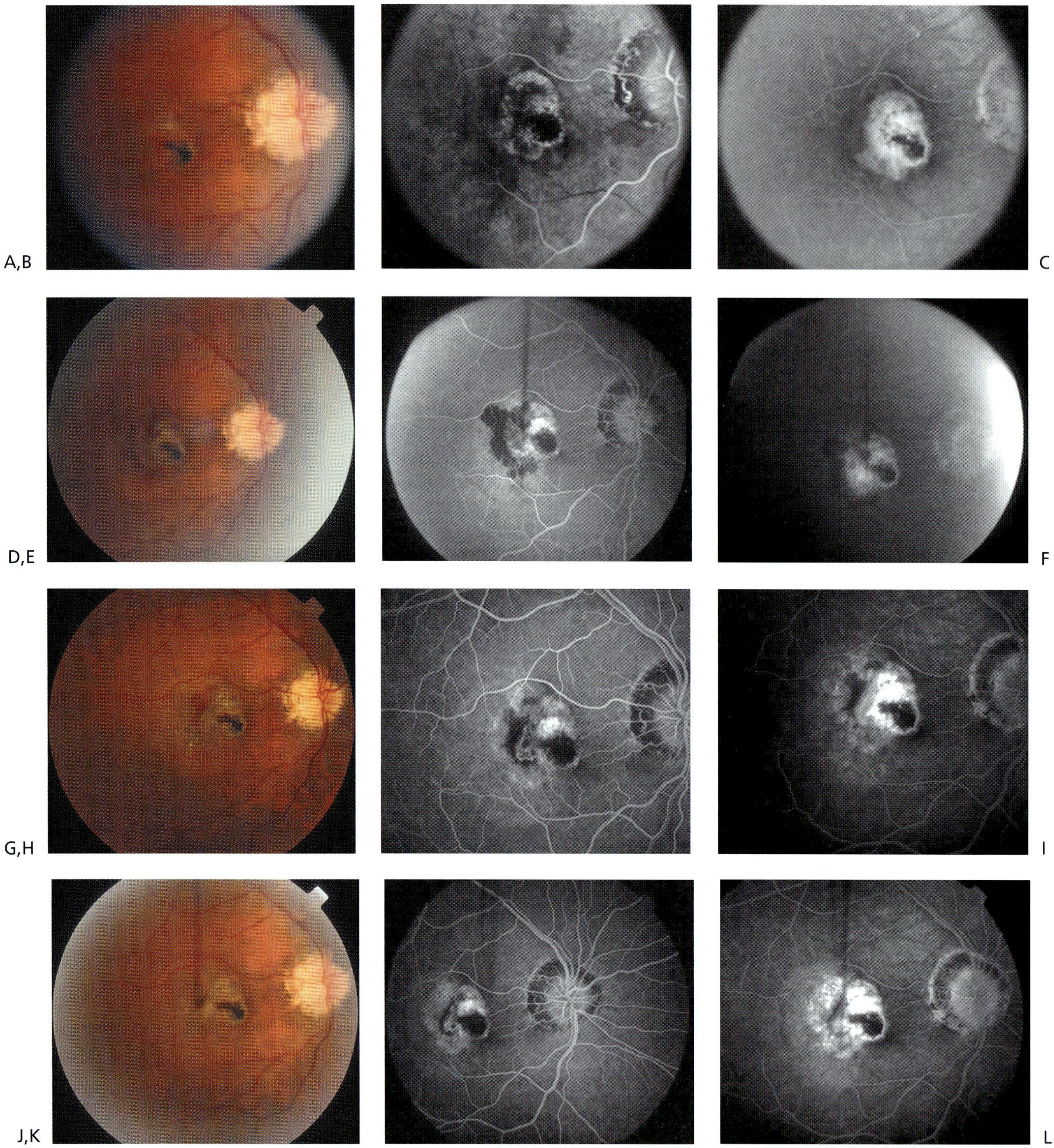

FIGURE 16.1. A patient with ocular histoplasmosis syndrome (OHS) and subfoveal CNV. **A through C:** Before treatment, this 48-year-old woman with evidence of a macular scar, peripapillary atrophy, and peripheral "histo" spots complained of decreasing vision and increasing distortion. Her baseline visual acuity was 20/50 with evidence of subfoveal CNV as shown by early hyperfluorescence and late fluorescein leakage and staining on her angiogram. She received verteporfin therapy. **D through F:** (1) Three-month follow up, 3 months post-PDT. Her visual acuity was 20/60 with evidence of a new submacular hemorrhage and persistent leakage from the CNV. A second treatment was given. **G through I:** (2) Six-month follow up, 3 months post-PDT. Visual acuity was worse at 20/60- with evidence of a new area of leakage by fluorescein angiography. A third treatment was administered. **J through L:** (3) Nine-month follow up, 3 months post-PDT. Visual acuity was slightly improved at 20/60 with no complaint of metamorphopsia. No treatment was recommended.

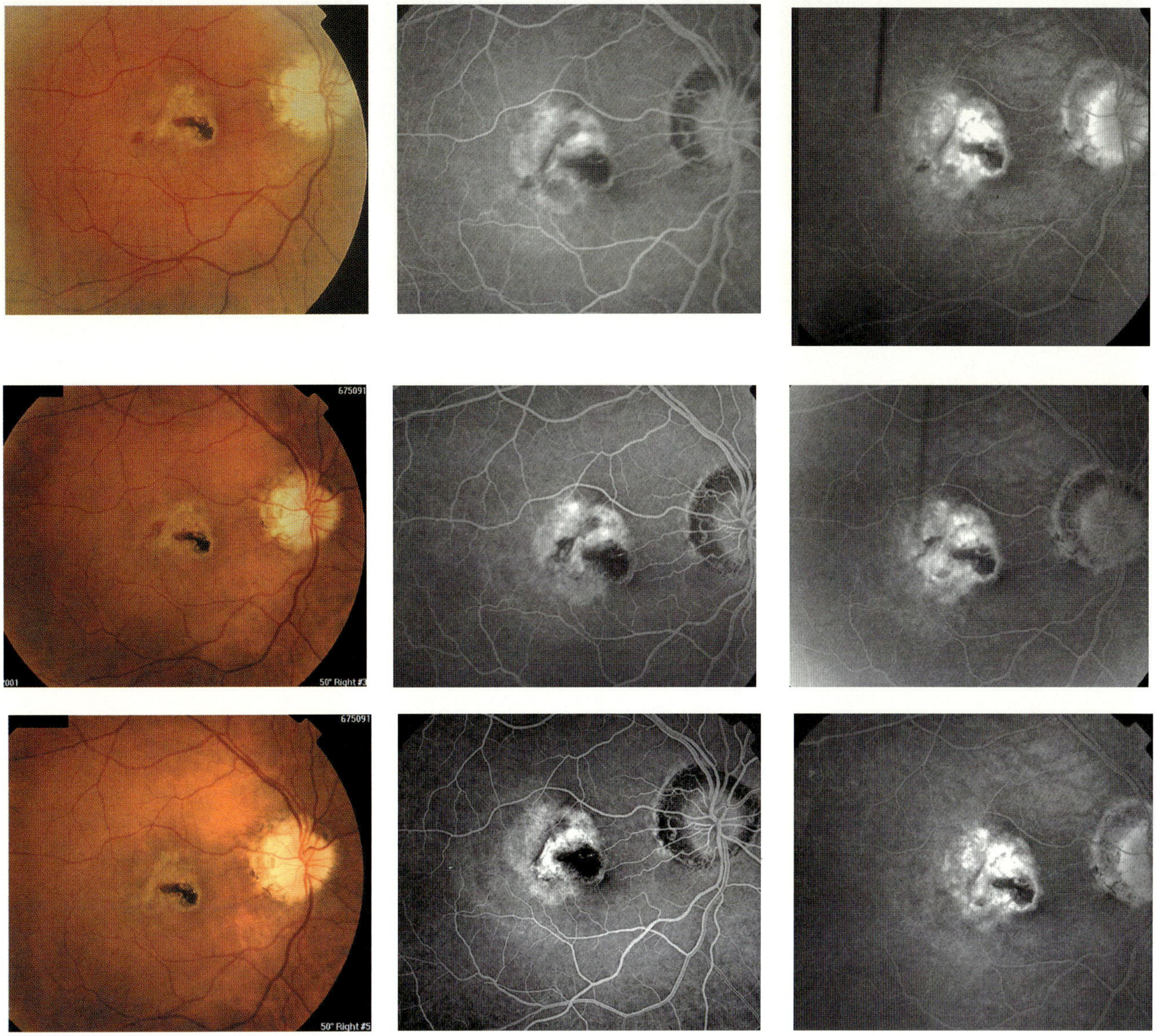

FIGURE 16.1 *(continued)*. M through O: (3) Twelve-month follow up, 6 months post-PDT. Visual acuity has improved to 20/30 with no evidence of leakage by fluorescein angiography. A small submacular hemorrhage was noted adjacent to the area of the CNV. No treatment was recommended. **P through R:** Sixteen-month follow up, 10 months post-PDT. Vision decreased to 20/50 with a small submacular hemorrhage and evidence of leakage on fluorescein angiography. A fourth treatment was recommended. **S through U:** (4) Nineteen-month follow up, 3 months post-PDT. Vision improved to 20/25 with no evidence of active CNV. She has been followed for an additional 6 months: Her vision remained stable at 20/25 and no additional treatments were necessary. This case is a good example of treatment every 3 months followed by cessation of therapy followed by recurrence of the CNV and the need to restart verteporfin therapy, resulting in excellent visual recovery therapy.

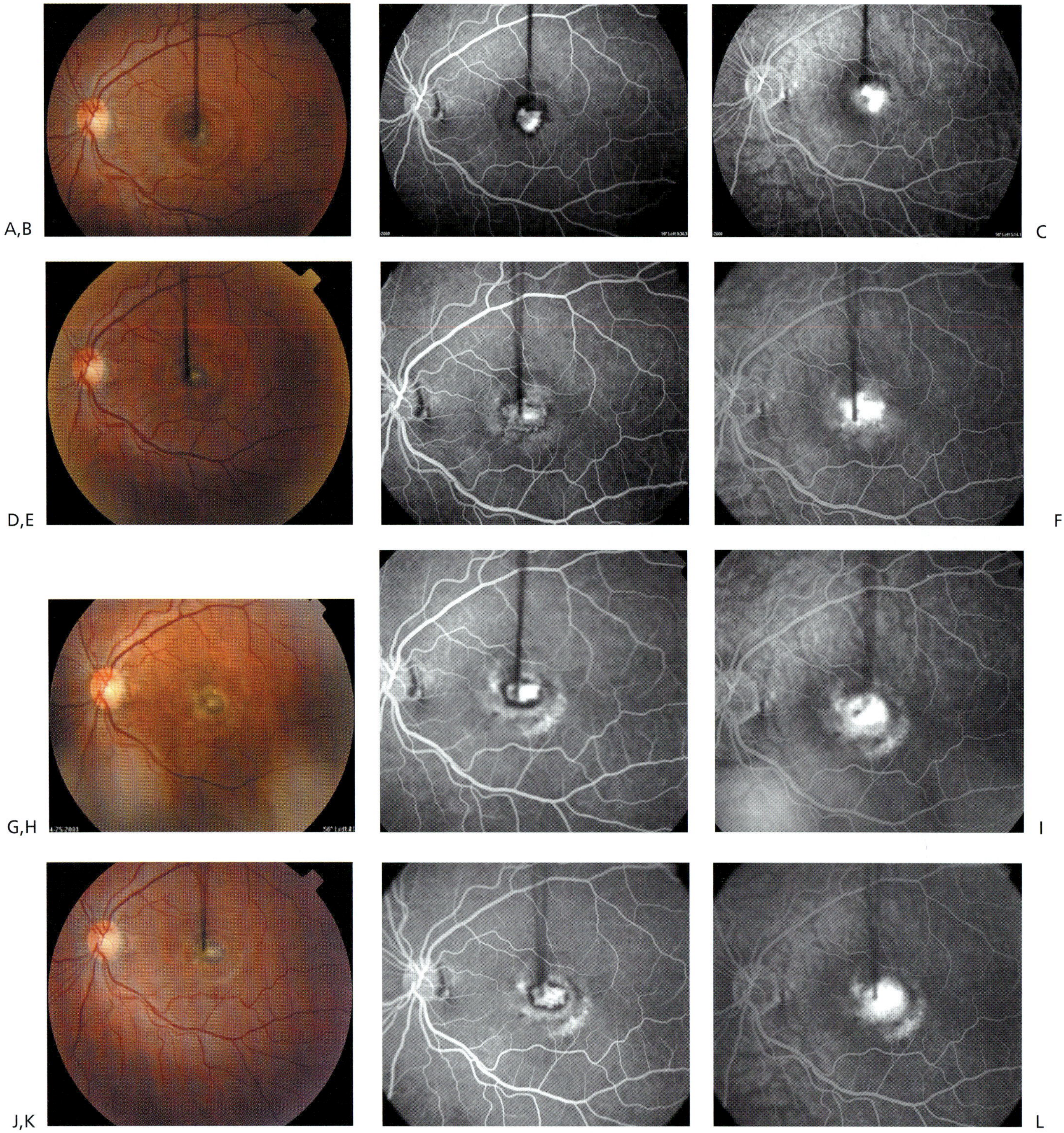

FIGURE 16.2. A patient with idiopathic subfoveal CNV. **A through C:** Before treatment, this 24-year-old woman complained of increasing distortion and worsening vision for several weeks. Her baseline visual acuity was 20/80 with evidence of classic subfoveal CNV as shown by early lacy hyperfluorescence and late fluorescein leakage and staining on her angiogram. She received verteporfin therapy. **D through F:** (1) Three-month follow up, 3 months post-PDT. Her visual acuity remained at 20/80 with evidence of persistent leakage from the CNV. A second treatment was given. **G through I:** (2) Six-month follow up, 3 months post-PDT. Visual acuity was stable at 20/80 with questionable leakage by fluorescein angiography. A third treatment was administered. **J through L:** (3) Nine-month follow up, 3 months post-PDT. Visual acuity improved at 20/50 with no complaint of metamorphopsia and no leakage on fluorescein angiography. Persistent fluorescein staining was evident. No treatment was recommended. She has been followed for a total of 18 months and has received no additional treatments. Her visual acuity fluctuates between 20/40 and 20/50. This case is a good example of continued visual acuity improvement once leakage from the CNV is stopped.

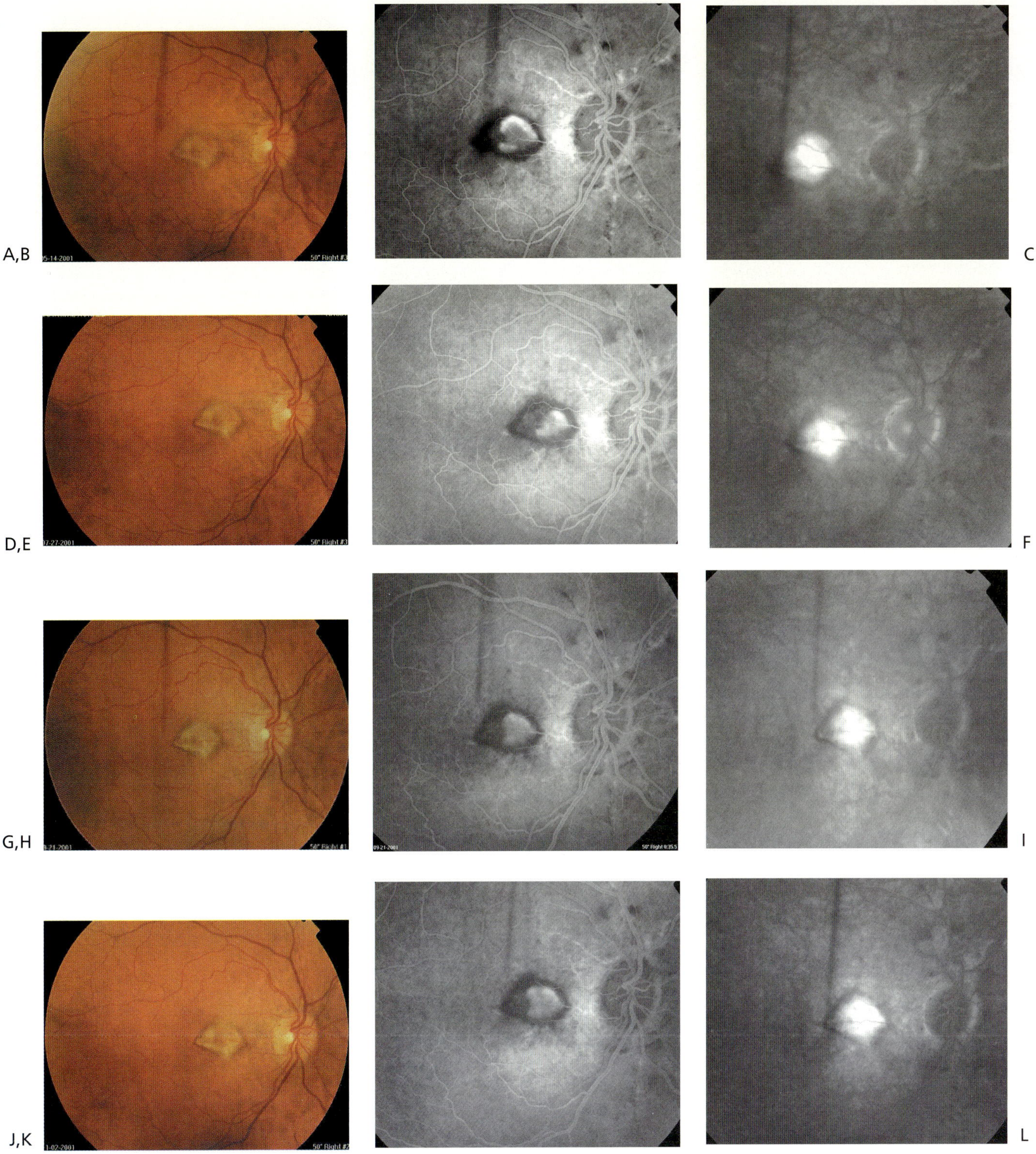

FIGURE 16.3. A patient with angioid streaks and subfoveal CNV. **A through C:** Before treatment, this 54-year-old man complained of increasing distortion and worsening vision for 2 months. His baseline visual acuity was 20/200 with evidence of classic subfoveal CNV as shown by early lacy hyperfluorescence and late fluorescein leakage and staining on his angiogram. He received verteporfin therapy. **D through F:** (1) Two-month follow up, 2 months post-PDT. His visual acuity remained at 20/200 with evidence of persistent leakage from the CNV. A second treatment was given. **G through I:** (2) Four-month follow up, 2 months post-PDT. Visual acuity was stable at 20/200 with questionable leakage by fluorescein angiography. A third treatment was administered. **J through L:** (3) Six-month follow up, 2 months post-PDT. Visual acuity improved slightly to 20/200+ with no complaint of metamorphopsia and no leakage on fluorescein angiography. Persistent fluorescein staining was evident. No treatment was recommended. He has been followed for 12 months and has received no additional treatments. His fluorescein angiogram remains unchanged and his vision has improved to 20/100. This case is a good example of aggressive early retreatments in a patient with CNV secondary to angioid streaks.

SUMMARY

A small open-label study of verteporfin therapy in OHS patients with subfoveal CNV strongly suggested a treatment benefit for this population. In contrast to the previous clinical trials, the OHS patients demonstrated an overall improvement in vision over a one-year period that has extended to 2 years. As a result of this study, the FDA has included subfoveal CNV in OHS as a labeled indication for verteporfin therapy. Verteporfin therapy of CNV secondary to causes other than AMD, pathologic myopia, and OHS have not been studied in a clinical trial setting, but the preliminary data from case reports and small case series look very encouraging, especially for CNV lesions that are small and predominantly classic or classic-only in composition. As clinical experience accumulates, these off-label applications of verteporfin therapy will continue to be reported and useful guidelines should evolve within the next few years.

REFERENCES

1. Sickenberg M, Schmidt-Erfurth U, Miller JW, et al. A preliminary study of photodynamic therapy using verteporfin for choroidal neovascularization in pathologic myopia, ocular histoplasmosis syndrome, angioid streaks, and idiopathic causes. *Arch Ophthalmol* 2000;118(3):327–336.
2. Saperstein DA, Rosenfeld PJ, Bressler NM, et al. Photodynamic therapy of subfoveal choroidal neovascularization with verteporfin in the ocular histoplasmosis syndrome: one-year results of an uncontrolled, prospective case series. *Ophthalmology* 2002; 109(8):1499–1505.
3. Treatment of Age-Related Macular Degeneration with Photodynamic Therapy (TAP) Study Group. Photodynamic therapy of subfoveal choroidal neovascularization in age-related macular degeneration with verteporfin: one-year results of 2 randomized clinical trials. *Arch Ophthalmol* 1999;117(10):1329–1345.
4. Miller JW, Schmidt-Erfurth U, Sickenberg M, et al. Photodynamic therapy with verteporfin for choroidal neovascularization caused by age-related macular degeneration: results of a single treatment in a phase 1 and 2 study. *Arch Ophthalmol* 1999;117 (9):1161–1173.
5. Schmidt-Erfurth U, Miller JW, Sickenberg M, et al. Photodynamic therapy with verteporfin for choroidal neovascularization caused by age-related macular degeneration: results of retreatments in a phase 1 and 2 study. *Arch Ophthalmol* 1999;117(9): 1177–1187.
6. Guidelines for using verteporfin (Visudyne) in photodynamic therapy to treat choroidal neovascularization due to age-related macular degeneration and other causes. *Retina* 2002;22(1):6–18.
7. Harding S. Photodynamic therapy in the treatment of subfoveal choroidal neovascularisation. *Eye* 2001;15:407–412.
8. Dantas MA, Slakter JS, Negrao S, et al. Photodynamic therapy with verteporfin in mallatia leventinese. *Ophthalmology* 2002; 109(2):296–301.
9. Potter MJ, Szabo SM, Chan EY, et al. Photodynamic therapy of a subretinal neovascular membrane in type 2A idiopathic juxtafoveolar retinal telangiectasis. *Am J Ophthalmol* 2002;133 (1):149–151.
10. Battaglia Parodi M, Da Pozzo S, Toto L, et al. Photodynamic therapy for choroidal neovascularization associated with choroidal osteoma. *Retina* 2001;21(6):660–661.
11. Barbazetto I, Schmidt-Erfurth U. Photodynamic therapy of choroidal hemangioma: two case reports. *Graefes Arch Clin Exp Ophthalmol* 2000;238(3):214–221.
12. Madreperla SA. Choroidal hemangioma treated with photodynamic therapy using verteporfin. *Arch Ophthalmol* 2001;119 (11):1606–1610.

17

VERTEPORFIN PHOTODYNAMIC THERAPY IN CLINICAL PRACTICE

GEORGE A. WILLIAMS
MARY E. MALMBERG

Age-related macular degeneration (AMD) represents the most common cause of visual loss in individuals greater than 50 years of age in North America and Europe. Epidemiologic and demographic studies demonstrate that the number of patients with visual complications from AMD will increase dramatically over the next two decades. The Beaver Dam Eye Study demonstrated that in a predominantly White population the prevalence of either neovascular AMD or geographic retinal pigment epithelial atrophy increased from 0.19% among people between 43 and 54 years of age to 7.1% among people 75 years of age or older (1). It is estimated from this and other studies (2) that 3 to 4 million people in the United States have AMD and that more than 200,000 new cases of choroidal neovascularization (CNV) develop each year. With the expectation that over the next 20 years the proportion of Americans 60 years of age or older will double, it is likely that visual loss from AMD will exceed the visual loss from combined effects of diabetic retinopathy and glaucoma early in the 21st century.

The advent of photodynamic therapy (PDT) with verteporfin as a proven treatment for some forms of CNV provides hope for many patients with AMD (3–5). Therefore, ophthalmologists who care for patients with AMD can anticipate an increase in the proportion of their practice dedicated to the management of AMD. A study by Margherio and colleagues suggests a significant increase in treatment for CNV from PDT (6). This study retrospectively reviewed 1,000 consecutive patients presenting with AMD to a referral-based retinal practice.

The following criteria were used for eligibility: 50 years of age or greater, drusen in either eye, and an absence of non-AMD causes for CNV such as pathologic myopia or angioid streaks. Each eligible patient was assessed for the following criteria: (a) neovascular AMD or non-neovascular AMD; (b) presence of subfoveal CNV; (c) presence of classic CNV; (d) presence of a predominantly classic CNV lesion; (e) presence of occult without classic CNV. A diagnosis of non-neovascular AMD was determined by clinical examination that always included biomicroscopy of the posterior pole with or without fluorescein angiography (FA). Neovascular AMD was diagnosed by clinical examination and then further categorized by FA. The worst eye determined the final categorization.

Of the 1,000 patients reviewed 526 (53%) had non-neovascular AMD and 474 (47%) had neovascular AMD. This reflects the referral bias expected in a tertiary practice. Of the 474 patients with neovascular AMD in at least one eye, 392 had subfoveal CNV. Of these, 392 patients with subfoveal CNV, 171 patients had predominantly classic CNV, 136 had occult without classic, and 85 were minimally classic. Therefore, based on the recommendations of the TAP study (3), 44% (171/392) patients with subfoveal CNV were eligible for PDT. Because this study was performed prior to the report of the VIP 24-month data (5), the contribution of treated occult without classic eyes was not considered. Therefore, patients were not classified by VIP criteria for evidence of disease progression as required by the VIP eligibility criteria. However, it seems reasonable to assume that the majority of the occult without classic patients were symptomatic, which was the reason for their referral. If a conservative estimate of 50% VIP eligibility in this group of occult without classic patients is assumed, another 63 patients become eligible for PDT. Therefore, 60% (235/392) patients with subfoveal CNV may be eligible for PDT. This is 2.4 times the number of patients eligible (99) for conventional thermal laser in this population. When the mean number of treatments necessary over the first 24 months of follow up is considered (5.4 for TAP, 5.0 for VIP), the increase in treatment volume is approximately 12-fold (2.4 × 5.0 = 12) beyond that expected with conventional laser surgery. The overall effect on a practice is considerably greater, however, when one considers the need for regular follow up with FA every 3 months and any additional post-treatment visits. This study, in conjunction with the demographic projections, suggests that the management of AMD with PDT will consume an increasing proportion of practice resources.

PRACTICE MANAGEMENT OF PHOTODYNAMIC THERAPY

The incorporation of PDT into a clinical practice presents multiple issues involving virtually all aspects of practice management. The challenge is to integrate PDT into clinical practice in an efficient and productive manner. The practice resources involved in PDT are considerable and include capital expenses, personnel, office space, angiography issues, unique billing issues, and physician time. Successful integration of PDT into clinical practice presents resource management issues not previously encountered by ophthalmologists.

Capital Expenses

Photodynamic therapy requires dedicated laser technology that can only be used for PDT. This unidimensional utility, unlike other lasers, limits the productivity of PDT lasers because they cannot be used to treat other disease processes. Previously, the Health Care Financing Administration, now Centers for Medicare and Medical Services (CMS), has estimated that ophthalmic lasers have a use rate of 50%. Although even this estimate is probably higher than the actual use for most practices, the use of PDT lasers is likely to be much lower. In our practice, we estimate the use of our busiest PDT laser to be 25% and our other PDT lasers to be less than 10%.

Either a portable laser unit or stationary laser unit is available from two manufacturers. The available laser units are comparable in their efficacy and facility, making laser selection a matter of personal preference and price. We have extensively used the lasers from both manufacturers and found them to be reliable and adequate. The portable units are smaller and can be removed from the slit-lamp to allow for non-PDT functioning. Their portability also allows them to be taken to different locations.

The two laser systems available are from Zeiss and Lumenis. The Zeiss Visulas 690S (Carl Zeiss, Inc., Thornwood, NY) can be either a fixed system with an integrated slit-lamp and wheelchair accessible table or a portable Visulink system that interfaces with a separate slit-lamp. The Coherent Opal Photoactivator and LaserLink adapter (Lumenis Inc., Santa Clara, CA) is a portable system that can interface with a variety of slit-lamps. Both the Zeiss and Lumenis systems have software that calculates the appropriate power based on the lesion size and delivery contact lens to provide the necessary energy of 50 J/cm^2 over 83 seconds. Because there is no visible treatment endpoint with PDT, both lasers have internal power measuring devices to assure the proper energy is being delivered.

Other capital expenses include supplies necessary for the intravenous infusion of verteporfin such as an infusion pump and intravenous catheters, lines, syringes, filters, and 5% dextrose. Novartis, the supplier of verteporfin, has an infusion kit containing the necessary supplies. Although convenient, this kit represents an additional expense.

The largest capital expense of PDT is the purchase of an inventory of the drug verteporfin. At current pricing, the cost to the practice is $1,350 per 15-mg vial of drug. A practice performing 10 PDT treatments a week incurs an expense of over $50,000 a month. An additional cost is the need for secure storage in a cool, dry place.

Personnel

The need for an intravenous infusion requires personnel skilled in drug preparation and intravenous access. This usually means a registered nurse (RN). Practices with a relatively low volume of PDT treatments may use an infusion service or a part-time nurse. However, as treatment volume increases, a full-time RN usually becomes necessary. The nurse is a critical component of the verteporfin therapy process providing not only drug preparation and intravenous access, but important preoperative and postoperative patient education beyond that provided by the ophthalmologist.

NURSING ISSUES IN PHOTODYNAMIC THERAPY

Patients arriving for their first PDT treatment are frequently apprehensive and concerned. Despite preoperative counseling by the physician, they often have misconceptions regarding the treatment and its expected outcome. Patients may presume that PDT is similar to other laser treatment they may have experienced. Some patients think that PDT treatment is similar to surgical procedures performed in a hospital operating room. The simple explanation that the patient need not undress and lie on an uncomfortable operating table in a cool room seems to start the process of relaxation and increases confidence in the process. Actually, patient education begins much earlier than the arrival at the office. Once it is determined that PDT is necessary, the nurse contacts the patient and an appointment is scheduled. At this initial phone contact, the nurse discusses the treatment and postoperative issues such as protection from phototoxicity. Protection when outside includes a wide-brimmed hat, sunglasses, gloves, and long-sleeved apparel, as well as long pants for 5 days following treatment. The office supplies sunglasses to each patient. The patient is also instructed to drink a quart or two of extra fluids over 24 to 36 hours prior to treatment. Increased hydration may be helpful in diminishing the incidence and severity of back pain, which occurs in approximately 2% of patients. A driver is required to bring the patient to and from the office. Any further questions the patient may have regarding PDT are answered at this time.

Once the appointment is made, a package of information is sent to each patient. The package includes a cover letter indicating the office location, parking facilities, and a contact phone number. There is also a pamphlet that answers the most commonly asked questions about PDT, a booklet explaining PDT in lay terms and a booklet on macular degeneration. Also included are maps for out-of-area patients. We also have returnable audiotapes and/or videotapes for those patients who have difficulty reading. For patient convenience, we include a copy of the consent form and post-treatment instructions. This allows the patient with visual impairment and their family to assimilate the information in their own home rather than feeling pressured to hurry through it at the office. This also allows the patient time to formulate questions prior to the appointment.

Patients and their families are encouraged to contact the office for questions or concerns about PDT.

The physician, nurse, and office staff must remain cognizant of the patients' emotional as well as physical status whenever working with patients receiving PDT. Every effort is made to put the patient at ease. The office is cheerful and is frequently decorated according to the current season or holiday to afford visual contrast. Plants and music help to soften the harsh clinic effect. Coffee and juice are available, and often there are cookies, candies, and other small snacks. This informal or "homey" atmosphere seems to help patients relax and feel more secure and comfortable.

After arriving at the office, and signing all the appropriate forms, the patient is measured for height and weight. The eye or eyes to be treated are dilated with 2.5% phenylephrine and 1% tropicamide. A wristband, indicating the use of a photosensitizing agent, is also placed. This is done so that in the unlikely event of mishap or emergency during the 5 days after treatment, medical personnel are alerted to avoid exposure to high-intensity lighting.

Using the height and weight, the nurse calculates the body surface area based on a nomogram of the Mosteller formula, and computes the appropriate drug dose. The correct dose of verteporfin (Visudyne) is 6 mg/m^2 of body surface area.

The physician reads the patient's FA prior to the arrival of the patient and measures the size of the lesion to be treated. This information is placed on the treatment record. The nurse then completes the calculation to determine the spot size of treatment, taking into consideration camera magnification and allowance for treatment of the margins. The calculations are recorded in the treatment record.

After pupillary dilatation, the patient is brought to the infusion room and seated in a dialysis type reclining chair. A family member or friend is encouraged to stay with the patient to offer a feeling of security and support. Again, all questions are addressed and the medical history reviewed. This time with the patient and family is helpful because the patients often express their concerns and misunderstandings of the treatment at this point.

The nurse must be flexible and sympathetic to the patient's needs and able to explain the disease process and treatment. Considerable time is spent emphasizing the need for safety measures following treatment.

A crucial step in PDT is to acquire venous access. Venipuncture is not a difficult procedure, but it requires practice to become proficient. Some patients are nervous about intravenous injections because of a previous adverse experience. Frequently, veins in the elderly are fragile and rupture easily. Perforating the skin can be enough to rupture fragile veins. For these patients or those with uncontrolled hypertension, one can sometimes avoid ruptured veins and subsequent hematoma, by keeping the tourniquet loose or by using hand pressure instead of a tourniquet. This results in less vessel wall tension during the venipuncture, reducing the potential for rupture and ensuing hematoma.

The antecubital fossa is the best location for the infusion of verteporfin as the veins are large, and readily accessible and easily cannulated. However, in the obese patient, antecubital veins may be deep and difficult to palpate. Veins in the forearm are frequently adequate for cannulation but tend to "roll," sometimes making cannulation difficult. The veins of last resort are those in the dorsum of the hand. Although the supplier of verteporfin (Novartis) does not recommend hand veins, they are sometimes the only veins available. However, they usually are small and there is a greater risk of nerve damage using these veins. Careful observation of the IV site is mandatory throughout the infusion.

Standard infusion equipment is necessary for infusing verteporfin. Angiocaths or butterfly needles of small-caliber (22-gauge) are less traumatic and usually well tolerated. Also used are 60-inch anesthesia extension tubing, a microdisc filter (1.2 μm), 10-cc syringes, and a 30-cc syringe. The filter and extension tubing are flushed with sterile water. The verteporfin is reconstituted with 7 cc sterile water to create a 2-mg/cc solution and the calculated dose withdrawn and added to enough 5% dextrose and water to make a total of 30 cc of infusing solution. The 30-cc syringe is then connected to an infusion pump and set for a rate of 3 cc/minute for 10 minutes.

A small percentage of patients (approximately 2%) experience back pain during the infusion of verteporfin. This generally starts in the low back or lower abdomen, radiating to the back. The pain often is described as pulsating in nature and may radiate across the hips and/or down one or both legs to the knees. The mechanism of this back pain is not clear. However, it is felt that increased hydration helps to decrease the intensity of pain and in some cases eliminate it altogether. The pain will abate within a few minutes of termination of the infusion with no residual effects.

If back pain begins, changing position from sitting to standing when symptoms first appear often decreases the intensity and duration of the back pain. Once the patient is standing, it is best to remain standing, as the discomfort tends to recur when the patient is reseated. The 60-inch extension tubing allows the patient the necessary mobility for standing. Slowing the time of infusion from 10 to 12 minutes may also decrease back pain. Not all patients have the back pain at each infusion. If the patient is unable to tolerate the pain, the infusion may be terminated early, keeping in mind that at least 50% of the infusion must be given to enable adequate treatment. Rarely is it necessary to terminate the infusion.

Infrequently, pain occurs around the shoulders, chest, upper abdomen, or thoracic spine. Patients report they feel as if they are having a heart attack with a tight band around the chest and associated difficulty in breathing. Therefore, it is necessary and prudent to have emergency equipment available. We have a crash kit and defibrillator in the infusion room. There should be someone available to assist and obtain additional help if needed. If there is a question of cardiovascular distress, the nurse should terminate the verteporfin infusion and summon the physician. Treatment of symptoms is begun, and together with the physician an assessment and determination is made as to whether to proceed or abort the treatment. Again, as with the low back pain, these symptoms usually subside within a few minutes of termination of the infusion without residual effect.

Following the infusion, a pressure dressing is applied to minimize the potential for bruising. There is a greater risk of phototoxicity at the injection site because of extravasation of drugs into the skin. This manifests as a painful reddened rash. When extravasation occurs, symptomatic treatment with ice and acetaminophen and covering the site are usually indicated.

Anesthetic drops are administered and the laser is appropriately set after completion of the infusion. The physician is notified at the termination of the infusion, indicating treatment must begin in 5 minutes. On arrival of the physician, the patient is comfortably positioned in a chair in front of the laser. If a visitor accompanies the patient during the laser therapy, protective eyewear is issued with instructions to wear it until the laser portion of the treatment is completed. The physician checks the calculations of the treatment record and verifies the laser settings. Following the laser, the nurse or other staff member escorts the patient to the waiting area.

Safety precautions are again reviewed, and avoidance of bright light exposure is emphasized to the patient and their family. Although the FDA suggests avoidance of light exposure for 5 days, in the TAP and VIP studies, 2 days was adequate. This is consistent with our clinical experience as well. Any final questions are answered, and the patient is given his or her next appointment. It is emphasized that the patient should contact the office immediately if there are any abrupt changes in vision prior to the next appointment.

Approximately 15 minutes after treatment, assuming the patient is in satisfactory condition, the patient is discharged home with a driver or family member. Patients may resume regular activities, diet, exercise, and medications following treatment.

Although the actual practice and performance of PDT is not difficult, many challenges are presented to the nurse. It is difficult to observe patients lose their independence as their visual loss progresses. They are often scared and depressed over their illness. A willingness to listen and empathize with their plight often enhances patients' willingness to continue with the multiple treatments usually necessary in PDT. Conversely, seeing patients improve or maintain visual function and regain some measure of independence is very gratifying.

UNITED STATES BILLING ISSUES

Since July 1, 2001, a national coverage policy from the Centers for Medicare and Medicaid Services (CMS), formerly the Health Care Financing Administration (HCFA), has been in effect to provide coverage and billing guidelines for ocular photodynamic therapy (OPT) (7). This national coverage decision (NCD) is binding on all Medicare carriers, intermediaries, peer review organizations, and other contractors including Medicare + Choice Organizations. It is not binding on non-CMS health care organizations.

The NCD states that OPT (PDT) is covered when used in conjunction with verteporfin only in patients with AMD with a diagnosis of neovascular AMD (ICD-9-CM 362.52) with a predominantly classic subfoveal choroidal neovascular lesion at the initial treatment as determined by FA. Subsequent retreatments require an FA demonstrating leakage but the lesion does not have to be predominantly classic. There are no requirements regarding visual acuity, lesion size, or number of retreatments. Coverage is also provided at carrier discretion for subfoveal choroidal neovascularization occurring in pathologic myopia (ICD-9 CM 362.16) or ocular histoplasmosis (ICD-9 CM 115.02, 115.12, 115.92). For patients meeting these criteria, CPT code 67221 with the description "Destruction of localized lesion of choroid (e.g., CNV); PDT (includes intravenous infusion)" should be billed with either the RT or LT modifier signifying treatment to either the right or left eye, respectively. When OPT is performed on both eyes on the same day, code 67225 should be submitted rather than using the −50 modifier for bilateral procedures. Therefore, when both eyes are treated, the first eye is billed with 67221 (RT or LT) and the second eye with 67225 (RT or LT).

The drug verteporfin is billed using HCFA Common Procedure Coding System (HCPCS) code J3395. Each of the preceding codes must be submitted on form HCFA-1500. At this time, many Medicare carriers cannot process PDT billings electronically creating some delay in reimbursement and increasing the cost of billing. The substantial fixed costs of PDT make accurate billing and tracking of receivable accounts critical.

The NCD has brought some order and uniformity to the billing process for OPT. However, it specifically precludes payment for occult CNV or for diseases other than AMD, pathologic myopia, and ocular histoplasmosis. Ophthalmologists may treat patients with lesions outside the NCD for whom they believe treatment is medically indicated and necessary. Because CMS will not pay for this indication, it is considered a noncovered benefit and the ophthalmologist can directly bill the patient if the patient has signed an advance beneficiary notice (ABN) prior to the treatment and CMS denies a submitted claim.

An ABN is necessary in order to charge a Medicare beneficiary for a service that is not covered by Medicare or if the physician has reason to believe the service will not be covered. The ABN should be used for patients who do not fulfill the criteria of the NCD. The ABN must be signed by the patient prior to the procedure and a claim must be submitted on the patient's behalf. The patient can be required to pay in advance, but if Medicare pays the claim (which it may do on a case-by-case basis), the patient's payment must be promptly refunded. The ABN program is currently undergoing revision. The latest information on ABN is available on the Vitreous Society website (*vitreoussociety.org*).

A potentially problematic issue is the question of post-treatment audits of PDT. Medicare carriers have the authority to request medical records for retrospective payment review. These medical records should include the FA and interpretation report and a report of the procedure including dosage of verteporfin. We also keep the verteporfin package insert in the file to further document the use of the drug.

The NCD requires that all patients undergoing PDT have a pretreatment FA within 30 days of the treatment. This angiogram must be available for review if an audit is requested. It is unclear what review criteria of the angiogram will be used to determine coverage eligibility. Furthermore, FA interpretation is not an absolute science (8). In the TAP investigation, despite a prestudy certification process, experienced clinical investigators were judged to be in error in 61/609 (10%) of eyes on retrospective review of the FA by the study photograph reading center. In addition only 90% of the eyes in the TAP investigation had definitely subfoveal CNV. Eligibility for coverage by Medicare is determined by the FA features for the initial treatment. Therefore, if treatment is denied, subsequent retreatments also will be denied. Because audits are rarely performed in a timely manner, it is conceivable that a patient may have received multiple retreatments based on the assumption that the original treatment was covered. The financial implications for a practice of such a denial are obvious.

The issue of Medicare copayments by the patient is particularly important in PDT. Ophthalmologists are required by HCFA to bill the patient for 20% of the Medicare allowable charge for all services and drugs. Failure to do so is a potential fraud and abuse violation. Medicare allows 95% of the average wholesale price as the allowable charge for verteporfin and reimburses the physician 80% of this allowable charge (approximately $1,220). Because the cost to the physician of verteporfin is $1,350, a loss occurs with each treatment if the copayment is not collected. When the allowable charge for the laser code 67221 (approximately $340) is added to the allowable charge for verteporfin, the patient has a 20% copayment of approximately $400 per treatment if no secondary coverage is available.

FLUORESCEIN ANGIOGRAPHY ISSUES

Photodynamic therapy and an increasing awareness of AMD mean an increase in the number of patients requiring FA. The need for routine follow-up angiography every 3 months further increases this demand. Therefore, practices must increase their photographic capabilities. For practices already operating at or near capacity, this may require the expense of additional photographers and cameras. Digital angiography avoids the time delay inherent to film-based angiography and many practices find it invaluable in enhancing photographic productivity. Newer digital camera systems have software capable of calculating lesion size.

VOLUME CONSIDERATIONS

The time constraints and requirements of PDT can be disruptive to a busy clinical practice. Our group has found it helpful to segregate PDT patients from the non-PDT patients in a separate area dedicated to PDT. This area has a separate waiting area with a receptionist responsible for patient check in, check out, and billing. An infusion room has two reclining chairs. The laser is in an adjacent room. This allows the nurse to prepare one patient for infusion while observing a second patient throughout the infusion. The physician can then be treating a third patient in the laser room. With this arrangement we can treat up to three patients an hour. We try to concentrate PDT treatments on specific days to minimize disruption of other clinical responsibilities. When possible, a single ophthalmologist is dedicated to performing only PDT-related responsibilities on these days.

Practices with lesser volume will not find it efficient to have dedicated PDT facilities or time, and will need to integrate PDT treatments into the regular clinic. If this is done, it is critical that physician access be maintained so that the ophthalmologist is available to address infusion-related issues and perform treatment at the correct time. This means that the ophthalmologist must see fewer non-PDT patients during this time. This decreased productivity represents another opportunity cost of PDT.

CONCLUSION

Photodynamic therapy is the most important therapeutic advance in the treatment of CNV to date. Ophthalmologists responsible for the treatment of patients with CNV must provide this service. The considerable costs of PDT require that both clinical care and practice management be optimized so that ophthalmologists can continue to provide this vision-saving therapy.

REFERENCES

1. Klein R, Klein BEK, Linton KLP. Prevalence of age-related macular degeneration: the Beaver Dam Eye Study. *Ophthalmology* 1992; 99:933–943.
2. Mitchell P, Smith W, Attebo K, et al. Prevalence of age-related maculopathy in Australia: the Blue Mountains Eye Study. *Ophthalmology* 1995;102:1450–1460.
3. Treatment of Age-Related Macular Degeneration with Photodynamic Therapy (TAP) Study Group. Photodynamic therapy of subfoveal choroidal neovascularization in age-related macular degeneration with verteporfin: one-year results of two randomized clinical trials. *Arch Ophthalmol* 1999;117:1329–1245.
4. Treatment of Age-Related Macular Degeneration with Photodynamic Therapy (TAP) Study Group. Photodynamic therapy of subfoveal choroidal neovascularization in age-related macular degeneration with verteporfin: two-year results of two randomized clinical trials. *Arch Ophthalmol* 2001;119:198–207.
5. Verteporfin in Photodynamic Therapy Study Group. Verteporfin therapy of subfoveal choroidal neovascularization in age-related macular degeneration. Two-year results of a randomized clinical trial including lesions with occult with no classic choroidal neovascularization—verteporfin in photodynamic therapy report 2. *Am J Ophthalmol* 2001;131:541–560.
6. Margherio RR, Margherio AR, De Santis M. Laser treatment with verteporfin therapy and its potential impact on retinal practices. *Retina* 2000;20:325–330.
7. Department of Health and Human Services Health Care Financing Administration. *Medical coverage issues manual.* Washington, DC: Department of Health and Human Services, 2001.
8. Kaiser RS, Berger JW, Williams GA, et al. Variability in fluorescein angiography interpretation for photodynamic therapy in age-related macular degeneration. *Retina* 2003;22:683–690.

18

INCIDENCE OF ELIGIBLE CASES IN CLINICAL PRACTICE

MAURO GOLDBAUM
JASON S. SLAKTER

Age-related macular degeneration (AMD) is the leading cause of legal blindness in people over 64 years old in the United States (1,2). Until recently, the only effective therapy for neovascular AMD, based on the Macular Photocoagulation Study Group (MPS), was fluorescein angiography (FA)–guided laser photocoagulation (3). The MPS group determined that only patients with classic or well-defined CNV were eligible for this therapy. In order to evaluate the potential benefits of laser photocoagulation on AMD, it was important to determine the frequency of classic membranes in patients with neovascular AMD. Freund and associates showed that only 13% of newly diagnosed patients with exudative maculopathy secondary to AMD present with classic CNV (4).

Photodynamic therapy (PDT) is a new treatment modality that has been proven to be effective for CNV. However, as for standard photocoagulation, PDT benefits only a group of patients who meet specific criteria. It would be useful to estimate the impact of this new treatment through the determination of the frequency of eligible patients.

ELIGIBILITY FOR PHOTODYNAMIC THERAPY

The efficacy of PDT using verteporfin (Visudyne, Novartis Pharmaceuticals, Basel, Switzerland) for CNV has been reported by the Treatment of Age-Related Macular Degeneration with Photodynamic Therapy (TAP) and the Verteporfin in Photodynamic Therapy (VIP) protocols (5–7).

The data showed a significantly improved outcome for patients with subfoveal CNV who underwent PDT over the placebo group. However, on angiographic subgroup analysis this beneficial effect appeared to be restricted to a selected group. This group presented with a CNV lesion that had a classic component corresponding to at least 50% of the total area of the lesion, or so-called predominantly classic CNV (5). After 24 months, the percentage of eyes with predominantly classic lesion that experienced a less than 15-letter loss was 59% in the treated group versus 31% in the placebo group (6). These differences on PDT efficacy based on different angiographic patterns of CNV are not well understood.

Pathologic myopic patients presented the best results with PDT. The percentage of eyes with a vision loss less than eight letters at 12 months was 72% in the treated group versus 44% in the placebo group (7). Subgroup analysis was not considered, but the vast majority of these patients tend to present with predominantly classic lesions. The effect of PDT with verteporfin on patients with other causes of CNV (e.g., histoplasmosis) is currently under investigation.

IMPACT OF PHOTODYNAMIC THERAPY

Age-related macular degeneration is the most common cause of CNV by far; therefore, the impact of PDT is mainly based on the incidence of neovascular AMD patients who meet the predominantly classic lesion criteria. Margherio and coworkers recently published on the frequency of different types of AMD (8). They performed a retrospective study on 1,000 consecutive records of new patients referred to a vitreoretinal referral practice during 1998. From 392 patients with subfoveal CNV, 171 (43.6%) presented with a predominantly classic lesion, 85 (21.7%) presented with a CNV lesion that was more than 0% but less than 50% classic (so-called minimally classic lesion), and 136 patients (34.7%) had a CNV with no classic component. These authors estimated the number of patients who would be eligible for PDT per year in the United States to be 84,000. The average number of treatments in 1 year is 3.4 per patient (5), which totals 286,000 applications of PDT per year in the United States alone.

A prospective study on the frequency of predominantly classic CNV was performed by the authors, also in a vitreoretinal referral practice (9). The authors studied all consecutive eyes that presented with newly diagnosed subfoveal CNV secondary to AMD during a 6-month period in 1999. Newly diagnosed CNV was considered to be the case with a maximum of a 3-month history of visual loss or metamorphopsia. The diagnosis of subfoveal CNV secondary to AMD was made based on clinical and angiographic findings as previously defined by MPS (10,11). In addition, stereoscopic color pictures were analyzed when the case required.

We measured the total area of the CNV and the partial area of each component of the lesion using measurement tools included in the digital imaging system. This is a somewhat different calculation of classic CNV composition than was used in the verteporfin therapy trials. The eyes were subdivided into four groups for this study (Fig. 18.1):

1. 100% classic CNV
2. CNV with 50% to 99% of a classic component
3. CNV with 1% to 49% of a classic component
4. CNV with no classic component

Eighty-three eyes of 83 patients with subfoveal CNV secondary to AMD were enrolled. Twelve eyes (14.5%) were diagnosed as 100% classic CNV, seven eyes (8.4%) were diagnosed as CNV with 50% to 99% of a classic component, 16 eyes (19.3%) were diagnosed as CNV with 1% to 49% of a classic component, and 48 eyes (57.8%) were classified as CNV with no classic component (Fig. 18.1). Predominantly classic CNV (lesions with >50% classic CNV) was found in 22.9% of the cases. Therefore, PDT with verteporfin would benefit almost 25% of the patients with subfoveal CNV based on the data from the TAP study (5,6).

In absolute numbers, the incidence of exudative maculopathy secondary to AMD is 200,000 new cases per year in the United States (12). Approximately 9% of these patients present with extrafoveal classic CNV (6). This means 18,000 patients are amenable to MPS laser photocoagulation. From the 186,000 patients, 22.9% or 42,600 patients are candidates for PDT with verteporfin. They need an average of 3.4 treatments per year (5), which amounts to almost 145,000 applications of PDT per year in the United States alone.

Certainly, treating 25% of the patients is not satisfactory. However, the number of patients with CNV secondary to AMD treatable with PDT is almost 2.4 times larger than it is with MPS laser photocoagulation, and the number of treatments with PDT is more than eight times the number of MPS laser applications.

OCCULT LESIONS

Occult lesions with no classic component remain controversial. The results of the TAP study suggested a potential benefit from PDT (5). However, this group of patients was not supposed to be enrolled according to the inclusion criteria. On the other hand, results of the VIP study demonstrated no effect of PDT for patients with this type of CNV at 12-month follow up (13). However, at 24 months, there was a significant difference in the rate of moderate and severe vision loss between the treatment and placebo groups (13). A detailed review of the VIP study has proposed that PDT with verteporfin is beneficial for a subgroup of occult lesions with no classic component (13). The most susceptible patients are the ones who present with smaller CNV

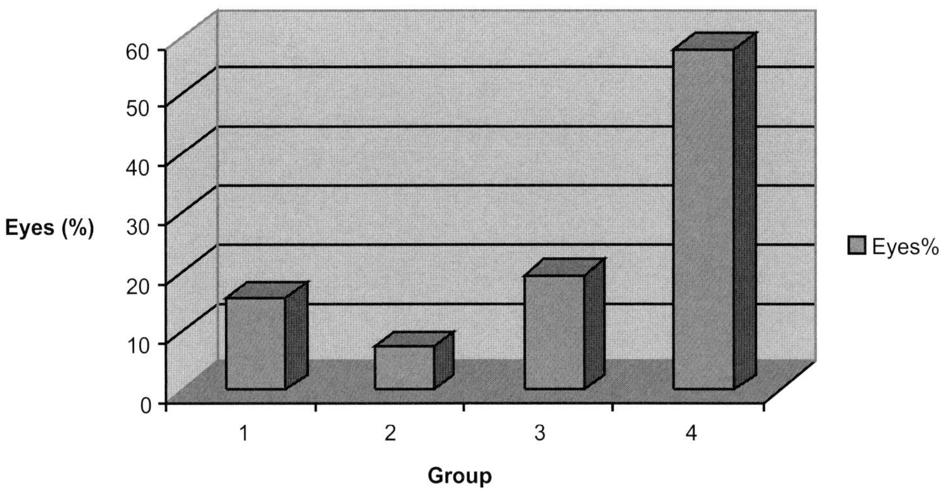

FIGURE 18.1. Distribution by angiographic morphology. Group 1: 100% classic CNV (14.5% of the eyes). Group 2: CNV with 50% to 99% of classic components (8.4% of the eyes). Group 3: CNV with 1% to 49% of classic components (19.3% of the eyes). Group 4: CNV with no classic components (57.8% of the eyes).

lesions (four disc areas or smaller) or lower levels of visual acuity at baseline (letter score less than 65, or approximately $20/50^{-1}$ with Snellen card).

In our study, 31 patients (64.6%) from the no-classic component had a CNV lesion smaller than four disc areas. Also, 32 patients (66.7%) from the no-classic component group presented visual acuity worse than $20/50^{-1}$. The presence of one condition or the other was detected in 44 patients (91.7%). This represents almost half of the patients with CNV secondary to AMD and, obviously, it enormously increases the number of patients who meet eligibility criteria for PDT. Together with the predominantly classic patients, we would be able to treat 75% of the patients with CNV secondary to AMD.

DIFFERENT FORMS OF CHOROIDAL NEOVASCULARIZATION

The studies of PDT with verteporfin for CNV treatment have followed concepts established by the MPS group (10,11). However, imaging advances have helped us study choroidal circulation since then. Because FA is the standard examination to subdivide CNV lesions, indocyanine green angiography (ICG) is useful to subcategorize occult CNV lesions (14). Different types and categories of CNV lesions have been described and suggested with the help of ICG angiography. Slakter and coworkers reported on retinal-choroidal anastomosis (RCA) in patients with occult CNV (15). Yannuzzi and colleagues used ICG angiography to reveal that 7.8% of elderly exudative maculopathy patients present with polypoidal choroidal neovascularization (P-CNV) (16). Without ICG, we suspected the diagnosis of RCA in eight (9.6%) patients in our study. At least one patient had a diagnosis of P-CNV. These numbers probably would increase using ICG angiography, but they represent at least 10% of patients who may have a different response to PDT. An ICG study of PDT patients may allow us to better understand the treatment differences of diverse types of occult CNV.

CHOROIDAL NEOVASCULARIZATION OF OTHER CAUSES

Choroidal neovascularization may be associated with etiologies other than AMD, such as presumed ocular histoplasmosis syndrome (POHS), pseudo-POHS, angioid streaks, myopia, or even idiopathic processes. Myopia is the most common among these (17). In a retrospective study with CNV patients younger than 59 years of age, high myopia was found in 62%, pseudo-POHS in 12%, angioid streaks in 5%, and no etiology in 17% (18). Obviously, these proportions vary based on epidemiologic characteristics (e.g., the incidence of histoplasmosis).

Choroidal neovascularization affects 5% to 10% of the myopic population, especially in eyes with degenerative myopia (more than six diopters with an axial length of more than 26 mm) (19,20). Hotchkiss and Fine reported that 40.7% of high myopic patients presented with CNV in their study (21). As with AMD, most of the CNV lesions in myopic patients involve the fovea. Seventy-four percent are subfoveal and almost all of the remaining are located within 100 to 300 μm of the fovea (22). Thus, a majority of patients with CNV secondary to pathologic myopia may benefit from verteporfin therapy.

SUMMARY

The results of the clinical trials involving PDT with verteporfin have clearly demonstrated that the nature of the neovascular lesion plays an important role in the outcome of therapy. As shown in this chapter, a majority of patients with CNV secondary to AMD (as well as other causes) have lesions that might benefit from verteporfin therapy.

REFERENCES

1. National Society to Prevent Blindness. *Visual problems in the United States: definitions, data sources, detailed data tables, analyses, interpretation.* New York: National Society to Prevent Blindness, 1980:1–46.
2. Tielsch JA. Vision problems in the U.S.: a report on blindness and visual impairment in adults age 40 and older. In: *Prevent blindness America.* Schaumburg, IL: Prevent Blindness, 1994.
3. Macular Photocoagulation Study Group. Argon laser photocoagulation for neovascular maculopathy: five year results from randomized clinical trials. *Arch Ophthalmol* 1991;109:1109–1114.
4. Freund KB, Yannuzzi LA, Sorenson JA. Age-related macular degeneration and choroidal neovascularization. *Am J Ophthalmol* 1993;115:786–791.
5. Treatment of Age-Related Macular Degeneration with Photodynamic Therapy (TAP) Study Group. Photodynamic therapy of subfoveal choroidal neovascularization in age-related macular degeneration with verteporfin: one-year results of 2 randomized clinical trials. *Arch Ophthalmol* 1999;117:1329–1345.
6. Treatment of Age-Related Macular Degeneration with Photodynamic Therapy (TAP) Study Group. Photodynamic therapy of subfoveal choroidal neovascularization in age-related macular degeneration with verteporfin: two-year results of 2 randomized clinical trials. *Arch Ophthalmol* 2001;119:198–207.
7. Verteporfin in Photodynamic Therapy Study Group. Photodynamic therapy of subfoveal choroidal neovascularization in pathologic myopia with verteporfin: 1-year results of a randomized clinical trial. *Ophthalmology* 2001;108:841–852.
8. Margherio RR, Margherio AR, DeSantis ME. Laser treatments with verteporfin therapy and its potential impact on retinal practices. *Retina* 2000;20:325–330.
9. Goldbaum M, Guyer DR, Freund KB, et al. Nature and frequency of newly diagnosed subfoveal choroidal neovascularization secondary to age-related macular degeneration. Submitted for publication.
10. Macular Photocoagulation Study Group. Subfoveal neovascular lesion in age-related macular degeneration: guidelines for evalua-

tion and treatment in the Macular Photocoagulation Study. *Arch Ophthalmol* 1991;109:1224–1257.

11. The International ARM Epidemiological Study Group. An international classification and grading system for age-related maculopathy and age-related macular degeneration. *Surv Ophthalmol* 1995;39:367–374.
12. Macular Photocoagulation Study Group. Five-year follow-up of fellow eyes of patients with age-related macular degeneration and unilateral extrafoveal choroidal neovascularization. *Arch Ophthalmol* 1993;111:1189–1199.
13. Verteporfin in Photodynamic Therapy Study Group. Verteporfin therapy of subfoveal choroidal neovascularization in age-related macular degeneration: two-year results of a randomized clinical trial including lesions with occult with no classic choroidal neovascularization. *Am J Ophthalmol* 2001;131:541–560.
14. Yannuzzi LA, Slakter JS, Sorenson JA, et al. Digital indocyanine green videoangiography and choroidal neovascularization. *Retina* 1992;12:191–223.
15. Slakter JS, Yannuzzi LA, Schneider U, et al. Retinal choroidal anastomoses and occult choroidal neovascularization in age-related macular degeneration. *Ophthalmology* 2000;107:742–753.
16. Yannuzzi LA, Wong DW, Sforzolini BS, et al. Polypoidal choroidal vasculopathy and neovascularized age-related macular degeneration. *Arch Ophthalmol* 1999;117:1503–1510.
17. Ballaco-Gabrieli C. Aetiopathogenesis of degenerative myopia: a hypothesis. *Ophthalmologica* 1982;185:199–294.
18. Cohen SY, Laroche A, Leguen Y, et al. Etiology of choroidal neovascularization in young patients. *Ophthalmology* 1996;103:1241–1244.
19. Campos R. La tache de Fuchs. In: *Problemes actuels D'Ophtalmologie.* Basel: Karger, 1957:363–364.
20. Curtin BJ, Karlin DB. Axial length measurements and fundus changes of the myopic eye. *Am J Ophthalmol* 1971;71:42–53.
21. Hotchkiss ML, Fine SL. Pathologic myopia and choroidal neovascularization. *Am J Ophthalmol* 1981;91:177–183.
22. Soubrane G, Pison J, Bornert P, et al. Néovaisseaux sous-rétiniens de la myopie dégénérative: résultats de la photocoagulation. *Bull Soc Ophtalmol Fr* 1986;86:269–272.

19

PHOTODYNAMIC THERAPY WITH TIN ETHYL ETIOPURPURIN

EDGAR LEE THOMAS
WENDY J. SNYDER

Age-related macular degeneration (AMD) is newly diagnosed in more than 84,000 people annually in the United States and is the leading cause of blindness in the aging population (1). Exudative (wet) AMD is marked by proliferating choroidal neovascularization (CNV) in the subretinal pigment epithelial space. When CNV occurs in the subfoveal space, fluid, blood, and lipid accumulates and ultimately disciform scarring results in severe central vision loss.

Thermal argon laser photocoagulation may be used to treat CNV. However, it produces full thickness destruction of the retina, including the overlying photoreceptors in the treatment area (2). The Macular Photocoagulation Study (MPS) demonstrated the efficacy of laser photocoagulation for subfoveal CNV for select cases, with a small but statistically significant difference in the level of visual acuity achieved several years after treatment, compared to the natural course of the disease (3). Many clinicians have found this treatment difficult to recommend because of the limited longevity of this patient population. Patients may not survive long enough to allow them to experience the full treatment benefit.

As early as 1987, the potential for photodynamic therapy (PDT) for the treatment of CNV in the eye was shown in an experimental animal model (4). Photodynamic therapy for CNV involves the systemic administration of a photoactive drug, which is subsequently activated at the treatment site by low power, nonthermal laser light of a wavelength specific for drug activation. Activation creates reactive oxygen species and free radicals that cause local cellular effects, including thrombosis in neovasculature, while sparing the overlying retina and potentially stabilizing or improving vision (5). In April, 2000, the United States Food and Drug Administration approved the first photodynamic therapy, verteporfin (Visudyne, Novartis Pharmaceuticals, Basel, Switzerland), for the treatment of predominantly classic (≥50%), subfoveal CNV-AMD. Published Phase III verteporfin data demonstrated a beneficial effect compared to placebo for the reduction of vision loss at 1 year for this subset of the CNV-AMD patient population (6,7).

SnET2 (tin ethyl etiopurpurin; Miravant Medical Technologies, Santa Barbara, CA) is another photoactive agent currently being evaluated for the treatment of subfoveal CNV in humans. Prior to the use of SnET2 CNV in AMD, approximately 400 patients had been treated in 16 nonophthalmologic clinical trials (8).

PHOTOSENSITIZER CHARACTERISTICS

SnET2 is a synthetic chlorin photosensitizer (Fig. 19.1). The primary absorption maxima of SnET2 are at 438 nm (159,000 $M^{-1}cm^{-1}$) and 664 (52,000, $M^{-1}cm^{-1}$) (Fig. 19.2).

SnET2 is a lipophilic photosensitizer formulated in a ready-to-use isotonic, isoosmotic lipid emulsion formulation. It is formulated at a concentration of approximately 1 mg/mL for intravenous (iv) administration based on body weight. The selected treatment wavelength of SnET2 in ophthalmic applications is 664 nm. In the treatment of CNV secondary to AMD, laser light at 664 nm from a 0.5 W diode laser is delivered to the fundus with a slit-lamp biomicroscope and slit-lamp adapter (Iridex Corp., Mountain View, CA). The irradiance ranged from 150 to 600 mW/cm^2 in preclinical studies with SnET2, whereas the irradiance was fixed at 600 mW/cm^2 in clinical studies.

PRECLINICAL STUDIES

Early preclinical studies were conducted with SnET2 in a series of ocular neovascularization models and glaucoma models.

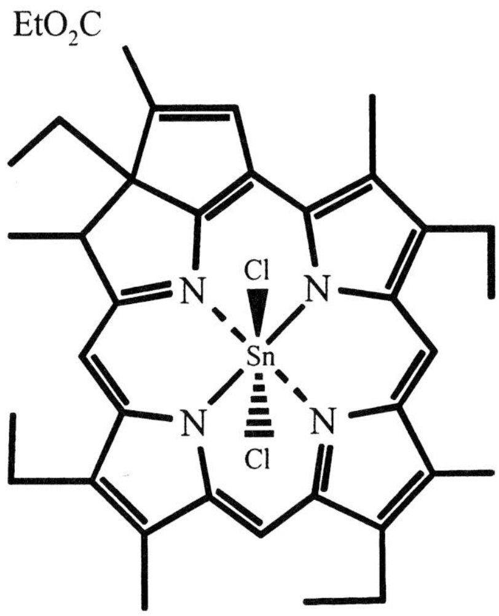

FIGURE 19.1. The chemical structure of tin ethyl etiopurpurin (SnET2).

CORNEAL NEOVASCULARIZATION

SnET2 was evaluated in a suture-induced corneal neovascularization model in Sprague Dawley rats (9). Placing a silk suture in the corneal stroma induced neovascularization. Fourteen days later, CNV developed and the suture was removed. SnET2 was intravenously administered at a dose 1.0 mg/kg with a slow bolus push. Approximately 10 minutes following SnET2 administration, low-power diode laser light (664 + 7 nm) was delivered to the cornea in a 3-mm diameter spot size. The light dose ranged from 10 to 25 J/cm^2 with an irradiance of 150 mW/cm^2. Fluorescein angiography (FA) and histopathology were used to evaluate the effect of SnET2-PDT on the neovascularization. Histopathology of the cornea was evaluated at 1, 7, 14, and 28 days following SnET2-PDT.

This study demonstrated the safe and effective treatment of CNV using SnET2-PDT. Persistent neovascular closure was seen at all light doses to 28 days. Light dose–dependent trends were noted. Partial neovascular closure was seen in approximately 70% of eyes at 28 days treated with 10 or 15 J/cm^2. Complete neovascular closure was seen in 33%, 10%, and 100% of eyes at 28 days treated with 10, 15, and 25 J/cm^2, respectively. Histopathology showed that adjacent ocular structures (e.g., iris, ciliary body, and retina) were normal.

NORMAL CHORIOCAPILLARIS

A series of studies was performed by Peyman and coworkers in pigmented rabbits to demonstrate occlusion of the

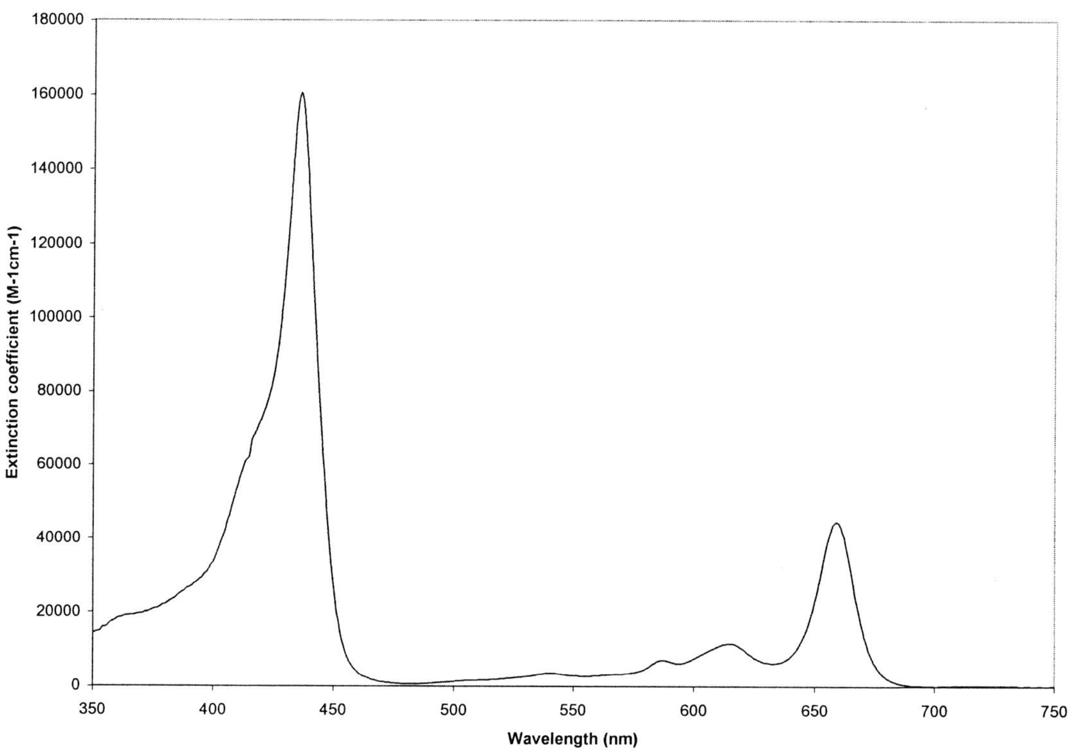

FIGURE 19.2. The absorption spectrum of SnET2 in 50:50 chloroform octanol; the absorption maxima are 438 nm (163,000 $M^{-1}cm^{-1}$), 540 nm (4,900 $M^{-1}cm^{-1}$), 587 nm (8,700 $M^{-1}cm^{-1}$), 616 nm (13,300 $M^{-1}cm^{-1}$), and 661 nm (52,000 $M^{-1}cm^{-1}$).

choriocapillaris following SnET2-PDT (10,11). In the initial study, the SnET2 dose was 0.5 and 1.0 mg/kg was followed by light treatment 15 to 45 minutes postadministration. Light was delivered to the fundus in a 1.5-mm diameter spot and 300 mW/cm^2 irradiance, light doses ranged from 5 to 20 J/cm^2 (10). Fluorescein angiography and histopathology were used at 1, 14, and 28 days following SnET2-PDT to demonstrate efficacy.

Occlusion of the choriocapillaris was seen at all SnET2 and light dose combinations. Occlusion of the choriocapillaris was observed at 5 J/cm^2, whereas the larger choroidal vessels remained perfused. The larger choroidal vessels also were occluded at 10 and 20 J/cm^2. Reperfusion was apparent at 14 days following PDT, and partial reperfusion was observed by 28 days. Histopathology at the lowest SnET2 and light dose combinations showed that occlusion of the choriocapillaris was achieved with minimal effects on the RPE, rods and cones, and neural retina. Disruption to the peripheral structures increased as the SnET2 and light dose combination increased. For example, disruption of the RPE, detachment of the rods and cones, and vacuolization of the rods and cones were all observed at higher drug and light dose combinations. The occlusion on the choriocapillaris with minimal effects on the surrounding tissues was primarily light dose–dependent.

A second study was conducted in this animal model to demonstrate the effect of the time interval on occlusion of the choriocapillaris (11). The SnET2 and light doses were fixed at 0.5 mg/kg and 20 J/cm^2, whereas the time interval ranged from 5 to 240 minutes between drug and light administration. Choriocapillaris occlusion was seen angiographically at time intervals to 20 minutes. Histopathology confirmed occlusion of the choriocapillaris with minimal damage to the overlying neural retina at these parameters. Fluorescein vesicle angiography demonstrated that occlusion was observed within 90 minutes after PDT treatment.

LASER-INDUCED CHOROIDAL NEOVASCULARIZATION

Cynomolgus monkeys with laser-induced CNV lesions were intravenously administered either 0.5 or 1.0 mg/kg SnET2 with a slow push (12). Laser light was delivered at irradiance levels of 150 – 600 mW/cm^2, 15 to 36 minutes following SnET2 injection. The light dose ranged from 20 to 75 J/cm^2. Angiography showed that 1.0 mg/kg of SnET2 and 25 to 75 J/cm^2 of laser light effectively closed CNV at 24 hours after PDT treatment.

CYCLODESTRUCTION

Pigmented rabbits were intravenously administered SnET2 to examine the distribution and efficacy of SnET2-PDT treatment in disrupting the ciliary processes (13). Within 24 hours, fluorescence microscopy showed that SnET2 was localized in the nonpigmented epithelium of the ciliary processes. SnET2-PDT treatment of the ciliary body was done at 24 hours post-SnET2 administration with a light dose of 50 or 100 J/cm^2. Histopathology demonstrated denudement of the ciliary body epithelium at the given drug and light dose combinations, suggesting that SnET2-PDT may be an effective method of cyclodestructive surgery.

FILTRATION SURGERY

SnET2 was administered both intravenously and subconjunctivally to rabbits prior to posterior lip sclerectomies to determine the antifibrotic efficacy of SnET2-PDT as an adjuvant to filtration surgery (14). Either 1 mg/kg SnET2 or 25 to 75 μg SnET2 (0.1 mL) were administered intravenously or subconjunctivally, respectively. The filtering region was irradiated with 30 J/cm^2 (100 mW/cm^2) 24 hours after iv administration or 3 hours following subconjunctival administration at the time of the filtration surgery. Intravenous doses of SnET2 did not show any antifibrotic responses or prolonged survival of the filtering bleb following surgery. SnET2-PDT with subconjunctival injections at all doses demonstrated prolonged survival of the filtering bleb to 4 weeks postsurgery.

SNET2 CLINICAL TRIALS

Doses of SnET2 of up to 1.6 mg/kg have been found to be safe and well tolerated in nonophthalmologic clinical trials of approximately 400 patients (15). Twenty-eight patients were initially treated and studied in a Phase I/II open-label, multicenter, dose escalation, 12-week trial. Doses of SnET2 of 0.25, 0.5, 0.75, and 1.0 mg/kg, were activated by 664-nm low power, nonthermal diode laser light (Iridex) at doses of 36, 72, and 108 J/cm^2 (Fig. 19.3). Twelve additional patients were subsequently treated with modifications in the light delivery procedure.

Ophthalmologic clinical trials for subfoveal choroidal neovascularization began with Phase I/II in 1997 with clinical study centers in Boston (Carmen A. Puliafito, New England Eye Center), New York City (Richard Rosen, New York Eye and Ear Infirmary), Baltimore (Robert P. Murphy, Glaser Murphy Retinal Treatment Center), and Beverly Hills (Edgar L. Thomas, Retina-Vitreous Associates). The initial trial included 28 patients using escalating drug and light doses. Doses of SnET2 were 0.25, 0.50, 0.75, and 1.0 mg/kg of body weight. Light doses of 36 (1 minute), 72 (2 minutes), and 108 (3 minutes) mJ/cm^2 were sequentially applied to the lesions with the escalating drug doses (Tables 19.1 and 19.2). The Iridex diode laser with a maximum

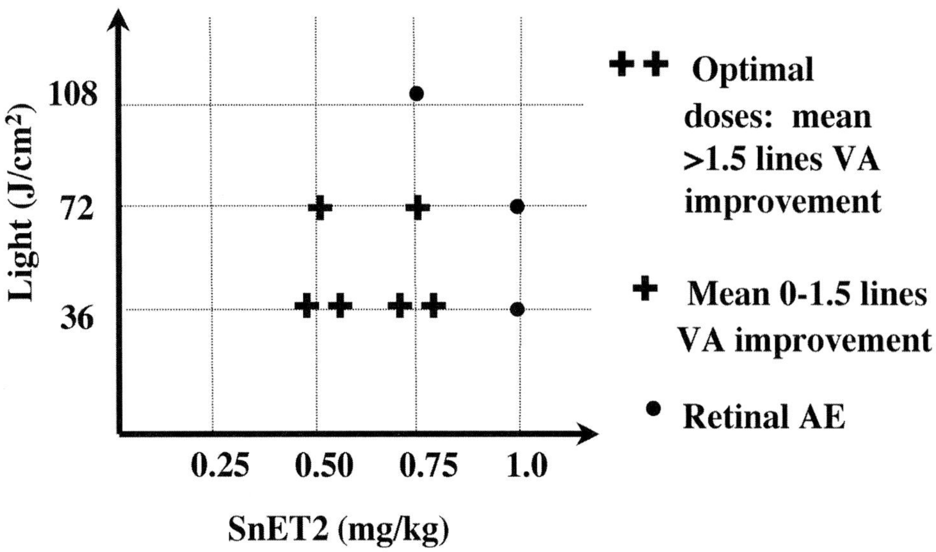

FIGURE 19.3. SnET2 Phase I/II dose escalation. Dose escalation efficacy/safety single plus sign (+) indicates moderate visual improvement. Double plus sign (++) indicates marked improvement in visual acuity. Enlarged dots (•) show toxicity seen angiographically.

spot size of 3,000 μm was applied using the Yanuzzi posterior pole lens.

Entry criteria were the presence of subfoveal CNV with at least some component of classic neovascularization: early, lacy, discrete, and vascular patterns of hyperfluorescence on FA without prior laser photocoagulation and visual acuity less than 20/100 using an ETDRS protocol refraction. End points chosen were closure of CNV complex on FA and change in ETDRS visual acuity over the initial 90 days following treatment. Response on FA was graded as complete if there was no evidence of fluorescence in the lesion; partial if there was diminution, but not absence, of fluorescence compared with baseline; or none if no evidence of change in fluorescence from baseline. An additional 12 patients were treated with a split and higher light doses. Four groups of three patients each received: (a) 0.5 mg/kg and light doses divided with 72 J/cm² of light followed at 60 minutes with 54 J/cm²; (b) 0.5 mg/kg and 126 J/cm²; (c) 0.75 mg/kg at 90 J/cm²; and (d) 0.75 mg/kg and 72 J/cm² followed by 36 J/cm² at 60 minutes. No difference in effect was seen with these varied light doses when compared to the light dose given at a single time setting. A total of 40 patients comprised the Phase I/II study.

Higher dose levels were not studied further because of increased microvascular changes on FA in the dose scheme 10 and 11 subgroups. Figure 19.3 shows the distribution of efficacy and toxicity of SnET2 dose/escalation of light and photosensitizer. The most efficacious SnET2 doses were in the intermediate range of the study at 0.50 and 0.75 mg/kg. The light dose at which these two doses were the most ben-

TABLE 19.1. SNET2 PHASE I/II TREATMENT SCHEME

Dose Scheme	Dose (mg/kg)	Minutes	Number (*n*)
1	0.25	1	3
2	0.25	2	3
3	0.50	1	3
4	0.50	2	3
5	0.50	3	3
6	0.75	1	3
7	0.75	2	3
8	0.75	3	3
9	1.0	1	3
10	1.0	2	1
11	1.0	3	0

PDT with SnET2
Edgar L. Thomas, M.D., and Wendy J. Synder, Ph.D.

TABLE 19.2. DIVIDED DOSE SNET2 PHASE I/II TREATMENT SCHEME

Dose	Light time 0	Light time 60 minutes	Number (*n*)
0.5 mg/kg	72 J/cm²	54 J/cm²	3
0.5 mg/kg	126 J/cm²	0	3
0.75 mg/kg	90 J/cm²	0	3
0.75 mg/kg	72 J/cm²	36 J/cm²	3

PDT with SnET2
Edgar L. Thomas, M.D., and Wendy J. Snyder, Ph.D.

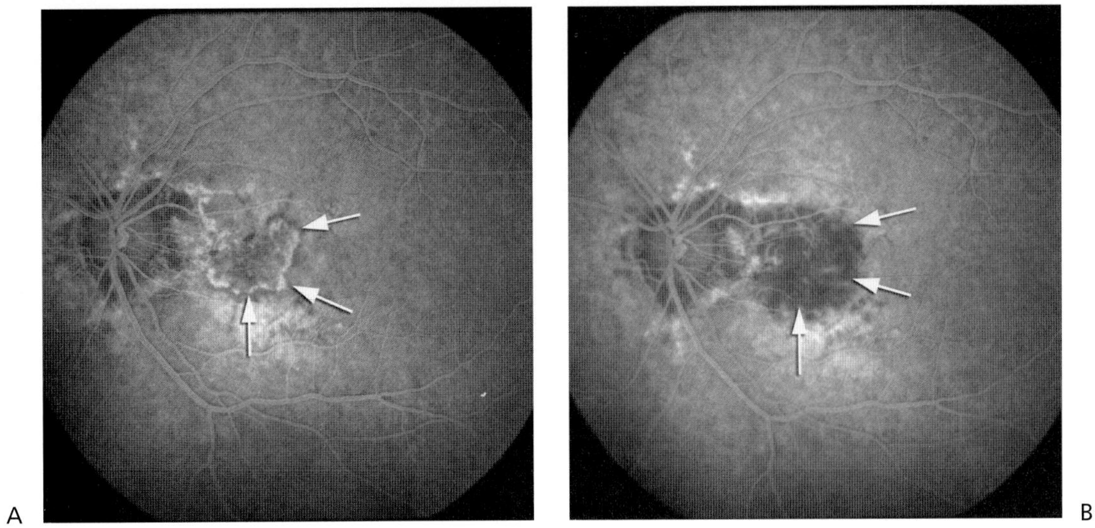

FIGURE 19.4. A: Early pretreatment fluorescein angiogram demonstrates lacy hyperfluorescence margin *(white arrows)* of the border of the classic choroidal neovascularization. **B:** Early posttreatment fluorescein angiogram shows absence (closure) of the lacy hyperfluorescence previously seen in Figure 19.4A, where the choroidal neovascularization was previously active *(white arrows).*

eficial in closing choroidal neovascular vessels was at 36 J/cm². These Phase I/II parameters were then used to design a multicenter, randomized, masked clinical trial in the United States.

These doses were chosen because the initial efficacy of SnET2 in the Phase I/II studies had shown a positive effect on visual acuities, with 1.9 lines improvement at 90 days with the 0.5-mg/kg dose, and 3.5 lines improvement with the 0.75-mg/kg dose. When compared to the MPS, the data are significantly better at the 90-day end point, than both the laser treated group and control untreated group. These data combined with the safety data supported the selection of these two dosing regimens for the Phase III study. A sequence of FA depicting the initial response to SnET2 is shown in Figure 19.4A, at baseline, and in Figure 19.4B at 2 weeks posttreatment. Discernible closure of the choroidal neovascular membrane is seen after treatment. No leakage or staining is noted over the central area where the membrane was prominent and the lace edges of the classic neovascular membrane are no longer visible.

PHASE III TRIAL

The SnET2 Phase III trial consists of two parallel, pivotal, prospective, multicentered, randomized, double-masked, placebo-controlled trials of 2 years total duration, with 933 patients at 60 centers in the United States. Institutional Review Board (IRB)/Ethics Committee approval was obtained. All patients were required to be 50 years of age or older and have subfoveal CNV caused by AMD. No lesions with clinically obvious glial or disciform-type scarring were eligible. Subretinal hemorrhage could not exceed 50% of the overall lesion. Baseline ETDRS visions must have been in a range of 15 to 60 letters read. Initial lesion size had to be equal to or less than 3.0 mm, and recurrent lesions could not be greater than 4.5 mm during the study. At entry, patients were randomized at 2:2:1 into one of three possible groups—0.5 mg/kg SnET2, 0.75 mg/kg SnET2, or placebo—all followed with a light dose of 36 J/cm². Two parallel clinical trials were approved and begun in 1998. The 2-year data collection end point was in December, 2001.

BASELINE DEMOGRAPHICS

Baseline demographic data were collected from eligible study participants, including gender, age, race, smoking history, diameter of lesion in study eye, ETDRS visual acuity, visual acuity strata, study eye (right or left), history of prior laser therapy in the fellow eye, menopausal status, weight, and height (16). The data were divided into the three groups according to the treatment assignments: placebo, 0.5, or 0.75 mg/kg. Mathematical analysis was conducted as appropriate for each category (e.g., percentage, mean, median, standard deviation, minimum, and maximum). No tests for statistical significance were done. The outcome measures for this analysis were: (a) the assessment of the equivalent distribution of the demographic parameters among the three data subgroups; (b) the determination whether or not the subgroups were well balanced; and (c) the assessment of the demographic and clinical profile of the total group as representative of the CNV-AMD patient population, within the predetermined entry criteria of the trial.

These groups represent the three randomization groups described in the preceding in the 2:2:1 schema. The overall average patient age in the study was 76.7 years with the standard deviation of + 7.28. The individual treatment groups were the placebo group (76.0 + 7.75 years), the 0.5-mg/kg group (77.0 + 7.15 years), and the 0.75-mg/kg group (76.6 + 7.18 years). This distribution of age is typical for the AMD population in the United States and shows an even distribution in each of the study groups. Almost 60% of the patients in the study groups were female, reflecting their statistically increased longevity. Menopausal status reflected the high prevalence of females in the study groups, approaching 55% of all patients in groups. Race distribution also was consistent with previous data, showing non-White patients making up less than 3.8% in the placebo group, 1.9% in the 0.5-mg/kg group, and 0.8% in the 0.75-mg/kg group. Smoking (epidemiology associated and probably causal for AMD) was prevalent in the past history of patients in all groups (17). In the placebo group, 16.9% were current smokers; in the 0.5-mg/kg group, 15.9% were current smokers; and in the 0.75-mg/kg group, 15.1% were current smokers. A much larger percentage of patients were former smokers: 49.2% in the placebo group, 50.0% in the 0.5-mg/kg group, and 45.2% in the 0.75-mg/kg group. Nonsmokers made up less than 17% in all groups.

Visual acuity, a critical component of efficacy of photodynamic therapy, was evaluated with ETDRS testing. The logarithmically based technique uses number of letters read rather than the more traditional Snellen acuities, therefore, it is ideal for evaluating treatment efficacy. Baseline levels of visual acuity were measured, with the placebo group showing a mean of 45.6 + 13.66 letters, the 0.5-mg/kg group 45.9 + 12.53, the 0.75-mg/kg group 45.4 + 12.51, and the total population averaging 45.7 + 12.74 letters. This distribution within the groups appears very consistent across the study groups. The visual acuity of patients in the SnET2 Phase III trial, compared to the verteporfin baseline acuity, represents better initial visual acuities, presumably because of the smaller lesion size chosen as an entry criterion.

Visual acuity strata for the groups also are important to review. Almost 60% of each group had an entry visual acuity of more than 45 letters on the ETDRS charts. The Snellen equivalent of 45 letters is approximately 20/120 vision. The placebo group was 59.0%, the 0.5-mg/kg group was 57.8%, and the 0.75-mg/kg group was 57.8%. Groups 1, 2, and 3 were between 31 and 45 letters, 24.0%, 25.0%, and 25.2%, respectively. All three groups had less than 20% of the eyes that were less than 31 letters. Prior laser photocoagulation had been performed in less than 20% of all fellow eyes in each of the study groups.

FLUORESCEIN ANGIOGRAPHIC CHARACTERISTICS AT BASELINE

Analysis of baseline angiographic findings from the Fundus Photographic Reading Center (FPRC) (University of Wisconsin–Madison) from the Phase III trial was reviewed (18). Angiographic analysis of baseline lesion characteristics was performed by the FPRC on 904 eyes. Eighty-six percent of eyes with evaluable CNV lesions had some area of classic CNV and 14% had no classic CNV. Fifty percent of lesions were greater than 50% classic CNV, 6% of those had evidence of occult CNV. Thirty-seven percent of lesions were less than 50% classic, 68% of those had evidence of occult CNV. Eighty percent of lesions had a baseline area of less than three standard disc areas (equivalent to the estimated area of the 3.0-mm laser spot on the retina in the average eye). Ninety-four percent of eyes had no evidence of fibrosis. Sixty-five percent of eyes had evidence of hemorrhage. Ninety-eight percent of eyes had evidence of leakage. Ninety-four percent of eyes had evidence of serous sensory retinal detachment.

The majority of the lesions in the trial demonstrated baseline angiographic characteristics consistent with study entry criteria:

1. 86.1% of lesions had some classic component.
2. 80.2% of lesions had area less than 3.0 disc areas (DAs) (approximately equivalent to the estimated area of the 3.0-mm laser spot on the retina in the average eye).
3. 94.0% had no evidence of fibrosis (in 97.9% of eyes, fibrosis was 0 to less than 0.5 DA).
4. 64.8% had some hemorrhage present (in 88.4% of cases, hemorrhage was 0 to less than 0.5 DA).

In addition, 97.7% had evidence of leakage and 93.6% had evidence of serous sensory retinal detachment, indicating active CNV. Nearly one half (49.5%) of the lesions were graded = 50% classic. Of these, 6.2% had evidence of any occult CNV. Of lesions graded less than 50% classic (36.6%), 68.0% had evidence of occult CNV. This descriptive analysis suggests that the majority of eyes met the entry criteria for lesion characteristics in the study, and represents a range of typical CNV lesions.

SUMMARY

These results indicate that SnET2 PDT of subfoveal CNV-AMD is safe and produces initial stabilization or improvement of visual acuity that may have persistent benefit. SnET2 could provide a significant addition to the armamentarium of treatments for CNV in ocular disease.

NOTE

As this volume goes to publication, SnET2 has completed two parallel, pivotal, multicenter, randomized, double-masked, placebo-controlled Phase III clinical trials. A New Drug Application (NDA) filing, followed by peer review publications, is expected in the United States in 2003.

REFERENCES

1. Margherio RR, Margherio AR, DeSantis ME. Laser treatment with verteporfin therapy and its potential impact on retinal practices. *Retina* 2000;20(4):325–330.
2. Thomas EL, Apple DJ, Swartz M, et al. Histopathology and ultrastructure of argon and krypton laser lesions in a human retina-choroid. *Retina* 1984;4:22–29.
3. Macular photocoagulation study group. Laser photocoagulation and subfoveal neovascular lesions of age-related macular degeneration: updated findings from two clinical trials. *Arch Ophthalmol* 1993;111:1200–1209.
4. Thomas EL, Langhofer M. Closure of experimental subretinal neovascular vessels with dihematoporphyrin ether augmented argon green laser photocoagulation. *Photochem Photobiol* 1987; 46:881–886.
5. Wu L, Murphy RP. Photodynamic therapy: a new approach to the treatment of choroidal neovascularization secondary to age-related macular degeneration. *Curr Opin Ophthalmol* 1999;10 (3):217–220.
6. Miller JW, Schmidt-Erfurth U, Sickenberg M, et al. Photodynamic therapy with verteporfin for choroidal neovascularization caused by age-related macular degeneration: results of a single treatment in a Phase 1 and Phase 2 study. *Arch Ophthalmol* 1999; 117:1161–1173.
7. Treatment of Age-Related Macular Degeneration with Photodynamic Therapy (TAP) Study Group. Photodynamic therapy of subfoveal choroidal neovascularization in age-related macular degeneration with verteporfin: one-year results of 2 randomized clinical trials. *Arch Ophthalmol* 1999;117:1329–1345.
8. Personal communication. Miravant Pharmaceuticals, Inc. Santa Barbara, CA.
9. Primbs GB, Casey R, Wamser K, et al. Photodynamic therapy for corneal neovascularization. *Ophthal Surg Lasers* 1998;29(10): 832–838.
10. Peyman GA, Moshfeghi DM, Moshfeghi A, et al. Photodynamic therapy for choriocapillaris using tin ethyl etiopurpurin (SnET2). *Ophthal Surg Lasers* 1997;28(5):409–417.
11. Moshfeghi DM, Peyman GA, Moshfeghi AA, et al. Ocular vascular thrombosis following tin ethyl etiopurpurin (SnET2) photodynamic therapy: time dependencies. *Ophthal Surg Lasers* 1998;29(8):663–668.
12. Baumal CR, Puliafito CA, Pieroth L, et al. Photodynamic therapy (PDT) of experimental choroidal neovascularization with tin ethyl etiopurpurin (SnET2). *Invest Ophthalmol Vis Sci* 1996; 37:S122.
13. Hill RA, Crean DH, Doiron DR, et al. Photodynamic therapy of the ciliary body with tin ethyl etiopurpurin and tin octaethyl benzochlorin in pigmented rabbits. *Ophthal Surg Lasers* 1997;28 (11):948–953.
14. Hill RA, Crean DH, Doiron DR, et al. Photodynamic therapy for antifibrosis in a rabbit model of filtration surgery. *Ophthal Surg Lasers* 1997;28(7):574–581.
15. Personal communication. Miravant Pharmaceuticals, Inc.
16. Thomas EL, Murphy RP, Tressler CS, et al. Photodynamic therapy with tin ethyl etiopurpurin (SnET2) of subfoveal choroidal neovascularization (CNV) in age-related maculopathy: study design and baseline characteristics. [ARVO Abstract] *Invest Ophthal Vis Sci* 2000;41(4):113(2828A).
17. Seddon JM, Willett WC, Speizer FE, et al. A prospective study of cigarette smoking and age-related macular degeneration in women. *JAMA* 1996;276(14):1141–1146.
18. Thomas EL, Li XY, Paciotti NM. Fluorescein angiographic characteristics of subfoveal choroidal neovascularization secondary to age-related maculopathy (CNV-AMD) in a pivotal phase III trial for SnET2-PDT. [ARVO Abstract] *Invest Ophthal Vis Sci* 2001;42(4):437(2352).

20

PHOTODYNAMIC THERAPY WITH LU-TEX: EARLY RESULTS

MARK S. BLUMENKRANZ
KATHRYN WOODBURN
JOAN W. MILLER
JASON S. SLAKTER

Monotexaphyrin lutetium (Optrin, Pharmacyclics, Inc., Sunnyvale, CA) is a member of a class of compounds called texaphyrins, which are water-soluble pentadentate metallo photosensitizers that have been shown to be of potential utility in the photodynamic therapy (PDT) of certain malignancies as well as atheromatous plaque (1,2). Monotexaphyrin lutetium has a molecular weight of 1,165.4 g/mol and broad absorption peaks at 474 and 732 nm with a characteristic fluorescence emission band centered at 750 nm (Fig. 20.1) (2). Based on these properties, as well as the demonstration of efficacy of another photodynamic agent, verteporfin studies—in both animal models (3) and Phase I, II, and III studies (4,5)—were undertaken in rabbits and primates to determine whether monotexaphyrin lutetium also might have utility in the treatment of choroidal neovascularization (CNV) in humans. These studies confirmed that the dye was able to be imaged within experimental CNV in rabbits and monkeys, and also was capable (in doses ranging from 2.0 to 4.0 mg/kg, and fluences of 50 to 150 J/cm^2) of producing photodynamic closure in a dose-dependent fashion (6–8).

Based on these preclinical studies, two Phase I/II studies were undertaken in conjunction with Pharmacyclics (Sunnyvale, CA) and Alcon Laboratories (Fort Worth, TX), at centers in Lausanne, Switzerland; Stanford, CA; New York City; and Boston, MA, to evaluate Lu-Tex.

SUBJECTS AND METHODS

In a preliminary study, using a final formulation of 2 mg/mL, with patients receiving between 0.5 and 4.0 mg/kg of drug by intravenous (iv) infusion and light fluences ranging from 50 to 150 J/cm^2, efficacy was established with evidence of dose-dependency both for drug and light. Doses of 3 mg/kg or greater and fluences of 100 J/cm^2 or greater were most effective, although they were associated with paresthesias in a significant proportion of patients (Alcon Laboratories and Michel Sickenberg, 1999, personal communication).

A prospective multicenter dose and light escalation trial was performed in the United States at three clinical centers using a 6-mg/mL formulation (Manhattan Eye and Ear Infirmary, Massachusetts Eye and Ear Infirmary, and Stanford University) on the basis of these preliminary data.

INCLUSION CRITERIA

1. Subfoveal CNV of any etiology in which the greatest linear dimension of the lesion measured less than 5,000 µm, and in which at least 50% of the lesion constituted either classic or occult neovascularization or some combination of both was required for entry. Visual acuity in the study eye was required to be logMar 0.3 (20/40) or worse, and visual acuity in the nonstudy eye logMar 1.7 (20/800) or better.
2. Hematologic, renal, and liver functions were required to be within normal limits.
3. Patients were required to be willing to use sun protection for proscribed study visits, including appropriate clothing and sunglasses for 14 days after treatment and return.

EXCLUSION CRITERIA

Any medical condition that precludes scheduled study visits for completion of the study, history of allergy or sensitivity to texaphyrin or porphyrin compounds, porphyria, allergy to fluorescein or indocyanine green (ICG) dye, uncontrolled

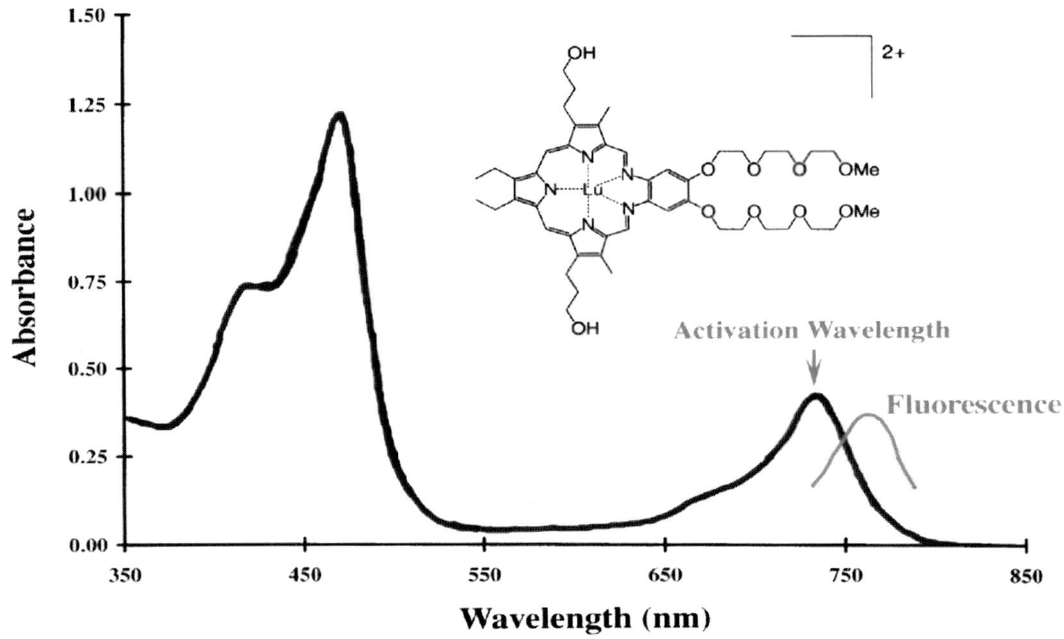

FIGURE 20.1. Structural formula and absorption and emission profile of monotexaphyrin lutetium.

hypertension, history of hepatitis, and use of anticoagulants were considered exclusion criteria. Ocular exclusion criteria included any ophthalmic disease that could worsen in the subsequent 24 months of follow up, preexisting retinal abnormalities that would compromise patient safety, intraocular surgery within 1 month prior to screening, a prior history of submacular surgery, pattern dystrophy, or retinal pigment epithelial tear. Patients eligible for conventional thermal laser treatment on the basis of Macular Photocoagulation Study guidelines, or subsequently, with verteporfin following approval, were required to sign a waiver stating that they were aware of the potential benefits of those therapies and willing to be enrolled in the current trial with that knowledge.

EVALUATION CRITERIA AND PROTOCOL

Patients meeting eligibility criteria underwent standardized pretreatment ICG and fluorescein angiography (FA), in addition to standardized visual acuity measurement with conversion to logMar acuity using a lighthouse Early Treatment Diabetic Retinopathy Study (ETDRS) 1 and 2 chart at 4 meters by a certified visual acuity examiner masked as to their treatment allocation at screening visit, day 7, and at least month 1. Fundus photography and FA were taken at the time of screening, and at days 7 and 30 with pharmacokinetic samples obtained on the day of treatment, day 1, and day 7.

Following determinations of the patient's weight, dosages ranging between 2 and 2.5 mg/kg were delivered via a 19-gauge needle attached to an iv line connected by iv tubing to a three-way stop clock preflushed with 5 to 10 cc of D_5W. The drug was prepared in a sterile fashion at a concentration of 6 mg/mL, withdrawn through a 0.45-µm filter, and administered as an iv infusion bolus with a constant infusion rate of approximately 1 L/h. Patients were monitored for at least 2 hours postinfusion and questioned with regard to the occurrence of any subjective adverse events, including ocular or back pain, pruritus, paresthesias, headache, or other ocular disturbance. Between 15 and 20 minutes following initiation of the iv injection of monotexaphyrin lutetium, patients underwent treatment with a monochromatic 732-nm diode laser coupled to a specialized slit-lamp delivery system optimized for activation of monotexaphyrin lutetium by Zeiss Instruments (Xena, Germany). The spot size varied from 1 to 6 mm in diameter, with a constant irradiance of 600 mW/cm^2 and a fluence ranging from 50 to 125 J/cm^2 dependent on the treatment allocation of the patient and calculated on the basis of the exposure time. Spot size was determined to be 1,000 µm larger than the greatest linear dimension of the lesion as measured by digital angiography in a manner comparable to that employed in the treatment of age-related macular degeneration with photodynamic therapy (TAP) and verteporfin in photodynamic therapy (VIP) trials (10). The treatment was immediately terminated in any patient experiencing an untoward effect, including evidence of allergy, severe ocular pain, or headache.

Determination of eligibility based on ocular systemic criteria as well as the angiographic evaluation were determined at each center by the principal investigator. The data were reviewed subsequently by the Digital Angiography Reading Center (DARC) at Manhattan Eye and Ear Infirmary. In selected patients, angiographic images with filters modified for Lu-Tex excitation and detection were taken on a specially modified Topcon 50 IA camera with Imagenet version 1.53 capture software and Windows 95 format. All images were transmitted to the centralized digital angiography reading center by telemetric methods in an unenhanced fashion in addition to standard transmittal of stereoscopic nondigital color fundus photographs of the disc and macula. The presence and extent of classic and occult CNV was assessed in disc areas and not used for purposes of allocating treatment group, but was reviewed in posttreatment stratification analysis.

Patients were subsequently evaluated when possible. Patients who subsequently demonstrated eligibility for verteporfin therapy following the initial 3-month follow-up period were permitted to receive verteporfin therapy subsequent to approval by the United States Food and Drug Administration (FDA) if they chose to do so. Treatment was carried out under the auspices of a clinical protocol submitted and approved by the FDA. In addition, the Institutional Review Board (IRB) was required to give approval at each participating center. Each patient enrolled in the study was offered and signed an informed consent in accordance with the recommendations guiding physicians and biomedical research involving human subjects adopted by the 18th World Medical Assembly (Helsinki, Finland, June, 1964, amended October, 1996).

RESULTS

Patient Demographics

A total of 54 patients, 26 men, ranging in age from 19 to 86 (mean age 66.9), and 28 women, ranging in age from 29 to 92 (mean age 66.3) were enrolled between September, 1999 and April 1, 2000. Forty-three patients had classic, occult, or mixed subfoveal CNV, arising from ARMD, and 11 patients had subfoveal neovascularization arising from other causes, including five with presumed ocular histoplasmosis/multifocal choroiditis, three with angioid streaks, two with pathologic myopia, and one with an old toxoplasmosis scar complicated by neovascularization. Patients underwent iv injection with 6 mg/L in volumes ranging from 16.2 to 36 mL (average 25 mL), corresponding to dosage range of 2.0 to 2.5 mg/kg. On average, light application was made 20 minutes following the initiation of iv injection, ranging from 15 to 29 minutes in 48 patients, with six patients having a light application between 30 and 45 minutes following administration of dye because of technical reasons.

TABLE 20.1. DISTRIBUTION OF DRUG DOSE AND LIGHT FLUENCE

Drug Dose (mg/kg)	Light Dose (J/cm^2)	Number of Patients
2.0	50	2
	65	18
	95	10
	125	17
2.5	125	7
	n = 54	

A total of 47 patients were treated with 2.0 mg/kg, of which two received 50 J/cm^2 of light, 18 received 65 J/cm^2, 10 received 95 J/cm^2, and 17 received 125 J/cm^2. The remaining seven patients received the combination of 2.5 mg/kg of drug, and 125 J/cm^2 of light (Table 20.1).

Angiographic evaluation of choroidal new vessel membrane closure and standardized visual acuity testing were undertaken at 1 week and 1 month following PDT (Tables 20.2, 20.3, 20.4, and 20.5).

One week following treatment, approximately one half of choroidal neovascular membranes treated with 50, 65, 95, or 125 J/cm^2 appeared totally or partially closed. Stratification analysis revealed 11 of 18 membranes fully or partially closed at 65 J/cm^2; six of 10 at 95 J/cm^2; and 18 of 24, respectively, with 125 J/cm^2. Partial or full closure was not achieved in either of two eyes treated with 50 J/cm^2. Therefore, overall, for the 54 patients treated, 35 (64.8%) were fully or partially closed at 1 week (Table 20.2).

This translated in visual terms to 53 of 54 (98%) patients losing fewer than three lines of vision at 1 week. Visual acuity was actually improved by two lines or greater in five patients. These data are summarized in Table 20.3.

TABLE 20.2. CHOROIDAL NEOVASCULARIZATION CLOSURE AT 1 WEEK

	J/cm^2			
Closure	50 (n = 2)	65 (n = 18)	95 (n = 10)	125 (n = 24)
None	2 (100%)	7 (38.9%)	4 (40%)	6 (25%)
Full or partial	0 (0%)	11 (61.1%)	6 (60%)	18 (75%)
				n = 54

TABLE 20.3. VISUAL ACUITY AT 1 WEEK

	J/cm²			
Visual Acuity Change	**50 (*n* = 2)**	**65 (*n* = 18)**	**95 (*n* = 10)**	**125 (*n* = 24)**
≥3 Line loss	0 (0%)	0 (0%)	0 (0%)	1 (4.2%)
<3 Line loss	2 (100%)	18 (100%)	10 (100%)	23 (95.8%)
				n = 54

By 1 month, of the eyes available for evaluation, 15 were from the 65 J/cm² group, 17 from the 125 J/cm² group, totaling 32 with gradable angiograms. Complete closure was only seen in 3% of these patients, including one of 15 treated with 65 J, and none of 17 patients treated with 125 J/cm². However, partial closure was still present in 40.6%, including six of 15 (40%) treated with 65 J/cm², and seven of 17 (41.1%) of those treated with 125 J/cm². Approximately 40.6% of all patients treated with 65 or 125 J and 2 or 2.5 mg/kg were closed at 1 month, constituting approximately a 13% absolute decline in the number of membranes either partially or totally closed at 1 week by 1 month.

Three of 39 (7.7%) had three lines or greater of vision loss, and the remainder 36 (92.3%), retained visual acuity within three lines of initial baseline. In this instance, the total number of patients studied at 1 month had a different denominator for vision testing and closure because seven more patients were available for visual acuity testing than angiography interpretation owing to technical factors (Tables 20.4 and 20.5).

Adverse events were commonly encountered, although mild and self-limited (Table 20.6). These included 16 of 47 (34%) of the 2 mg/kg patients developing paresthesias involving the fingers or lips, and six of seven patients (85.7%) receiving 2.5 mg. Although there appeared to be frequent yellowing and some nonselective damage to the normal choriocapillaris, including mild serous fluid exudation on the first posttreatment day, by 1 week following therapy, only one patient treated with 2 mg/kg of 65 J/cm² (5.5%) demonstrated a serous retinal detachment. Another patient developed a similar complication when receiving 2.0 mg/kg with 125 J/cm². Periocular aching was encountered in six of 24 (25%) patients receiving 125 J/cm², but only in two of 30 (6.6%) patients receiving lower doses of 50 to 95 J/cm². No patients developed cutaneous phototoxicity or retinal vascular closure. No patients developed severe or disabling chest or back pain, which has been described previously with verteporfin therapy (5). However, review of the angiograms by the central reading center suggested that 24 of 43 (56%) demonstrated some evidence of transient choroidal leakage during some period following the treatment, and 10 of 43 (23%) some degree of late choroidal pigmentation as a presumed sequela of this.

DISCUSSION

This drug and light dose escalation study employing 2 to 2.5 mg/kg of monotexaphyrin lutetium, and 50 to 125 J/cm² 732-nm monochromatic laser light optimized for Lu-Tex activation demonstrated that monotexaphyrin

TABLE 20.4. CHOROIDAL NEOVASCULARIZATION CLOSURE AT 1 MONTH

	J/cm²	
Closure	**65 (*n* = 15)**	**125 (*n* = 17)**
None (59.4%)	9 (60%)	10 (58.9%)
Full or partial (40.6%)	6 (40%)	7 (41.1%)
n = 32 Available for angiographic interpretation		

TABLE 20.5. VISUAL ACUITY AT 1 MONTH

	J/cm²	
Visual Acuity Change	**65 (*n* = 15)**	**125 (*n* = 24)**
≥3 Line loss (7.7%)	0 (0%)	3 (12.5%)
<3 Line loss (92.3%)	15 (100%)	21 (87.5%)
n = 39 Available patients		

TABLE 20.6. ADVERSE EVENTS

Adverse Event	Frequency
Paresthesias	2.0 mg: 16/47 (34%) 2.5 mg: 6/7 (85.7%)
Transient retinal damage at 1 week or greater	2.0 mg/65 J/cm² Serous detachment (n = 1) (5.5%) 2.0 mg/125 J/cm² Serous detachment (n = 1) (4.2%)
Eye discomfort	125 J/cm²: 6/24 (25%) 50, 65, 95 J/cm²; 2/30 (6.6%)
No cases of cutaneous phytotoxicity or retinal vessel closure	

lutetium is capable of closing subfoveal CNV under certain conditions. Because this was a Phase I/II dose ranging study without a control or placebo group, no comment can be made with regard to the efficacy of this form of treatment, either on the basis of visual acuity or angiographic choroidal neovascular membrane closure over the long term. However, it does appear that the drug in dosages of 2.0 mg or greater and 65 J/cm^2 or greater is capable of selectively closing CNV, although generally to a partial rather than complete degree. In this study, no attempt was made to limit patients only to those with greater than 50% classic CNV because of the uncertainty of assumptions regarding the mechanism of action of drug, as well as the demonstration of another effective form of therapy in this selected group of patients during the course of the performance of this study. However, it can be inferred by the relatively high incidence of mild presumed drug-related adverse events (paresthesias in 34% to 86% of the patients treated with 2 or 2.5 mg/kg) that the safety profile of the drug is not as favorable as that of verteporfin, which is not associated with paresthesias to a significant degree, but may result in lower back pain in up to approximately 2.5% of patients and 3.5% photosensitivity reactions. Neither of those two problems was seen in these Lu-Tex patients. No attempt was made in this study to stratify patients prospectively between those with greater than and less than 50% classic CNV. The principal end point in this study was visual acuity and not angiographic closure of choroidal new vessels at 1 week and 1 month. Therefore, no precise comparison can be made with the TAP and VIP trials, which evaluated visual acuity and angiographic closure at 12 and 24 months, including a provision for retreatment to occur at 3-month intervals provided that angiographic leakage occurred during interval visits (3,6).

In the Phase I/II study of verteporfin by Miller and coworkers, Regimens 2 and 4, which were found to be most favorable, included a dosage of verteporfin of 6 mg/m^2, and duration of infusion of 10 minutes followed by light fluences of 50 to 100 J/cm^2 (5). Light fluences higher than this caused some nonselective damage to the pigment epithelium and choriocapillaris in some patients. In that study at 1 week following therapy, 68% to 78% of patients in Regimens 2 and 4 (corresponding roughly to those subsequently selected for Phase III study) achieved stabilization of visual acuity at 1 week. Greater than three lines of visual loss occurred in approximately 5% to 9% of patients at 1 week analogous to this study in which approximately 2% of patients also lost greater than three lines of vision at 1 week. Angiographic closure rates for patients 1 and 4 weeks following treatment Regimens 2 and 4 with verteporfin appeared somewhat higher than with monotexaphyrin lutetium. There was an absence of all fluorescein leakage from classic CNV 1 week following treatment in 2% to 100% of patients, depending on the regimen used. Leakage typically reappeared after 1 month in most patients. There did not appear to be a dose–response relationship in the ability to stop fluorescein leakage from classic CNV in Regimen 4, in which absence of leakage was seen in 100% of 21 patients following verteporfin therapy. Conversely, in the current study, higher light fluences appeared to be more effective in closure than lower fluences, although closure rates generally were lower.

In the current study, an attempt was made subsequent to initial enrollment to classify angiographic closure by the reading center in 31 of the 54 patients enrolled who were felt to have some component of classic subfoveal CNV. Two of thirty-one were judged to have complete closure, and five of 31 had greater than 50% closure of the classic component. This contrasts with 11 of 31, who demonstrated less than 50% closure at 1 week, and eight of 31 possible progression and/or nonspecific damage simulating progression.

In some patients, clear-cut photodynamic closure of normal choriocapillaris was obtained at the same time as incomplete closure of components of classic neovascularization within the lesion complex (Fig. 20.2). Figure 20.2 A and B demonstrates the early and late fluorescein frames of a patient with a large predominantly classic choroidal neovascular membrane prior to photodynamic therapy with Lu-Tex. Figure 20.2 C and D demonstrates the early and late frames of the same patient one week following photodynamic therapy with Lu-Tex. Note the circular area of hypofluorescence surrounding the lesion (Fig. 20.2 C), confirming the presence of photodynamic closure of normal choriocapillaris. Additionally, there appears to be reduction in the amount of initial fluorescence from the choroidal neovascularization itself in the early frame, although there is still a considerable degree of late leakage corresponding to the center of the hypofluorescent circle (Fig. 20.2 D), indi-

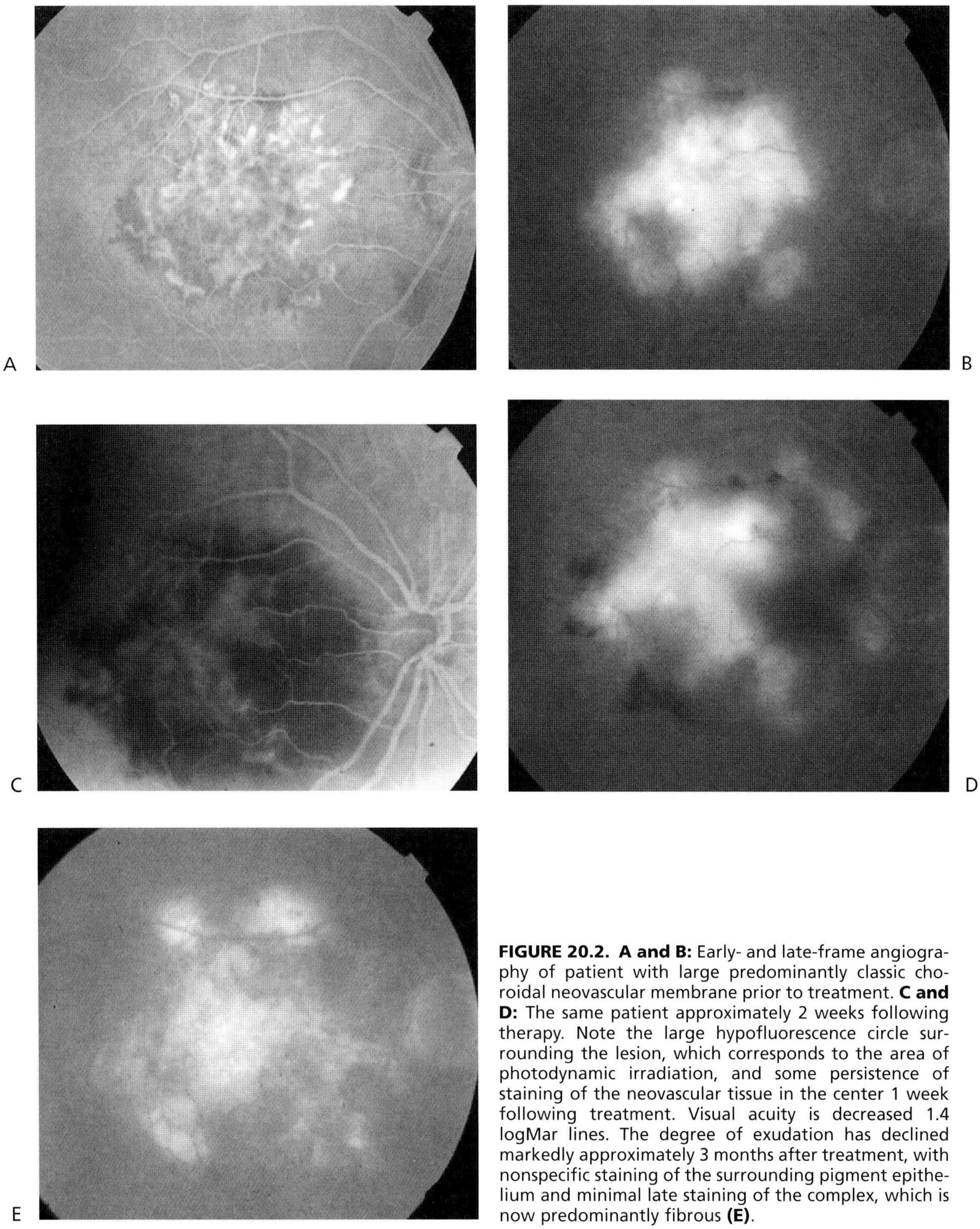

FIGURE 20.2. A and B: Early- and late-frame angiography of patient with large predominantly classic choroidal neovascular membrane prior to treatment. **C and D:** The same patient approximately 2 weeks following therapy. Note the large hypofluorescence circle surrounding the lesion, which corresponds to the area of photodynamic irradiation, and some persistence of staining of the neovascular tissue in the center 1 week following treatment. Visual acuity is decreased 1.4 logMar lines. The degree of exudation has declined markedly approximately 3 months after treatment, with nonspecific staining of the surrounding pigment epithelium and minimal late staining of the complex, which is now predominantly fibrous **(E)**.

cating some degree of non-selectivity in the presence of an obvious therapuetic effect. Three months later visual acuity remained at its pretreatment level of logMar 0.56, corresponding to roughly 20/70 despite the presence of obvious circular pigmentary disturbance, late staining consistent with the combination of mild RPE/choriocapillaris injury, and central fibrous scar in this 72 year-old woman (Fig. 20.2E). This suggests that the selectivity of the drug was less than that for verteporfin, at least in the dosage and fluence levels included in this study when light application occurred 15 to 20 minutes following administration. It is possible that selectivity for this drug might differ with a different dosage, fluence, or timing regimen. However, in prior primate studies, treatment parameters suggest a relative degree of comparability between human and primate new vessel closure similar to that seen in primate and human studies for verteporfin (4,7,8).

In selected patients, imaging with specialized filters optimized for excitation and capture of emitted fluorescence from monotexaphyrin lutetium was performed immediately following drug administration, and prior to photodynamic activation (6–8). In Figure 20.3, the fluorescence pattern of a patient with classic CNV is compared in Figure 20.3A following fluorescein injection with that seen following administration of Lu-Tex in Figure 20.3B, but prior to PDT with Lu-Tex. Figure 20.4 A and B demonstrates a predominantly classic choroidal neovascular membrane surrounded by a rim of hemorrhage in a 56-year-old woman with multifocal choroiditis. There appears to be mild RPE decompensation secondary to chronic serous exudation surrounding the lesion. Two weeks following treatment there appears to be closure of the classic component of the CNV centrally, but a large surrounding zone of hypoperfusion of the choriocapillaris in the early frames of the angiogram associated with progressive late staining consistent with photodynamic injury to the choriocapillaris and secondary exudative response (Fig. 20.4 C and D). One month later, the central choroidal neovascular membrane still appears to be hypoperfused, although there is mottling of the surrounding retinal pigment epithelium with less exudation but more staining of damaged pigment epithelium and choriocapillaris. The visual acuity has improved from log Mar 1.16 to 0.82 (approximately 20/125) by 1 week (Fig. 20.4 E and F).

The development of a mottled circular lesion associated with RPE disturbance and late staining was not universally associated with a decline in visual acuity. Such a lesion, which resembles the moderately atrophic scar following transpupillary thermal therapy (TTT) in some respects, was associated with reduction in degree of late staining and visual improvement in some instances (10).

In one instance, a 48-year-old man presenting with with a predominantly classic recurrence of choroidal neovascularization (Fig. 20.5A) and initial visual acuity of logMar .56

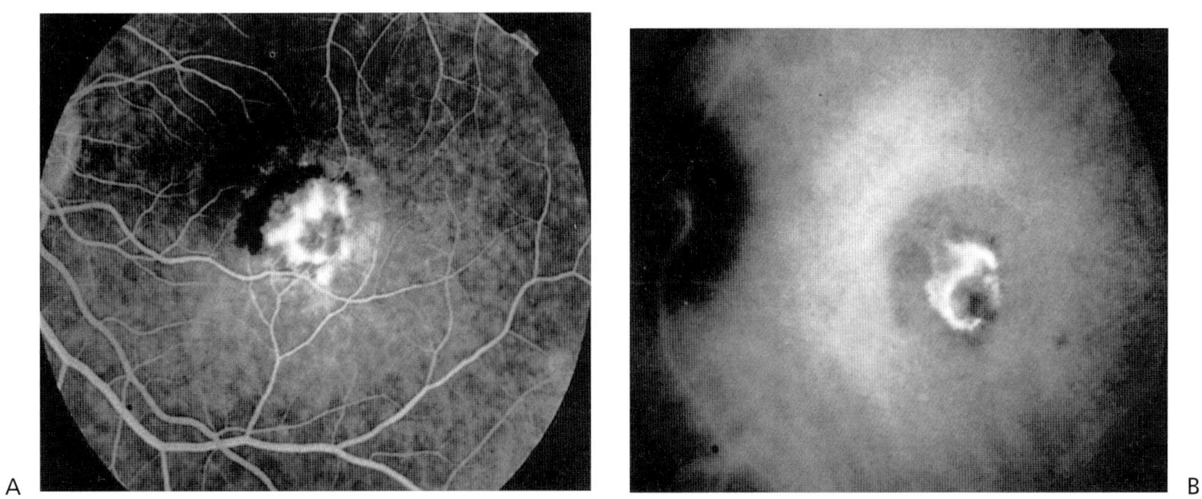

FIGURE 20.3. A: A 29-year-old woman with subfoveal choroidal neovascular membrane secondary to histoplasmosis demonstrates a typical pattern of leakage with surrounding blockage because of hemorrhage on the superonasal edge of the lesion. **B:** The same patient seen in late frames of Lu-Tex angiography in which the blockage from blood associated with FA is ameliorated by imaging at 750 nm. Note the biolocalization of Lu-Tex, which fluoresces to a greater degree within the lesion than in the surrounding normal choroid, as well as the subtle surrounding hypofluorescent zone corresponding to abnormal choriocapillaris and pigment epithelium. The Lu-Tex angiogram appears to more accurately predict the margins of the lesion relevant to the application of the photodynamic irradiation than the fluorescein angiogram and emphasizes the potential utility of photodynamic angiography as an aid in treatment planning.

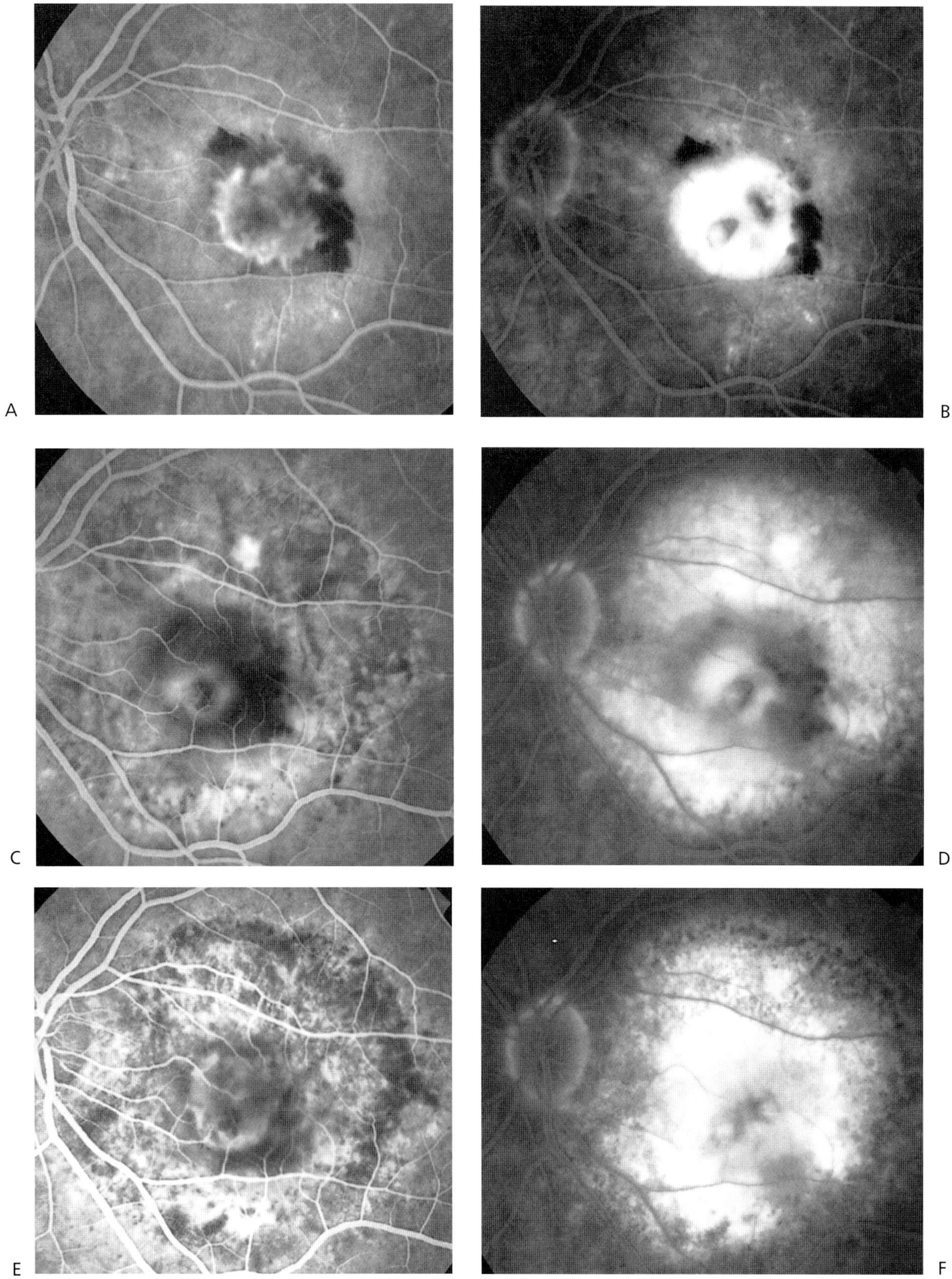
A
B
C
D
E
F

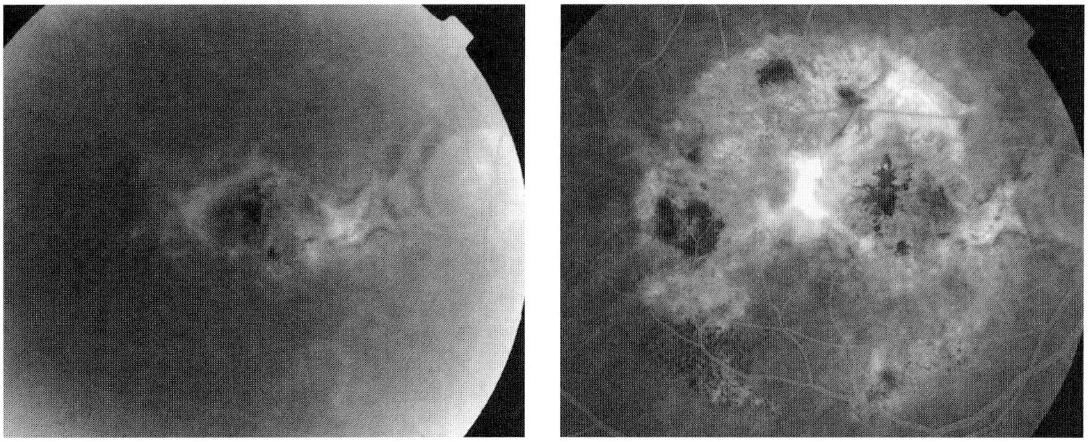

A B

FIGURE 20.5. A: A 48-year-old patient with subfoveal CNV extending from peripapillary net. **B:** Following treatment with Lu-Tex, there is similar nonspecific late staining of the circular zone of the retinal pigment epithelium and choriocapillaris corresponding to the circle of photodynamic irradiation. Visual acuity is in excess of 20/50 and stable despite the presence of retinal pigment epithelium mottling transmission fluorescence and late staining of fibrous tissue.

(approximately 20/70) underwent Lu-Tex PDT for subfoveal CNV associated extension from a juxtapapillary neovascular membrane. Despite the fact that the patient developed a large circular mottled pigment epithelial scar with late staining as well as persistence of some fibrous tissue, which stained in the late frames of the angiogram (Fig. 20.5B), visual acuity actually improved to the level of 20/40 after 1 year of follow up. This indicates that alterations induced in the surrounding pigment epithelium as well as changes in the permeability of choroidal neovascular tissue in response to PDT may play a role in the final visual acuity independent of the development and/or persistence of fibrous or fibrovascular tissue in subretinal and subpigment epithelial space (Figs. 20.5 A and B).

SUMMARY

Monotexaphyrin lutetium (Optrin), a novel synthetic water-soluble photosensitizing agent, is capable of producing photodynamic closure of subfoveal CNV in humans. Preliminary studies using a formulation with a lower concentration of drug (2 mg/mL) suggest that doses of 3 mg/kg or greater and light levels of 100 J/cm^2 or greater are most effective, although they are associated with potential undesirable side effects including paresthesias and ocular pain. Subsequent studies using a different formulation in the United States of 6 mg/mL suggest that dosages higher than 2.0 mg/mL are also capable of producing photodynamic closure of subfoveal CNV, although closure often is partial. Approximately 60% to 70% of patients achieve partial or full closure of a combination of classic and occult neovascularization, but only approximately 15% of patients achieve complete closure at dosages of 2.0 mg/kg and fluences of 95 to 125 J/cm^2. It remains uncertain whether or not better closure rates could be achieved by a different formulation of drug or a different combination of timing of light administration. Employing the parameters specified in the current trial, there appears to be some degree of nonspecific damage to surrounding normal choroid and pigment epithelium 1 week following therapy in up to 56% of patients, associated with later pigmentary changes in up to 23%, although this is not necessarily correlated with reduced visual function. Compared with verteporfin, and

←

FIGURE 20.4. A and B: A 56-year-old woman with predominantly classic CNV and surrounding subretinal hemorrhage associated with multifocal choroiditis demonstrates a typical pattern of early and late leakage on initial pretreatment of fluorescein angiogram. **C and D:** Approximately 10 days following treatment with a relatively large spot, the classic component of the choroidal neovascular membrane is mostly closed, although there is extensive staining associated with photodynamic injury to the surrounding pigment epithelium and choriocapillaris. There may be an early retinal choroidal anastomosis forming at the center of the classic component of the CNV associated with some late staining in that region. **E and F:** One month later, much of the exudative subretinal fluid is dried up and the central scar remains relatively hypofluorescent, although there is remodeling in the surrounding pigment epithelium and choriocapillaris. Visual acuity after initially improving 1 week following treatment has declined from logMar 1.16 to 1.46 1 month following treatment.

taking into account differences in trial design and other factors, Lu-Tex appears to be less effective in closing classic CNV than verteporfin and more likely to be associated with adverse events, including paresthesias and nonspecific damage to surrounding normal pigment epithelium, although it has potential advantages with regard to its suitability as an agent for photodynamic angiography.

REFERENCES

1. Young S, Woodburn K, Wright M, et al. Lutetium texaphyrin (PCI–0123): a near-infrared water-soluble photosensitizer. *Photochem Photobiol* 1996;63:896–897.
2. Sessler JL, Hemmi G, Mody TD, et al. Texaphyrins: synthesis and applications. *Chem Res* 1994;27:43–50.
3. Miller J, Walsh A, Kramer M, et al. Photodynamic therapy of experimental choroidal neovascularization using lipoprotein-delivered benzoporphyrin. *Arch Ophthalmol* 1995;113:810–818.
4. Miller J, Schmidt-Erfurth U, Sickenberg M, et al. Photodynamic therapy with verteporfin for choroidal neovascularization caused by age-related macular degeneration results of a single treatment in a phase 1 and 2 study. *Arch Ophthalmol* 1999;117:1161–1173.
5. Photodynamic therapy of subfoveal choroidal neovascularization in age-related macular degeneration with verteporfin. One-year results of two randomized clinical trials. *Arch Ophthalmol* 1999;117:1329–1345.
6. Blumenkranz M, Woodburn K, Qing F, et al. Lutetium texaphyrin (Lutex): A potential new agent for ocular fundus angiography and photodynamic therapy. *Am J Ophthalmol* 2000;129: 353–362.
7. Graham K, Arbour J, Connolly E, et al. Digital angiography using lutetium texaphyrin in a monkey model of choroidal neovascularization. *Invest Ophthalmol Vis Sci* 1999(Suppl);40:S402.
8. Arbour J, Connolly E, Graham K, et al. Photodynamic therapy of experimental choroidal neovascularization in a monkey model using iv infusion of lutetium texaphyrin. *Invest Ophthalmol Vis Sci* 1999;40:S401.
9. Photodynamic therapy of subfoveal choroidal neovascularization in pathologic myopia with verteporfin. One year results of a randomized clinical trial. *Ophthalmology* 2001;108:841–852.
10. Reichel E, Berrocal A, Ip M, et al. Transpupillary thermotherapy of occult subfoveal choroidal neovascularization in patients with age-related macular degeneration. *Ophthalmology* 1999;106: 1908–1914.

21

ANGIOGRAPHY WITH VERTEPORFIN

DEEBA HUSAIN
MICHAL KRAMER
EVANGELOS S. GRAGOUDAS
JOAN W. MILLER

The human retinal and choroidal vessels are currently imaged with fluorescein angiography (FA) and indocyanine green (ICG) angiography. Fluorescein angiography provides a good visualization of retinal vessels, but the choroidal vasculature is not well seen. Indocyanine green angiography provides better visualization of the large choroidal vessels. Both of these techniques image small vessels rather poorly.

Verteporfin or liposomal benzoporphyrin derivative (BPD) has an absorption/excitation spectrum between 350 and 690 nm (with absorption maximum at 354, 418, 574, 626, and 688 nm). This enables visualization of smaller choroidal vessels. Verteporfin selectively accumulates in CNV; therefore, it can image and localize new vessels better than the currently available angiography modalities.

Angiography using photosensitizers provides timing information, indicating the timing of localization of the dye to CNV and its clearance from retinal vessels. Angiography of normal iris vessels and rubeosis iridis also can be performed with verteporfin.

Sodium fluorescein and indocyanine green are the two dyes used to image the fundus in a clinical setting. Sodium fluorescein has peak excitation at 465 to 590 nm and peak emission at 420 to 430 nm, and provides good visualization of the retinal vasculature (1). The pigment in the retinal pigment epithelium and choroid blocks vascular fluorescence and does not allow visualization of choroidal vessels (1). Fluorescein also leaks from fenestrated vessels such as choriocapillaris and provides background fluorescence; however, it obscures the view of the deeper choroidal vessels. Classic CNV are visualized with fluorescein during imaging; however, the borders of the membrane are not well delineated in the later frames because of dye leakage (Fig. 21.1). Additionally, the presence of blood or fibrous tissue obscures the view of the lesion during FA.

Indocyanine green has an absorption and emission spectrum in the range of 800 nm, and these longer and near infrared wavelengths enable deeper tissue penetration, and visualization of deeper choroidal vessels (Fig. 21.2) (2,3). The smaller choroidal vessels and classic CNV are poorly visualized by this technique. An ICG scanning laser ophthalmoscope (SLO) can image some neovascular membranes that are occult or ill defined as well as smaller choroidal vessels.

Conversely, use of both FA and ICG does not provide adequate information about the smaller choroidal vessels and CNV that are ill defined and occult. Alternative dyes might provide improved visualization. Verteporfin is a liposomal preparation of benzoporphyrin derivative. It is a synthetic chlorinlike porphyrin, which is a lipophilic photosensitizer with a molecular weight of 718.81. It has absorption/excitation spectrum (Fig. 21.3) between 350 and 690 nm (with absorption maximum at 354, 418, 574, 626, and 628 nm) (4,5). Fluorescence emission of verteporfin for excitation below 650 nm occurs in a narrow band, with a maximum at 690 nm (5). Therefore, imaging with this dye allows visualization of smaller choroidal vessels.

Verteporfin is a liposomal preparation of benzoporphyrin derivative. When in circulation in the blood it partitions rapidly into the lipoprotein fraction of plasma. Ninety percent of verteporfin is recovered within the lipoprotein fraction in 1 hour. Thirty-five percent of the dye is bound to low-density lipoproteins (LDL) (6). It has been shown that tumors accumulate LDL-associated photosensitizer (7). Neovascular tissues may have increased LDL receptors in the proliferating endothelium and increased LDL transport across the endothelium of permeable vessels (8,9). This may be one explanation for the accumulation of lipoprotein-associated photosensitizer in CNV (10).

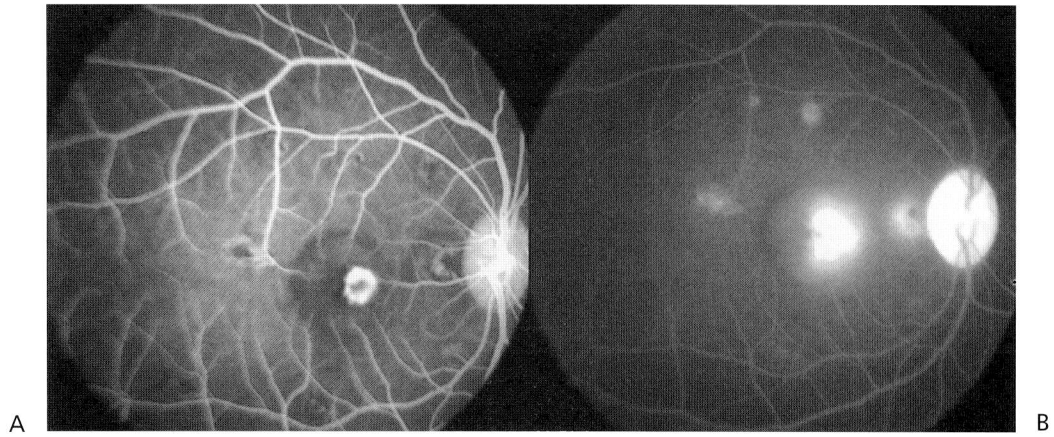

FIGURE 21.1. A: Early phase fluorescein angiogram of the CNV model showing hyperfluorescence in the area of experimental CNV. B: Late-phase fluorescein angiogram of the CNV model showing leakage in the area of experimental CNV.

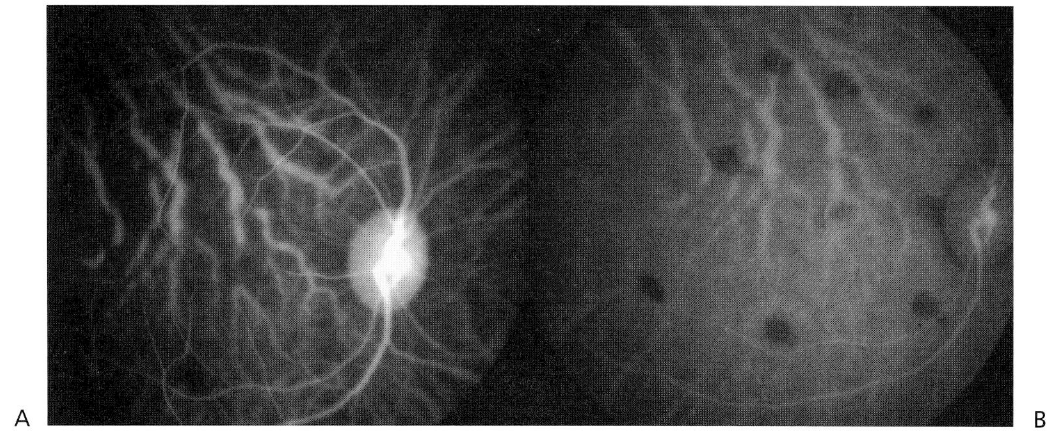

FIGURE 21.2. A: Early-phase (9-second) indocyanine green (ICG) angiography of the monkey eye, showing dye in the small and large choroidal vessels and retinal vessels. No significant fluorescence is seen in the area of CNV. B: Late-phase (37-minute) ICG angiography of the monkey eye, showing some persistent dye in the large choroidal and retinal vessels and a faint hyperfluorescent rim in the area of the experimental CNV.

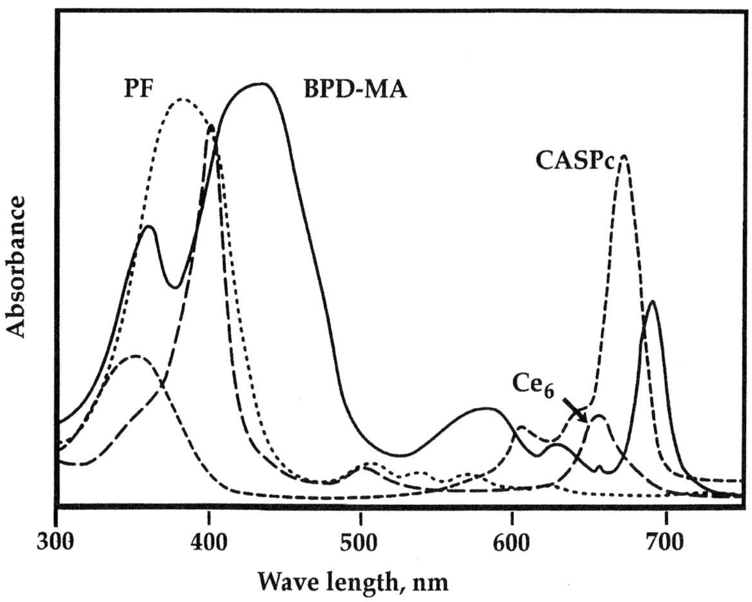

FIGURE 21.3. Absorption spectra of selected photosensitizers that have been used in photodynamic therapy. BPD-MA, benzoporphyrin derivative monoacid; CASPc, chloroaluminum sulfonated phthalocyanine; Ce6, chlorine 6; PF, photofrin. (From: Lui H, Anderson RR. Photodynamic therapy in dermatology: recent developments. *Dermatol Clin* 1993;11:1–13, with permission.)

IMAGING TECHNIQUE

Angiography with verteporfin was performed at our laboratory on experimental choroidal CNV, and normal retina and choroid in the cynomolgus monkey. Choroidal neovascularization was created using the argon laser injury model (11) and imaging was performed 4 weeks after induction of CNV. Verteporfin was injected intravenously over 30 seconds in doses of 0.5, 1, and 2 mg/kg.

The filters used for verteporfin angiography were based on *in vivo* confirmation by spectrofluorometry of the published excitation and emission spectra (12). The spectral band centered at 580 nm was used for excitation (half width: 60 nm), and fluorescence was detected through a barrier filter centered at 695 nm (half width: 50 nm). Following intravenous (iv) injection of verteporfin, angiography was performed using a Topcon Ophthalmic Imaging Systems (Paramus, NJ) 50-VT fundus camera fitted with the excitation and barrier filters. The digital images were captured with a Kodak Megaplus Digital camera (Kodak, Rochester, NY), and then stored by the Topcon Ophthalmic Imaging System Digital Angiography System. A 50-degree field centered on the posterior pole was used. Images were taken at 1-second intervals for the first minute after dye injection, followed by 5 minute-, 15 minute-, and 30-minute intervals for 2 hours.

Iris angiography (13) was performed with 2 mg/kg of verteporfin, injected intravenously over 30 seconds in the cynomolgus monkey. Photographs were taken with a TRC 50 IA fundus camera (Topcon) mounted with an adapter containing an achromatic lens with a focal length of 25.4 m (Newport PACO 22) (14). Photographs were taken every 2 to 3 seconds for the first 30 seconds; then at 45 seconds; then at 1, 2, 3, 5, 7, 10, 15, 30, 45, and 60 minutes.

IMAGING WITH VERTEPORFIN

Normal Retina and Choroid

Verteporfin angiography resulted in sharp images of retinal and choroidal vessels. Transit phase was 9 to 15 seconds after iv injection of the dye. The arterial phase in the retinal vessels was seen at 9 seconds, followed by venous laminar flow around 10 seconds. Complete venous filling was seen by 15 seconds. Fluorescence intensity increased during the first 20 to 30 seconds. The retinal vessel fluorescence faded 5 to 17 minutes and completely disappeared 20 to 60 minutes after dye injection.

The appearance of choroidal vessel fluorescence was found to be coincidental with retinal vessel fluorescence, varying from 7 to 15 seconds. The details of small choroidal vessels appeared to increase during the first minute after verteporfin injection. The fluorescence faded variably from 70 to 360 seconds. Faint background fluorescence appeared at 15 to 20 minutes and lasted throughout the 2-hour study.

Choroidal Neovascularization

Angiography with verteporfin allowed clear imaging of CNV (10). Transit phase, lasting from 9 to 14 seconds, showed hyperfluorescence surrounded by hypofluorescence in the area of CNV (Fig. 21.4). The details of the neovascular membranes were apparent in 5 to 30 minutes and they had a fanlike or pinwheel appearance with good delineation of the borders. Starting at 30 to 50 minutes the borders of the membranes became fuzzy, indicating mild leakage of the dye (Fig. 21.4). The contrast between the CNV and background increased as the study progressed.

Verteporfin angiography in the experimental primate model, did not show any side effects, despite using bolus iv

A B

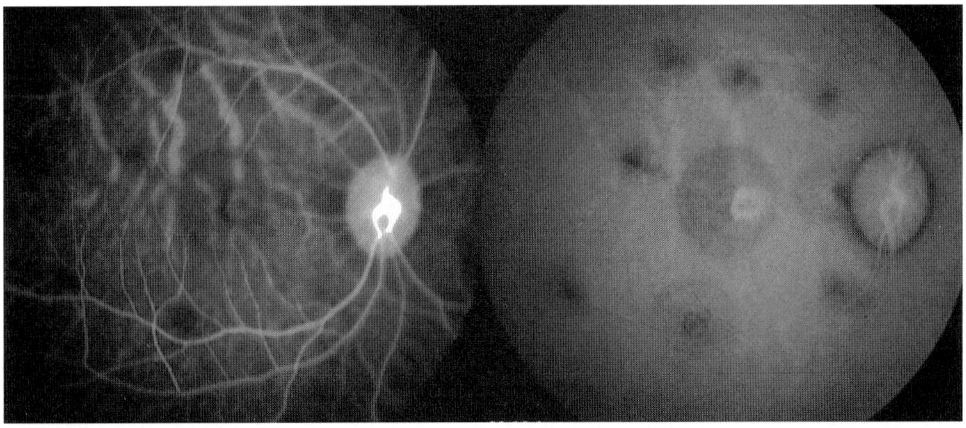

FIGURE 21.4. A: Early-phase (13-second) benzoporphyrin derivative (BPD) (verteporfin) angiography of the monkey eye, showing dye in the small and large retinal and choroidal vessels and early hyperfluorescence of the experimental CNV. **B:** Late-phase (33-minute) BPD (verteporfin) angiography of the monkey eye, showing some persistent dye in the retinal vessels and bright hyperfluorescence of the experimental CNV.

administration. The retinal irradiance produced by the flash of light of 580 nm, exposure 3 seconds, on the digital angiography system with maximum flash energy of 300 mW, was measured at 5 mJ/cm^2. According to ANSI guidelines for light safety (15), the maximum permissible number of exposures at that energy is 55. Thus, the light levels we used to perform verteporfin angiography are safe for humans. During the Phase I/II clinical trials of verteporfin for PDT of CNV, angiography also was performed on patients with CNV. Verteporfin was injected at a dose of 12 mg/m^2 over 15 minutes. Fluorescent images were seen with the slow injection, but the quality of images were poor. Improving the imaging of CNV in patients requires a more rapid injection of dye.

Iris Angiography

Verteporfin angiography of normal iris vessels demonstrated fluorescence between 6 and 10 seconds, starting from the iris root and filling toward the pupillary border (13). The transit phase lasted 10 to 20 seconds, with some increased fluorescence at 2 to 3 minutes. Verteporfin imaged deeper normal iris vessels, which demonstrated some tortuosity. The fluorescence decreased progressively and was substantially reduced by 7 to 10 minutes.

Verteporfin imaging of iris neovascularization showed large corkscrew mostly radial vessels, filling the iris root to the pupillary border. These vessels were visualized at 45 seconds to 1 minute. Vessel density appeared to be greater in eyes with rubeosis than in those with normal iris. The late phase of the angiogram showed minimal leakage of the dye. This hyperfluorescence faded by 20 to 30 minutes (Chapter 9).

CONCLUSION

The currently available imaging techniques do not optimally image smaller choroidal vessels and ill-defined and occult CNV. Fluorescein angiography images retinal vessels and classic CNV, and ICG-A images larger choroidal vessels. Verteporfin, which is currently United States Food and Drug Administration–approved for PDT of CNV (16,17) can image details of smaller choroidal vessels. Verteporfin accumulates in the neovascular tissue. It has been demonstrated that areas of CNV show early hyperfluorescence surrounded by hypofluorescence in the transit phase. Fanlike patterns of choroidal new vessels with clear delineation of the borders are seen as the study progresses. There is minimal blurring of the CNV border in the late phase of the study, indicating mild leakage of the dye. The study of the fluorescent pattern in the experimental model of CNV with verteporfin helped to determine the time of PDT after dye injection. The optimal time for PDT is when there is good fluorescence in the CNV and after the dye has cleared from the retinal circulation in order to avoid damage to retinal vessels.

Adding excitation and barrier filters on the existing digital angiography imaging systems for FA and ICG easily permits imaging with verteporfin. Good images have been obtained using 580 nm for excitation and 695 nm for the barrier filter. There are several reasons for selecting 580 nm excitation filter.

1. This wavelength has limited penetration in the choroid because absorption by blood is substantial for wavelengths less than 580 nm. This minimizes the bright background fluorescence, which is detrimental to high-contrast visualization of deeper vessels.
2. Shorter wavelengths are absorbed by natural chromophores, such as hemoglobin, melanin, macular pigment, and lens. This effect may be even more pronounced because the potential use of this dye is more common in elderly patients with cataract and macular degeneration.
3. The longer wavelength absorption is located closer to the emission peak, and it would be technically difficult to design filters with adequate rejection without losing either excitation or emission light.

Verteporfin angiography has advantage over FA in delineating CNV because FA leaks rapidly; therefore, it does not well define the borders of classic CNV. Verteporfin also has the potential of imaging occult CNV, because it accumulates in neovascular tissue and shows only mild leakage compared to fluorescein. Verteporfin also has an advantage over ICG, because ICG images CNV as an area of hyperfluorescence surrounded by hypofluorescence, with no details of the CNV vascular pattern and no well-defined borders, whereas verteporfin angiography gives better quality images that well define the choroidal neovascular pattern and its borders. Also, it accumulates in both occult and classic CNV. Verteporfin angiography may be helpful for the treatment of CNV. First, it demarcates the borders, thus defining the area of treatment. Second, it helps in choosing the most appropriate time for treatment after dye injection. In the later phases of the angiogram, verteporfin accumulates in CNV while the retinal vessels are cleared of the dye, which allows for selective treatment of the CNV while preventing any damage to retinal vessels.

REFERENCES

1. Delori F, Castany M, Webb R. Fluorescence characteristics of sodium fluorescein in plasma and whole blood. *Exp Eye Res* 1978; 27:417–425.
2. Benson R, Kues H. Fluorescence properties of indocyanine green as related to angiography. *Phys Med Biol* 1978;23:159–163.
3. Yannuzzi L, Slakter J, Sorenson J, et al. Digital indocyanine green videoangiography and choroidal neovascularization. *Retina* 1992; 12:191–223.
4. Richter AM, Waterfield E, Jain AK, et al. In vitro evaluation of phototoxic properties of four structurally related benzoporphyrin derivatives. *Photochem Photobiol* 1990;52:495–500.

5. Kessel D. In vitro photosensitization with a benzoporphyrin derivative. *Photochem Photobiol* 1989;49:579–582.
6. Allison B, Pritchard P, Richter A, et al. The plasma distribution of benzoporphyrin derivative and the effects of plasma lipoproteins on its biodistribution. *Photochem Photobiol* 1990;52: 501–507.
7. Richter AM, Waterfield E, Jain AK, et al. Liposomal delivery of a photosensitizer, benzoporphyrin derivative monoacid ring A (BPD), to tumor tissue in a mouse tumor model. *Photochem Photobiol* 1993;57:1000–1006.
8. Fogelman AM, Berliner JA, Van Lenten BJ, et al. Lipoprotein receptors and endothelial cells. *Semin Thromb Hemos* 1988;14: 206–209.
9. Rutledge JC, Curry FRE, Lenz JF, et al. Low density lipoprotein transport across a microvascular endothelial barrier after permeability is increased. *Circ Res* 1990;66:486–495.
10. Husain D, Kramer M, Kenny AG, et al. Effects of photodynamic therapy using Verteporfin on experimental choroidal neovascularization and normal retina and choroids up to 7 weeks after treatment. *Invest Ophthalmol Vis Sci* 1999;40(10):2322–2331.
11. Miller JW, Walsh AW, Kramer M, et al. Photodynamic therapy of experimental choroidal neovascularization using liposomal delivered benzoporphyrin. *Arch Ophthalmol* 1995;113:810–818.
12. Delori F. Spectrophotometer for noninvasive measurement of intrinsic fluorescence and reflectance of ocular fundus. *Appl Optics* 1994;33:7439–7452.
13. Husain D, Miller JW, Kenney AG, et al. Photodynamic therapy and digital angiography of experimental iris neovascularization using liposomal benzoporphyrin derivative. *Ophthalmology* 1997; 104(8):1242–1250.
14. D'Anna SA, Hochheimer BF, Joondeph HC, et al. Fluorescein angiography of heavily pigmented iris and new dyes for iris angiography. *Arch Ophthalmol* 1983;101:289–293.
15. ANSI. American national standard for safe use of lasers. *ANSI 136.1-1993 (revision of ANSI 136.1, 1986).* Orlando, FL: TLIO America, 1993.
16. Treatment of Age-Related Macular Degeneration with Photodynamic Therapy (TAP) Study Group. Photodynamic therapy of subfoveal choroidal neovascularization in age related macular degeneration with Verteporfin: one-year results of 2 randomized clinical trials. *Arch Ophthalmol* 1999;117(10):1329–1345.
17. Verteporfin in Photodynamic Therapy Study Group. Verteporfin therapy of subfoveal choroidal neovascularization in age related macular degeneration: two year results of a randomized clinical trial including lesions with no classic choroidal neovascularization. *Am J Ophthalmol* 2001;131(5):541–560.

22

ANGIOGRAPHY WITH LU-TEX

KENNETH B. GRAHAM
J. DANIEL ARBOUR
MARK S. BLUMENKRANZ
EVANGELOS S. GRAGOUDAS
JOAN W. MILLER

Photodynamic therapy (PDT) has been a major advance in the treatment of age-related macular degeneration (AMD) (1–4). However, the localization of the currently used photosensitizers to the neovascular complex is estimated from fluorescein angiography (FA) (5,6). This may explain why some lesions respond well to PDT, whereas others do not despite appearing identical on FA. It is known from angiographic studies that the speed and degree of photosensitizer localization to the choroidal neovascularization (CNV) depends on a number of individual parameters, such as cardiac output, rate of choroidal blood flow, protein binding of dye, and lesion composition (7,8). The localization and time of maximal accumulation to the CNV can be determined with a photosensitizer that can form angiographic images (9). This allows more selective damage to the CNV while avoiding surrounding normal tissue.

LUTETIUM TEXAPHYRIN

Lutetium texaphyrin (Lu-Tex, Pharmacyclics, Inc., Sunnyvale, CA) is a water-soluble photosensitizer that may be used for angiography. Lu-Tex (Fig. 22.1) is a member of the class of compounds called texaphyrins (10). The texaphyrins are synthetic water-soluble tripyrrolic pentaaza-expanded porphyrins with the ability to exhibit strong absorption in the 730 to 770 nm range and efficiently generate singlet oxygen (11). Lu-Tex has a molecular weight of 1,165.4 g/mol and broad absorption at 474 and 732 nm (Fig. 22.2). The fluorescence emission of Lu-Tex is intense and centers at 750 nm, where the signal is not obstructed by the presence of endogenous chromophores (12). Lu-Tex is an ideal photosensitizer in many ways. Lu-Tex is retained in the vasculature of tumor models while leaving surrounding normal vessels unharmed (13). The intracellular localization of Lu-Tex has been shown to be in the lysosome by confocal laser scanning microscopy. Photodynamic therapy with Lu-Tex induces apoptosis, as shown by gel electrophoresis in mammary sarcoma cells (7,12). In addition, Lu-Tex has been used in clinical trials for solid malignancies and for peripheral atherosclerotic disease with no significant systemic skin photosensitization (10,14,15).

For angiography with Lu-Tex, the excitation filters could use either of Lu-Tex's two absorption peaks (Fig. 22.2). However, it has been shown that the optimal filter combination is with the 474-nm peak for best absorption (16). This allows good separation from the fluorescence peak of Lu-Tex at 750 nm, thus eliminating the potential for pseudofluorescence artifact.

LU-TEX ANGIOGRAPHY IN RABBITS

With the appropriate excitation and barrier filters for the specific absorbance and emission peaks of Lu-Tex, high-resolution digital images are possible. This has been demonstrated in rabbits (17). Figure 22.3 shows the rabbit medullary ray and choroidal vasculature with fluorescein and Lu-Tex angiography. The Lu-Tex angiogram shows greater resolution of the choroidal vasculature compared to the FA. Fluorescein demonstrates the laser-induced vasculitis with early leakage and late obscuration of the vessel margins. Lu-Tex has better delineation of the vessel margins because of its higher molecular weight and stronger affinity for plasma proteins.

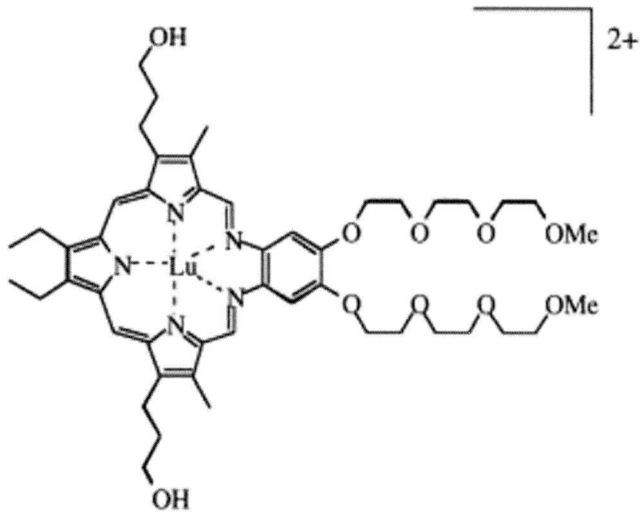

FIGURE 22.1. Structure of lutetium texaphyrin (Lu-Tex). (From: Blumenkranz M. Lutetium texaphyrin (Lu-Tex): a potential new agent for ocular fundus angiography and photodynamic therapy. *Am J Ophthamol* 2000;129:354, with permission from Elsevier Science.)

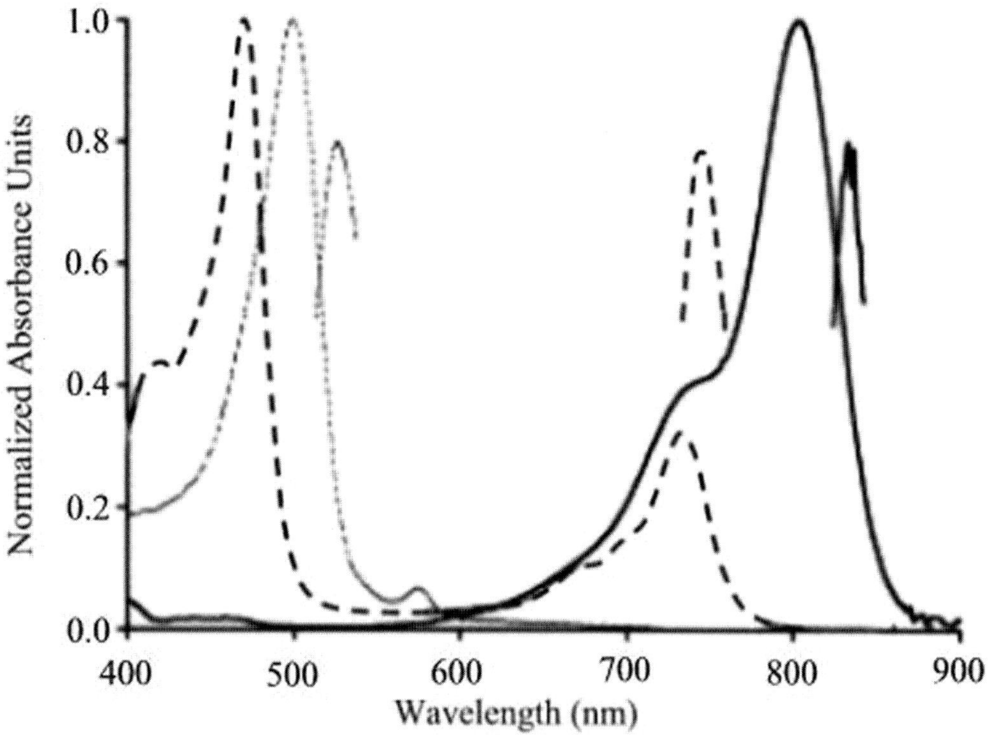

FIGURE 22.2. Composite normalized absorption spectra of Lu-Tex *(long dashed line),* fluorescein *(dotted line),* and indocyanine green *(solid black line).* The respective fluorescein emission spectrum of each dye is shown at 80%. (From: Blumenkranz M. Lutetium texaphyrin (Lu-Tex): a potential new agent for ocular fundus angiography and photodynamic therapy. *Am J Ophthamol* 2000;129:356, with permission from Elsevier Science.)

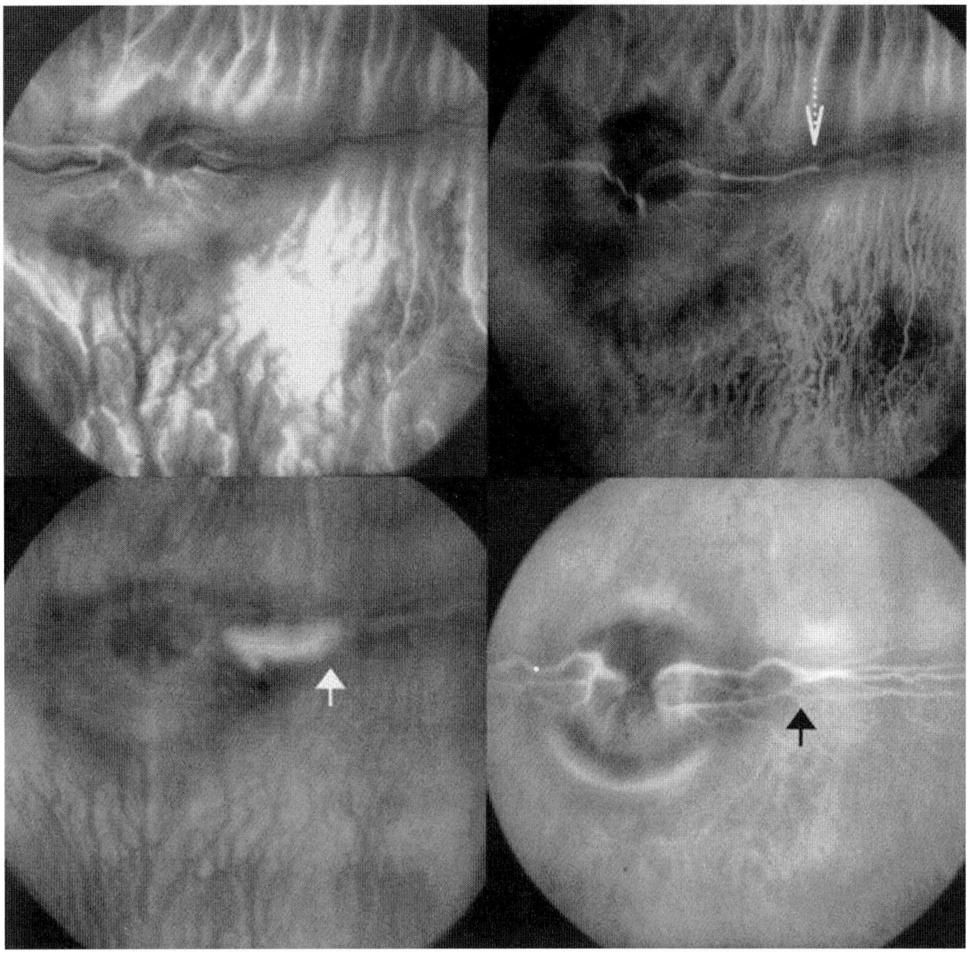

FIGURE 22.3. Laser-induced thermal vasculitis of the rabbit medullary ray vessel. Early- and late-phase fluorescein **(left top and bottom)** and Lu-Tex **(right top and bottom)** angiograms of the choroidal vascular bed and medullary ray vessels. **Top right:** The point of vascular constriction *(white arrow)* is shown in the Lu-Tex angiogram. **Bottom right:** The corresponding area of staining in late frame *(black arrow)*. **Bottom left:** In contrast, a late fluorescein study of a comparable region of vasculitis *(white arrow)* shows extensive fluorescein extravasation. (From: Blumenkranz M. Lutetium texaphyrin (Lu-Tex): a potential new agent for ocular fundus angiography and photodynamic therapy. *Am J Ophthamol* 2000;129:357, with permission from Elsevier Science.)

LU-TEX ANGIOGRAPHY IN MONKEYS

Similar findings are seen with Lu-Tex angiography in monkeys. Choroidal neovascularization may be induced in monkey eyes using a laser injury model (18,19). The CNV is formed by placing seven to nine high-intensity argon green laser photocoagulation spots between the major temporal arcade vessels. The monkeys are then followed weekly for 2 to 3 weeks with fundus photography and FA (16). Figure 22.4 shows the FA of CNV in the left eye of a cynomolgus monkey. There is progressive staining and leakage of fluorescein from the CNV. In contrast, Figure 22.5 shows the Lu-Tex angiogram (6 mg/kg of Lu-Tex) of the same monkey eye. At 25 seconds, Lu-Tex shows maximal fluorescence of the retinal vessels and early fluorescence of the CNV. By 6 minutes, Lu-Tex has started to clear from the retina vessels and increased fluorescence of the CNV. As the angiogram progresses to 40 minutes, there is a slow decrease of Lu-Tex fluorescence from the CNV with minimal leakage into the subretinal space. By 2 hours, Lu-Tex has cleared from the retinal and choroidal vessels, but remains partially in the CNV.

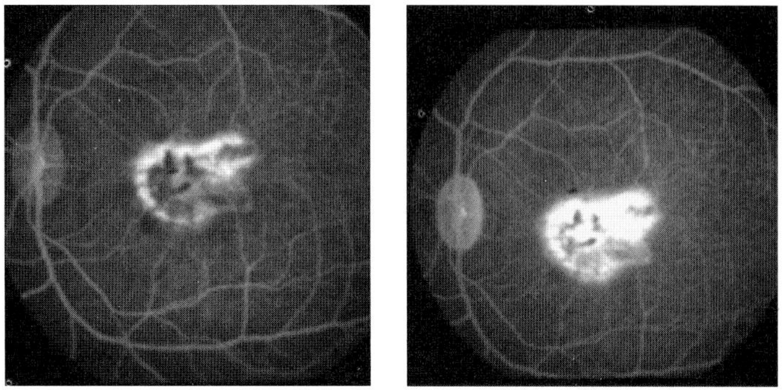

A B

FIGURE 22.4. Fluorescein angiogram of a monkey eye with a laser-induced choroidal neovascular membrane (CNV). **A:** There is staining of the CNV at 1.7 minutes. **B:** There is progressive staining and leakage of fluorescein from the CNV at 6.5 minutes.

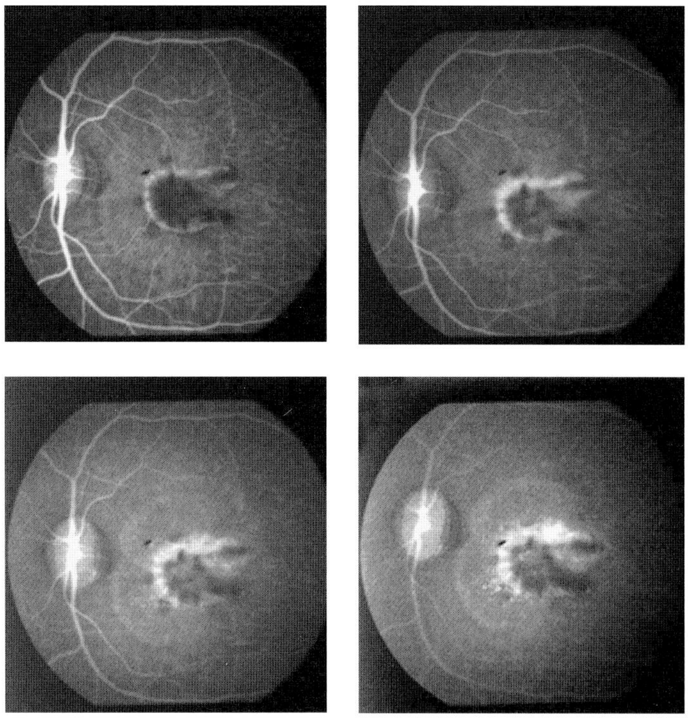

A B C D

FIGURE 22.5. Digital angiography using 6 mg/kg of Lu-Tex in the same monkey eye as Figure 22.4. **A:** There is a peak fluorescence from the retinal vessels and early staining of the CNV at 25 seconds post-Lu-Tex injection. **B:** There is maximal fluorescence of the CNV by 6 minutes. **C:** There is a slow decrease of CNV fluorescence at 40 minutes, with minimal leakage of Lu-Tex into the subretinal fluid. **D:** The fluorescence of the choroidal and retinal vessels is diminished, but remains in the CNV at 2 hours.

OVERVIEW

Fluorescein angiography is the current standard for PDT (6). However, the lower absorption and emission wavelengths of fluorescein cause the light to be absorbed and scattered by the pigment layers of the fundus (20). Thus, there is poor visualization of the choroid and choriocapillaris, where CNV originates. In addition, fluorescein has a lower binding affinity for plasma albumin, rapidly leaks from abnormal vessels, and produces a diffuse background fluorescence (21). Thus, FA gives only an estimate of the extent of the disease.

Indocyanine green (ICG) has a longer wavelength for absorption and emission (Fig. 22.2). This allows better visualization of the deep choroidal vessels. Indocyanine green has a higher binding affinity for plasma protein. However, optical imaging with ICG is limited by inferior diffraction-limited resolution of small vascular structures (22). Indocyanine green has been used in conjunction with laser with limited success at closure of the CNV (23).

In contrast, Lu-Tex has an emission between that of fluorescein and ICG (Fig. 22.2). The shorter wavelength of Lu-Tex is not limited by diffraction. This allows Lu-Tex to image both the retinal and choroidal vasculature. In addition, Lu-Tex has a high binding affinity for plasma proteins, similar to ICG (17). As a result, there is minimal leakage of Lu-Tex from the CNV, providing better localization of the active neovascularization. In contrast to ICG, Lu-Tex is an efficient generator of singlet oxygen (24). Therefore, Lu-Tex may prove to be a valuable tool in the treatment of AMD. We may be better equipped to selectively damage the CNV with a photosensitizer that has the ability to form angiographic images.

REFERENCES

1. Miller JW, Walsh AW, Kramer M, et al. Photodynamic therapy of experimental choroidal neovascularization using lipoprotein-delivered benzoporphyrin. *Arch Ophthalmol* 1995;113(6):810–818.
2. Kramer M, Miller JW, Michaud N, et al. Liposomal benzoporphyrin derivative verteporfin photodynamic therapy. Selective treatment of choroidal neovascularization in monkeys. *Ophthalmology* 1996;103(3):427–438.
3. Husain D, Miller JW, Michaud N, et al. Intravenous infusion of liposomal benzoporphyrin derivative for photodynamic therapy of experimental choroidal neovascularization. *Arch Ophthalmol* 1996;114(8):978–985.
4. Miller H, Miller B. Photodynamic therapy of subretinal neovascularization in the monkey eye. *Arch Ophthalmol* 1993;111(6):855–860.
5. Treatment of age-related macular degeneration with photodynamic therapy (TAP) Study Group. Photodynamic therapy of subfoveal choroidal neovascularization in age-related macular degeneration with verteporfin: one-year results of 2 randomized clinical trials. *Arch Ophthalmol* 1999;117(10):1329–1345.
6. Bressler NM. Photodynamic therapy of subfoveal choroidal neovascularization in age-related macular degeneration with verteporfin: two-year results of 2 randomized clinical trials. *Arch Ophthalmol* 2001;119(2):198–207.
7. Woodburn KW, Fan Q, Miles DR, et al. Localization and efficacy analysis of the phototherapeutic lutetium texaphyrin (PCI-0123) in the murine EMT6 sarcoma model. *Photochem Photobiol* 1997;65(3):410–415.
8. Haimovici R, Kramer M, Miller JW, et al. Localization of lipoprotein-delivered benzoporphyrin derivative in the rabbit eye. *Curr Eye Res* 1997;16(2):83–90.
9. Kramer M, et al. Imaging of experimental choroidal neovascularization (CNV) using liposomal benzoporphyrin derivative monoacid (BPD-MA) angiography. *Invest Ophthalmol Vis Sci* 1995;36(Suppl):S236.
10. Young SW, Woodburn KW, Wright M, et al. Lutetium texaphyrin (PCI-0123): a near-infrared, water-soluble photosensitizer. *Photochem Photobiol* 1996;63(6):892–897.
11. Sessler JL, Miller RA. Texaphyrins: new drugs with diverse clinical applications in radiation and photodynamic therapy. *Biochem Pharmacol* 2000;59(7):733–739.
12. Woodburn KW, Fan Q, Kessel D, et al. Phototherapy of cancer and atheromatous plaque with texaphyrins. *J Clin Laser Med Surg* 1996;14(5):343–348.
13. Fingar VH, et al. Assessment of selected damage to tumor vasculature after PDT. *Photochem Photobiol* 1998;67S:25S.
14. Wieman T, et al. Phase I photodynamic trial with lutetium texaphyrin (PCI-0123) in patients with metastatic cancer. *Photochem Photobiol* 1996;64:80S.
15. Rockson SG, Kramer P, Razavi M, et al. Photoangioplasty for human peripheral atherosclerosis: results of a phase I trial of photodynamic therapy with motexafin lutetium (Antrin). *Circulation* 2000;102(19):2322–2324.
16. Graham KB, et al. Digital angiography using lutetium texaphyrin in a monkey model of choroidal neovascularization (ARVO abstract 2117). *Invest Ophthalmol Vis Sci* 1999;40: S402.
17. Blumenkranz MS, et al. Lutetium texaphyrin (Lu-Tex): a potential new agent for ocular fundus angiography and photodynamic therapy. *Am J Ophthalmol* 2000;129(3):353–362.
18. Ryan SJ. Subretinal neovascularization. Natural history of an experimental model. *Arch Ophthalmol* 1982;100(11):1804–1809.
19. Ohkuma H, Ryan SJ. Experimental subretinal neovascularization in the monkey. Permeability of new vessels. *Arch Ophthalmol* 1983;101(7):1102–1110.
20. Archer D, Krill AE, Newell FW. Fluorescein studies of normal choroidal circulation. *Am J Ophthalmol* 1970;69(4):543–554.
21. Bloome MA. Fluorescein angiography: risks. *Vision Res* 1980;20(12):1083–1097.
22. Benson RC, Kues HA. Fluorescence properties of indocyanine green as related to angiography. *Phys Med Biol* 1978;23(1):159–163.
23. Guyer DR, Duker JS, Puliafito CA. Indocyanine green angiography and dye-enhanced diode laser photocoagulation. *Semin Ophthalmol* 1992;7(3):172–176.
24. Bilgin MD, al Akhras MA, Khalili M, et al. Photosensitization of red blood cell hemolysis by lutetium texaphyrin. *Photochem Photobiol* 2000;72(1):121–127.

23

FUTURE DIRECTIONS IN PHOTODYNAMIC THERAPY

JOAN W. MILLER

We have moved into an exciting era in photodynamic therapy (PDT). This old technology is finally coming into its own with the widespread introduction of verteporfin PDT as a treatment for choroidal neovascularization (CNV). Ophthalmologic applications have led to a resurgence of interest in PDT as an effective treatment modality for other medical conditions. The application of PDT in ophthalmology is expanding and improvements to current technology are being pursued actively.

Verteporfin PDT has been approved by health authorities around the world for treatment of CNV in age-related macular degeneration (AMD), pathologic myopia, and ocular histoplasmosis syndrome (1–7). Choroidal neovascularization secondary to other conditions, including angioid streaks, choroiditis, trauma, choroidal osteoma, juxtafoveal telangiectasis, choroidal rupture, and retinal degenerations such as mallatia leventinese and fundus flavimaculatus have been treated and reported (1,8–15). Neovascularization elsewhere in the eye also may benefit from PDT, as predicted by preclinical experiments in the treatment of iris neovascularization and CNV (16). Ocular tumors represent another application and success has been reported in the treatment of choroidal hemangiomas by a number of authors (17–23). Retinal capillary angiomas may be treated when they do not overly the optic nerve (24–26). Small choroidal melanomas in the macula may be another important application of PDT, and work by Young and others justifies this approach (27,28).

Other photosensitizers are being pursued for application in ophthalmology. Tin etiopurpurin showed promise in experimental studies and early clinical trials, but did not meet the primary vision outcome in multicenter, randomized trials (29–31). Similarly, lutetium texaphyrin appeared to be effective in preclinical models, but could not be used effectively without side effects in clinical trials (32–34). Other photosensitizers that are still being studied include the phthalocyanines and chlorins such as NPe6 and ATX-S10Na. Additional studies and particularly clinical trials will demonstrate whether these photosensitizers will prove beneficial and add to our clinical therapy.

Angiography using photosensitizers may prove to be an important diagnostic and therapeutic tool. Angiography using verteporfin provides imaging of small choroidal vessels and CNV with spectral characteristics between fluorescein and indocyanine green (ICG) (35). Other photosensitizers, particularly those with absorption and emission peaks in the longer wavelengths, may be similarly useful (36). In addition, angiography using photosensitizers provides important dosimetry information, allowing one to determine the optimal time to apply light for PDT of the tissue of interest (37,38). In the case of CNV, angiography indicates clearance of verteporfin from retinal vessels by 15 minutes after drug injection, and localization to CNV at 15 to 30 minutes after injection. To date, angiography has been limited in patients. In the case of verteporfin, the use of an infusion rather than rapid intravenous administration yielded poor-quality images. Lu-Tex angiography in patients did yield some useful images but has not been pursued because Lu-Tex PDT has not. It may prove useful to perform angiography with photosensitizers in order to determine any differences in localization prior to PDT, based on cardiac output, or the nature of the CNV, such as differences in flow characteristics.

Antiangiogenic therapy is another approach to ocular neovascular disorders as well as for tumors. Combination therapy of PDT and antiangiogenic agents may yield improved results over either one alone. One needs to consider the various molecules involved in neovascularization in thinking about combining PDT and antiangiogenic therapy. These include a vast array of growth factors, cytokines, and other molecules. We have begun investigating several of these as potential adjuncts to PDT.

Early *in vitro* studies by our group demonstrated a synergistic effect of PDT and antiangiogenic therapy on microvascular endothelial cells with no effect on retinal cells (39). Photodynamic therapy was performed with Lu-Tex and angiostatin, an antiangiogenic plasminogen fragment, treating bovine retinal capillary endothelial cells and human retinal pigment epithelial cells. This work was repeated using verteporfin PDT with similar findings, and more recently confirmed *in vivo* in a rat model of CNV.

Vascular endothelial growth factor (VEGF) is a growth factor that appears to play an important role in ocular neovascularization. VEGF expression has been correlated with neovascularization in experimental iris, retinal, and choroidal neovascularization (40–42). In addition, VEGF expression has been demonstrated in clinical specimens of diabetic retinopathy and neovascular AMD (40,43,44).

RhuFabV2 is a recombinant humanized monoclonal antibody fragment produced by Genentech (San Francisco, CA) and directed against VEGF. Although a full-length anti-VEGF antibody administered intravitreally prevented experimental iris neovascularization, the full length antibody at 150 kDa is too large to cross from the vitreous cavity to the RPE and choroid after intravitreal injection (45). The rhuFabV2 fragment, with a molecular weight of 48 kDa has been shown to penetrate the retina after intravitreal injection.

First, we showed that intravitreal rhuFabV2 inhibits experimental CNV in the laser-injury model, comparing eyes receiving rhuFabV2 with eyes receiving vehicle (46). We then designed a series of experiments to demonstrate the safety and efficacy of intravitreal rhuFabV2 combined with verteporfin PDT using the laser injury CNV model in the monkey (47). Weekly treatments were initiated 14 days after laser injury. We used paired eyes in which one eye received intravitreal rhuFabV2 plus verteporfin PDT and one received intravitreal vehicle plus verteporfin PDT. The intravitreal injections were performed every 2 weeks and PDT was performed every 2 weeks for a total of three treatments. Three groups were studied varying the order of intravitreal injections and PDT. Outcome measures of inflammation and angiographic leakage were assessed weekly, with follow-up through 2 weeks after the third PDT. Angiographic grading was performed by masked graders using standard angiograms.

A very mild anterior chamber reaction following rhuFabV2 injection was noted in the previous study by Krzystolik and coworkers; this diminished with subsequent injections. In examining the paired eyes, there appeared to be less leakage at day 21, and at day 42 when combination therapy was used rather than PDT alone. Leakage in the PDT-alone eye and not the combination therapy eye occurred in four pairs of eyes at day 21 and two pairs of eyes at day 42. However, in no pairs was leakage seen in only the combination rhuFabV2/PDT eye. Histologically, eyes treated with PDT only typically showed a fibrovascular scar with a few open capillaries, but eyes treated with combination rhuFabV2 and PDT showed only a fibrous scar. These preclinical results show that rhuFabV2 intravitreal injection plus verteporfin PDT is safe and appears to result in a greater reduction in angiographic leakage from CNV than PDT alone. There was transient ocular inflammation with the initial injection of rhuFabV2 but this does not appear to be clinically significant.

Currently two molecules directed against VEGF are being pursued in clinical trials. RhuFabV2, described in the preceding section and produced by Genentech, is in Phase III trials for neovascular AMD. EYE001 (Macugen), an anti-VEGF aptamer produced by Eyetech Pharmaceuticals (New York, NY), has completed Phase I/II trials and is currently in Phase III clinical trials for neovascular AMD alone, and in combination with verteporfin PDT. Preliminary results are promising with both molecules.

Combination therapy using antiangiogenic agent rhuFabV2 or angiostatin, and verteporfin PDT led to decreased angiographic leakage from experimental CNV compared to PDT treatment alone. One explanation for the synergistic response on proliferating endothelium is the induction of apoptosis by the antiangiogenic agents, making the cells more susceptible to PDT-induced apoptosis. Other combination agents to be considered include other anti-VEGF agents; angiostatic steroids, including anecortave acetate; endostatin; and integrin antagonists. The timing and frequency of combination therapy needs to be elaborated further.

Combination therapy of antiangiogenic agents and PDT also may prove to be beneficial for ocular tumors. Retinal capillary angiomas have been demonstrated to be VEGF-dependent, and combination therapy of anti-VEGF agents and PDT to decrease growth and leakage of vessels could be a great advance over our current therapy (48,49). Other tumors that could be treated include choroidal hemangiomas, retinoblastomas, and choroidal melanomas.

Another approach to improving PDT has been to target the photosensitizer more directly to the neovascular endothelium. One strategy is to bind the photosensitizer to a targeting molecule directed at binding sites on the CNV endothelium, such as VEGF receptors or integrins. We selected a peptide ATWLPPR in our first series of experiments that has been shown to bind specifically to the VEGFR2 receptor (also known as KDR or FLK-1). This peptide completely inhibits VEGF binding to VEGFR2 (50,51). We produced a targeted verteporfin by binding verteporfin to a polyvinyl alcohol (PVA) linker and then to the homing peptide ATWLPPR. We used verteporfin-PVA for controls. This is a large but untargeted commercially available verteporfin. We performed these experiments in the laser-injury CNV model in the rat, for which we have worked out the dosimetry for verteporfin PDT (52).

We found that PDT using both targeted verteporfin and verteporfin-PVA were effective in CNV closure. Prior to PDT, FA in the rat model showed hyperfluorescence and leakage of the experimental CNV. There was no perfusion or leakage from CNV 1 day following treatment with targeted verteporfin. We found that both large molecules were more efficient than unbound verteporfin in achieving CNV closure.

We also performed PDT to normal retina and choroid again to assess selectivity. We found that there was no angiographic change 1 day after PDT using VEGFR2-targeted PDT. Histologically, the VEGFR2-targeted treated eye showed preserved retina and very minimal changes to RPE. Treatment of normal retina and choroid using the verteporfin-PVA control showed hyperfluorescence on angiography and retinal damage on light microscopy.

In summary, the targeted verteporfin and verteporfin PVA were both more efficient at CNV closure than unbound verteporfin. VEGFR2-targeted verteporfin PDT appeared to be selective when normal retina and choroid were treated, resulting in choriocapillaris closure with minimal effect on RPE or neurosensory retina. In contrast, treatment with the verteporfin-PVA control showed nonselective retinal damage. These positive findings will be pursued further in experimental models and hopefully will warrant clinical investigation in the future. In addition, other homing molecules may be developed with even greater selectivity to neovascular endothelium.

Another strategy to improve PDT is to modulate the tissue response following treatment. With this strategy one would seek to increase the injury to the cells targeted for PDT while decreasing any injury to adjacent cells. Modulators of apoptosis may be used to achieve this selective tissue effect. In preliminary studies our group demonstrated that both microvascular cells and retinal cells undergo apoptosis after PDT, but may use different pathways (39). This could allow one to modify the response of these cells in different directions to increase or decrease the apoptotic response.

Agents to be used in conjunction with PDT, including antiangiogenic and apoptosis modulators, will need to be delivered on a more chronic basis. Systemic delivery has proved to be problematic for many of these agents, and local delivery is probably preferred. Intravitreal delivery for retinal and choroidal diseases may be reasonable but carries a long-term cumulative risk of endophthalmitis and retinal detachment. We are investigating trans-scleral delivery of agents using both passive and active devices for less invasive, long-term delivery of drugs to treat retinal and choroidal diseases (53).

In conclusion, PDT represents an important first step in the treatment of ocular disorders. However, there is room for improvement and some of the strategies being pursued have been described. Improved selectivity through targeting of photosensitizers, along with combination therapy of antiangiogenic agents and apoptosis modulators, may improve efficacy and recurrence rates as well as selectivity. Local, long-term, minimally invasive drug delivery strategies will improve the tolerability and safety of our therapies. Ultimately, our goal is to develop safe and effective strategies to preserve and improve vision in these devastating diseases.

REFERENCES

1. Sickenberg M, Schmidt-Erfurth U, Miller JW, et al. A preliminary study of photodynamic therapy using verteporfin for choroidal neovascularization in pathologic myopia, ocular histoplasmosis syndrome, angioid streaks, and idiopathic causes. *Arch Ophthalmol* 2000;118(3):327–336.
2. Saperstein DA, Rosenfeld PJ, Bressler NM, et al. Photodynamic therapy of subfoveal choroidal neovascularization with verteporfin in the ocular histoplasmosis syndrome. One-year results of an uncontrolled, prospective case series. *Ophthalmology* 2002; 109(8):1499–1505.
3. Verteporfin in Photodynamic Therapy (VIP) Study Group. Photodynamic therapy of subfoveal choroidal neovascularization in pathologic myopia with verteporfin. One-year results of a randomized clinical trial. *Ophthalmology* 2001;108:841–852.
4. Verteporfin in Photodynamic Therapy (VIP) Study Group. Photodynamic therapy of "early-onset" and occult subfoveal choroidal neovascularization in age-related macular degeneration with verteporfin. One-year results of a randomized clinical trial. *Am J Ophthalmol* 2002;131:541–560.
5. Treatment of Age-Related Macular Degeneration with Photodynamic Therapy (TAP) Study Group. Verteporfin (Visudyne) therapy of subfoveal choroidal neovascularization in age-related macular degeneration. One year results of two randomized clinical trials. *Arch Ophthalmol* 1999;117:1329–1345.
6. Treatment of Age-Related Macular Degeneration with Photodynamic Therapy (TAP) Study Group. Photodynamic therapy of subfoveal choroidal neovascularization in age-related macular degeneration with verteporfin. Two-year vision results of two randomized clinical trials. *Arch Ophthalmol* 2001;119:198–207.
7. Treatment of Age-Related Macular Degeneration with Photodynamic Therapy (TAP) Study Group. Photodynamic therapy of subfoveal choroidal neovascularization in age-related macular degeneration with verteporfin. Guidelines for using verteporfin (Visudyne) in photodynamic therapy to treat choroidal neovascularization. *Retina* 2002;22:6–18.
8. Potter MJ, Szabo SM, Chan EY, et al. Photodynamic therapy of a subretinal neovascular membrane in type 2A idiopathic juxtafoveolar retinal telangiectasis. *Am J Ophthalmol* 2002;133 (1):149–151.
9. Battaglia Parodi M, Da Pozzo S, Toto L, et al. Photodynamic therapy for choroidal neovascularization associated with choroidal osteoma. *Retina* 2001;21(6):660–661.
10. Dantas MA, Slakter JS, Negrao S, et al. Photodynamic therapy with verteporfin in mallatia leventinese. *Ophthalmology* 2002; 109(2):296–301.
11. Valmaggia C, Niederberger H, Helbig H. Photodynamic therapy for choroidal neovascularization in fundus flavimaculatus. *Retina* 2002;22(1):111–113.
12. Coquelet P, Postelmans L, Snyers B, et al. Successful photodynamic therapy combined with laser photocoagulation in three eyes with classic subfoveal choroidal neovascularisation affecting two patients with multifocal choroiditis: case reports. *Bull Soc Belge Ophtalmol* 2002(283):69–73.
13. Spaide RF, Freund KB, Slakter J, et al. Treatment of subfoveal choroidal neovascularization associated with multifocal choroiditis and panuveitis with photodynamic therapy. *Retina* 2002;22 (5):545–549.
14. Shaikh S, Ruby AJ, Williams GA. Photodynamic therapy using verteporfin for choroidal neovascularization in angioid streaks. *Am J Ophthalmol* 2003;135(1):1–6.
15. Karacorlu M, Karacorlu S, Ozdemir H, et al. Photodynamic therapy with verteporfin for choroidal neovascularization in patients with angioid streaks. *Am J Ophthalmol* 2002;134(3): 360–366.

16. Husain D, Miller J, Kenney A, et al. Photodynamic therapy and digital angiography of experimental iris neovascularization using liposomal benzoporphyrin derivative. *Ophthalmology* 1997;104: 1242–1250.
17. Robertson DM. Photodynamic therapy for choroidal hemangioma associated with serous retinal detachment. *Arch Ophthalmol* 2002;120(9):1155–1161.
18. Barbazetto I, Schmidt-Erfurth U. Photodynamic therapy of choroidal hemangioma: two case reports. *Graefes Arch Clin Exp Ophthalmol* 2000;238(3):214–221.
19. Kjeka O, Krohn J. Photodynamic therapy of circumscribed choroidal haemangioma. *Acta Ophthalmol Scand* 2002;80(5):557–558.
20. Landau IM, Steen B, Seregard S. Photodynamic therapy for circumscribed choroidal haemangioma. *Acta Ophthalmol Scand* 2002;80(5):531–536.
21. Madreperla SA. Choroidal hemangioma treated with photodynamic therapy using verteporfin. *Arch Ophthalmol* 2001;119 (11):1606–1610.
22. Schmidt-Erfurth UM, Michels S, Kusserow C, et al. Photodynamic therapy for symptomatic choroidal hemangioma: visual and anatomic results. *Ophthalmology* 2002;109(12):2284–2294.
23. Sheidow TG, Harbour JW. Photodynamic therapy for circumscribed choroidal hemangioma. *Can J Ophthalmol* 2002;37(5): 314–317.
24. Schmidt-Erfurth U, Hasan T, Schomacker K, et al. In vivo uptake of liposomal benzoporphyrin Derivative and photothrombosis in experimental corneal neovascularization. *Lasers Surg Med* 1995;17:178–188.
25. Atebara NH. Retinal capillary hemangioma treated with verteporfin photodynamic therapy. *Am J Ophthalmol* 2002;134(5): 788–790.
26. Schmidt-Erfurth UM, Kusserow C, Barbazetto IA, et al. Benefits and complications of photodynamic therapy of papillary capillary hemangiomas. *Ophthalmology* 2002;109(7):1256–1266.
27. Kim R, Hu L, Foster S, et al. Photodynamic therapy of pigmented choroidal melanomas of greater than 3mm thickness. *Ophthalmology* 1996;103:2029–2036.
28. Young L, Howard M, Hu L, et al. Photodynamic therapy of pigmented choroidal melanomas using a liposomal preparation of benzoporphyrin derivative. *Arch Ophthalmol* 1996;114:186–192.
29. Peyman GA, Moshfeghi DM, Moshfeghi A, et al. Photodynamic therapy for choriocapillaris using tin ethyl etiopurpurin (SnET2). *Ophthalmic Surg Lasers* 1997;28(5):409–417.
30. Baumal C, Puliafito C, Pieroth L, et al. Photodynamic therapy (PDT) of experimental choroidal neovascularization with tin ethyl etiopurpurin. *Invest Ophthalmol Vis Sci* 1996;37:S122.
31. Wu L, Murphy RP. Photodynamic therapy: a new approach to the treatment of choroidal neovascularization secondary to age-related macular degeneration. *Curr Opin Ophthalmol* 1999; 10(3):217–220.
32. Arbour J, Graham K, Carson D, et al. Photodynamic therapy of experimental choroidal neovascularization in a monkey model using intravenous infusion of lutetium texaphyrin. *Invest Ophthalmol Vis Sci* 1999;40:S401.
33. Blumenkranz MS, Woodburn KW, Qing F, et al. Lutetium texaphyrin (Lu-Tex): a potential new agent for ocular fundus angiography and photodynamic therapy. *Am J Ophthalmol* 2000;129 (3):353–362.
34. Woodburn KW, Engelman CJ, Blumenkranz MS. Photodynamic therapy for choroidal neovascularization: a review. *Retina* 2002;22(4):391–405.
35. Kramer M, Kenney A, Delori F, et al. Imaging of experimental choroidal neovascularization (CNV) using liposomal benzoporphyrin derivative monoacid (BPD-MA) angiography. *Invest Ophthalmol Vis Sci* 1995;36:S236.
36. Blumenkranz M, Woodburn K, Verdooner S. Lutex texaphyrin angiography: a new method for the evaluation and treatment of retinal and choroidal vascular disorders. *Invest Ophthal Vis Sci* 1998;39:S468.
37. Graham K, Arbour J, Connolly E, et al. Digital angiography using lutetium texaphyrin in a monkey model of choroidal neovascularization. *Invest Ophthal Vis Sci* 1999;40:S402.
38. Arbour J, Connolly E, Palmer J, et al. Digital angiography of CNV in the monkey using benzoporphyrin, phthalocyanine, and rose bengal. *Invest Ophthal Vis Sci* 1998;39:S590.
39. Renno R, Delori F, Holzer R, et al. Photodynamic therapy using Lutex induces apoptosis in vitro, and its effect is potentiated by angiostatin in retinal capillary endothelial cells. *Invest Ophthal Vis Sci* 2000;41:3963–3971.
40. Miller JW, Adamis AP, Shima D, et al. Vascular endothelial growth factor/vascular permeability factor is temporally and spatially correlated with ocular angiogenesis in a primate model. *Am J Pathol* 1994;145(3):574–584.
41. Pierce EA, Avery R, Foley E, et al. Vascular endothelial growth factor/vascular permeability factor expression in a mouse model of retinal neovascularization. *Proc Natl Acad Sci USA* 1995;92: 905–909.
42. Husain D, Ryan A, Cuthbertson R, et al. Vascular endothelial growth factor (VEGF) expression is correlated with choroidal neovascularization in a monkey model. *Invest Ophthal Vis Sci* 1997;38:S501.
43. Aiello L, Avery R, Arrigg P, et al. Vascular endothelial growth factor in ocular fluid of patients with diabetic retinopathy and other retinal disorders. *N Engl J Med* 1994;331(22):1480–1487.
44. Kvanta A, Algvere P, Berglin L, et al. Subfoveal fibrovascular membranes in age-related macular degeneration express vascular endothelial growth factor. *Invest Ophthalmol Vis Sci* 1996;37: 1929–1934.
45. Adamis A, Shima D, Tolentino M, et al. Inhibition of VEGF prevent ocular neovascularization in a non-human primate. *Arch Ophthalmol* 1996;114:66–71.
46. Krzystolik M, Afsahari M, Adamis A, et al. Intravitreal anti-VEGF Antibody Fragment (rhuFab VEGF) prevents experimental choroidal neovascularization. *Arch Ophthalmol* 2002;120: 143–152.
47. Gauthier D, Husain D, Kim I, et al. Safety and efficacy of intravitreal injection or rhuFabVEGF in combination with verteporfin PDT on experimental choroidal neovascularization. *Invest Ophthalmol Vis Sci* 2002.
48. Chan CC, Vortmeyer AO, Chew EY, et al. VHL gene deletion and enhanced VEGF gene expression detected in the stromal cells of retinal angioma. *Arch Ophthalmol* 1999;117(5):625–630.
49. Aiello LP, George DJ, Cahill MT, et al. Rapid and durable recovery of visual function in a patient with von Hippel-Lindau syndrome after systemic therapy with vascular endothelial growth factor receptor inhibitor su5416. *Ophthalmology* 2002;109(9): 1745–1751.
50. Binetruy-Tournaire R, Demangel C, Malavaud B, et al. Identification of a peptide blocking vascular endothelial growth factor (VEGF)-mediated angiogenesis. *Embo J* 2000;19(7):1525–1533.
51. Renno R, Terada Y, Haddadin M, et al. Selective targeting of verteporfin to choroidal neovascularization mediated by a homing peptide to VEGF-R2. *Invest Ophthalmol Vis Sci* 2002.
52. Zacks D, Ezra E, Terada Y, et al. Verteporfin photodynamic therapy in the rat model of choroidal neovascularization: angiographic and histologic characterization. *Invest Ophthamol Vis Sci* 2002;43:2384–2391.
53. Ambati J, Gragoudas ES, Miller JW, et al. Transscleral delivery of bioactive protein to the choroid and retina. *Invest Ophthalmol Vis Sci* 2000;41:1186–1191.

SUBJECT INDEX

Page numbers followed by "f" indicate a figure; page numbers followed by "t" indicate a table.